ANNUAL REVIEW OF
PHARMACOLOGY
AND TOXICOLOGY

ANNUAL REVIEW OF PHARMACOLOGY AND TOXICOLOGY

VOLUME 26, 1986

ROBERT GEORGE, *Co-editor*

University of California School of Medicine, Los Angeles

RONALD OKUN, *Co-editor*

University of California School of Medicine, Los Angeles

ARTHUR K. CHO, *Associate Editor*

University of California School of Medicine, Los Angeles

ANNUAL REVIEWS INC.   4139 EL CAMINO WAY   PALO ALTO, CALIFORNIA 94306 USA

ANNUAL REVIEWS INC.
Palo Alto, California, USA

International Standard Serial Number: 0362–1642
International Standard Book Number: 0–8243–0426-8
Library of Congress Catalog Card Number: 61–5649

Typesetting by Kachina Typesetting Inc., Tempe, Arizona; John Olson, President
Typesetting coordinator, Jeannie Kaarle

PRINTED AND BOUND IN THE UNITED STATES OF AMERICA

Annual Review of Pharmacology and Toxicology
Volume 26, 1986

CONTENTS

SOME RELATED ARTICLES IN OTHER *ANNUAL REVIEWS*

From the *Annual Review of Medicine,* Volume 37 (1986):

Clinical Pharmacology of Nicotine, Neal L. Benowitz

Aluminum and Renal Osteodystrophy, Henry G. Nebeker and Jack W. Coburn

Action and Toxicity of Cyclosporine, William M. Bennett and Douglas J. Norman

Use of Beta Adrenoceptor Blockade During and After Acute Myocardial Infarction, Peter Sleight

Treatment of Hypercholesterolemia, John P. Kane and Richard J. Havel

From the *Annual Review of Neuroscience,* Volume 9 (1986):

Neurotransmitter Receptor Mapping by Autoradiography and Other Methods, Michael J. Kuhar, Errol B. De Souza, and James Unnerstall

The Molecular Neurobiology of the Acetylcholine Receptor, Michael P. McCarthy, Julie P. Earnest, Ellen F. Young, Seunghyon Choe, and Robert M. Stroud

Inactivation and Metabolism of Neuropeptides, Jeffrey F. McKelvy and Shmaryahu Blumberg

Histamine as a Neuroregulator, George D. Prell and Jack Peter Green

From the *Annual Review of Physiology,* Volume 48 (1986):

Mediation by Corticotropin Releasing Factor (CRF) of Adenohypophysial Hormone Secretion, Catherine L. Rivier and Paul M. Plotsky

Mechanism of Thyrotropin Releasing Hormone Stimulation of Pituitary Hormone Secretion, Marvin C. Gershengorn

Endogenous Opioid Peptides and Hypothalamo-Pituitary Function, Trevor A. Howlett and Lesley H. Rees

Somatostatin Mediation of Adenohypophysial Secretion, Yogesh C. Patel and Coimbatore B. Srikant

Growth Hormone Releasing Hormone, Marie C. Gelato and George R. Merriam

Neurotransmitters in Temperature Control, J. M. Lipton and Wesley G. Clark

Neuronal Receptors, Solomon H. Snyder

ANNUAL REVIEWS INC. is a nonprofit scientific publisher established to promote the advancement of the sciences. Beginning in 1932 with the *Annual Review of Biochemistry*, the Company has pursued as its principal function the publication of high quality, reasonably priced *Annual Review* volumes. The volumes are organized by Editors and Editorial Committees who invite qualified authors to contribute critical articles reviewing significant developments within each major discipline. The Editor-in-Chief invites those interested in serving as future Editorial Committee members to communicate directly with him. Annual Reviews Inc. is administered by a Board of Directors, whose members serve without compensation.

ANNUAL REVIEWS OF		SPECIAL PUBLICATIONS
Anthropology	Medicine	Annual Reviews Reprints:
Astronomy and Astrophysics	Microbiology	Cell Membranes, 1975–1977
Biochemistry	Neuroscience	Cell Membranes, 1978–1980
Biophysics and Biophysical Chemistry	Nuclear and Particle Science	Immunology, 1977–1979
Cell Biology	Nutrition	
Earth and Planetary Sciences	Pharmacology and Toxicology	Excitement and Fascination
Ecology and Systematics	Physical Chemistry	of Science, Vols. 1 and 2
Energy	Physiology	
Entomology	Phytopathology	History of Entomology
Fluid Mechanics	Plant Physiology	
Genetics	Psychology	Intelligence and Affectivity,
Immunology	Public Health	by Jean Piaget
Materials Science	Sociology	Telescopes for the 1980s

For the convenience of readers, a detachable order form/envelope is bound into the back of this volume.

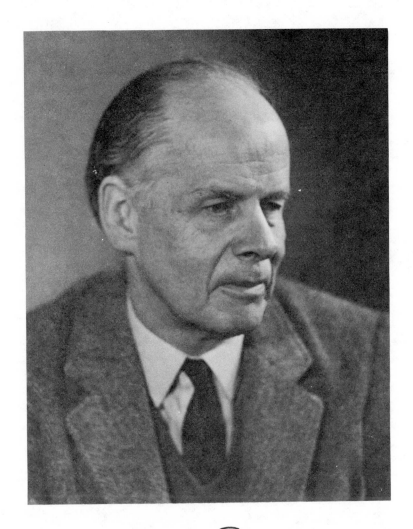

William Paton.

Ann. Rev. Pharmacol. and Toxicol. 1986. 26:1–22

ON BECOMING AND BEING A PHARMACOLOGIST

W. D. M. Paton

Oxford University, 13 Staverton Road, Oxford, OX2 6XH, United Kingdom

FINDING THE SUBJECT

Like others of my generation, I found my vocation of pharmacology by chance, having originally intended to go into academic medicine. In the 1930's, medical students received teaching in the actions of drugs, but the days of undergraduate degrees or later course work in pharmacology lay far in the future. So I was essentially self-taught, with all the freedom, but also the ignorances of the autodidact. Indeed for much of my life I have been among those with a similar background, not a few of whom would say that they were not "really" pharmacologists, but physiologists, biochemists, pathologists, chemists, or some other species. It was therefore not surprising that there was a good deal of discussion, on faculty boards and elsewhere, about the nature of the subject. I came to recognize that it is the sign of a newly developing discipline to be mildly obsessed with what it "really" is, and to be concerned with establishing an identity. Toxicology is going through something of the same process today. The resistance of established subjects to the emergence of new ones is an old story—going back at least to the opposition to the formation of the Geological Society by Sir Joseph Banks (president of the Royal Society) in the last century. Physicists and chemists seemed lucky; they did not need to ask such questions, which had been settled long before, but could get on with the work.

Nor was some discussion about the nature of the discipline unjustified. Pharmacology has a taproot stretching back into the remote past of man's attempts at healing; but it also has more modern roots. So pharmacology did not lack for those ready to explain that it was "only" a branch or application of physiology, medicine, chemistry, or biochemistry. Like any other discipline, pharmacology needs constantly to renew its vision. For me, the character of the

1

subject seemed obvious and most of the formal definitions failed to express what it was that caught my own imagination. Before giving my own definition, let me mention how I was caught.

I suppose it was chance that, at the end of my medical residency, after qualifying in medicine during the London "blitz", I had a fifth attack of pneumonia (following a checkered pulmonary childhood). Medical investigation thereafter pronounced me unfit for military service, and also cast doubt on my capacity to do the residencies required for a career in medicine. The immediate outcome, after I failed to get a job at the Brompton Hospital, was that I took a post as a pathologist in a tuberculosis sanatorium. There was a brief training by a London pathologist, Dr. S. R. Gloyne. (It is somewhat ironic that his main life's work was trying to persuade an unbelieving world that asbestos damaged the lungs.) As was customary at that time, I was then on my own, doing sedimentation rates, blood counts, and culturing sputum or pleural fluid for tubercle bacilli. Occasionally I prepared lung biopsy specimens to assess the presence of cancer cells, and Gloyne would check my conclusions. The work was interesting, but my superintendent was an abrasive character, and I did not get on with him. By chance, a nephew of the then Secretary of the Medical Research Council was also on the staff. It was through him that, for the third time, I was offered a job at the National Institute for Medical Research at Hampstead. I had put previous offers aside, wishing to do clinical work of some kind. But now the offer was a relief and I accepted. On my last night at the sanatorium, I told my superintendent what I thought of him, which I had been too naïve to do before. He beamed all over, for he was one of those that like to challenge others; he then said he hoped to start a tuberculosis research unit at the hospital, and asked me to stay on and start it. I refused, but that was perhaps my first adult lesson in distinguishing between appearance and reality.

So off I went to work under G. L. Brown in Sir Henry Dale's old laboratory, joining in their wartime work on diving and submarine problems. I will say a word about the laboratory later. For the moment it will suffice to say that when peace came, the laboratory turned back to its old activities, and I began to turn into a respiratory physiologist. But then F. C. MacIntosh, the second in command, was asked by another member of the Institute, R. K. Callow, to look at the toxicity of an antibiotic that his group had isolated, named licheniformin. MacIntosh asked me to join him, and we started by testing the hydrochloride for its effect on the blood pressure of a cat under chloralose. It produced a quite characteristic response: no action for around 30 seconds and then an abrupt but fairly transient fall in blood pressure, often marked by a tachycardia during the recovery phase. It was a fascinating picture; for the initial latent period meant that the drug had no direct vasodilator action or cardiodepressant action, yet when the fall came, it was as abrupt as that produced by an equidepressant dose of histamine or acetylcholine. What was going on? In itself the simple tracing pointed to the answer: that the drug released a vasodilator from the periphery, which, on recirculation, produced the fall in pressure. It could hardly be other than histamine if it was to persist long enough in the blood. A sample of blood taken from the animal at the nadir of the blood pressure produced an abrupt fall, of 5 to 10 second latency, due to a substance with histamine's properties. J. A. B. Gray and I later verified the circulation times involved.

So licheniformin turned out to be a histamine liberator (1), and I had had the good fortune to see a new, clean, surprisingly specific pharmacological response, which was in itself rather attractive as a tracing. When we went on to find that the same pattern was displayed by any dibasic compound in which the basic groups (amine, amidine, isothiourea, guanidine) were separated by around 6 or more carbon atoms, I was fascinated. A clean action caused by a specific chemical structure opened a new world. I have sketched elsewhere (2) how the follow-up led to the work with Nora Zaimis on the methonium compounds (3). Phenyl biguanide and Compound 48/80 were other dividends. The point, however, is that the fish was caught. That experience and what it led to is the basis of my own definition of pharmacology:

> If physiology is concerned with the function, anatomy with the structure, and biochemistry with the chemistry of the living body, then pharmacology is concerned with the changes in function, structure, and chemical properties of the body brought about by chemical substances. In the same way, pathology is concerned with the changes brought about by disease. For pharmacology there results a particularly close relationship with chemistry; and the work may lead quite naturally, with no especial stress on practicality, to therapeutic application, or (in the case of adverse actions) to toxicology.

Such a pattern seems to me both to do justice to what catches the imagination of those working in the different fields, as well as showing how they all belong to one family.

Do such definitions matter? Most of the time not. But in the recruitment of new blood, it is useful to have some shorthand description; and when it comes to higher policy, the nonscientific administrator is liable to define pharmacology, just from its etymology, as "the science of drugs", with a resulting difficulty in distinguishing it from pharmacy.

Competition for funds, or simple enthusiasm for a subject, often leads to exaggerated claims for a particular discipline, and to the view that other subjects are inferior or merely applications of it. (Sentences containing "merely" or "only" should always be viewed with deep skepticism.) I like to reduce such claims to an absurdity. Let us start with pharmacology;

> which may be said to be merely applied physiology;
> which is, of course, merely an embodiment of biochemistry;
> which is merely chemistry in one development;
> which is merely the working out of certain physical principles;
> which is merely the body of particular solutions of certain mathematical equations.

But mathematics is only a branch of logic, as Bertrand Russell and his peers established, so that philosophy is the fundamental basis of it all.

Yet we know today that philosophical ideas are culturally determined, not absolute, so that sociology is the central discipline.

But sociological thinking must be merely a function of psychological process.

Such processes are, of course, no more than exercises in the pharmacology of the central nervous system.

The whirligig is complete.

Pharmacology, then, can take its own place. There is no one science central to all the others, as various scientific chauvinists would have us believe.

It is equally untrue to real life to say that "all science is one". That suggests a sort of homogenized intellectual mayonnaise, with no differentiation. One can, of course, trace relationships, as indeed I have just done. But each scientist seems to find something particular that catches his imagination. The disciplines that become separate, for the time being, are those areas that seem to fire enough people, are attractive enough to the young, and are worth meeting for, thus creating a kind of mental center of gravity. One need not be exclusive, but can move between one center of gravity and another.

If one asks, when did pharmacology begin, perhaps one can place the start in the remote past of *materia medica,* or with Magendie's first analysis of the action of a drug, or with the founding of chairs and societies, or with the therapeutic explosion from the 1930s onwards (4). But historically, the Stockholm Congress in 1961 now seems to me one of the watersheds. Börje Uvnäs had asked me to join its organizing committee; and there followed a fascinating discussion of the program to be developed in pharmacology's first independent international meeting. It was a critical moment. That meeting might have fallen apart into its biochemical, physiological, chemical, pathological, toxicological groupings. But it did not; the great and marvelous fact was that despite misgivings it fell triumphantly together. The establishment of pharmacology as an independent discipline, a center of gravity in its own right, was certain from then on.

As for my research on diving, I can see now that it too had a pharmacological component. For instance, there had been operational reports of what was called "shallow water black-out", and one of our concerns was the risk to a diver (and also to those in a sunken submarine) of becoming unconscious through CO_2 accumulation. It had previously been thought that respiratory stimulation would always provide sufficient warning, but we had found that if sufficient oxygen was present to remove any hypoxic drive, as was normally the case in diving, then CO_2 could produce unconsciousness readily (even pleasantly) without gross respiratory stimulation. It fell to me to run the O_2/CO_2 mixture breathing experiments to define the range of individual sensitivity.

All the members of the laboratory "blacked out" in their turn, as did any unwary visitors, such as B. H. C. Matthews and D. G. Evans. Judging by subsequent careers, a few minutes of 10–20% CO_2 has no long-term toxicity. But the experiments led to reading about anesthesia. Then G. L. Brown asked me to join him in advising some civil engineers on compressed air work, which resulted in collaboration with D. N. Walder and others on "bends". So an interest in high pressure biology was implanted that survived even when wartime work was all wound up. That interest produced, with E. B. Smith, a colleague in physical chemistry, the Oxford High Pressure Group; and the research still, in the problems presented by the "rapture of the deeps" and the High Pressure Neurological Syndrome, has its pharmacological flavor.

For those whom it suits, pharmacology is a lovely subject, carrying one quite naturally from the molecular level to the whole man, using any and every skill one possesses, intellectually demanding yet with practical usefulness round the corner, not yet too sophisticated technically, and still young and fresh enough for the simpleminded to be able to contribute.

"F4"

Sir Henry Dale's laboratory, the Division of Physiology and Pharmacology, in the National Institute for Medical Research in Hampstead, was one of the classic laboratories. It deserves study in its own right, and I hope that those who worked there have left some account. A latecomer like myself, though deeply influenced by it, can only give a hint of what it must have been like in its prime.

The fourth laboratory on the first floor, it was, in 1944, a large communal laboratory. If one's own experiment was not going too well, or there was a waiting period, one could look at someone else's. The storage cupboards full of equipment reached up to a high ceiling. That ceiling was stained from the overflows in the organic chemistry laboratory above. When we rolled cylinders of gas on the floor, to make new mixtures to breathe in the diving experiments, protests would come from readers in the rather beautiful Georgian-style library below. A small side room contained a bicycle ergometer used for studies at controlled oxygen consumption. The laboratory was entered from a corridor that ran the length of the building, and there was a small office, a small workshop with a lathe and hand-tools, and a lavatory immediately across the corridor. One of the pleasures was that if one went out into the corridor one was only too likely to bump into someone from one of the other laboratories.

The main laboratory was simply laid out: There was a long window bench looking out over the tennis court and other grounds, the Institute's main workshop, and the shed housing J. S. Haldane's old compression chamber, recently transferred from the Lister Institute; desks, arranged according to the inhabitants and needs of the moment; operating tables and kymographs; an old watercentrifuge with a balance for its cups and a stern notice from the head technician above it: "Near enough is not good enough"; paper-smoking and varnishing cabinets in one corner, adapted during wartime to accommodate a Haldane gas-analysis apparatus; a refrigerator, oven, waterpumps, and so on.

At lunchtime we could join other members of the Institute in the lunch room at the top of the building and then go through to the coffee room, which had a balcony looking south over the rest of London. Towards the end of the War, when the time of the "doodlebugs" came, one could see the defensive barrage balloons on the Downs. Across the road outside the Institute was the pub, the "Hollybush", where one could take a visitor after work in the evening or have some celebration.

Between 1944 and 1949, when the Institute moved to Mill Hill, H. B. Barlow, J. A. B. Gray, B. D. Burns, and W. L. M. Perry were other members of staff; M. Goffart, J. L. Malcolm, A. Sand, M. Vianna Dias, and Nora Zaimis were our honored visiting workers.

The head technician, L. W. Collison, had been Dale's personal technician, and was of kindred quality. Not greatly educated, of rather gloomy appearance, formal, courteous, tough, a stern disciplinarian, yet as determined to stand up for his staff's rights as for his own, he was intrinsically very kind, and a man of the highest standards. These he displayed in his preparation for experiments, in his construction of exquisitely delicate Brodie bellows for sensitive plethysmography, and above all in his preparation and mounting of smoked drum tracings for publication. Many of the classical tracings in the *Journal of Physiology,* establishing the theory of chemical transmission, attest to his artistry.

How does one pin down the intangibles that create a successful laboratory? You were expected to stand on your own feet. Yet there was every kind of support by advice, criticism, personal help, and (most notably) general pleasure at any progress you made. No feasible experiment, if you wanted to try it out, was barred. The range of equipment available and the little workshop across the corridor made it easy to develop a new technique. But perhaps the secret lay in the two at the top, both of whom had shared in the *anni mirabiles* of chemical transmission before the War. G. L. Brown ran the laboratory on a very light rein and gave the laboratory high spirits and a wonderfully deft experimental skill—he was a joy to watch. F. C. MacIntosh exhibited a depth of thought and an unquenchable considerateness in everything he said and did. It is impossible to set down what one owes them.

INTO A WIDER WORLD

In 1949, with the move of the National Institute to Mill Hill, G. L. Brown went to the chair of Physiology at University College, F. C. MacIntosh to that at McGill, and W. Feldberg took over "F4", establishing its ethos in a new environment. We worked together on histamine release from skin; devising a perfused skin preparation and learning how to write papers with him were equal delights. (To describe our consumption of cigarillos would, today, doubtless count as pornography.) There was also collaboration with Burns (on endplate depolarization), with Perry (on ganglia), and with new recruits such as W. W. Douglas (on anticholinesterase effects) and M. Schachter (on the effect of antihistamines on the release of histamine), as well as writing papers with Nora Zaimis.

The Director, Sir Charles Harington, was always slightly irritated at comparison with the Hampstead days; yet W. A. H. Rushton's remark, that "moving to a larger laboratory is like an adiabatic expansion: the particles become more distant from each other, and the temperature falls", seemed to have some truth. One bumped into members of other sections less often. Yet it was, in fact, during a corridor conversation that Albert Neuberger remarked to me that he felt his work was not going very well, and perhaps he ought to move. A year later, a chair at St. Mary's and a burst of new work thereafter showed his wisdom.

I am not quite sure what generates this restlessness, which I was feeling, too. The wish to be one's own master does not seem sufficient cause, when one has so much freedom and such facilities. Perhaps, for an experimentalist, it is more the wish to have a shot at doing a new experiment, to head a department oneself. For me, it led in 1952 to a Readership in Applied Pharmacology at University College Hospital, joined by J. W. Thompson, under two professors, M. L. Rosenheim in Medicine and F. R. Winton in Pharmacology. The laboratory was embedded in the Medical Unit, with an additional small room across the road in University College, and £200 a year running expenses. Our formal responsibility was to help Heinz Schild with his practical class in the College, and to give a course of 20 lectures bridging the basic pharmacology taught by Schild and the therapeutics lectures by physicians (that also fell to me to organize). It was quite a challenge to produce a complete lecture course after life at an institute. Work on histamine release went on, and John and I had an interesting time with A. Goldberg testing porphobilinogen, which had been recently isolated from patients with porphyria by R. G. Westall, to see if it was a possible causal agent of their symptoms. Unfortunately it proved rather inactive.

After two years, however, a serpent appeared in the Eden, namely C. A. Keele, with an invitation from the Royal College of Surgeons to start a new department of pharmacology there, for postgraduate teaching. By then I had had many contacts with anesthetists and physicians over the use of the methonium compounds and it seemed to me self-evident that no undergraduate course could possibly equip a medical student with all the basic knowledge he needed in his career—there was too great an annual flow of new drugs and new procedures involving totally new principles. So the idea of postgraduate education, of teaching those already experienced in medical practice who wanted to be updated, made sense. So did the idea of fuller laboratory resources.

In this academic experiment, John Thompson (now in Newcastle), John Vane, and John Gardiner (now in Hong Kong) joined me. I couldn't have asked for anything better than to start a new laboratory with such colleagues. It is remarkable to me now, when academic tenure is so much discussed, that it seemed to matter little to us that I was losing tenure and they were not receiving it. There was only enough money for the new laboratory for 5 years, and its continuance depended on our success. We were lucky with our research fellows and associated staff, all from the clinical world: J. G. Murray, E. Marley, G. C. Clark, and J. P. Payne, later to occupy chairs of surgery, pharmacology, surgery, and anesthesiology, respectively. Of our visitors, B. B. Gaitonde went on to head the Haffkine Institute, and Emile Savini to chairs in France. It was a very happy time, and it was the best interaction of "basic" and "clinical" science I have ever had. That the department did indeed continue, under Gustav Born, John Vane, and Graham Lewis, has always pleased me.

The Royal College of Surgeons broadened my life, but the effect was nothing compared to that of the move to Oxford in 1959. As an Oxford graduate, one was "imprinted" by the University and one's old college; but the experience of an undergraduate, "the toad beneath the harrow", and of one of the dons, the "harrow" itself, is very different. It is too much to describe here, and indeed, it is still in process.

But there are two things from my time at Oxford that I like to mention. The first arises when aspersions are cast on the academic standing of pharmacology. Then I like to recall that in 1962, out of an established staff of six, four were Fellows of the Royal Society: E. Bulbring, H. Blaschko, H. R. Ing, and myself. That is in part a tribute to my predecessor, J. H. Burn, but it seems to me also to show that quality is not impossible even to a small science. Other departments can make equivalent claims.

Second, I have concluded from 25 years at an undergraduate university, as well as from seeing many other forms of research life, that no research institution keeps its freshness and vigor, unless it is continually rinsed through by exposure to new youthful minds. The undergraduate can be infuriating, lazy, stupid, and rude (and also charming, hardworking, intelligent, and courteous). No doubt he feels the same about his seniors. But there is something uniquely invigorating in being obliged to interest minds quite new to a subject, and to respond to the naïve, sometimes foolish, but essentially unspoiled vision of it that they have. New centers of research, free from the "burden" of teaching and the associated tasks, can flourish for a time. But follow their progress over the years, and you will see the complacent inward look developing—unless some wise person has contrived a youthful revivifying stream.

RATE THEORY REVISITED

I am sometimes asked what I think about rate theory today. The question always drives me back to the mental puzzles that evoked it.

The idea of rate theory germinated around 1955. The immediate stimulus was an invitation to give a paper on the mechanism of neuromuscular block at the World Congress of Anesthesiologists in Scheveningen that year. The two types of agents, depolarizing and nondepolarizing, that Eleanor Zaimis and I had distinguished operationally in some detail, were familiar. But examples were accumulating of block of an intermediate type, such as what she called "dual block". Bovet had contrasted "pachycurares" and "leptocurares" corresponding (for example), to tubocurarine and decamethonium, thus emphasizing the role of molecular shape. But the intermediate type of response, with typically stimulant phenomena followed by apparently simple curare-like block, was found even with a "leptocurare" like tridecamethonium. I included in my paper (5) a crude estimate of polarity of the various agents (the ratio of C atoms to N atoms), and suggested that when the ratio rose above 8 to 10, a transition occurred from depolarizing to intermediate type. It therefore seemed to be progressive hydrophobicity that caused the development of a curare-like component of action. The survey suggested that "drugs with some measure of hydrocarbon loading may (through their lipoid affinity) develop an attachment to the membrane of a kind different from, additional to, and interfering with, the attachment which leads to endplate activation. For instance, it might be essential, for normal activation, that a chemical bond be rapidly made and broken, or that the molecule has to move across or through the membrane; fixation of the molecule by its hydrocarbon content to adjacent lipoid regions of the membrane could well interfere with such a process".

But the problem of dual block was not the only stimulus. The work on the methonium compounds had raised in an especially acute form the question of how it was possible that structures so closely alike as hexamethonium and decamethonium could not merely act selectively on different effector organs, but act in totally different ways. Work with W. L. M. Perry had revealed the action of nicotine on the ganglion also to be of intermediate type, with depolarizing block passing over to a nondepolarized hexamethonium-like state; and on the guinea-pig ileum the self-block and bell-shaped dose-response curve were not well understood. Study of the anaphylactic spasm of sensitized ileum, and the extent to which it could be imitated with histamine, also raised some puzzles. Finally, there was a long-standing wish to describe the time course of recovery from neuromuscular blocking agents, ever since our finding, during potency comparisons of decamethonium with tubocurarine, that after apparently complete recovery of a muscle twitch from tubocurarine there might still be enough tubocurarine left to antagonize the action of decamethonium.

I was, however, at that time almost totally ignorant of receptor theory (what there was of it), and had just started a notebook devoted to the subject. It is hard today to understand the paucity of knowledge about, and the almost antagonistic attitude to, the receptor concept at that time. For a start, my greatest help was Haldane's 1930 book on enzymes, to which I turned after initial study of adsorption isotherms in a textbook of physical chemistry. In due course I found Gaddum's 1926 paper, then Clark's monograph of 1937, and Gaddum's formulation of competitive antagonism in the same year. Then there was Schild's pA notation in 1947 and 1949. But there were also a number of papers incompatible with Gaddum's formulation, and in the background were, for instance, the critical remarks by Dale in 1945 of the whole receptor concept, and a conspicuous lack of any direct evidence for it. In 1954 there began a long series of papers by Ariens and his colleagues, developing for drug action a framework comparable to that available for enzyme kinetics. By hindsight, these could have helped me; but at the time the multiplicity of possible models presented, with a growing number of disposable parameters, left me rather confused. I found myself more at home with R. P. Stephenson's work published in 1956. But although his introduction of the concept of efficacy seemed a real advance, it did nothing to answer my question of why some drugs are stimulant, some antagonistic, and some intermediate. To say that efficacy was high, low, or medium just restated the problem.

I think it is unlikely that I would have gone much further had not a bronchial episode led to a period in bed, around 1956. For something to do, I started working through for myself the equations that a bimolecular type of reaction may lead to, particularly seeking formulations that would be experimentally testable. I looked for patterns that could explain the bell-shaped dose response curve of nicotine on the gut, that would give some physical interpretation of efficacy, that would explain the transition from stimulation to relaxation with intermediate-type drugs, and that would help to analyze the time course of blocking agents in the body. Haldane and Briggs' analysis of the results of a two-point attachment, with a bell-shaped substrate concentration-velocity curve interested me very much, and I was carried far out of my depth in trying to extend it and its kinetics. I made rather little progress. When the thought finally occurred that receptor excitation might be a function of rate of association of drug with receptor, it seemed almost magical how many of the questions it solved. If activation of the receptor required that a high rate of drug turnover continually releases receptors for fresh associations, then the characteristic sequence (stimulation then block) of intermediate drug action followed naturally, drug-receptor dissociation rate could provide the independently measurable index of efficacy, and the slowing of dissociation by hydrophobic bonding explained the shift from stimulation to block with increased hydrophobic loading in homologous series.

It was quite a busy time in other ways. There was the move to the Royal College of Surgeons in 1954. From 1951 to 1957 I was secretary of the Physiological Society. In 1959 I moved to Oxford. Most of my experiments were performed in the evening and it shows. There is not nearly enough replication in the paper that I finally wrote (6). It would have been wiser, too, to have separated more distinctly the various themes in that paper. I felt the phenomena of nonspecific desensitization of smooth muscle were important, that they showed that nonreceptor effects could be great and needed to be controlled, and that they seemed to provide an immediate explanation of the existence of spare receptors (for they meant that receptor occupancy would not always be the rate-limiting step). This last point, however, was really a separate issue.

I would treat the ion exchange model differently today. There is no evidence that it plays any role, although I still wonder about the fate of counter ions to charged groupings in the receptor in the presence of an interacting drug. The model was only suggested, because it seemed to me necessary to give some illustrative example of a possible quantal mechanism. MacIntosh and I had considered an ion-exchange mechanism for the action of histamine liberators, with the bases exchanging with histamine in the tissues. So, in my reading round the subject of neuromuscular block, I had noticed Ing and Wright's suggestion of an ion exchange by alkylammonium salts at the neuromuscular junction. It was a simple concept that had stuck in the memory. Finally I was impressed with the evidence about loss of potassium as a result of agonist action. But again, it was a side issue.

Rate theory had its first exposure to the British Pharmacological Society in July 1959. Then, in 1961, I was asked to present the paper before publication at a meeting of the Royal Society, which I did, loaded up with analgesics. The President, H. W. Florey, asked Gaddum, who was present, if he thought the theory was sound, and Gaddum replied that he thought there might be something to it. Bernard Katz asked what quantal mechanism I envisaged. I could only repeat my working analogy, that the drug-receptor interaction was more akin to the playing of a piano (where a finger that is not rapidly withdrawn interferes with the flow of sound), than it is to the playing of an organ. That weekend I went into Hammersmith Hospital for a bilateral antro-ethmoidostomy. One of my pleasantest memories was at a meeting of the British Pharmacological Society around that time, at which John Vane, describing an experimental set-up, referred to "what I understand we must now call an isolated piano bath".

What does one think of the theory now? I think it helped to promote interest in receptor studies, particularly on the kinetic side. I still find its economy conceptually attractive, requiring as it does only two rate constants and one other constant to couple the receptor to the effector. So far, I see no other independently testable interpretation of efficacy. As a possible model it does not seem to mislead the student, since most of its consequences for the general pattern of drug action are quite sound: agonists do wash out quickly; for equiactive doses, antagonists do usually take longer to act and to pass off, the more potent they are; decline of antagonism can be measured, and changes in receptor occupancy do follow an exponential course. With partial agonists, agonism is prompt and then antagonism follows; hydrophobic loading does generally favor antagonist rather than agonist action.

I was very disappointed that the measurement of the rate constants of drug receptor interaction has proved so difficult, particularly with smooth muscle, where the range of values seems wider (and thus potentially more informative) than with striated muscle. It was ironical that it was our own work at Oxford (7) showing how the relatively large uptake of drug by the receptor created a large reserve of drug, that led to the possibility that the kinetics were diffusion, not receptor, controlled, as Douglas Waud had come to suspect and Thron and Waud then showed (8). No way was found to distinguish the two possibilities. I was back in the old position, unable to find a definitive, objective, independent sign of efficacy.

It is pleasing that agonist action has now turned out to be quantal, and it seems likely to be linked to receptor turnover. But it seems uncertain how the quantum originates, whether from the allosteric behavior of the receptor or from some aspect involving the drug molecule too. It was also interesting that an identical theory was formulated within gustatory physiology, quite independently, but for similar reasons.

My guess, however, is that the deeper understanding of the kinetics of drug action is not going to come through the formulation of drug-receptor equations, but from qualitatively new observations. Patch-clamping and conductance-channel biophysics, molecular engineering, and ultramicroscopy offer fascinating openings. I have suspected that our formulations will prove far too simple, ever since seeing some of D. C. Phillips' X ray crystallographic pictures of the interaction of a number of different substrates with lysozyme. With each substrate, the interacting regions were subtly different. Presumably the same is true with drugs interacting with receptors, and the reactions that we blithely represent by a single equation, $D + R \rightleftharpoons DR$, are in fact all different.

ON DOING WHAT YOU ARE ASKED TO DO, AND THE STIMULATED ILEUM

I have already mentioned two lines of research that followed on an "outside" stimulus—histamine liberation and rate theory. This is an important phenomenon, weakening the concept of the autonomous scientist in his ivory tower; even in research he seems to need stirring up from time to time. A third example was an invitation to talk on the pharmacology of the small intestine at a Gordon Conference, presumably because of my ganglionic work. I knew little about the gut, and found considerable doubt in the literature even as to the transmitters. So I began to search for some way of making a "neuroeffector" preparation out of a strip of intestine, on which one could do analyses comparable to those on striated muscle or ganglionic preparations. N. Ambache had found that a strip of gut would twitch if an electric stimulus was applied to its surface. But one then finds that the point of excitation moves and is undefined. It was then that I recalled some old experiments by Rushton, dealing with Lapicque's chronaxie theory of curare action, and Du Bois Reymond's cosine law: that excitation of a nerve in an electric field is in proportion to the cosine of the angle between nerve and field. Suppose one placed an electrode in the lumen of the gut, another outside, and created a field between them. The field would now be defined, independent of gut movement. But would the nerve networks of Auerbach's plexus be at an angle to be excited? The first experiment, in my office-cum-laboratory at the College of Surgeons, is still vivid. I set up the Trendelenburg preparation used to study peristalsis; my only piece of platinum, soldered to a lead, was threaded into the lumen. An alligator clip, dipping into the outer bath fluid, provided the other electrode. It worked like a bomb, with shocks as short as 50 μsec. I had, in a few moments, both a new neuroeffector test-bed (9), and something to say in New Hampshire. G. L. Brown, when he heard about it, was very amused, and called it the "electric clyster" in a mock eighteenth century poem. He also sponsored it for a demonstration at a Royal Society soirée, at which Fellows were able to do an Otto Loewi-type experiment for themselves: they took fluid from one bath holding an eserinised strip of intestine, with or without stimulation, and tested it for acetylcholine content on a second comparable strip arranged for assay.

    The guinea-pig ileum longitudinal muscle is a great gift to the pharmacologist. It has low spontaneous activity (unlike rabbit or rat); nicely graded responses (not too many tight junctions); is highly sensitive to a very wide range of stimulants; is tough, if properly handled, and capable of hours of reproducible behavior. A further bonus appeared later when I did electron microscopy on it, and found that Auerbach's plexus lay on the surface of the longitudinal muscle, not penetrating into it. As a result, after Humphrey Rang had shown how to separate strips of longitudinal muscle, Aboo Zar was able to produce acutely denervated strips simply by pulling them off the plexus (10). I know nothing quite like these preparations in physiological pharmacology. Normally, to denervate one cuts a nerve and then waits for it to degenerate; but during that time profound changes take place in the postsynaptic structure, so that one does not have a perfect control. The longitudinal muscle of guinea-pig ileum, with its diffusive type of transmission, is the only tissue I know of that allows you rigorously to compare innervated and totally denervated muscle. This was particularly important at the time for making absolutely certain that the acetyl-choline released came from nervous tissue, not muscle. I had found that morphine inhibited the ileum twitch without affecting the response to acetyl-choline and reduced ACh output (11), I was now confident in the conclusion that morphine was acting on nervous tissue and that the ileum could be used as a "paradigm of the brain."

The preparation has proved admirable for teaching. The coaxial method of stimulation was only necessary when stimulator power was limited, and simple field stimulation proved to work admirably. Particularly enjoyable was the collaboration with Sylvester Vizi on the effect of catecholamines on transmitter output, opening up a profitable presynaptic vein (12). So has been its use in identifying and assaying opioid peptides and drugs. Perhaps every scientist should be asked to talk on something about which he is ignorant, every five to ten years or so.

COMMITTEES

In my best, or worst, year, I counted service on 72 committees that met at least once, and sometimes ten to twenty times, in that year. I am sure there are others with a similar experience. It seems too many, yet none of them was trivial. The most severe critics were those who wanted me to serve on a seventy-third. Is there anything to say about it, except to warn?

It does require a decision at some stage in one's life. When the invitation first comes, it is not unflattering to find that somebody actually wants your services. Most people would agree that democracy, with continually changing com-mittees, is in the end better than dictatorship or oligarchy. There is, too, the opportunity both to be more "in the know" and to have some influence. Most people find a small dose of one or the other attractive enough to exchange for a little research time or some leisure. In the event, you do indeed lose time, and it can be trying to spend hours awarding money to others to do experiments you would like to be doing yourself. Some say discouragingly that such work is "all right for those that like it". It is a great simplification when you grasp that the only valid reason for doing anything is that it is the right thing for you to do. There is in the end a genuine satisfaction in seeing work progressing that you helped to forward. Even more important, and a reflection of the fact that shared endeavor is the most potent source of friendship, are the friends you make. So, if advice were wanted whether or not to undertake such work, the heart of it must be the importance of diagnosing one's own capacities and values. It proves to be a balance between one's own work on one side, and, on the other, new friendships while forwarding the work of others. Not a very obvious choice. I recall a famous remark by F. M. R. Walshe, the great neurologist at University College Hospital, a Catholic and vigorous controversialist for whom I served as house officer. After seeing a pair of outpatient twins he said, "I wish one could baptize one twin and use the other as a control". (If we could live a second life, would we go back to do the controls to the choices we have made?)

Nevertheless, committee work can certainly go too far. I suspect that pharmacology may be especially vulnerable. The pool of trained pharmacologists is in any case not very large. The academic part has to teach doctors, physiologists, pharmacologists, biochemists, chemists, and pharmacists. It has to attract students, arm them with an undergraduate training, introduce them to research, and then supply them to industry as new recruits to an extent that the other preclinical sciences are not called upon to do, proportionate to their total numbers. It must also supply the research leaders for industry. In the United Kingdom, I reckon that industry has taken away from academic life men who would have filled about a third of the professoriate. (By and large industry does not repay to academia its training and recruitment debt, despite the great scientific contributions of industrial pharmacologists.) That brain drain cannot strengthen the remaining pool to whom it chiefly falls to provide the general servicing (and defense) of pharmacology in its private and public functions. Finally, the sheer usefulness of pharmacology frequently brings its practitioners into practical affairs and issues that call for expert advice.

It would be better if the work was shared more widely. Committees might more often invite younger scientists to serve, instead of relying largely on older people. This would widen the decision-making base, and keep the decision process nearer to the front line of new knowledge, the true source of freshness and invigoration. Getting the right balance between age and youth is quite an art. It is wrong to burden the young while they are still establishing themselves, and while they are in a particularly fruitful phase. They also may lack patience. The old often have a mass of useful case history to call on, and have seen many "experiments" tried. Yet there is a tendency for old men to fight old battles; and while sometimes those battles are over issues that are still alive, too often the arena has moved elsewhere. I can see no rules, except perhaps to prefer for service those who are a shade reluctant to serve.

Secondly, it would be interesting to try building into the standing orders of any committee a terminating rule, that it must be disbanded after three years unless a really strong positive case for its continuance is made.

Thirdly, when a statutory committee simply must meet, it should be expeditious. My best example is my old "boss", G. L. Brown, whom I saw get through a statutory faculty board meeting at University College in 1.5 minutes flat, having accomplished all the required business.

CHOOSING AND JUDGING

Among the most important of committees are those concerned with making choices over appointments and awarding grants. I must have been involved in making hundreds, if not thousands, of such choices. Some years ago I was suddenly struck with repugnance at the whole procedure; and I wished never to make a judgment on another scientist again, nor have it in my power to influence his career in any way. Unfortunately one cannot responsibly just contract out. I suspect it was a reaction that was shared by others, for a general movement has occurred toward examining the efficiency of the decisions made by grant-giving bodies, and toward testing the validity of peer review.

For some time I have made little lists, as opportunity offers, of two things. One was of the names of those whom I had helped to choose for positions, together with their competitors' names. The other was of unforeseeable events (for example an unexpected death of someone in a key position, or a surprise career decision). Taking the approach of the naive empiricist, as opposed to that of the a priori thinker, I hoped that the first list would allow me to look back and see how wise a choice had been and that the second would enable me to test how far decisions seen in hindsight as incorrect could be understood as partly inevitable.

I cannot pretend to any great enlightenment. One thing that struck me was the mind's resistance to the idea that events indeed cannot be foreseen. My list of unpredictables has now lost all the impact each item had at the time it was entered; the choices now seem historically inevitable. Among the protective mechanisms of our minds there is something that rejects uncertainty and the cautious suspension of belief that an awareness of uncertainty requires. Since then, I have been struck by the rarity with which, for instance, journalists are willing to suspend judgment. In public utterance, the "all-or-none" law operates, with premature polarization and sharp antithesis clouding the possibility of any intermediate ground on public issues. Perhaps that is one reason why the scientist may find public affairs difficult.

A second thought was really a question, and it arises from the teaching and examining of students too. What is the proper time span for judging academic and professional performance? Should the competence of a medical student be judged by performance in an examination, in the first residency, after 10 years practice, or by the mortality rate among his patients throughout his life? Is a professor chosen for what he will do immediately, in five years, or over his whole career? Does one judge by the latest work of an individual, by the integral over his whole career thus far, or by some extrapolation into the future based on previous work?

Discussion of such questions does not prove very useful. One tends perhaps to favor that way of assessment that would put the best light on one's own work. But I do share the general suspicion of publication lists. The enormous growth of multi-author papers, and the breaking up of work into multiple papers, has made bibliographies extremely hard to interpret, and time rarely allows the reading of them. Yet if one sets them aside, what evidence is one to use? Referees are often flatly contradictory of each other and themselves need refereeing. It is only a matter of luck if there is an authority on the topic in one's decision group.

I believe, however, that for career choices at least, there is information that could be better used. Among the signs of peer trust and confidence are: the appointment of an individual to editorial boards, or to some office in a society, or to be a representative of some sort, or to be an examiner, or to be an organizer of some meeting or event. Success with graduate students is another sign. In each of these situations, other scientists are entrusting some part of their own concerns to another individual. It is true that none of these tests directly measure, say, creativity. But it is also true that people do not entrust matters of these kinds to the ignorant, foolish, or unresourceful. If one looks back at office-bearers and editorial boards and the like, it seems to me that many of those whose research I have admired do indeed appear among the names.

I would not wholly abandon the Citation Index type of approach, provided one restricts oneself to well-refereed journals of substance, and corrects for self-citation. But I would also like a Scientific Service Index, which records those activities where a scientist has been chosen by his peers. My only gloomy thought is that, once established, the Law of Indeterminacy (that the act of observing a phenomenon itself changes the phenomenon) would operate, as it has begun to do with the Citation Index.

More important, now that we are so much in one another's hands, is to keep thinking about assessment. It is common enough for bodies to look backward at their successes. It will take more courage to extract the rejections and the alternative policies not adopted, and to examine the failures. A good clinical trial notes adverse reactions and deaths, as well as benefits and survivals. Why should one assess one's own past choices less rigorously?

THE SOCIAL RESPONSIBILITY OF SCIENTISTS

Do scientists have, by virtue of their skills and knowledge, any particular social duty outside their science? It is a sign of the times that the question would, today, almost always be interpreted politically, although it is equally valid at the level of individual action on behalf of other individuals. The answers are immensely varied, and the causes taken up equally so, whether nuclear war, preservation of endangered species, pollution in all its facets, holistic medicine, or civil liberties. There would likewise be no agreement about the range over which the scientist speaks with particular authority, and where with no more than any citizen's. He may like to claim an objectivity conferred on him by training and practice, but the nonscientist does not always find this convincing.

For my own part, I have been pushed out of the purely academic path over two issues. In each case what got under my skin was what seemed to me, to quote a phrase of my grandfather's, "suppressio veri and suggestio falsi". The first was the antivivisection movement. Soon after I had qualified in 1942, I saw an advertisement by an antivivisection society on a hoarding near our flat in London. It claimed to give the number of children dying from diphtheria over a term of years, who had been vaccinated against the disease. None of the other relevant figures, about numbers at risk and the fate of the unvaccinated, were given. It stuck in my mind. Perhaps it prepared me for joint work while secretary of the Physiological Society, later as Chairman of the British Research Defense Society, and later still for writing "Man and Mouse" (13). Such tasks took time away from the laboratory; yet how could anyone who has seen what medicine can do as a result of animal experimentation, who then sees that work traduced, fail to defend it?

There may be a trace of genetic predisposition here—I am very proud of my grandfather. David Macdonald was a Presbyterian minister in Derby in 1901, when Stephen Coleridge, the leading antivivisectionist of his day, came to lecture on animal experimentation. My grandfather, who was interested in science and bought *Nature* every week to circulate round his parish, did not like the style of what he heard. He criticized it vigorously at the meeting, citing Ferrier, Keith, and Spencer Wells, and then wrote to the local paper referring to "suppressio veri" and "suggestio falsi" and saying that no lover of truth could support Mr. Coleridge's society. Coleridge then launched a suit for libel, demanding a public apology, damages and costs. Although David Macdonald was a poor man, he refused these. He had always been friendly with the local doctors, and in due course they came to his rescue, bringing in Lauder Brunton and Victor Horsley. When the case came up, David Macdonald needed to do no more than show that there had been no personal attack; after 30 minutes, the jury asked if they needed to hear any more, returned a not guilty verdict and said the case should never have been brought. It remains an exceptional case to my knowledge, of a member of the church putting himself at risk for the world of science. A gentle, affectionate man, he retired to the Scottish Highlands, and died after overtiring himself in the mountains. One of his sayings was: "You should not criticize people unless you have been in the same position and done better."

The other "outside" activity has to do with drug dependence. Work with morphine led me in 1966 to attend a meeting on adolescent drug dependence, where I heard about cannabis use for the first time. Two points were of interest. One was Dr. Rasor's remark that 95% of his New York heroin users had also used cannabis, but only 30–50% had used other drugs like amphetamine, alcohol, and barbiturates. The other point was the flat contradiction of one psychiatrist by another as to the reasons for cannabis use. So I went away to look up this curious material. What I found did not seem to correspond at all with some of the assertions being made (about harmlessness, lack of after-effects, nonaddictiveness, power to improve mental function, and the like). As

I then began to see the effects in students, my overwhelming feeling was that a vulnerable generation had been gulled. I felt some duty at least to publicize more of the original information, rather than allowing secondary and tertiary citations appear to be the sum of information available. This led to a good deal of lecturing (14) and some writing, and the discovery of Gabriel Nahas as an ally. E. W. Gill, R. G. Pertwee, and I started some work, which later was extended with mass spectrometry under David Harvey. No one can be happy about the incidence and effects of drug dependence today. But now, three satellite conferences (15) and many symposia and reviews later, there is at last some solid information, and the subject is no longer so briskly brushed under the carpet of sociological bromides.

As always, the work brought new friends. It also proved interesting in new ways, because of the political and media dimensions. It is irksome at first to find oneself classified by the antivivisectionist activists with slave traders and Nazi war criminals or by the "pot lobby" with Commissioner Anslinger. One learns the edge behind the advice "If you can't stand the heat, get out of the kitchen". But it is also fascinating to learn to what extent the dictum that "the medium is the message" is true. There is no doubt that a truly effective publicity campaign can both induce a widespread belief in quite erroneous or misleading ideas, and also cause not so much the rejection but the discounting of evidence. But only for a time. In the end, evidence wins through. Perhaps the tendency of the human mind to question everything is ultimately a very great protection. For it means that even if false ideas become current (e.g. that millions of animal experiments are done in the cosmetics industry, or that one cannot develop tolerance to or dependency on cannabis), once such ideas become in any sense orthodoxy, they become themselves subject to doubt and scrutiny. Then the evidence begins to make its mark. But there is, of course, a price, paid by the continuance of unnecessary ignorance, and the suffering of its victims.

EMPIRICAL AND A PRIORI THINKING

As the trajectory of a pharmacologist's life moves from the laboratory to the committee world and back again, inevitably patterns appear. One is the division between those who have done experiments and those who have not. It correlates closely with the division between those with an empirical habit of mind and those whose approach is a priori. I suspect it is what really underlies C. P. Snow's two cultures. Most of the time we inhabit both worlds, but sometimes one meets each mode of thought in all its purity.

The a priori mode of thought needs some defense, if one is writing for scientists, for it seems so absurd to the scientifically trained not to learn from experience all that one possibly can. But there is more to it than that. It is only too familiar a sight to find the conclusions drawn from some body of empirical evidence being bitterly disputed. The onlooker soon appreciates the adage about "lies, damn lies, and statistics". If someone then says, in effect, that there are a limited number of possibilities, that all the outcomes can be envisaged (using imagination, intelligence, experience, and wide reading), and that simply by reflecting on these one can reach rational decisions, it can be attractive and cogent. The empiricist himself uses such methods in deciding if something is "plausible". (The weakness is that in fact all possible outcomes cannot be envisaged.) If the approach is combined with skill in presentation, a powerful a priori case can be built up. It is here that training in the humanities or in law is so powerful; for it is a training that takes a vast range of human experience as its raw material, and teaches how to think deeply and argue cogently about it. Yet, in the end, one must see it as dealing entirely with the given. The facts of a case simply serve, not to suggest further inquiry, but to identify the category of previous thought and analysis to be applied. It can then be quite a battle to get new evidence sought for or considered.

The experimenter has ultimately a different approach. He knows that there are still things not known, which are also not deducible, and that they are out there waiting to be discovered, by the method of deliberate experiment. That method is easy to write about, but not so easy to acquire. I reckon that I did not really learn what it was about until I had been at Hampstead for around six months. There seems to be a similar interval with my graduate students, before they move from making the observations they feel they "ought" to make, to trusting what they actually see with their own eyes and having the confidence to act on it. A little later comes the marvelous time when they actually make a discovery, however minute, of something that was not known before. It is then that the feeling for when something is proved or not proved begins to grow.

Philosophically, of course, some argue that nothing is ever proved. So let us put it a little more practically: that the empiricist learns that, with the right procedures, he can reach conclusions on which both he and others seem to be able to build, conclusions that are not dependent on his own prejudice, nor on his own powers of advocacy, but which remain true when the experiment is in the hands of others. At that moment, he joins the community of experimental scientists, a community spread over the world among his contemporaries, and reaching back in time through the centuries and forward into the future. We are not just of the same family as our colleagues of today, but also of Ehrlich and Dale and Cushny and Abel and Stephen Hales and Robert Hooke and Robert Boyle.

The lesson of the experimental method is not pain-free, for it is accompanied by repeated demonstrations of how wrong one's ideas had been, of one's experimental inadequacies, of one's stupidity in framing rational possibilities. But once learned, the reward is great. Today, relativism underlies a great deal of thinking; and it often seems fair and cautious to believe that there is no certain answer to some question. Yet if that leads on to the conclusion that it is never possible to say whether or not this or that "is the case", the outlook is depressing indeed; for then force would be the only way to settle uncertain questions. But the experimenter who finds that he can confirm another person's findings, or has his own unexpected results verified in another laboratory, begins to have some confidence that there is a world where something objective exists, that movement forward in some sense, however modest, is possible.

The empiricist's danger may be that of too great an attachment to the latest evidence. But he should be an optimist; for he knows there is more to find, and in that finding, new opportunities are born.

SOME CONCLUSIONS

By the time one retires, any generalizations one might make are of small use. Looking back, I think it was only rarely that I actually took advice; example was a much commoner source of information. At the same time, there are a few points that, if asked, I like to hint at.

The first is the importance of keeping your nerve. There are always ups and downs; but there are always new and unexpected opportunities. My own career allowed me several opportunities to take the road that clearly suited me; and others have told me the same. So one can make mistaken choices, and yet have other chances. I think, too, that the saying is right that "the main difficulty is almost always muddle not malice". Conspiracy theory seems to me historically inaccurate in almost every case; and it can waste a lot of time and emotion.

A second point is the importance of "self-diagnosis", of discovering where your real interests and skills lie. It is not easy, for at the start one does not know the options, and once you are launched there are plenty of pressures from others to do this or that. One useful measure is to discover what your mind turns to when it is "free-coasting", i.e. when there are no pressures on it, nothing is expected of you, and you are even a little bored. A similar test is to recognize those activities where time seems to disappear. Charles Morgan puts it romantically in "The Judge's Story": "ask yourself in what work, what company, what loyalty your own voice is clear and in what muffled. By that answer rule your life". One's mind has a "grain", and it is better to work along it.

A third point is distinguishing between the various meanings of the superlative case of the adjective "good". One meaning is simply "very good". A second meaning is "the best". This has the interesting feature of being a function of the surroundings. The level is set by the competition. While competition may be a potent stimulus, it may also be virtually absent. The paradox may then arise of the "best" not even being particularly "good". This is the weakness of relying totally on the competitive impulse. Finally comes "the best possible", where both the competition and that internal impulse to do yet better are both drawn upon. Here is where the new ground is broken. Words-worth describes it, in his passage on the bust of Newton in King's College Chapel, as "the prism and silent face, the marble index of a mind voyaging through strange seas of thought alone." That level is for only a few, but perhaps L. W. Collison's notice in F4, mentioned earlier, "Near enough is not good enough", was in the same spirit.

Lastly, accuracy is a quality that can be most helpful. It need not be restricted to measurement. Sometimes a situation can get complicated, with allowances here, and compensating severity there. If one sets aside all the adjustments, and simply tries, at the start, to make as accurate a description or diagnosis or account as possible, it can release a cramp. Everyone respects accuracy; and once the initial ground is clear, solutions become easier to find. None of these matters are easy; but a strategy that seeks to begin with accuracy is off to a good start.

Literature Cited

1. MacIntosh, F. C., Paton, W. D. M. 1949. The liberation of histamine by certain organic bases. *J. Physiol.* 109:190–219

2. Paton, W. D. M. 1982. Hexamethonium: contribution to symposium honouring Sir John McMichael. *Br. J. Clin. Pharmacol.* 13:7–14

3. Paton, W. D. M., Zaimis, E. J. 1952. The Methonium Compounds. *Pharmacol. Rev.* 4:219–53

4. Paton, W. D. M. 1963. The early days of pharmacology, with special reference to the nineteenth century. In *Chemistry in the Service of Medicine*, ed. F. N. L. Poynter, pp. 73–88. London: Pitman

5. Paton, W. D. M. 1956. Mode of action of neuromuscular blocking agents. *Br. J. Anaesth.* 28:470–80

6. Paton, W. D. M. 1961. A theory of drug action based on the rate of drug-receptor association. *Proc. R. Soc. London Ser. B.* 154:21–69

7. Paton, W. D. M., Rang, H. P. 1965. The uptake of atropine and related drugs by intestinal smooth muscle of the guinea-pig in relation to acetylcholine receptors. *Proc. R. Soc. London Ser. B.* 163:1–34

8. Waud, D. R. 1968. Pharmacological receptors. *Phamacol. Rev.* 20:49–88

9. Paton, W. D. M. 1954. The response of the guinea-pig ileum to electrical stimulation by co-axial electrodes. *J. Physiol.* 127:40–41P

10. Paton, W. D. M., Zar, M. A. 1968. The origin of acetylcholine released from guinea-pig intestine and longitudinal muscle strips. *J. Physiol.* 194:13–33

11. Paton, W. D. M. 1957. The action of morphine and related substances on contraction and on acetylcholine output of coaxially stimulated guinea-pig ileum. *Br. J. Pharmacol.* 12:119–27

12. Paton, W. D. M., Vizi, E. S. 1969. The inhibitory action of noradrenaline and adrenaline on acetylcholine output by guinea-pig ileum longitudinal muscle strip. *Br. J. Pharmacol.* 35:10–28

13. Paton, W. D. M. 1984. *Man and mouse: animals in medical research.* Oxford/New York: Oxford Univ. Press. 174 pp.

14. Paton, W. D. M. 1968. Drug dependence—a socio-pharmacological assessment. Public lecture to British Association, Dundee, *Adv. Sci.* 25:200–12

15. Paton, W. D. M., Nahas, G. G., Braude, M., Jardillier, J. C., Harvey, D. J., eds. 1979. *Marihuana: Biological Effects: analysis, metabolism, cellular responses, reproduction and brain.* Oxford/New York: Pergamon 777 pp.

Ann. Rev. Pharmacol. Toxicol. 1986. 26:23–37

CURRENT ANTIDEPRESSANTS[1]

Leo E. Hollister

Departments of Medicine, Psychiatry and Pharmacology, Stanford University School of Medicine and Department of Medicine, Veterans Administration Medical Center, Palo Alto, California 94304

INTRODUCTION

Depression is very likely a heterogeneous disorder (Table 1). According to the current classification of the Diagnostic and Statistical Manual (DSM-III), several diagnoses are possible, based on the presence or absence of mania as well as the severity of the depression (1). A classification that uses somewhat older nomenclature has the advantage of offering some practical guides to treatment (2). Many other classifications are possible and the nomenclature is constantly changing.

Prior to the late 1950s, depression was treated primarily with electroconvulsive therapy and psychotherapy. The advent of effective antidepressants changed practice, so that presently drug therapy is the main modality of treatment (3). Specific types of psychotherapy may be useful alone for patients with mild depressions and may be adjunctive to drug treatment in more severe depressions. Severe depressions that constitute suicidal risk or that are refractory to drugs should be treated with electroconvulsive therapy. I shall review the current drugs used for treating depression, limiting them to those used in the United States and focusing on the newer antidepressants.

DRUGS AS TOOLS FOR UNDERSTANDING PATHOGENESIS

Drugs have been valuable tools for understanding the pathogenesis of depression. The early discovery that reserpine evoked depressive reactions led to the so-called amine hypothesis of depression. Because reserpine depleted stores of biogenic amines (e.g. norepinephrine, serotonin, and dopamine) from nerve endings, depression was associated with a depletion of biogenic amines (4).

[1]The US Government has the right to retain a nonexclusive, royalty-free license in and to any copyright covering this paper.

Table 1   Classification of depression

Source	Classification	Characteristics	Reference
DSM-III (1980)	Bipolar	Mixed manic, depressed	(1)
	Major Depressions (Unipolar)	Single or recurrent episodes	
	Others	Cyclothymic disorders, Dysthymic disorders (depressive neurosis), Atypical bipolar, Atypical depression, Schizo-affective adjustment disorder with depression	
Hollister Trichotomous Classification (1978)	Reactive	Secondary to psychosocial loss, physical illness, other psychiatric disorders—nonspecific treatment	(2)
	Endogenous	Genetic-biochemical basis; Occurs in any epoch of life—antidepressants specifically useful	
	Manic-depressive	Typically cyclic depression and mania but one or the other manifestation may predominate—most stabilized patients treated with lithium, treat depression or mania with antidepressants or antipsychotics, respectively	

Additional evidence for the amine hypothesis came from knowledge of the action of clinically effective antidepressant drugs. Virtually all types of antidepressants act by increasing the amount of aminergic neurotransmitter in the synapse (5). Although greatest attention has been paid to the biogenic amines norepinephrine and serotonin, the action of some of the newer drugs has raised the possibility that dopamine may also play a role.

Each of the various types of antidepressants acts in different ways to increase the amount of aminergic neurotransmitter at the synapse. Tricyclics block the amine pump, the "off switch" of aminergic neurotransmission. Such an action presumably permits a longer sojourn of neurotransmitter at the receptor site. Monoamine oxidase inhibitors block a major degradative pathway for the amine neurotransmitters, which presumably permits more amines to accumulate presynaptically and more to be released. Sympathomimetics also block the amine pump, but are thought to act primarily by increasing the release of catecholaminergic neurotransmitters (6).

Most of the newer antidepressants also act by one or another of these mechanisms, as well as by acting as direct receptor agonists or antagonists. For

Table 2   The action of tricyclic antidepressants on various receptors in the brain [a]

Receptor	Effect of tricyclic antidepressant
Beta-2-adrenoreceptor	Down-regulation due to increased concentration of noradrenaline
Serotonin-1-receptor	Functional significance unknown
Serotonin-2-receptor	Down-regulation due to increased concentration of serotonin
Muscarinic acetylcholine receptor	Blocked Many anticholinergic side effects ? sedation
Alpha-1-adrenoreceptor	Blocked Orthostatic hypotension Sedation
Alpha-2-adrenoreceptor	Presynaptic down-regulation due to increased concentration of noradrenaline Less inhibiton of noradrenaline release
Histamine-1-receptor	Antagonized Sedation
Histamine-2-receptor	Antagonized ? consequences
Dopamine autoreceptor	Unknown; weak action

[a]Source: Potter W.Z. (5).

a long while the increase of aminergic neurotransmitter in the synapse was thought to increase postsynaptic responses in a deficient system. Such conclusions were based on short-term studies. Clinically, however, drugs are given long-term, which is deemed necessary for their full antidepressant action. When long-term administration of antidepressants is studied in animals, and the postsynaptic consequences are measured by the generation of cyclic AMP, a subsensitivity of the postsynaptic receptor is observed (7, 8). Thus, thinking about the consequences of increased aminergic neurotransmission produced by antidepressants has made a 180 degree turn. The evidence is now strong that the original theory was incorrect.

It appears that most classes of clinically effective antidepressants lead to decreased sensitivity of postsynaptic beta-adrenoreceptors. These include selective uptake inhibitors of both norepinephrine and serotonin, blockers of the uptake of both amines, monoamine oxidase inhibitors, and some drugs that block uptake of neither neurotransmitter. Electroconvulsive therapy likewise decreases receptor sensitivity. In addition, tricyclic antidepressants, the most widely studied class, act on a number of receptors, as shown in Table 2. More of these receptor actions elicit unwanted effects than contribute to the therapeutic actions (9).

As both serotonin and norepinephrine seem to be involved in depression, an attempt has been made to reconcile the two-neurotransmitter theory of depression with the decreased sensitivity of β receptors. It is assumed that the final common denominator of antidepressant action is an augmentation of norepinephrine release with consequent down-regulation of beta-receptors. Serotonin, however, plays a permissive role in this process, acting at the level of the receptor. Block of serotonin synthesis in animals pretreated with parachlorphenylalanine (PCPA), a tryptophan hydroxylase inhibitor, negates the down-regulation of receptors that normally follows treatment with desipramine. PCPA also blocks the clinical effects of antidepressants. A similar distribution of norepinephrine and serotonin terminals in the cortex provides an anatomical basis for the interdependence of the two aminergic systems. Thus, the debate over which neurotransmitter is most involved in depression seems to have been resolved: both are involved, but norepinephrine represents the final common pathway (10).

DRUGS FOR TREATING DEPRESSION

The number of drugs available for treating depression has been growing rapidly. The original group was exemplified by the tricyclic antidepressants, the monoamine oxidase inhibitors and, to a lesser extent, the sympathomimetic amines and lithium. This group might be referred to as "first-generation" antidepressants. During the past several years, a number of other drugs, usually chemically and sometimes pharmacologically different from these other classes, have been introduced. These drugs are often called "second-generation" antidepressants.

"First-Generation" Antidepressants

TRICYCLICS   Chemical structures of some of the most commonly used tricyclics are shown in Figure 1. Slight modifications occur either in the ring structure or side chain. Even though slight, these chemical alterations provide pharmacological differences among the various tricyclics.

Imipramine   This drug was the first antidepressant, discovered as such fortuitously in the clinic. Its pharmacokinetic properties, as well as those of some other antidepressants, are shown in Table 3. The major metabolic pathway is demethylation, which leads to formation of desipramine, an active metabolite. The amount of desipramine in steady-state conditions actually exceeds that of the parent compound in most patients. Desipramine may be further oxidized to active metabolites, but the extent of their contribution to therapeutic effects is uncertain (11). Imipramine blocks the amine pump both for norepinephrine and serotonin; desipramine specifically blocks uptake of norepinephrine. The net

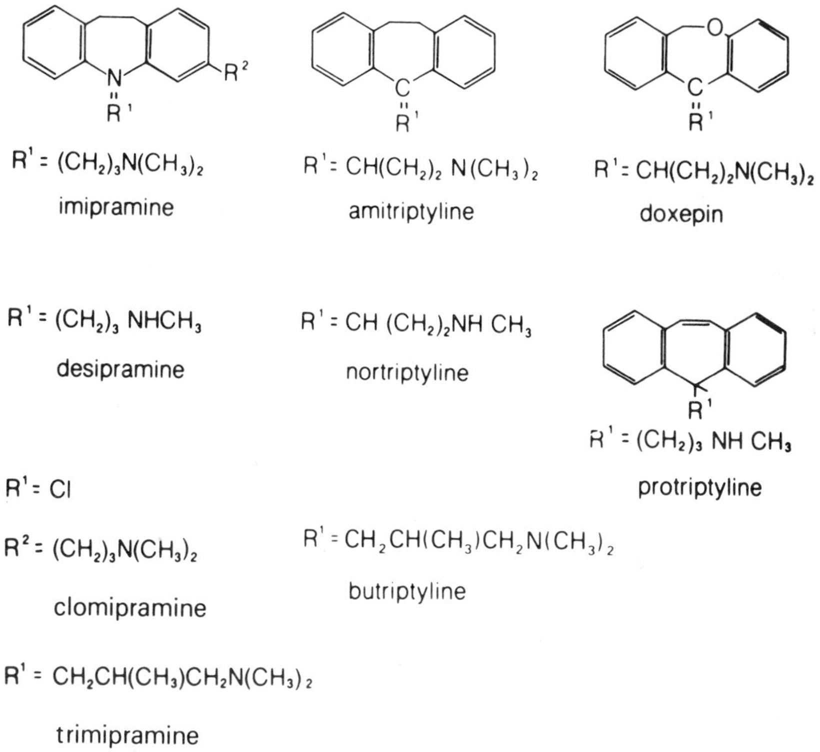

R' = (CH₂)₃N(CH₃)₂

imipramine

R' = CH(CH₂)₂ N(CH₃)₂

amitriptyline

R' = CH(CH₂)₂N(CH₃)₂

doxepin

R' = (CH₂)₃ NHCH₃

desipramine

R' = CH (CH₂)₂NH CH₃

nortriptyline

R' = (CH₂)₃ NH CH₃

protriptyline

R' = Cl

R² = (CH₂)₃N(CH₃)₂

clomipramine

R' = CH₂CH(CH₃)CH₂N(CH₃)₂

butriptyline

R' = CH₂CH(CH₃)CH₂N(CH₃)₂

trimipramine

Figure 1 Structural relationships among various tricyclic antidepressants. Major differences are in minor changes in the ring or side chain.

effect is that imipramine blocks uptake of norepinephrine more than of seroto-nin. Moderate sedative and anticholinergic effects may be troublesome to some patients. Alpha-adrenoreceptor blocking actions may be greater than those of most other tricyclics, which predisposes to orthostatic hypotension. Imip-ramine is a membrane-active local anesthetic (as are other tricyclics), which gives it both antiarrhythmic as well as arrhythmogenic actions. Usual doses of the drug are 75 and 300 mg/day.

Desipramine   A metabolite of imipramine, this drug is used as a separate entity. A quicker onset of action than the parent drug was postulated, but that contention has been difficult to prove. Desipramine has fewer sedative, anti-cholinergic, and alpha-adrenoreceptor blocking actions than most other tricy-clics. Patients who cannot tolerate the unwanted effects produced by these pharmacological actions may tolerate desipramine better. Doses are similar to those for imipramine.

Table 3 Pharmacokinetic parameters of various antidepressants

Drug	Bioavailability (%)	Protein binding (%)	Plasma $t_{1/2}$ (hr)	Metabolites in plasma	Volume of distribution (l/kg)	Therapeutic plasma concentrations (ng.ml)
Imipramine	29–77	88–93	6–20	Desipramine usually more; active	20–40	>180 total
Amitriptyline	31–61	82–96	31–46	Nortriptyline; usually less, active	—	>200 total
Nortriptyline	46–79	93	18–28	10-Hydroxy; 3–4 times as abundant; ? activity	21–57	50–150
Desipramine	—	70–90	14–62	2-Hydroxy metabolite	22–59	145
Protriptyline	—	—	55–124	None active	19–26	70–170
Clomipramine	—	—	22–84	Desmethyl metabolite predominant; active	7–20	80–100
Doxepin	13–45	—	8–24	Desmethyl; active	9–33	—
Amoxapine	—	—	—	9-Hydroxy; 3–10 times as abundant; active	—	200–400
Alprazolam	—	65–75	6–27	? hydroxy	0.65–1.44	—
Maprotiline	66–75	88	21–25	Desmethylated, active	15–28	200–300
Trazodone	—	—	8	m-Chlorophenyl-piperazine; active	—	—
Buproprion	—	85	11–14	? Active	—	25–100
Nomifensine	—	—	2–4	? Active	—	—

Amitriptyline   This tricyclic was the most widely used until recently. A demethylated metabolite, nortriptyline, is generally not as abundant as the parent drug. Although amitriptyline in vitro has a selective action in blocking uptake of serotonin, nortriptyline has a mixed action. The net result is that amitriptyline has a mixed effect, predominantly on serotonin. Amitriptyline is probably the most sedative and most anticholinergic of all tricyclics; it is often used when sedation is desired (12). Doses are usually 75–300 mg/day.

Nortriptyline   A metabolite of amitriptyline, this drug is also used as a separate entity. During the first pass through the liver it is extensively metabolized to 10-hydroxy-nortriptyline, which is far more abundant than the parent compound. The exact amount of activity contributed by the metabolite is unknown. Relatively fewer sedative and anticholinergic actions occur with nortriptyline than with the parent drug. Doses of nortriptyline have usually been lower than for the other tricyclics, although the basis of such conservatism has not been established.

Doxepin   The strong sedative effects of this drug have been the basis for its promotion as an antianxiety as well as an antidepressant drug. A demethylated metabolite also contributes to its action. Doxepin itself has a relatively weak action in blocking the amine pump, despite the fact that it is generally thought to be equally effective as an antidepressant. Doses are similar to those of other tricyclics.

Protriptyline   This drug has been one of the least popular tricyclics, and has not been widely promoted. Some clinicians believe that it has a stimulating action; it is certainly the least sedative tricyclic. Some anticholinergic action remains. Protriptyline may be a reasonable alternative for patients who become overly sedated by the other tricyclics. Doses are considerably lower than those of other tricyclics, generally 10–40 mg/day.

Others   Butriptyline and trimipramine are isobutyl side-chain modifications of amitriptyline and imipramine, respectively. They differ little from the prototype drugs. Clomipramine is a chlorinated ring-substituted homolog of imipramine. Just why this modification provides a presumed specific efficacy for obsessive-compulsive patients is unclear. Doses of these drugs are similar to those of other tricyclics.

MONOAMINE OXIDASE (MAO) INHIBITORS   MAO inhibitors are classified as hydrazides (-C-N-N-configuration) and nonhydrazides. The structures of some MAO inhibitors are shown in Figure 2.

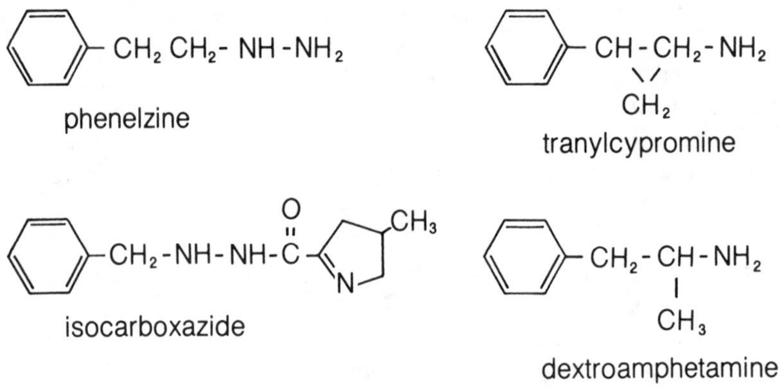

phenelzine: $CH_2 CH_2 - NH - NH_2$

tranylcypromine: $CH - CH_2 - NH_2$ with CH_2

isocarboxazide: $CH_2 - NH - NH - C$ (with O) CH_3, N

dextroamphetamine: $CH_2 - CH - NH_2$ with CH_3

Figure 2 Structural relationships among MAO inhibitors. Note the close chemical relationship between tranylcypromine and dextroamphetamine.

Phenelzine   This drug has been the most durable MAO inhibitor and is the only one currently promoted in the United States. At least 80% inhibition of monoamine oxidase must be obtained for optimal clinical effects. Doses of 1 mg/kg/day are usually necessary to obtain such inhibition, but the process takes time and so does the regeneration of the enzyme (13). Improvement in patients may not be evident until two or more weeks of treatment. When the drug is stopped, the enzyme is not regenerated for another two weeks. Tricyclics should not be added or replaced in the treatment program for at least that period. The converse sequence of the MAO inhibitor following tricyclics can usually be done with no delay. Usual doses of phenelzine are 45–90 mg/day.

Isocarboxazide   This MAO inhibitor is neither widely used nor promoted and has been less well studied than the others. Usual doses are 20–50 mg/day.

Tranylcypromine   The chemical structure of this nonhydrazide MAO inhibitor is similar to that of dextroamphetamine. It retains some of the sympathomimetic actions of the latter drug but is a much more potent inhibitor of monoamine oxidase. Usual doses are 10–30 mg/day.

SYMPATHOMIMETICS   These drugs are used only in rare patients. Occasionally, they produce benefit in patients who have been resistant to the other antidepressants.

Dextroamphetamine   The structure of this compound is shown in Figure 2. Insomnia and loss of appetite limit its use in some patients although stimulation and appetite suppression may be desirable effects for others. Some patients require substantial doses to obtain benefit but show little evidence of tolerance or dependence with prolonged treatment. Usual doses are 10–30 mg/day, with some patients requiring as much as 60 mg/day. Methylphenidate, an amphetamine surrogate, is even less commonly used and has no special advantages.

LITHIUM   Although lithium carbonate has been reported to be useful for treating acute depressions that appear not to be part of manic-depressive disorder, it is seldom used as a sole treatment. More likely it may be added to a tricyclic when the latter provides inadequate remission (14). Its use in preventing recurrences of depression, whether unipolar (endogenous) or bipolar (associated with manic episodes) is well documented. However, in a unipolar patient who has responded to a conventional antidepressant it is usually easier to continue or maintain the patient on that drug than it is to switch to lithium.

"Second-Generation" Antidepressants

The enthusiasm with which these drugs have been received stems from the several problems that remain with the "first-generation" drugs. First, only about 60–65% of depressed patients are helped and many do not attain a full remission of symptoms. Second, the clinical response to first-generation drugs may be delayed. This delay may be more a consequence of the slow induction of treatment mandated by the side effects of these drugs. Thus, it is more likely a pharmacokinetic than a pharmacodynamic phenomenon. Third, the numerous side effects of first-generation antidepressants may make it impossible to treat some patients with fully effective doses or may lead to noncompliance with treatment on the part of others. Finally, tricyclics in particular are potentially lethal when taken in overdose. The paradox is that one must prescribe such drugs to a group of patients with the highest risk of suicide.

Although it has not been claimed that the newer antidepressants are more effective overall than the tricyclics with which they are usually compared, they do assert three advantages: (*a*) a more rapid onset of action, (*b*) more tolerable side effects, (*c*) greater safety when taken in overdose (15).

Four of these drugs are currently on the market in the United States and more are expected soon. The variety of chemical structures of these drugs is shown in Figure 3.

Amoxapine   Amoxapine is a demethylated metabolite of the antipsychotic, loxapine. It is further metabolized to hydroxy metabolites, which are 3–10 times as abundant as the parent drug and which probably account for the antidepressant activity (16). The net effect is more blockade of uptake of norepinephrine than of serotonin. The anticholinergic action is weak. The dopamine-receptor blocking action of loxapine is retained to a somewhat lesser degree in amoxapine, which also has some antipsychotic activity. This combined action may be especially suitable for patients with psychotic or agitated

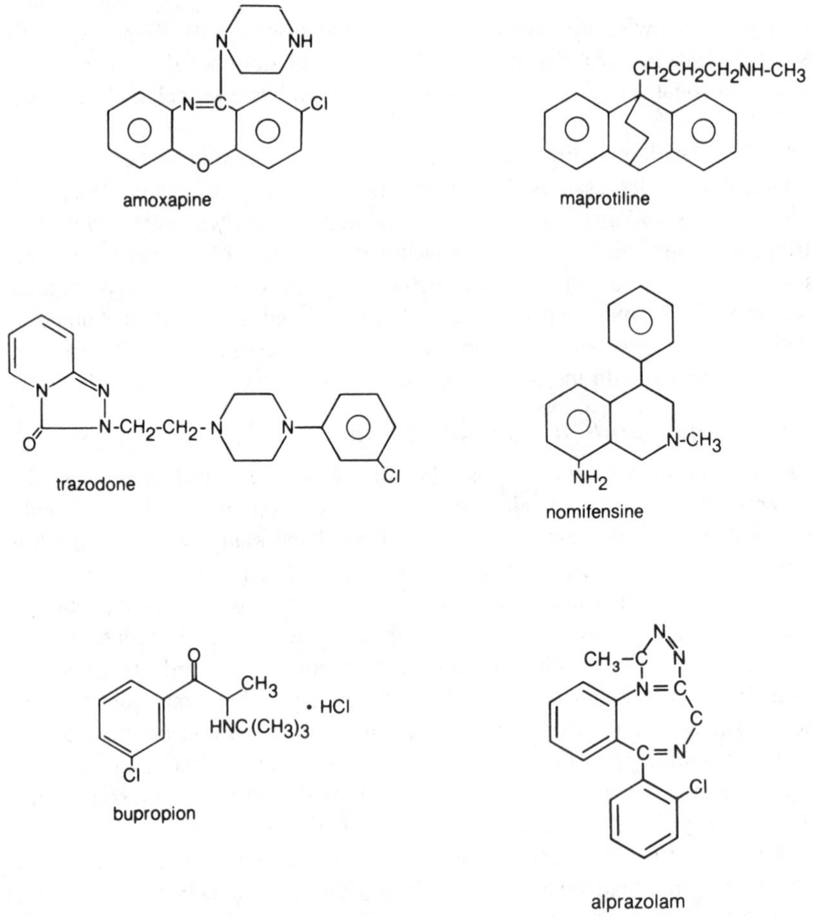

amoxapine

maprotiline

trazodone

nomifensine

bupropion

alprazolam

Figure 3   Structures of "second-generation" antidepressants. A variety of structures are involved.

depressions. However, it may also lead to extrapyramidal syndromes and hyperprolactinemia with sexual disturbances in men and amenorrhea-galactorrhea in women. Although the drug has less cardiotoxic action than tricyclics in overdoses, it produces seizures that are difficult to control, with an attendant fatality rate. Usual doses are 150–300 mg/day.

The claim for a more rapid onset of action is not substantiated and is further offset by an apparent tolerance to the therapeutic effects that may develop in some patients after an initial response. Not only are the usual sedative and anticholinergic side effects of tricyclics as common with this drug, but it also adds some of the side effects of antipsychotics. Severe neurotoxicity, which occurs after overdoses, makes it at least as dangerous as those tricyclics with predominant cardiotoxicity. In summary, amoxapine offers very little.

Maprotiline   A two-carbon bridge across the central ring of the 6-6-6 three-ring structure of this drug creates a fourth ring, making it a tetracyclic compound (17). The side chain is the same monodemethylated aminopropyl sidechain found in desipramine, creating a rather similar structural geometry. The primary action of the drug is to block uptake of norepinephrine; it also has less sedative or anticholinergic action than amitriptyline, the drug against which it has most often been compared. Had it been compared with desipramine, which it resembles both in structure and in major mode of action, it is likely that no differences in these side effects would have been noted. The drug had a decade of use in other countries before arriving in the U.S. and was well recognized to cause seizures, even within the range of therapeutic doses. These are usually 100–300 mg/day.

Whether maprotiline has a faster onset of action has not been adequately tested. It seems to offer nothing new in its mechanism of action nor fewer sedative and anticholinergic side effects as compared with desipramine. Seizures occur at therapeutic doses far more often than with tricyclics. Skin rashes also seem to be more frequent. Overdoses are about as dangerous as with tricyclics. The drug offers little advantage over desipramine. Oxaprotiline, an active metabolite, is under clinical investigation but should not be much different.

Trazodone   Although frequently described as a triazolopyridine compound, trazodone is more properly described as a phenylpiperazine. In this respect it resembles chemically oxypertine, a drug that has been used both as an antipsychotic and as an antianxiety agent. Pharmacologically, it is complicated (18). Some doses act as a serotonin receptor antagonist, while others act both as a serotonin agonist and as an uptake inhibitor. It may also increase release of norepinephrine by blocking alpha-2 adrenoreceptors. The exact mode of its therapeutic action is unknown, although presumably it works mainly as a serotonergic drug. An active metabolite, m-chlorophenylpiperazine, is formed; but it is not clear to what extent it may contribute to the antidepressant effect. Although clinically it has appeared to be as effective as the tricyclics against which it has been compared, results have often been spotty. Some patients obtain much relief, while others derive no benefit. The same dichotomy applies to its sedative effects. These limit doses in some patients while others are not at all bothered. Skin rashes seem to be more common than expected. Rare instances of short runs of ventricular tachycardia and priapism have occurred. The usual daily doses are 150–400 mg.

No claim is made for a more rapid onset of action, which is difficult to prove at best. The anticholinergic side effects of tricyclics are definitely fewer with this drug, but sedation can be troublesome. Overdoses have been managed easily with no apparent cardiotoxicity, despite the ventricular tachycardia reported with therapeutic doses. If one were more confident about its therapeutic efficacy, which has been called into question, it might have some advantages (19).

Nomifensine A phenylisoquinoline derivative, nomifensine has been marketed in numerous countries around the world during the past several years and has been given to millions of patients. Despite this extensive clinical experience, it is a new drug in the United States. Abundant evidence suggests that nomifensine is a potent inhibitor of both dopamine and norepinephrine uptake (20). The neuropharmacological profile of the drug has been thought to lie between that of amphetamine and imipramine (21). In man, the EEG profile of the drug resembles that of desipramine (22). The latter observation is consonant with the fact that no amphetamine-like stimulation could be found in volunteer subjects given single doses (23). Almost every study agrees that nomifensine has little antimuscarinic action.

Most of the drug in plasma is in the form of a conjugate; numerous metabolites have been described. The $t_{1/2}$ of unchanged drug is 2–4 hours, but the clinical span of action is much longer, possibly due to an active metabolite.

The lack of effects of the drug on blood pressure, cardiac conduction times, and EKG in normal subjects, as well as the lack of significant cardiovascular complications following overdose, have made it more suitable than tricyclics for patients with cardiovascular disease (24). Another advantage over conventional antidepressants is a notable lack of psychomotor impairment (25). Side effects such as dry mouth, headache, and dizziness are so common that they are difficult to evaluate when reported for any drug. On the other hand, nausea, vomiting, or restlessness might be expected consequences of an increase in dopaminergic activity, whatever the mechanism. Excitation, delirium, stereotyped movements, and dyskinesia have been rarely reported but are plausible. In general, the drug has tended to produce fewer minor side effects than the tricyclics with which it has been compared. A sizable number of patients treated with the drug, perhaps as many as 1%, experience drug fever early in the course of treatment. The significance of this immune response to the drug remains to be seen.

No claim has been made for a more rapid onset of action. Clinically, the drug is as efficacious as the conventional antidepressants against which it has been compared, offering the notable advantage of a diminished number of the common side effects related to sedation and to anticholinergic actions. Overdoses of nomifensine have been marked by drowsiness, tremor, tachycardia, and obtunded consciousness. No convulsions, cardiac arrhythmias, or EKG changes have been noted. All side effects have been easily managed. If more experience with the drug in the United States confirms its efficacy and safety, nomifensine may represent a true advance in antidepressant drug treatment.

Several other new drugs may soon be available as treatments for depression.

Buproprion   Buproprion has a phenethylamine structure that superficially resembles that of amphetamine or methoxamine. Chemical modifications on the ring and side chain have markedly changed its spectrum of pharmacological actions. The chlorine atom on the ring protects against rapid metabolism; the tertiary alkyl group is not readily dealkylated, avoiding pressor activity; the aminoketo group confers lipid solubility (26).

The exact mode of action of buproprion is unclear. It seems definitely to require the presence of intact dopamine neurons in the brain. An early study suggested that the drug acted primarily as a dopamine uptake inhibitor (27). It has little effect on norepinephrine uptake, no anticholinergic actions, and no inhibiting effects on monoamine oxidase. Chronic treatment produced neither down-regulation of beta-adrenoreceptors nor of dopamine receptors. It is possible that its major pharmacological effects may be mediated by an active metabolite.

Dry mouth is the most common side effect. Rashes may occur in 1–2% of patients. Anorexia and mild agitation may also be observed. Seizures have occurred with high doses (600–750 mg/day), which are no longer recommended; usual daily doses are 300–450 mg. Orthostatic hypotension or other cardiovascular effects have been notably absent during clinical drug trials.

Buproprion is of interest because it appears to work primarily through dopaminergic mechanisms, raising the possibility that this neurotransmitter may also be relevant to the pathogenesis of depression. A more rapid onset of action than that of conventional antidepressants has not been documented. The drug also lacks most of the sedative, anticholinergic, and cardiovascular side effects of tricyclic antidepressants, although it is equally effective. Overdoses of from 900–3000 mg have been easily managed without any cardiovascular problems. This drug will be exceedingly interesting to watch as it is used in clinical practice.

Alprazolam   Alprazolam was one of a series of triazolobenzodiazepines synthesized in 1971. By 1973 the first report of its clinical use in anxious patients had appeared (28). Clinical observations suggested that it might also be useful for treating depression, and the first report on the use appeared in 1976. More recently, it has been thought to be useful for treating patients with panic attacks and agoraphobia.

Alprazolam exhibits the same profile of pharmacological activities as most other benzodiazepines (29). These actions would certainly justify its use as an antianxiety drug but do not explain why it should be different from other benzodiazepines in being an effective antidepressant. The efficacy of the drug in depression rests largely on a multiclinic trial that compared alprazolam (159 patients) with imipramine (146 patients) and placebo (131 patients). These patients met the standard research diagnostic criteria for depression. After 42 days of treatment, both active drugs produced more improvement in depression than placebo but were not different overall. Drowsiness was more often found in alprazolam-treated patients and dry mouth in those treated with imipramine (30). Although the drug is not officially labeled for use as an antidepressant, many clinicians are using it. Clinical consensus at the moment is that the drug may be useful in mildly depressed patients who are outpatients but that it is not fully effective in severe depressives.

About the only side effects that have been noted with alprazolam relate to its action on the central nervous system. Drowsiness has been the most common complaint. Yet even the frequency and intensity of this side effect seem to be less than from comparable doses of other benzodiazepines. Some of the studies of the drug in depressed patients have used doses up to 10 mg/day (equivalent perhaps to 100 mg/day of diazepam). Thus, it is possible that should patients being treated with such doses be suddenly withdrawn from the drug, an abstinence syndrome would follow.

Alprazolam, if it really is a major antidepressant, would seem to have many advantages over the others. The major drawback is the slow withdrawal of the drug that may be needed to avoid abstinence syndromes.

CONCLUSIONS

The physician has available an increasing number of antidepressant drugs. None are clearly superior overall. Because some patients respond to one drug and not to another, however, the increasing selection of antidepressants provides additional opportunities for successful treatment. The problem for the pharmacologist is to reconcile apparent differences in the modes of action of these drugs with their common property of antidepressant effect. As we learn more about how drugs act in treating depression, we can postulate new theories about the condition's biological bases.

Literature Cited

1. *Diagnostic and Statistical Manual of Mental Disorders* (DSM-III). 1980. Washington, DC: American Psychiatric Association, pp. 205–24
2. Hollister, L. E. 1983. *Clinical Pharmacology of Psychotherapeutic Drugs,* pp. 71–2 New York: Churchill-Livingstone 2nd ed.
3. Hollister, L. E. 1978. Treatment of depression with drugs. *Ann. Intern. Med.* 89:78–84
4. Garver, D. L., Davis, J. M. 1979. Biogenic amine hypothesis of affective disorders. *Life Sci.* 24:383–94
5. Potter, W. Z. 1984. Psychotherapeutic drugs and biogenic amines. Current concepts and therapeutic implications. *Drugs* 28:127–43

6. Sugrue, M. F. 1983. Do antidepressants possess a common mechanism of action? *Biochem. Pharmacol.* 12:1811–17
7. Vetulani, J., Sulser, F. 1975. Action of various antidepressant treatments reduces reactivity of noradrenergic cyclic AMP-generating system in limbic forebrain. *Nature* 257:495–96
8. Bannerjee, S. P., Kung, L. S., Riggi, S. J., Ghanda, S. K. 1977. Development of b-adrenergic receptor subsensitivity by antidepressants. *Nature* 268:445–56
9. Richelson, E. 1979. Tricyclic antidepressants and neurotransmitter receptors. *Psychiatr. Ann.* 9:195–96
10. Sulser, F. 1984. Antidepressant treatments and regulation of norepinephrine receptor-coupled adenylate cyclase sys-

tems in the brain. *Adv. Biochem. Psychopharmacol.* 39:249–61
11. Sutfin, T. A., De Vane, L., Jusko, W. J. 1984. The analysis and disposition of imipramine and its active metabolites in man. *Psychopharmacology* 82:310–17
12. Blackwell, B. 1984. Antidepressant drugs. In *Meyler's Side Effects of Drugs,* ed. M. N. G. Dukes, pp. 24–61. Amsterdam: Elsevier
13. Robinson, D. S., Nies, A., Ravaris, C. L., Ives, J. O., Bartlett, D. 1978. Clinical pharmacology of phenelzine. *Arch. Gen. Psychiatry* 35:629–35
14. De Montigny, C., Grunberg, F., Mayer, A., Deschens, J-P. 1981. Lithium induces rapid relief of depression in tricyclic antidepressant non-responders. *Brit. J. Psychiatry* 138:252–56
15. Coccaro, E. F., Siever, L. J. 1985. Second generation antidepressants: A comparative review. *J. Clin. Psychopharmacol.* 25:241–60
16. Jue, S. G., Dawson, G. W., Brogden, R. N. 1982. Amoxapine: A review of its pharmacology and efficacy in depressed states. *Drugs* 24:1–23
17. Wells, B. G., Gelenberg, A. J. 1981. Chemistry, pharmacology, pharmacokinetics, adverse effects and efficacy of the antidepressant, maprotiline hydrochloride. *Pharmacotherapy* 1:121–39
18. Clements-Jewery, S., Robson, P. A., Chidley, L. J. 1980. Biochemical investigations into the mode of action of trazodone. *Neuropharmacology* 19:1165–73
19. Klein, H. E., Muller, N. 1985. Trazodone in endogenous depressed patients: A negative report and a critical evaluation of the pertaining literature. *Prog. Neuro-Psychopharmacol. Biol. Psychiatr.* 9:173–86
20. Randrup, A., Braestrup, C. 1977. Uptake inhibition of biogenic amines by newer antidepressant drugs: relevance to the dopamine hypothesis of depression. *Psychopharmacology* 53:309–14
21. Spencer, P. S. J. 1977. Review of the pharmacology of existing antidepressants. *Brit. J. Clin. Pharmacol.* 4:57S–68S
22. Saletu, B., Bruenberger, J., Linzmayer, L., Taeuber, K. 1982. The pharmacokinetics of nomifensine. Comparison of pharmacokinetics and pharmacodynamics using computer pharmaco-EEG. *Int. Pharmacopsychiatr.* 7(Suppl.1): 43–72
23. Hamilton, M. J., Smith, P. R., Peck, A. M. 1982. Buproprion, nomifensine and dexamphetamine on performance, subjective feelings, autonomic variables and EEG in healthy volunteers. *Brit. J. Clin. Pharmacol.* 14:153P
24. Burrows, G. D., Vohra, J., Dumovic, P., Scoggins, B. A., Davies, B. 1978. Cardiological effects of nomifensine, a new antidepressant. *Med. J. Aust.* 1:341–43
25. Wittenborn, J. R. 1977. Contrasts in antidepressant medications. *Brit. J. Clin. Pharmacol.* 4:153S–56S
26. Soroko, F. E., Mehta, N. B., Maxwell, R. A., Ferris, R. M., Schroeder, D. H. 1977. Buproprion hydrochloride. A novel antidepressant agent. *J. Pharm. Pharmacol.* 29:767–70
27. Cooper, B. R., Hester, T. J., Maxwell, R. A. 1980. Behavioral and biochemical effects of the antidepressant buproprion (Wellbutrin): evidence for selective blockade of dopamine uptake in vivo. *J. Pharmacol. Exp. Ther.* 215:127–34
28. Itil, T. M., Polvan, N., Egilmez, S., Saletu, B., Maraso, J. 1973. Anxiolytic effects of a new triazolobenzodiazepine, U-31,889. *Curr. Ther. Res. Clin. Exp.* 15:225–38
29. Rudzik, A. D., Hester, J. B., Tang, A. H., Straw, R. N., Frils, W. 1973. Triazolobenzodiazepines, new class of central nervous system depressant compounds. In *The Benzodiazepines* ed. S. Garattini, E. Mussini, L. O. Randall, pp. 285–97. New York: Raven Press
30. Feighner, J. P., Aden, G. C., Fabre, L. F., Rickels, K., Smith, W. T. 1983. Comparison of alprazolam, imipramine and placebo in the treatment of depression. *J. Am. Med. Assoc.* 249:3057–64

Ann. Rev. Pharmacol. Toxicol. 1986. 26:39–58

THE BIOLOGICAL BASIS AND MEASUREMENT OF THRESHOLDS

W. N. Aldridge

Toxicology Unit, Medical Research Council Laboratories, Woodmansterne Road, Carshalton, Surrey, SM5 4EF, United Kingdom

"𝖂𝖆𝖘 𝖎𝖋𝖙 𝖉𝖆𝖘 𝖓𝖎𝖙 𝖌𝖎𝖋𝖋𝖙 𝖎𝖋𝖙 ᷓ 𝖆𝖑𝖑𝖊 𝖉𝖎𝖓𝖌 𝖋𝖎𝖓𝖉 𝖌𝖎𝖋𝖋𝖙/𝖛𝖓𝖉 𝖓𝖎𝖉)𝖙𝖘 𝖔𝖇𝖓 𝖌𝖎𝖋𝖋𝖙/𝖆𝖑𝖑𝖊𝖎𝖓 𝖉𝖎𝖊 𝖉𝖔𝖋𝖎𝖘 𝖒𝖆𝖈𝖇𝖙 𝖉𝖆𝖘 𝖊𝖎𝖓 𝖉𝖎𝖓𝖌 𝖐𝖊𝖎𝖓 𝖌𝖎𝖋𝖙 𝖎𝖋𝖙." (1)

"What is it that is not poison? All things are poisons and none that are not. Only the dose decides that a thing is not poisonous". (2)

INTRODUCTION

The above famous statement was made by Paracelsus in 1538 in reply to the criticism by academic medical men about his use of poisons to treat the sick. In his *Defensiones* he illuminates the fundamental issue that the distinction between poisonous and nonpoisonous substances is not real; the dose can move a substance from being nonpoisonous (and sometimes even beneficial) to poisonous. The thresholds for such and other actions depend on measurement. For example the auditory threshold, i.e. the least intensity at which a given sound can be perceived, is defined as an intensity of sound emitted. As knowledge of biological mechanisms increases, it may be possible to show that when a sound is emitted but not perceived, several steps in the complex process of hearing have been activated but the whole process not completed. In a similar way, as mechanisms of toxicity become established in molecular terms, possibilities emerge for answering the question of whether a threshold actually exists and explaining it in biological terms.

39

0362-1642/86/0415-0039$02.00

Single molecules of a macromolecule (such as an enzyme or a receptor) are either active or inactive, although the activity or properties of the macromolecule are sometimes changed; e.g. acetylcholine on the nicotinic receptor (3), the regulation of enzymes by formation or breakdown of the phosphoenzyme (4), or the blocking of an enzyme catalytic center such as acetylcholinesterase by reaction with organophosphorus compounds (5, 6). Thus the control of metabolism and function is often entirely analogous at the molecular level to the perturbation of physiological systems by inhibitors and toxins. The occupancy of certain crucial sites in some parts of the macromolecule in vivo and whether this measurable change in activity becomes translated into a clinical or other response define the threshold question.

The above comments concern acute phenomena. When occupancy by a toxin of a catalytic site or receptor is maintained, the plasticity of biological systems is such that the primary response may become neutralized. Thus, if rats are exposed to an organophosphorus compound over a long period of time during which the acetylcholinesterase is inhibited in the brain, the initial rise in the concentration of acetylcholine is followed by a reduction to normal concentrations (7), i.e. the system adapts to the changed circumstances, presumably by producing less acetylcholine.

Toxicologists are mainly concerned with thresholds of chronic rather than acute exposure to chemicals. It is vital to know whether acute exposure leads to chronic toxicity or disease or whether chronic exposure will eventually lead to an accumulation of individual undetectable effects until clinical signs or syndromes appear. An empirical approach to such questions leads to the impossible philosophical conundrum of proving a negative. However, as knowledge of mechanisms increases one can ask more fundamental questions. For example, if after administration of a toxic chemical a degree of reaction with a relevant receptor or target can be measured, does this lead to disease?

For practical purposes many methods for the determination of threshold or no-effect levels depend on mathematical models of varying complexity. However, as noted by the European Chemical Industry Ecology and Toxicology Center, "the use of generalised mathematical schemes for deriving safety factors is to be depreciated because they cannot accommodate the wide variation in animal and human response and the variable quality and quantity of much of the data available. There is no alternative to the use of expert scientific judgement in this matter on a case by case basis" (8).

Invoking expert scientific judgment implies that an exact answer to the question cannot be given. The purpose of this paper is to emphasize the kind of biological information required for a logical approach to the problem. This includes measures of received dose rather than the concentration in the environment external to the animal or human, and knowledge of mechanisms derived from experimental studies on animals.

MECHANISMS OF TOXICITY

Although toxicity to a mammal is observed as clinical signs and symptoms of dysfunction, we can now subdivide the whole poisoning process into several well-defined aspects (9; Figure 1).

After entry of the chemical by several routes, the toxicity process is represented as four interconnecting compartments: They are in order from left to right: 1. all systems that influence the *delivery* of the chemical or a metabolically derived toxic derivative to its site(s) of action; 2. the interaction (called the *early reactions*) of the proximal toxin with targets (analogous often to pharmacological receptors) that are usually, but not exclusively, macromolecules; 3. the induction following the early (primary) reaction(s) of a cascade of *biochemical and physiological changes;* 4. the *consequences to the organism* that are seen as clinical signs, symptoms, or syndromes, which may range from serious impairments of function (as seen in many neuropathies) to minor skin conditions. This scheme can be extended ad infinitum with many details of toxic processes. In its present form, however, it concentrates the mind on four aspects of the toxic process that must often be studied using different experimental approaches.

The question of whether a threshold exists can now be refined and extended. Instead of asking whether a given dose leads to clinical signs of disease, one can ask whether a given degree of reaction with the target leads to clinical signs; whether a given reaction with the target causes biochemical, physiological, or

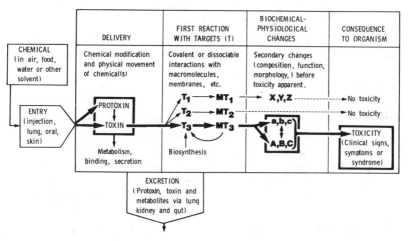

Figure 1   Scheme for developing toxicity due to chemicals. Heavy lines/letters = toxicity, light lines = less or no toxicity. T_1, T_2, T_3 = targets; MT_1, MT_2, MT_3 = modified targets. A, B, C, X, Y, Z, a, b, c = independent or linked changes. Acute or chronic toxicity differ by the time in one or more phases. Adapted from (9).

morphological changes; and what the relationships are between such changes and the clinical signs.

The identification of the relevant target is a vital component of such an approach and is a rate-limiting step in the progress of research. The development of sensitive analytical methods and the ability to produce monoclonal antibodies by the new techniques of molecular biology have, in principle, solved most problems of measuring how extensively chemicals react with their targets. Comparison of the properties of such proteins, (produced in quantity by bacteria separated by cloning techniques) with the same protein present in vivo, and perhaps attached to membrane, will aid in this process. Comparison of the properties of the target from the experimental animal with properties of the target from man (using postmortem material) is also possible. In the experimental animal it should prove increasingly possible to relate the degree of reaction of the chemical with the target (which is a measure of tissue or cell dose) to subsequent biological events.

EXPOSURE AND MEASUREMENT OF IN VIVO DOSE OF TOXIC CHEMICAL

Research on animals to produce information about the effects on man of exposure to chemicals is based on the premise that laboratory animals' component parts (enzymes, macromolecules, membranes, etc) are similar to man's, but that major differences lie in the relationships among the parts and their quantitative and kinetic properties. Major interspecies differences in sensitivity to a chemical are often due to great differences in the processes shown in the delivery section of Figure 1. Rapid metabolism and/or excretion of the toxin are often major factors. As shown in Figure 1, excretion may result from the early reactions phase. Covalent interaction results in the breakdown of the toxic chemical. Thus if the interaction does not result in toxicity (cf Figure 1), the process may be regarded as detoxification. Such a process has been experimentally demonstrated in the rat for the reaction of carboxylesterase and the highly toxic organophosphorus compound, Soman (10). Binding of chemicals to plasma proteins has been much studied and provides a depot of the chemicals and also increases the dose necessary to cause toxicity by reducing the circulating concentration of compound. An example of this is the influence on toxicity of the binding of trimethyltin to rat hemoglobin but not to the hemoglobin from other species [(11); see conclusions section].

An accurate measure of absorbed dose is a requirement for using the results of laboratory animal studies to predict quantitative effects in man. As a measure of received dose of organophosphorus compounds, the activities of acetylcholinesterase in erythrocytes and NTE in leucocytes are useful in acute and chronic poisoning.

One of the most helpful developments is the use of hemoglobin as a protein containing amino acid residues with a reactivity for many substances: Hemoglobin also has a long life in man (120 days). Thus exposure can be estimated some time after the event. The theoretical basis for its use has been well discussed (12–18), and the methodology for the measurement of specific adducts in hemoglobin has been worked out (12, 19, 20). The principle of the method has much potential for monitoring received or absorbed doses resulting from exposure of humans and laboratory animals. Problems remain to be solved and the interpretation of results is difficult for electrophiles of a wide range of reactivity produced in vivo by metabolic activation from inactive compounds. The use of the information for risk assessment also continues to provoke much discussion. Other possibilities are the use of other proteins to directly measure tissue-dose in experimental animals and the use of a very recent development employing a modified and more sensitive Edman degradation method that does not require hydrolysis of the hemoglobin. This latter method also has some potential, where the nature of the exposure is unknown, to identify the resultant adducts (21).

Although the main thrust of these developments concerns genotoxic agents, methods could be developed for other chemicals causing other types of toxicity.

TYPES OF REACTION OF CHEMICALS WITH MACROMOLECULES

Reactions with targets such as those shown in the early reactions section of Figure 1 are of two types, reversible and covalent.

REVERSIBLE INTERACTION
M is regenerated from M·AB when the concentration of AB is lowered by other processes. There is no destruction of AB in the reaction.

M = Macromolecule

AB = Chemical

$$M + AB \underset{k_{-1}}{\overset{k_{+1}}{\rightleftharpoons}} M{\cdot}AB \overset{k_{+2}}{\longrightarrow} B + MA \overset{k_{+3}}{\longrightarrow} M + A$$

COVALENT INTERACTION

When 1 mol MA is formed, 1 mol of AB is broken down. M is regenerated from MA by another reaction (k_{+3}). One reaction cycle results in the breakdown of 1 mol of AB into the products A and B.

The reaction mechanisms have consequences for the toxic process. It is probable that for some reactions the time during which the target is modified is an important factor in the development of toxicity. For example the development of morphological change in the cerebellum after methylmercury poisoning in rats seems to depend not only on the concentration of the methylmercury in the brain but also on the length of time it is there (22). Development of signs of poisoning may also depend on the speed at which the target is modified (23, 24).

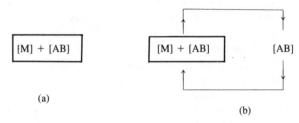

(a)

(b)

Affinity constants or reaction rates are almost always measured in vitro with the macromolecule (enzyme or receptor) and the ligand or reactive chemical in a small volume (cf (a) above). Under these circumstances the molar concentration of the macromolecular component can approach that of the chemical reactant, i.e. $[AB] \cong [M]$ and AB (mol)$\cong$M (mol). The relationship between the degree of reaction and concentration of reactant $[AB]$ will have a different slope from that when $[AB] >> [M]$. In vivo the macromolecule is often perfused with a large volume containing $[AB]$ and under these circumstances the determining feature is that the quantity of AB (mol) $>>$ M (mol). Even for extremely toxic substances this condition applies. For example the amount of acetylcholinesterase in rat brain is approximately 100 pmol (calculated from an acetylcholinesterase activity in rat brain of 30 μmol/min/brain and a catalytic center activity of 295,000/min). The toxicity of the nerve gas Soman to rats is 80 μg/kg when given subcutaneously (10); this is 88 nmol/200g rat, an excess approaching 10^3 over the 100 pmol amount of acetylcholinesterase.

It seems probable that AB (mol) $>>$ M (mol) will be the normal condition, and the degree of reaction in vivo will be linearly related to the dose administered. Reaction of metabolites of trans-4-dimethylaminostilbine in rats with the protein and nucleic acids of a variety of tissues, as well as hemoglobin, have been shown to relate linearly to doses over a range of 5×10^{-10}–3.5×10^{-5} mol/kg (15, 25, 26).

EXAMPLES OF VARIOUS NEUROTOXIC CHEMICALS

In the following pages I use examples of chemicals that cause neurotoxicity to demonstrate how knowledge of mechanisms of toxicity influences views about thresholds (a dose just below that producing a response). These thresholds concern not only clinical signs but also other obligatory steps following from the early and primary reaction of the chemical with the target (cf Figure 1).

Wherever possible, I discuss methods to measure in vivo dose and how the results of experimental studies can be linked to observations in man.

Organophosphorus Compounds (Acute Toxicity)

It has long been known that the acetylcholinesterase of erythrocytes is similar to that of brain, and exposure may be monitored by its measurement (27). The threshold for untoward effects has been discovered empirically in man by routine measurements performed during the medical supervision of the spraymen engaged in World Health Organization spraying programs to control vector-borne disease. Since most organophosphorus compounds are uncharged and lipid soluble they penetrate all tissues including the brain. It is known that dimethylphosphorylated acetylcholinesterase is relatively unstable; it spontaneously reactivates to yield the parent active enzyme and, at a slower rate, changes to a stable monomethylphosphorylated enzyme known as aged enzyme (28). After a day of spraying, these reactions occur, and the activity of acetylcholinesterase the next day is a measurement of aged enzyme (29). If the dose absorbed each day is repeated then the aged enzyme also increases from day to day. Because both the mechanisms of reaction of organophosphorus compounds with acetylcholinesterase and the properties of the phosphorylated enzyme are known, the spraying operation can be conducted safely. Such knowledge and monitoring procedures have allowed large numbers of patients infected with *Schistosoma hematobium* to be treated completely safely by the oral administration of metrifonate (O,O-dimethyl 2,2,2-trichloro-1-hydroxyethyl phosphonate) (29). Few or no untoward effects were seen (30, 31).

Thus the target involved in the acute toxicity of organophosphorus compounds is known, a similar target is present in an accessible tissue (erythrocytes), reaction of the target with the chemical (inhibition of enzyme activity) can be measured, and in animals this may be related to clinical signs or acetylcholine concentrations in nerve tissue. This allows the threshold to be defined. The properties of the target may be compared between animal and man and the threshold established in man.

The dose of organophosphorus compound that produces symptoms may of course be different in various species. Metrifonate is not an inhibitor of acetylcholinesterase but breaks down spontaneously to dichlorvos, a very active inhibitor. In Table 1 it is shown that 15–20 times as much metrifonate is required in the hamster as is required to produce the same inhibition in man. This difference is probably due to a more rapid disposal of the active inhibitor dichlorvos in the hamster (Nordgren, I., unpublished, 1985) than in man (32). Thus although the threshold for clinical effect, expressed in terms of percentage inhibition of acetylcholinesterase, is the same in hamsters and man, the dose

Table 1   Inhibition of erythrocyte cholinesterase in hamsters and man after treatment with metrifonate.

Metrifonate oral dose (mg/kg)	Acetylcholinesterase (% of control)	
	Human[a]	Hamster[b]
7.5	80	—
10	50	—
12.5	65	—
7.5–60	—	100
120	—	94
150	—	68
200	—	47

[a]Taken from (21)
[b]Unpublished results W. N. Aldridge & B. W. Street 1984. Biomolecular rate constants for inhibition of acetylcholinesterases by dichlorvos are for hamsters (1.26 × $10^5 M^{-1} min^{-1}$) and for human 1.17 × $10^5 M^{-1} min^{-1}$ (28)

administered to achieve this inhibition is 15–20 times as high in hamster as in man.

Organophosphorus Compounds (Chronic Delayed Neuropathy)

Some organophosphorus compounds produce a condition known as delayed neuropathy. Signs of this axonal neuropathy take 10–30 days to appear in animals and man; the early primary reaction is with a membrane-bound neuropathy target esterase (NTE) present in the peripheral and central nervous tissue (33–35). The structure-activity relationships for a large number of organophosphorus compounds are known, and all take part in the reaction scheme shown in Figure 2. For the development of delayed neuropathy, 70–80% of NTE must be phosphorylated or phosphonylated followed by the removal of one of the groups attached to phosphorus (aging reaction). If the aging reaction does not occur, even though the esterase activity of NTE is inhibited, delayed neuropathy does not develop. The aging reaction cannot on chemical grounds occur when NTE is phosphinylated (both R^1 and R^2 directly linked to phosphorus), carbamylated, or sulfonylated (36) (cf Figure 2). Animals pretreated with the above three classes of compounds in doses sufficient to inhibit NTE by 70% do not develop delayed neuropathy. If an organophosphorus compound able to cause delayed neuropathy is administered to such pretreated animals, the animals are protected and no disease occurs.

When NTE is phosphinylated or sulfonylated, hen esterase activity slowly reappears with a half-life of 4.5–5.0 days (Figure 3), presumably due to resynthesis of new enzyme. When a hen is dosed with phenylbenzylcarbamate, the carbamylated NTE is unstable and reactivates (cf. Types of Reaction of

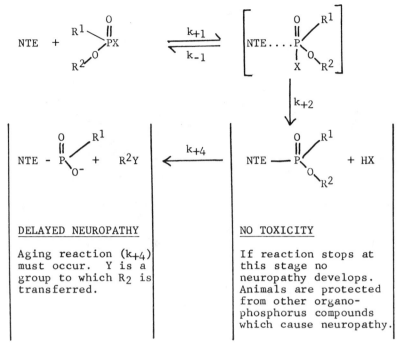

Figure 2   Reactions necessary for initiation of delayed neuropathy by organophosphorus compounds. R^1 may be linked to P either directly or via O, S, or N. R^2 must be linked to P by O, S, or N. Chemical evidence for aging has only been provided for transfer of R^2 of R^2O to $Y(k_{+4})$ and not for R^2S- or R^2NH- (43).

Chemicals with Macromolecules) with a half-life of approximately 6 hr (Figure 3). Hens pretreated with any of the compounds shown in Figure 3 are protected until NTE inhibition is reduced to 28–35%—i.e. the animals are protected until approximately 70% of the catalytic centers are unoccupied and able to be phosphorylated followed by aging after treatment with a neuropathic organophosphorus compound (36, 37).

These observations prove that NTE is the primary target involved in the reaction with certain neuropathic organophosphorus compounds. Biochemical/physiological changes following the primary reaction and the appearance of clinical signs of neuropathy (at 10–14 days in the hen and 14–30 days in man) have not been defined, and the nature of the biological cascade in this "silent" period is unknown. The threshold of 70–80% inhibition or phosphorylation of NTE in hens after an acute dose is now well established (38).

Three questions may be asked: (*a*) How can information obtained in the hen be applied to man? (*b*) What is the threshold with chronic doses? (*c*) How can humans be monitored for toxicologically significant exposure?

Having established the properties of NTE in the hens, we can examine the

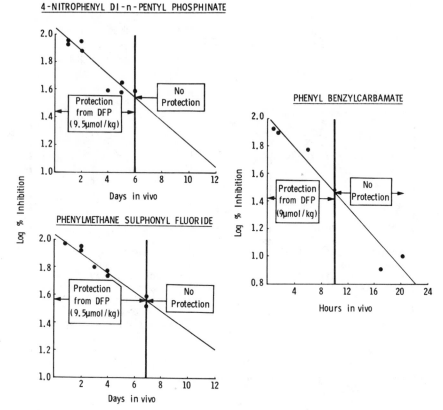

Figure 3   Protection of hens from delayed neuropathy by pretreatment with various compounds. DFP is diisopropylphosphorofluoridate. Inhibition of neuropathy target esterase (NTE) is plotted as percentage of the maximum inhibition measured. Data from (36, 37).

enzyme from human tissue. Except for minor differences, hen and human NTE are similar (39, 40). Since there may be major differences in the rates and routes of metabolic disposal of organophosphorus compounds in hens and humans it is not possible to predict from in vitro inhibition studies of NTE the effective dose in the two species. Comparison of the relative inhibitory power of the proximal inhibitory organophosphorus compounds against those of acetylcholinesterase and NTE in microsomes from hen and human brain give a good indication of human susceptibility to this chronic toxicity relative to acute toxicity (40, 41). Measurement of acetylcholinesterase and NTE after dosing a few hens also indicates the potential or lack of potential for delayed neuropathy of the compound. After such experiments have been done it will be possible to predict whether humans suffering from acute poisoning will develop delayed neuropathy later.

Much of the experimental work on delayed neuropathy has been done with single or at most a few doses of organophosphorus compounds. Does the threshold of 70% inhibition of NTE apply for chronic administration, or is there an accumulation of morphological changes with lower inhibition? Hens were maintained on a daily dose of mono-2-methylphenyl diphenyl phosphate such that a steady-state 50% inhibition of NTE was obtained for 10 weeks (42). No neuropathy was found. Raising the dose, after 50% inhibition had been maintained for several weeks, to produce 70–90% inhibition resulted in neuropathy 10 days later (42). These experiments show that an acute dose of approximately 50 mg/kg produces neuropathy whereas a total of 175 mg/kg given over 10 weeks in daily doses does not; measurement of the inhibition of NTE shows that the toxic chemical was delivered to the target. Thus, for hens, it appears that the threshold is approximately the same in terms of degree of reaction with NTE for both acute and chronic doses.

NTE, defined by its sensitivity to organophosphorus compounds, is a B-esterase. It seems, however, to be a unique B-esterase; when it ages the released group is attached to a neighboring group (43). This transferred group has been characterized by its volatility after treatment with alkali (43, 44). Other phosphorylated esterases when they age release the group into the medium. Using this unique characteristic NTE been identified in tissues other than those of the central and peripheral (45) nervous system and particularly in spleen, placenta, thymus, and circulating leucocytes (35, 46–50). The determination of NTE activity in leucocytes in hens (42) and humans (51, 52) is related to the previous dose of active inhibitor and takes into account the bioactivation of inactive precursors and detoxification. Although the method requires more validation, it could provide a valid monitoring procedure in cases of occupational, accidental, or intentional exposure.

Acrylamide (Peripheral Neuropathy)

Acrylamide causes a peripheral neuropathy in many species of animal (53), including man (54). Acrylamide in rats is an uncharged and highly water soluble compound that mixes uniformly with the body water. It reacts with cysteine residues in hemoglobin to produce stable adducts (55), and a method has recently been developed for their measurement (56). The macromolecular target in the early primary reaction that leads to peripheral neuropathy is unknown. It is uncertain whether the proximal toxin is acrylamide or metabolite (57). Nevertheless in an occupational exposure it should be possible to examine those exposed for clinical signs, to determine cysteine adducts in hemoglobin and to calculate the integrated dose of acrylamide absorbed. A threshold for clinical peripheral neuropathy may thus be established in both man and other animals. Similar studies to define a threshold dose in relation to morphological findings (58, 59) would enable us to establish, in animals, the relationship between dose received and discrete morphological findings or clinical signs of toxicity.

2,5-Hexanedione (Hydrocarbon Neuropathy)

It has now been established that the predominantly peripheral neuropathy caused in rats by hexane, 2-hexanol, 2-hexanone (methyl n-butyl ketone), and 2,5-hexanediol result from metabolism in vivo to a common proximal toxin, 2,5-hexanedione (60, 61; cf Figure 4). Methyl n-butyl ketone causes a similar neuropathy in man (62, 63) and it is metabolized to 2,5-hexanedione. The morphological characteristics have been well described (64, 65) and it has been shown that 2,5-hexanedione, acrylamide, and organophosphorus compounds produce different patterns of morphological change (66). The structural deter-

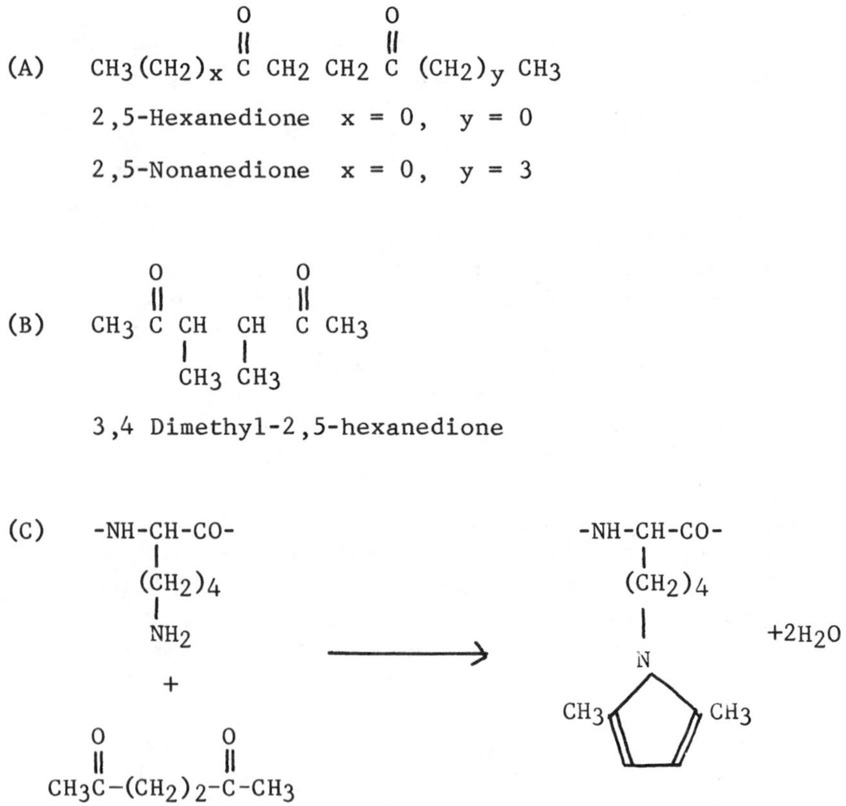

(A) $CH_3(CH_2)_x \overset{\overset{\text{O}}{\|}}{C} CH_2\ CH_2\ \overset{\overset{\text{O}}{\|}}{C} (CH_2)_y\ CH_3$

2,5-Hexanedione   x = 0,   y = 0

2,5-Nonanedione   x = 0,   y = 3

(B) $CH_3\ \overset{\overset{\text{O}}{\|}}{C}\ \underset{\underset{CH_3}{|}}{CH}\ \underset{\underset{CH_3}{|}}{CH}\ \overset{\overset{\text{O}}{\|}}{C}\ CH_3$

3,4 Dimethyl-2,5-hexanedione

(C)   -NH-CH-CO-   -NH-CH-CO-
          | |
        (CH₂)₄   (CH₂)₄
          | | +2H₂O
        NH₂   N
                          ⟶
          +   CH₃⟨   ⟩CH₃
     $CH_3\overset{\overset{\text{O}}{\|}}{C}-(CH_2)_2-\overset{\overset{\text{O}}{\|}}{C}-CH_3$

Figure 4   Neuropathy caused by 1,4-diketones. (A) Structural requirements in diketones; (B) 3,4-dimethyl-2,5-hexanedione, which reacts with primary amines faster than 2,5-hexanedione, and is 20–30 times more neuropathic (73); (C) postulated reaction of 2,5-hexanedione with amino group in lysine to form a 2,5-dimethylpyrrole derivative (72, 74).

minant within 2,5-hexanedione essential for the production of neuropathy is two oxygen atoms (of the keto groups) separated by four carbons (Figure 4). Other compounds with longer carbon chains that contain this grouping or can be metabolized to such a structure are also neuropathic (67–71). Thus, although the complete structural requirements for neuropathic potential have not been worked out, e.g. whether x in Figure 4 can be more than 0, the requirement for the 1,4-diketone grouping seems absolute.

The requirement for a 1,4-diketone structure has been utilized to formulate a chemical hypothesis that involves reaction with primary amino groups (presumably in proteins) to form a stable 6-membered pyrrole ring adduct (72). Other diketones with the keto groups in the 1,3-, 1,2-, or 1,5- positions are not neuropathic (68). The hypothesis has also received support from the observation that a 3,4-dimethyl substitution in 2,5-hexanedione increases reactivity with amino groups to form a pyrrole and also decreases the dose required to produce a neuropathy like that produced by 2,5-hexanedione (73, 74). Precisely which macromolecules react with 2,5-hexanedione and initiate the toxicity is not known, but they may well be neurofilaments, which accumulate at the nodes of Ranvier as an early event in the developing neuropathy (64). It is possible that after the primary reaction with amino groups in the neurofilament protein, the pyrrole adduct auto-oxidizes to form a cross-linking reactive center (74).

Comparative dose-response relationships have been worked out for 2,5-hexanedione and several compounds metabolized to it (Table 2). Even though the circulating concentrations of 2,5-hexanedione differ by a factor of 8, the doses required to produce neuropathy are remarkably similar (*last column*, Table 2). This is surprising for a compound with a disposal half-life in plasma of approximately 6 hr (60). If reaction with neurofilaments is a primary event an explanation may be available. Passage of neurofilaments down the axon is part

Table 2 Relative neurotoxicity of various compounds in relation to their conversion to 2,5-hexanedione[a]

Compound	Time to clinical end point (days)	No. of doses	2,5-Hexanedione: Peak serum concentration (μmol/ml;B)	Dose (A × B)
2,5-Hexanedione	17	13	4.59±0.79	59.7±10.3
5-Hydroxy-2-hexanone	22	16	2.56±0.41	41.0± 6.6
2,5-Hexanediol	29	21	1.92±0.47	40.3± 9.9
Methyl n-butyl ketone	56	40	0.89±0.10	35.6± 4.0
2-Hexanol	83	61	0.60±0.05	36.6± 3.0

[a]Data from (60). Rats were dosed orally with 6.6 mmol of each compound per kg for 5 days a week.

of the slow component of axonal transport that moves down the nerve at 1–2 mm per day (75, 76). Passage down some long nerves may take up to 50 days and during repeated exposure 2,5-hexanedione would have opportunity to react with neurofilaments over a long period; this could be the explanation for its apparent cumulative behavior. Thus the threshold is likely to be low—certainly much less than 0.6 μmol/ml—and is determined by the life of a particular organelle. Factors such as repair on its way down the nerve or resynthesis of new protein will affect this threshold.

2,5-Hexanedione has also been shown to react with proteins in the erythrocyte (presumably mainly hemoglobin, the most abundant protein), and the pyrrole adducts can be determined (74, 77). No experimental work has been published on the stability of these pyrrole adducts, i.e. whether they are like alkylated adducts and persist for the life of the erythrocyte. Further experimental work and examination of those exposed should allow determination of the dose-response relationships and the threshold dose in experimental animals and man. The long life of hemoglobin and its disposal when it becomes "old", rather than the first-order turnover process seen for most proteins, probably show many kinetic similarities to the slow passage of neurofilaments down a nerve axon with their disposal at the end (78, 79). Both of the above processes have a kinetic analogue in the relationship between methylmercury in blood and the progression of the methylmercury down the hair as it grows (79a).

Carcinogenic and Mutagenic Chemicals

Carcinogenesis is not considered in detail here because it has often been reviewed (80). As new information is obtained on the mechanisms involved in the multistaged process leading from initiation to tumor (e.g. information on promotion, oncogenes, etc), it may be possible to consider thresholds for weak carcinogens. This is in contrast with a complete and strong carcinogen, such as diethylnitrosamine, which shows the characteristic of extending the time required for detection of liver tumors as its dose is reduced. In other words the fundamental absence of a threshold is indicated (81).

On general grounds it seems probable that some as yet incompletely defined modification by chemicals of the DNA template in a cell, leading to nonlethal mutation, is a process that has no threshold. Initiation requiring chemical modification in the DNA in principle could also be brought about by changes in the repair-synthesis system where a one-to-one molecular relationship between DNA and enzyme occurs; for example, the influence of beryllium on the fidelity of DNA synthesis (82). The results of long-term animal experiments, indicating chemically induced increased incidence of tumors in the progeny after pre- or postnatal exposure of rats to nitrosoureas, urethane, or Xrays, should provoke much thought and attention (83–87).

CONCLUSIONS

The intent of this paper is to consider the existence of threshold from a fundamental biological standpoint and not to concentrate on the practical problems of those who have to set limits of exposure for populations. In this context attempts to decide, in a particular case, whether in principle a threshold exists, are separate from the problem of devising sound methods to test whether it does.

When a biological function that depends on the collaborative action of a large number of the same macromolecules such as receptors or enzymes is deranged then it seems probable that a threshold exists. The action of a number of molecules of a receptor or enzyme could be prevented or modified without any demonstrable change in biological function. However, when biological function is dependent on the action of one molecule such as DNA or those molecules (enzymes) associated with it in a one-to-one molecular relationship, then the existence of a threshold seems fundamentally unlikely. Acceptance of this view, of course, means that exposure to most toxic chemicals at low concentrations for a lifetime will be harmless. In contrast, for those chemicals causing genetic changes this seems unlikely. Such statements ignore questions of risk involving the slope of dose-response curves (which need not be constant over the whole dose range) or the differing susceptibility of individuals. Practical decisions have to be made even though the risk is not zero.

As knowledge of mechanisms of toxicity of chemicals is extended it will become clear that different facets of the toxic process have different thresholds. For example when inhibition of an enzyme results in defined symptoms the thresholds for these two measurable parameters will be different. In general if we move from right to left in Figure 1, from the clinical signs towards measurement of circulating toxin, several thresholds occur at lower concentrations of toxin. These dose-response relationships can be worked out in laboratory animals and will provide the scientific background for the interpretation of the often limited data (dose and clinical signs) available for man.

An illustration of this principle is shown by the action of trimethyltin which causes neuronal necrosis in rats only in the hippocampus, amygdaloid, or pyriform cortex (88, 89). The dose required to cause these effects is higher in rats than in such other species as the marmoset, hamster, and gerbil (11). This is undoubtedly due to the binding of trimethyltin to rat hemoglobin only, so that 70% of the administered dose is sequestered in an inactive form. The concentrations of trimethyltin in brain associated with neuronal necrosis in the above four species are similar (11) and there is no evidence of selective accumulation in the affected areas (89). It is thus possible to predict the dose that will be required to produce such lesions in man (11). Neuronal necrosis in rats and other species of experimental animals is preceded by aggression (88), and this has been seen in some of the reported cases of poisoning in man (90–92). Even with considerable neuronal necrosis in rats, after a recovery period it is difficult to detect behavioral abnormalities (88), but deficiencies in memory and problem solving have been found (93, 94). Poisoned men who showed severe symptoms have subsequently been pronounced clinically normal (90–92). In this instance detailed information about the dose-response curve, threshold for neuronal necrosis, and early behavioral changes would provide a sound basis for predicting (a) what concentrations will not cause permanent loss of neurons in man, and (b) the relationship of these levels to initial symptoms. When the biochemical basis for its action is known another dose-response and threshold may be measured.

In these and similar studies the measurement of received or absorbed dose is vital. The increasing sophistication of detection, identification, and quantitation techniques now available allows such measurements. For covalently reactive chemicals the measurement of hemoglobin adducts has proved valuable and can be extended.

Literature Cited

1. Theophrastus Bombastus von Hohen-heim gen. Paracelsus, Aug 24, 1538. *Epistola dedicatora St. Veit/Karnten; Sieben Defensionen oder Sieben Schutz-, Schirm- und Trutzreden. Dritte Defension*
2. Henschler, D. 1973. Toxicological problems relating to changes in the environment. *Angew. Chem. Internat. Ed. Eng.* 12:274–83
3. Raftery, M. A., Conti-Tronconi, B. M., Dunn, S. M. J., Crawford, R. D., Middlemas, D. 1984. The nicotinic acetylcholine receptor: its structure, multiple binding sites and cation transport properties. *Fundam. Appl. Toxicol.* 4:S34–S51
4. Krebs, E. G., Beavo, J. A. 1979. Phosphorylation-dephosphorylation of enzymes. *Ann. Rev. Biochem.* 48:923–59
5. Aldridge, W. N., Reiner, E. 1972. *Enzyme inhibitors as substrates: Interactions of esterases with esters of organophosphorus and carbamic acids.* Amsterdam: Elsevier. 328 pp.
6. Aldridge, W. N. 1981. Organophosphorus compounds: molecular basis for their biological properties. *Sci. Prog. Oxford* 67:131–47
7. Blair, D., Dix, K. M., Hunt, P. F., Thorpe, E., Stevenson, D. E., Walker, A. I. T. 1976. Dichlorvos—A 2 year inhalation carcinogenesis study in rats. *Arch. Toxicol.* 35:281–94

8. Turner, L., ed. Considerations regarding the extrapolation of biological data in deriving occupational exposure limits. *Tech. Rep. No. 10* Brussels: Eur. Chem. Indust. Ecol. & Toxicol. Cent., 21 pp.
9. Aldridge, W. N. 1981. Mechanisms of toxicity. New concepts are required in toxicology. *Trends Pharmacol. Sci.* 2:228–31
10. Sterri, S. H. 1981. Factors modifying the toxicity of organophosphorus compounds including dichlorvos. *Acta Pharmacol. Toxicol.* 49(Suppl. V):67–71
11. Brown, A. W., Verschoyle, R. D., Street, B. W., Aldridge, W. N., Grindley, H. 1984. The neurotoxicity of trimethyltin chloride in hamsters, gerbils and marmosets. *J. Appl. Toxicol.* 4:12–21
12. Ehrenberg, L., Hiescha, K. D., Osterman-Golkar, S., Wennberg, I. 1974. Evaluation of genetic risk of alkylating agents: tissue dose in the mouse from air contaminated with ethylene oxide. *Mutat. Res.* 24:83–103
13. Osterman-Golkar, S., Ehrenberg, L., Segerback, D., Hallstrom, I. 1976. Evaluation of genetic risks of alkylating agents: II. Haemoglobin as a dose monitor. *Mutat. Res.* 34:1–10
14. Ehrenberg, L., Moustacchi, E., Osterman-Golkar, S., Ekman, G. 1983. Dosimetry of genotoxic agents and dose-

response relationships of their effects. *Mutat. Res.* 123:121–82

15. Neumann, H. G. 1984. Analysis of haemoglobin as a dose monitor of alkylating and acylating agents. *Arch. Toxicol.* 56:1–6

16. Hayes, A. W., Schnell, R. C., Miya, T. S., eds. 1983. Symposium on *Biological Monitors of Exposure to covalently binding chemicals*. In *Development in the Science and Practice of Toxicology*, pp. 245–318. Amsterdam: Elsevier. 614 pp.

17. Osterman-Golkar, S., Bailey, E., Farmer, P., Gorf, S., Lamb, J. 1984. Monitoring exposure to propylene oxide through the determination of haemoglobin alkylation. *Scand. J. Work Environ. Health.* 10:99–102

18. Osterman-Golkar, S., Farmer, P. B., Segerback, D., Bailey, E., Calleman, C. J., et al. 1983. Dosimetry of ethylene oxide in the rat by quantitation of alkylated histidine in haemoglobin. *Teratogenesis, Carcinogenesis & Mutagenesis* 3:395–405

19. Farmer, P. B., Bailey, E., Lamb, J. H., Connors, T. A. 1980. Approach to the quantitation of alkylated amino acids in haemoglobin by gas chromatography-mass spectrometry. *Biomed. Mass. Spectrom.* 7:41–46

20. Farmer, P. B., Gorf, S. M., Bailey, E. 1982. Determination of hydroxypropylhistidine in haemoglobin as a measure of exposure to propylene oxide using high resolution gas chromatography-mass spectrometry. *Biomed. Mass. Spectrom.* 9:69–71

21. Tornqvist, M., Mowrer, J., Jensen, S., Ehrenberg, L. 1985. Determination of human haemoglobin adducts by a modified Edman degradation method. *Anal. Biochem.* In press

22. Magos, L., Peristianis, G. C., Snowden, R. T. 1978. Post exposure preventative treatment of methylmercury intoxication in rats with dimercaptosuccinic acid. *Toxicol. Appl. Pharmacol.* 45:463–75

23. Barnes, J. M. 1975. Assessing hazards from prolonged and repeated exposure to low doses of toxic substances. *Br. Med. Bull.* 31:196–200

24. Paton, W. D. M. 1961. A theory of drug action based on the rate of drug-receptor combination. *Proc. R. Soc. London Ser. B*:154:21–69

25. Neumann, H. G. 1980. Dose-response relationship in the primary lesion of strong electrophilic carcinogens. *Arch. Toxicol.* 3:69–77(Suppl.)

26. Neumann, H. G., Gangler, B. J. M., Taupp, W. 1978. The metabolic activation of trans 4-dimethylaminostilbene after oral administration of doses ranging from 0.025–250 μmol/kg. In *Proc. 1st Int. Congr. Toxicol.*, ed. G. L. Plaa, W. A. M. Duncan, pp. 177–190. New York/ London: Academic, 670 pp.

27. Vandekar, M. 1980. Minimising occupational exposure to pesticides: cholinesterase determination and organophosphorus poisoning. *Residue Rev.* 75:67–79

28. Skrinjaric-Spoljar, M., Simeon, V., Reiner, E. 1973. Spontaneous reactivation and aging of dimethyl phosphorylated acetylcholinesterase and cholinesterase. *Biochim. Biophys. Acta* 315:363–69

29. Aldridge, W. N. 1980. Acetylcholinesterase and other esterase inhibitors. In *Enzyme Inhibitors as Drugs*, ed. M. Sandler, pp. 115–125. London: Macmillan. 285 pp.

30. Davis, A., Bailey, D. R. 1969. Metrifonate in urinary schistosomiasis. *Bull. WHO* 41:209–24

31. Plestina, R., Davis, A., Bailey, D. R. 1972. Effect of metrifonate on blood cholinesterases in children during the treatment of schistosomiasis. *Bull. WHO* 46:747–59

32. Nordgren, I., Holmstedt, B., Bengtsson, E., Finkel, Y. 1980. Plasma levels of metrifonate and dichlorvos during treatment of schistosomiasis with bilarcil. *Am. J. Trop. Med. Hyg.* 29:426–30

33. Johnson, M. K. 1975. Organophosphorus esters causing delayed neurotoxic effects. Mechanism of action and structure-activity studies. *Arch. Toxicol.* 34:259–88

34. Johnson, M. K. 1975. The delayed neuropathy caused by some organophosphorus esters: mechanism and challenge. *CRC Crit. Rev. Toxicol.* 3:289–316

35. Johnson, M. K. 1982. The target for initiation of delayed neurotoxicity by organophosphorus esters: biochemical studies and toxicological applications. *Rev. Biochem. Toxicol.* 4:141–212

36. Johnson, M. K. 1974. The primary biochemical lesion leading to the delayed neurotoxic effects of some organophosphorus esters. *J. Neurochem.* 23:785–89

37. Johnson, M. K. 1970. Organophosphorus and other inhibitors of brain neurotoxic esterase and the development of delayed neuropathy in hens. *Biochem. J.* 120:523–31

38. Johnson, M. K., Lotti, M. 1980. Delayed neurotoxicity caused by chronic feeding of organophosphates requires a high point of inhibition of neurotoxic esterase. *Toxicol. Lett.* 5:99–102

39. Lotti, M., Johnson, M. K. 1980. Neurotoxic esterase in human nervous tissue. *J. Neurochem.* 34:747–49

40. Lotti, M., Johnson, M. K. 1978. Neurotoxicity of organophosphorus pesticides: predictions can be based on in vitro studies with hen and human tissue. *Arch. Toxicol.* 41:215–21

41. Lotti, M., Ferrara, S. D., Caroldi, S., Sinigaglia, F. 1981. Enzyme studies with human and hen autopsy tissue suggest O-methoate does not cause delayed neuropathy in man. *Arch. Toxicol.* 48:265–70

42. Lotti, M., Johnson, M. K. 1980. Repeated small doses of a neurotoxic organophosphate. Monitoring of neurotoxic esterase in brain and spinal cord. *Arch. Toxicol.* 45:263–71

43. Clothier, B., Johnson, M. K. 1979. Rapid aging of neurotoxic esterase after inhibition by di-*iso*propyl phosphorofluoridate. *Biochem. J.* 177:549–58

44. Williams, D. G., Johnson, M. K. 1981. Gel-electrophoretic identification of hen brain neurotoxic esterase, labelled with tritiated di-*iso*propyl phosphorofluoridate. *Biochem. J.* 199:323–33

45. Caroldi, S., Lotti, M. 1982. Neurotoxic esterase in peripheral nerve: assay, inhibition and rate of synthesis. *Toxicol. Appl. Pharmacol.* 15:498–501

46. Dudek, B. R., Richardson, R. J. 1980. Human leucocyte neurotoxic esterase. Potential biomonitor for neurotoxic organophosphorus compounds. *19th Ann. Meeting Soc. Toxicol.*, Abstr. No. 433

47. Gurba, P. E., Richardson, R. J. 1983. Partial characterisation of neurotoxic esterase of human placenta. *Toxicol. Lett.* 15:13–17

48. Dudek, B. R., Richardson, R. J. 1982. Evidence for the existence of neurotoxic esterase in neural and lymphatic tissue of the adult hen. *Biochem. Pharmacol.* 31:1117–21

49. Sprague, G. L., Bickford, A. A. 1981. Effect of multiple di-*iso*propylfluorophosphate injections in hens: a behavioural, biochemical and histological investigation. *J. Toxicol. Environ. Health.* 8:973–88

50. Richardson, R. J., Dudek, B. R. 1978. Occurrence of neurotoxic esterase in various tissues of the hen. *Toxicol. Appl. Pharmacol.* 45:269–70

51. Lotti, M., Becker, C. E., Aminoff, M. J., Woodrow, J. E., Sieber, J. N., et al. 1983. Occupational exposure to the cotton defoliants DEF and merphos. A rational approach to monitoring organo-

phosphorus-induced delayed neurotoxicity. *J. Occup. Med.* 25:517–22

52. Lotti, M. 1983. Lymphocyte neurotoxic esterase. A biochemical monitor of organophosphorus induced delayed neurotoxicity in man. *Adv. Biosci.* 46:101–8

53. McCollister, D. D., Oyen, F., Rowe, V. K. 1964. Toxicology of acrylamide. *Toxicol. Appl. Pharmacol.* 6:172–81

54. LeQuesne, P. M. 1980. Acrylamide. In *Experimental and Clinical Neurotoxicology*, ed. P. S. Spencer, H. H. Schaumburg, pp. 309–25. Baltimore/London: Williams & Wilkins, 929 pp.

55. Hashimoto, K., Aldridge, W. N. 1970. Biochemical studies on acrylamide, a neurotoxic agent. *Biochem. Pharmacol.* 19:2591–604

56. Bailey, E., Farmer, P. B. 1985. The interaction of acrylamide with cysteine residues in haemoglobin. *Human Toxicol.* In press

57. Acrylamide. In *Environmental Health Criteria 1985*, Vol. 49. Geneva: WHO. pp. 1–121

58. Cavanagh, J. B. 1982. The pathokinetics of acrylamide intoxication: A reassessment of the problem. *Neuropathol. Appl. Neurobiol.* 8:315–36

59. Cavanagh, J. B., Gysbers, M. F. 1983. Ultrastructural features of the Purkinje cell damage caused by acrylamide in the rat: A new phenomenon in cellular neuropathology. *J. Neurocytol.* 12:413–37

60. DiVincenzo, G. D., Krasavage, W. J., O'Donoghue, J. L. 1980. Role of metabolism in hexacarbon neuropathy. In *The Scientific Basis of Toxicity Assessment*, ed. H. Witschi, pp. 183–200. Amsterdam: Elsevier/North Holland Biomedical. 329 pp.

61. Spencer, P. S., Schaumburg, H. H. 1975. Experimental neuropathy produced by 2,5-hexanedione—a major metabolite of the neurotoxic industrial solvent methyl n-butyl ketone. *J. Neurol. Neurosurg. Psychiatry* 38:771–75

62. Allen, N. 1980. Identification of methyl n-butyl ketone as the causative agent. See Ref. 54, pp. 834–45

63. Allen, N., Mendell, J. R., Billimaier, D. J., Fontaine, R. E., O'Neill, J. 1975. Toxic neuropathy due to methyl n-butyl ketone. *Arch. Neurol.* 32:209–18

64. Jones, H. B., Cavanagh, J. B. 1983. Distortion of the nodes of Ranvier from axonal distension by filamentous masses in hexacarbon intoxication. *J. Neurocytol.* 12:439–58

65. Jones, H. B., Cavanagh, J. B. 1983. Cytochemical staining characteristics of peripheral nodes of Ranvier in hexacar-

bon intoxication. *J. Neurocytol.* 12:459–73

66. Cavanagh, J. B. 1982. Mechanisms of axon degeneration in three toxic 'neuropathies': organophosphorus, acrylamide and hexacarbon compared. *Recent Adv. Neuropathol.* 2:213–42

67. Shifman, M. A., Graham, D. G., Priest, J. W., Bouldin, J. W. 1981. The neurotoxicity of 5-nonanone: preliminary report. *Toxicol. Lett.* 8:283–88

68. O'Donoghue, J. L., Krasavage, W. J. 1979. The structure-activity relationships of aliphatic diketones and their potential neurotoxicity. *Toxicol. Appl. Pharmacol.* 48:A55

69. O'Donoghue, J. L., Krasavage, W. J., DiVincenzo, G. D., Ziegler, D. A. 1982. Commercial grade methyl heptyl ketone (5-methyl-2-octanone) neurotoxicity: contribution of 5-nonanone. *Toxicol. Appl. Pharmacol.* 62:307–16

70. O'Donoghue, J. L., Krasavage, W. J. 1979. Hexacarbon neuropathy. A γ-diketone neuropathy. *J. Neuropathol. Exp. Neurol.* 38:333

71. Spencer, P. S., Bischoff, M. C., Schaumburg, H. H. 1978. On the specific molecular configuration of neurotoxic aliphatic hexacarbon compounds causing central peripheral distal axonopathy. *Toxicol. Appl. Pharmacol.* 44:17–28

72. DeCaprio, A. P., Olajos, E. J., Weber, P. 1982. Covalent binding of a neurotoxic hexane metabolite: conversion of primary amines to substituted pyrrole adducts by 2,4-hexanedione. *Toxicol. Appl. Pharmacol.* 65:440–50

73. Anthony, D. C., Boekelheide, K., Graham, D. G. 1983. The effect of 3,4-dimethyl substitution on the neurotoxicity of 2,5-hexanedione. 1. Accelerated clinical neuropathy is accompanied by more proximal axonal swelling. *Toxicol. Appl. Pharmacol.* 71:362–71

74. Anthony, D. C., Boekelheide, K., Anderson, C. W., Graham, D. G. 1983. The effect of 3,4-dimethyl substitution on the neurotoxicity of 2,5-hexanedione. 2. Dimethyl substitution accelerates pyrrole formation and protein cross linking. *Toxicol. Appl. Pharmacol.* 71:372–82

75. Lasek, R. J. 1981. Cytoskeletons and the architecture of nervous system. *Neurosci. Res. Program. Bull.* 19:7–31

76. Hoffman, P. N., Lasek, R. J. 1975. The slow component of axonal transport. Identification of major structural polypeptides of the axon and their generality among mammalian neurons. *J. Cell Biol.* 66:351–66

77. Mattocks, A. R., White, I. N. H. 1970. Estimation of metabolites of pyrrolizidine alkaloids in animal tissues. *Anal. Biochem.* 38:529–35

78. Roots, B. I., Bondar, R. L. 1977. Neurofilamentous changes in goldfish (*Carassius Auratus* L.) brain in relation to environmental temperature. *J. Neuropathol. Exp. Neurol.* 36:453–64

79. Roots, B. I. 1983. Neurofilament accumulation induced in synapses by leupeptin. *Science* 221:971–72

79a. Clarkson, T. W., Marsh, D. O. 1982. Mercury toxicity in man. In *Clinical, Biochemical, and Nutritional Aspects of Trace Elements.* pp. 549–68. New York: Alan R. Liss

80. Christian, M. S., ed. 1985. Cancer and the Environment. Possible mechanisms of thresholds for carcinogens and other toxic substances. *J. Am. Coll. Toxicol.* 2:1–321

81. Schmahl, D. 1979. Problems of dose-response studies in chemical carcinogenesis with special reference to N-nitroso compounds. *CRC Crit. Rev. Toxicol.* 6:257–81

82. Skilleter, D. N. 1984. Biochemical properties of beryllium potentially relevant to its carcinogenicity. *Toxicol. Environ. Chem. Rev.* 7:213–28

83. Tomatis, L., Cabral, J. R. P., Likhachev, A. J., Ponomarkov, V. 1981. Increased cancer incidence in the progeny of male rats exposed to ethylnitrosourea before mating. *Int. J. Cancer* 28:475–78

84. Cabral, J. R. P., Tomatis, L., Likhachev, A. J., Ponomarkov, V., Enzeby, B. 1983. Prenatal exposure to ethylnitrosourea (ENU) and its effect on four successive generations. *Toxicologist* 3(136):34 (Abstr).

85. Nomura, T. 1982. Parental exposure to X-rays and chemicals induces heritable tumours and anomalies in mice. *Nature* 296:575–77

86. Tomatis, L., Hilfrich, J., Turosov, V. 1975. The occurrence of tumours in F_1, F_2 and F_3 descendents of BD rats exposed to N-nitrosomethylurea during pregnancy. *Int. J. Cancer* 15:385–90

87. Tomatis, L., Ponomarkov, V., Turusov, V. 1977. Effects of ethylnitrosourea administration during pregnancy on three subsequent generations of BDVI rats. *Int. J. Cancer* 19:240–48

88. Brown, A. W., Aldridge, W. N., Street, B. W., Verschoyle, R. D. 1979. The behavioural and neuropathologic sequellae of intoxication by trimethyltin compounds in the rat. *Am. J. Pathol.* 97:59–82

89. Aldridge, W. N. 1985. The toxicology and biological properties of organotin compounds. In *Tin as a Vital Nutrient: Implications in Cancer Prophylaxis and Other Physiological Processes,* ed. N. Cardarelli. Boca Raton, Florida: CRC Press. In press

90. Ross, W. D., Emmett, E. A., Steiner, J., Tureen, R. 1981. Neurotoxic effects of occupational exposure to organotins. *Am. J. Psychiatry* 138:1092–95

91. Fortemps, E., Amand, G., Bourboir, A., Lauwerys, R., Laterre, E. C. 1979. Trimethyl poisoning: report of two cases. *Int. Arch. Occup. Environ. Health* 41:1–6

92. Ray, C., Reinecke, H. J., Besser, R. 1984. Methyltin intoxication in six men: toxicologic and clinical aspects. *Vet. Hum. Toxicol.* 26:121–22

93. Walsh, T. J., Miller, D. B., Dyer, R. S. 1982. Trimethyltin, a selective limbic system neurotoxicant impairs radical arm maze performance. *Neurobehav. Toxicol. Teratol.* 4:177–83

94. Swarzwelder, H. S., Hepler, J., Holahan, W., King, S. E., Leverenz, H. A., et al 1982. Impaired maze performance in the rat caused by trimethyltin treatment: problem-solving deficits and perseveration. *Neurobehav. Toxicol. Teratol.* 4:169–76

Ann. Rev. Pharmacol. Toxicol. 1986. 26:59–77

OPIOID PEPTIDE PROCESSING AND RECEPTOR SELECTIVITY

Volker Höllt

Department of Neuropharmacology, Max-Planck-Institut für Psychiatrie, Am Klopfer-spitz 18 A, D- 8033 Planegg-Martinsried, West Germany

INTRODUCTION

Since the discovery of the enkephalins in 1975, an increasing number of larger opioid peptides, which contain the sequence of either met-enkephalin or leu-enkephalin at their N-terminus, have been isolated. All these opioid peptides belong to one of three peptide families, each deriving from a distinct precursor molecule: Proopiomelanorcortin (POMC), the common precursor for β-endorphin, ACTH, and additional MSH-containing peptides; proenkephalin A, the common precursor for met- and leu-enkephalin and several larger enkephalin-containing peptides (e.g. peptide E, peptide F) and proenkephalin B (prodynorphin), another precursor for leu-enkephalin and for larger opioid peptides (e.g. the dynorphins, neo-endorphins and leumorphin). The structures of these precursor molecules of several species have been determined using recombinant DNA techniques [reviewed by Numa (1)].

The precise proteolytic processing of POMC has been analyzed in pituitary cells and described in recent reviews (2–5). Similarly, the processing of proenkephalin A in the bovine adrenal medulla has been extensively reviewed recently (6, 7). Less is known about the processing of proenkephalin B [pro-dynorphin, summarized in (8)]. Moreover, the proteolytic fragmentation of all three opioid peptide precursors within the central nervous system is still poorly understood.

In addition to the multiplicity of opioid peptides, there is pharmacological evidence for multiple opioid receptors. Martin et al (9) classified opioid receptors in terms of their effects in whole animals as being morphine-like (μ), ketocyclazocine-like (κ), and N-allylnormetazocine-like (σ). The pharmacological characterization of opioid receptors by the use of isolated tissues such as

59

0362-1642/86/0415-0059$02.00

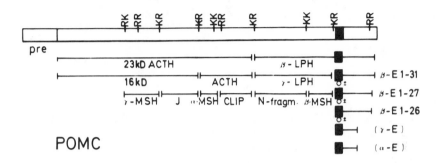

POMC

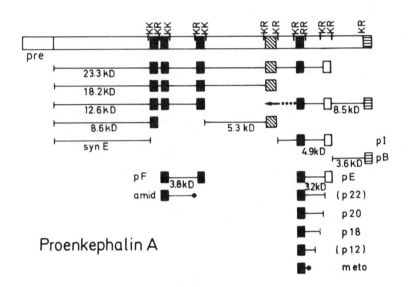

Proenkephalin A

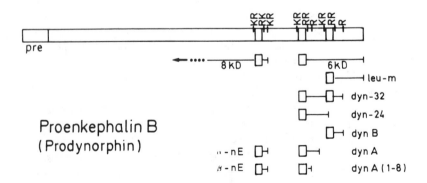

Proenkephalin B
(Prodynorphin)

the guinea-pig ileum and the vasa deferentia of the mouse, rat, and rabbit has led to the observation that, in addition to interacting with the μ- and κ-types of opioid receptors, the opioids can interact with δ- (10) and ε- receptors [(11); reviewed in (12)]. In this review an attempt is made to summarize the literature describing the various products of processing of the three opioid precursors and their selectivity for the different classes of opioid receptors.

THE PROOPIOMELANOCORTIN (POMC) SYSTEM
Processing Products

The structure of bovine POMC, together with its major processing products, is shown schematically in Figure 1 (13). Each of the peptides in the precursor molecule is bounded by pairs of basic amino acid residues, which represent the sites of proteolytic processing (14). The major source of POMC production is the pituitary. Studies of biosynthesis have revealed that the processing of POMC in the intermediate lobe of rats is different from that in the anterior lobe (3, 5). In general, POMC undergoes more cleavages and its products more posttranslational modifications in the intermediate lobe than in the anterior pituitary. There is little or no β-lipotropin in the intermediate pituitary. β-Endorphin is posttranslationally modified by α-N-acetylation which leads to a complete loss of its activity at opioid receptors. In addition, it is shortened at its C-terminus by 4 or 5 amino acids. Thus, N-α-acetyl-β-endorphin 1–27, and N-acetyl-β-endorphin 1–26 are major end products in the processing of POMC in the intermediate pituitary of rats (2, 3). In contrast, β-lipotropin is a major POMC end product in the anterior pituitary. Its concentrations are about twofold higher than those of β-endorphin 1–31, which is not posttranslationally modified. Differential processing in the anterior and intermediate pituitary lobes also exists for the ACTH domain of POMC. Whereas ACTH 1–39 is the major product in the anterior lobe, this peptide undergoes further proteolysis

---

← ⎯⎯

Figure 1   Opioid peptide precursors and processing products. Data are derived from the following references: POMC (1–3, 5, 13, 24), proenkephalin A (1, 6, 7, 41, 47–60), proenkephalin B (1, 86–95, 99). The presence of modifications in the nonlipotropin portion of POMC has been omitted for simplicity. Upward marks indicate cleavage at basic amino acids (K = lysine, R = arginine). Abbreviations are: POMC = proopiomelanocortin; ACTH = corticotropin; LPH = lipotropin; MSH = melanotropin; CLIP = corticotropin-like intermediate lobe peptide; J = joining peptide; α, β, γ-E = α, β, γ-endorphin; kD = kilodaltons; syn E = synenkephalin; pB, E, F, I = peptide B, E, F, I; p22, 20, 18, 12 = BAM-22P, -20P, -18P, -12P; amid = amidorphin; meto = metorphamide; dyn = dynorphin; leu-m = leumorphin; nE = neoendorphin; pre = signal sequence. ■ = met-enkephalin, □ = leu-enkephalin; ⊟ = met-enk-arg-phe, ⊠ = met-enk-arg-gly-leu; ● = amido group, ○ = N-α-acetyl-residue; ← indicates that the N-terminus of the peptide is not precisely defined.

and posttranslational processing in the intermediate pituitary. After acetylation and amidation, the major end product of POMC is α-MSH. In addition to acetylation and amidation, many posttranslational modifications occur in the non-β-lipotropin portion of POMC that are not discussed here (4, 5).

Processing of POMC in the brain appears to be similar to that found in the intermediate pituitary. In general, immunoreactive material of a molecular size similar to that of β-endorphin and α-MSH is the predominant POMC product in the brains of rats and humans (15, 16). However, N-acetylation of β-endorphin seems much less pronounced in the brain than in the intermediate pituitary. Some authors (17, 18) were not able to detect N-acetyl-β-endorphin and α-MSH in rat brain. Other groups found N-acetylated variants in several brain regions of rats, although to a varying degree (19–21). In some brain regions the acetylated forms of β-endorphin and α-MSH were the predominant POMC products (3, 21). Moreover, cleavage at the carboxyl terminus of β-endorphin appears to occur in the brain. This is indicated by the detection of acetylated and nonacetylated forms of β-endorphin 1–26 and β-endorphin 1–27 (3).

Shorter cleavage products of β-endorphin such as α-endorphin (β-endorphin 1–16) and γ-endorphin (β-endorphin 1–17) have been isolated from pituitary tissue. These peptides do not, however, seem to be true processing products of POMC in the pituitary as indicated by pulse-labelling studies (2). Similarly, met-enkephalin is not a processing product of POMC in the pituitary (2).

γ-Endorphin and α-endorphin and their des-tyrosine forms have been found in brain extracts (22). It is still unclear whether these peptides might be extraction artifacts or degradation products resulting from the extracellular proteolysis of β-endorphin.

POMC has recently been biosynthesized in the hypothalamus of the rat (23). Liotta et al found some differences in the processing of POMC in brain as compared to that in the pituitary. Whereas β-lipotropin is first cleaved from its precursor to yield a biosynthetic intermediate termed 23 kD ACTH (24) in both pituitary lobes, at least part of POMC in the hypothalamus appears to undergo a primary cleavage that removes all or part of the N-terminal fragment. This indicates an altered order of processing (23). As in the intermediate pituitary, hypothalamic POMC was processed into molecules of sizes similar to those of β-endorphin and α-MSH. In contrast to the peptides of the intermediate pituitary, these peptides were physicochemically similar to des-acetyl α-MSH and authentic rat β-endorphin 1–31, indicating that no major acetylation of POMC products occurs in the hypothalamus.

Receptor Selectivity

Although β-endorphin was discovered almost 10 years ago, its receptor selectivity characteristics have not yet been fully clarified. In guinea-pig brain β-endorphin shows a slight binding selectivity for μ- over δ-receptor sites, with negligible affinity for κ-sites (25). It exhibits no opioid activity on the rabbit vas deferens, a preparation proposed to have κ-opioid receptors only (12, 26–28). In the mouse vas deferens, however, β-endorphin shows no selectivity for μ-over κ- or δ-receptors as revealed in receptor inactivation experiments using a site-directed alkylating agent (29). It is possible, however, that β-endorphin interacts with ε-receptors in the mouse vas deferens. Moreover, there is increasing evidence that, in addition to μ- and δ-sites, β-endorphin interacts with a distinct population of binding sites in brain [putative ε-sites that differ from classical μ-, δ-, and κ-sites (30–33a)]. ε-Receptors occur in high abundance in the rat vas deferens (11). In this preparation, β-endorphin 1–27 is slightly more potent than its parent peptide β-endorphin 1–31. Further C-terminally shortened cleavage products, such as γ-endorphin (β-endorphin 1–17), α-endorphin (β-endorphin 1–16), and met-enkephalin (β-endorphin 1–5) are considerably less potent than β-endorphin 1–31 in the rat vas deferens (11). Although part of this potency difference may be attributed to the preferential inactivation of the shorter peptides by enzymatic degradation (33b), there appears to exist an intrinsically high potency of β-endorphin 1–31 and its processing product β-endorphin 1–27 on this preparation. Structure-activity studies revealed that the activation of the ε-receptors in the rat vas deferens requires large β-endorphin sequences (at least β-endorphin 1–21) (11, 33b, 34).

Similar observations have been made in binding studies using ^{3}H-β-endorphin as ligand. Met-enkephalin, α-, and γ-endorphin had considerably lower binding affinities than β-endorphin 1–31 and β-endorphin 1–27 (32). Thus, a C-terminally extended long peptide chain in β-endorphin as compared to met-enkephalin appears to increase the selectivity and potency for putative ε-receptors, and increases the resistance to degrading enzymes. On the other hand, modification of the N-terminus by acetylation virtually abolishes binding and opioid activity in the various preparations (3, 31).

Of a wide variety of endogenous opioid peptides tested, β-endorphin has been shown to be the most potent peptide in inducing analgesia after intracerebroventricular injection in mice (35). Interestingly, the complete carboxyterminal end of β-endorphin is necessary for full analgesic potency. Thus, the processing product β-endorphin 1–27 is much less analgesically active than β-endorphin 1–31 (3, 36). Furthermore, β-endorphin 1–27 even antagonizes the analgesic effect of β-endorphin 1–31 when coinjected into the brains of mice (36). Therefore, it has been suggested that the C-terminal processing of the parent peptide may produce a physiologically important antagonist of β-endorphin (36). However, no evidence of an antagonist action of β-endorphin 1–27 or other β-endorphin fragments was found in isolated tissue preparations (34). Moreover, the dramatic loss of analgesic activity of the C-terminally shortened peptide as compared to β-endorphin 1–31 was not reflected by similar changes in the affinity to either μ-, δ-, or ε-receptors (11) in isolated tissues or in its binding properties to rat brain membranes (32). Thus, the functional significance of the C-terminal processing of β-endorphin in terms of altered opioid activity is not yet clear. Recent investigations, however, indicated that β-endorphin 1–31 might possess a second biologically active sequence at its C-terminus which activates the complement-binding system (37). β-Endorphin 1–27 is inactive in this system. Moreover, β-endorphin has been demonstrated to bind to lymphocytes through its C-terminal fragment, (38) and there is increasing evidence that the C-terminal portion of β-endorphin may influence the immune system by a nonopioid mechanism (39). Moreover, a dipeptide that is probably released by C-terminal processing of β-endorphin 1–31 (glycyl-glutamine) has recently been isolated from pituitary tissue and shown to possess properties characteristic of neurotransmitters (40).

In summary, β-endorphin 1–31 and β-endorphin 1–27 are processing end products in the pituitary and also in the brain. These peptides interact preferentially with μ-, δ-, and ε-, but not κ-opioid receptors. N-acetylation of these peptides in the intermediate pituitary (and possibly also in the brain) abolishes the opioid activities of these peptides and may be regarded as a physiological inactivation mechanism. C-terminal processing may, however, have a regulatory function in abolishing interactions of β-endorphin 1–31 with the immune system.

THE PROENKEPHALIN A SYSTEM

Processing Products

The structure of bovine proenkephalin A together with its major processing products is given in Figure 1 (41). Assuming that paired basic amino acids are processing signals, the structure of proenkephalin A suggests potential cleavage into four copies of met-enkephalin and one copy each of leu-enkephalin, the heptapeptide met-enkephalin-arg-phe (met-enk-arg-phe), and the octapeptide met-enk-arg-gly-leu. In addition, however, a wide variety of larger enkephalin-containing peptides have been isolated from bovine adrenal medulla (6, 7). The same copies of enkephalin and extended peptides are contained in human proenkephalin A (1, 42) and in rat (43–45). However, in *Xenopus laevis* proenkephalin A contains only met-enkephalin and extended sequences, but no leu-enkephalin (46).

In the bovine adrenal medulla proenkephalin A processing appears to occur predominantly at the C-terminus, since the majority of isolated enkephalin-containing precursor peptides possess the N-terminus of proenkephalin A [23.3 kD (47), 18.2 kD (48), 12.6 kD, 8.6 kD (49)]. In contrast, only two peptides that contain the intact C-terminus of proenkephalin A [peptide B (3.6 kD) (50) and an 8.5-kD peptide (51)] have also been described. In addition, several enkephalin-containing peptides have been isolated that are derived from the mid-portions of the precursor. One is 5.3 kD (52); another, peptide I, is 4.9 kD (50).

There is a series of peptides that contain the sequence of met-enkephalin at its N-terminus and thus exhibit opioid activity. One such example is peptide F (53), a 3.8-kD peptide containing two met-enkephalin sequences, one at its N- and another at its C-terminus. A carboxy-terminally amidated peptide comprising the first 26 amino acids of peptide F has recently been isolated and named amidorphin (54). Peptide E is a 3.2-kD peptide possessing the sequence of met-enkephalin at its N-terminus and that of leu-enkephalin at its C-terminus (55). Several carboxy-terminally shortened peptides of peptide E have been isolated: BAM-22P (56), BAM-20P (56), BAM-18P (57), BAM-12P (58), and a carboxy-terminally amidated octapeptide corresponding to the first 8 amino acids of peptide E. This last peptide has been named metorphamide or adrenorphin (59, 60). Most of these peptides appear to be processed by cleavage at pairs of basic amino acids. Exceptions are BAM-22P and BAM-12P. It has therefore been claimed that these peptides are products of nonspecific proteolysis (7).

The generation of metorphamide (59) involves proteolytic cleavage at a single arginine amino acid—a cleavage site that exists in several peptide precursors (4). Furthermore, the C-terminal glycine residue is converted into an amino group by a specific amidating enzyme (61, 62). Similar mechanisms exist for the conversion of peptide F (1–27) into amidorphin (54).

There is strong evidence that proenkephalin A in bovine brain is similar or identical to that found in the adrenal medulla. Liston et al (63) isolated a 10-kD peptide from bovine caudate nucleus, the sequence of which is identical to residues 1–70 of adrenal medullary proenkephalin A. This peptide contains no opioid sequences and has been termed synenkephalin. Moreover, using antibodies against peptides from the adrenal medulla, immunoreactive peptides with the chromatographic properties of met-enk-arg-phe (64, 65), met-enk-arg-gly-leu (65), BAM-12P (66), BAM-22P (51, 67), peptide F (67), amidorphin (54), metorphamide (59), and BAM-18P (57) have been found in bovine brain. Moreover, proenkephalin A mRNA in bovine adrenal medulla and in various bovine brain areas has been shown to have the same size of about 1400 nucleotides (68, 69).

On the other hand, there is increasing evidence that processing of pro-enkephalin A in the adrenal medulla is different from that in the bovine brain. In the adrenal medulla the initial cleaving occurs near the carboxyl-termini, liberating large intermediates of 8.6–23.3 kD with intact N-termini (Figure 1). In the supraoptic nucleus, however, initial processing steps appear to involve the removal of the N-terminal fragment (70). The high-molecular-weight enkephalin-containing peptides are predominant in the supraoptic nucleus, whereas the neurohypophysis almost exclusively contains free enkephalins. This indicates an almost complete processing of proenkephalin A along the hypothalamo-neurohypophyseal pathway (70).

In general, the processing of proenkephalin A appears to be more complete in the brain than in the adrenal medulla. Thus, the bovine adrenal medulla contains high amounts of high-molecular-weight enkephalin-containing peptides and relatively low amounts of free enkephalins (7). In the brain, however, free enkephalins are the predominant processing products of proenkephalin A.

In addition, peptides of higher molecular weight reacting with antibodies against BAM-22P, peptide F, met-enk-arg-phe, and met-enk-arg-gly-leu are more abundant in the adrenal medulla than in bovine hypothalamus or striatum (65, 67). In particular, in human brain tissue very low amounts of larger peptides reacting with antibodies directed against BAM-22P, BAM-12P, met-enk-arg-phe, and met-enk-arg-gly-leu have been found (71). This indicates that neuronal proenkephalin A is processed very rapidly in the brain and that the processing intermediates do not accumulate to any significant extent.

However, species differences may exist, since substantial amounts of proenkephalin A precursor and high-molecular-weight intermediates have been found in striatal tissue of rats and guinea pigs (72). Moreover, putative processing products of higher molecular weight appear to be present in some rat brain areas when antibodies directed against met-enk-arg-phe (73), or met-enk-arg-gly-leu (74) have been used.

The distribution of proenkephalin A–derived peptides in rats has been extensively investigated by immunohistochemical studies. An anatomical description of the widespread distribution of the proenkephalin A system in the brain is beyond the scope of this chapter and the reader is referred to a recent review by Watson et al (75).

An important problem is whether or not leu-enkephalin, present in a single copy in proenkephalin A, derives from this precursor or from proenkephalin B (prodynorphin), in which it is present in three copies.

The ratio of leu-enkephalin to met-enk-arg-phe or to met-enk-arg-gly-leu, putative processing end products also present as single copies in proenkephalin A, has been found to be about 1 : 1 in many areas of the rat brain (76, 77). This indicates that leu-enkephalin might predominantly arise from the processing of proenkephalin A with no major contribution of leu-enkephalin by proenkephalin B (prodynorphin). However, in certain regions, such as the substantia nigra, leu-enkephalin is derived from proenkephalin B (77). Thus, leu-enkephalin in the brain can be derived from either proenkephalin A or B, indicating regional differences in the processing rates of the precursor molecules.

As compared with met-enk-arg-phe the levels of metorphamide (adrenorphin = met-enk-arg-arg-val-NH2) were very low in the rat brain (78, 79). In addition, there was no correlation between the distributional patterns of metor-phamide (adrenorphin) and met-enk-arg-phe, implying that the amidated peptide is generated from proenkephalin A in a way distinct from that by which met-enk-arg-phe is formed in each region of the brain.

Interestingly, the highest concentration of the amidated octapeptide has been found in the olfactory bulb where other opioid peptides have been found in negligible amounts (78). This unique distributional pattern suggests that this peptide might have specialized physiological functions distinct from those of other opioid peptides.

A major processing product of proenkephalin A in the rat brain appears to be BAM-18P. This peptide has been shown to occur in higher concentrations in the hypothalamus than metorphamide (adrenorphin), BAM-12P, BAM-22P, and peptide E (57).

Receptor Selectivity

As revealed by binding studies, met-enkephalin and leu-enkephalin possess a high selectivity for δ binding sites in guinea-pig brain (10, 25) and mouse brain (28, 80). The heptapeptide met-enk-arg-phe and the octapeptide met-enk-arg-gly-leu have comparable affinities for μ- and δ- opioid receptors with lower affinities for κ-sites [reviewed in (12)]. The larger opioid peptides derived from the peptide E domain of proenkephalin A (peptide E, BAM-22P, BAM-12P) show high affinity and selectivity for μ-sites; in addition, they have high affinities for κ-sites—about 40–50% of the affinities for the μ-sites. In contrast, the affinity for δ-sites is low (28, 80, 81). The binding selectivity of metorphamide (59) is similar to that of the above peptides, indicating that the site selectivity does not markedly change when peptide E is processed to metorphamide. In contrast, peptide F exhibits an about 100-fold lower affinity for μ-sites than the peptides of the peptide E domain. Moreover, peptide F does not have any preferential affinity for any of the three types of binding sites tested (28, 80, 81).

In general, this binding selectivity is confirmed by the pharmacological selectivity of the opioid peptides in various bioassays. The "μ-selective" pattern of pharmacological activity of the peptide E–derived peptides is indicated by the high potency of this peptide in the guinea-pig ileum compared to the low potency of these peptides in the mouse vas deferens (55, 56, 59, 81, 82).

The interaction of the peptide E–derived peptides with functional κ-receptors is indicated by their high activity on the rabbit vas deferens—a preparation that has been shown to exclusively contain opioid κ-receptors (27, 28, 59, 82). Also, peptide E, BAM-22P, and BAM-12P appear to interact with κ-opioid receptors in the mouse vas deferens as revealed in experiments using a site-directed alkylating agent (29).

In contrast, the smaller opioid products of proenkephalin A (met-enkephalin, leu-enkephalin, met-enk-arg-phe, and met-enk-arg-gly-leu) exhibit a clear selectivity for δ-opioid receptors in the mouse vas deferens (29, 83). The octapeptide met-enk-arg-gly-leu appears also to interact with κ-opioid receptors as evidenced in the mouse vas deferens rendered cross-tolerant to κ-opioid receptor agonists (84).

Peptide F is not active on the rabbit vas deferens, and exhibits a low potency on the guinea pig ileum and mouse vas deferens (27, 55, 82), indicating that it does not have any particular affinity at μ-, κ, and δ-opioid receptors.

However, peptide F and the larger peptides of the peptide E domain (peptide E, BAM-22P) show a substantial potency on the rat vas deferens, indicating that they interact with putative ε-receptors (82, 85). Moreover, these peptides elicit a pronounced analgesia after injection into the mouse brain (34). It is noteworthy that the relative potencies of the above peptides on the rat vas deferens, i.e. on putative ε-receptors correlate well with their analgesic potencies in mice (82). This suggests that the ε-receptor may play a role in analgesia.

In conclusion, the enkephalins are not the ultimate products of proenkephalin A in many areas of the brain. A wide variety of larger carboxy-terminally extended peptides possessing different receptor selectivities have been identified. The peptides of the peptide E domain are potent agonists at μ-, κ-, and ε-receptors, whereas peptide F exhibits substantial potency at ε-receptors only. Complete processing of proenkephalin A into the enkephalins, the heptapeptide, and the octapeptide, is associated with a change in the receptor selectivity towards δ-opioid receptors.

THE PROENKEPHALIN B (PRODYNORPHIN) SYSTEM

Processing Products

The structure of porcine proenkephalin B (prodynorphin) has been deduced from cloned DNA sequences complementary to hypothalamic mRNA (86). It contains three leu-enke-phalin sequences each flanked by pairs of basic amino acids (Figure 1). If, however, lys-arg pairs were the only processing signals, proenkephalin B would be cleaved into three larger opioid peptides: β-neoendorphin (87), dynorphin A (88, 89), and leumorphin (90). However, several other peptides derived from proenkephalin B have been identified, indicating that enzymes with more complex specifications are involved. The pro-lys bond at the carboxy-terminus of β-neoendorphin is often resistant to proteolysis, and the larger decapeptide [α-neoendorphin, (91)] is a major processing product. Moreover, cleavage at dibasic residues is not obligatory but may also occur where single arginines exist. Thus, the formation of dynorphin B [rimorphin, (92, 93)] results from a cleavage between threonine-13 and arginine-14 of leumorphin. By a similar cleavage, dynorphin A (1–8)

(94, 95) is formed from dynorphin A. This type of cleavage appears to occur frequently, and the smaller peptides are thus more abundant than the larger ones in many areas of the brain (96–98). In addition, several larger peptides have been identified as putative processing products: A 4-kD peptide containing dynorphin A at the N-terminus and dynorphin B at the C-terminal end has been isolated [dynorphin 32 (92)]. Dynorphin 24 contains dynorphin A with a C-terminal extension of lys-arg and the sequence of leu-enkephalin (92). There is also evidence for a 6-kD peptide comprising dynorphin A and leumorphin (99). In addition, 8-kD peptides representing N-terminally extended forms of α- and/or β-neoendorphin have been found in the adenohypophysis of rats (100, 101).

Proenkephalin B–derived peptides are most abundant in the neural lobe of the rat pituitary. They are colocalized with vasopressin in neurons originating in the magnocellular nuclei of the hypothalamus (102, 103).

Several products of proenkephalin B have been found in the posterior pituitary including the 6-kD peptide, dynorphin 32, dynorphin A, dynorphin A(1–8), α-neoendorphin, β-neoendorphin, and dynorphin B (97–99, 104).

There is also some evidence that leu-enkephalin is a processing product of proenkephalin B in the rat posterior pituitary. Osmotic stimuli such as salt-loading concomitantly decrease dynorphin A and leu-enkephalin levels in the posterior pituitary but have no effect upon met-enkephalin levels (105, 106).

Part of the leu-enkephalin in the rat posterior/intermediate pituitary, but not in the brain, can undergo N-acetylation (107). N-acetyl-leu-enkephalin is devoid of opioid activity. Dynorphin A and its high-molecular-weight forms, however, are not acetylated. On the other hand, a minor portion of dynorphin A (1–8) appears to be α-N-acetylated, suggesting that N-acetylation may occur during the late stages of proenkephalin B processing (104).

In contrast to the processing of proenkephalin B in the posterior pituitary, differential processing of proenkephalin B appears to occur in the anterior lobe. A putative end product in this lobe is a 6-kD dynorphin peptide containing the C-terminal part of proenkephalin B with the sequence of dynorphin A at its N-terminus. This peptide shows opioid activity (97, 99, 101). There is no evidence for the further processing of the 6-kD peptide into dynorphin A, leumorphin, or dynorphin B in the adenohypophysis of rats. On the other hand, α-neoendorphin and β-neoendorphin are processing products in this lobe. In addition, large N-terminally extended (non-opioid) forms of α- and β-neoendorphin have been found with a molecular size of about 8 kD (100, 101).

The distribution of the various proenkephalin B–derived peptides has been extensively studied in many areas of rat (96–98, 100, 108) and human (71, 100, 109, 110) brain. These studies strongly suggest that proenkephalin B is differentially processed in the various brain areas (96–98, 108). Whereas dynorphin A and dynorphin A (1–8) occur in about equal amounts in the posterior pituitary, dynorphin A (1–8) is the predominant peptide in the brain. The ratio of dynorphin A(1–8) to dynorphin A is particularly high in the striatum and the midbrain (96, 98, 111).

Similarly, the molar ratio of α-neoendorphin to β-neoendorphin differs in various brain regions (112). In two thirds of 100 microdissected brain areas, α-neoendorphin is more abundant than β-neoendorphin (113). This indicates regional differences in the activity of enzymes that remove the C-terminal lysine of α-neoendorphin. The best candidates for such enzymes are post-proline cleaving enzymes, which exist in the brain (114).

Although dynorphin B is abundant within the rat brain, the presence of leumorphin in brain is still a matter of controversy (97, 98, 115). Suda et al used an efficient extraction method, and reported the existence of substantial amounts of leumorphin in human striatum (110).

A striatonigral pathway in rat brain containing very dense collections of fibers and terminals reacting with antibodies directed to dynorphin A (1–13) has been identified (116). The cell bodies of these fibers are located in the head of the caudate nucleus (117). The substantia nigra has one of the highest concentrations of dynorphins and neoendorphins within the central nervous system of rat (77) and man (109). Deafferentation of the globus pallidus results in a concomitant decrease in the levels of leu-enkephalin and dynorphin B, but not of met-enk-arg-gly-leu (77). This experiment provides evidence for processing of proenkephalin B into leu-enkephalin and for a distinct anatomical location of the proenkephalin A and proenkephalin B systems in the brain. On the other hand, there is also evidence for colocalization of both systems such as in medullary neurons of the rat (118).

Leu-enkephalin, which can derive from proenkephalin A and proenkephalin B, may undergo further posttranslational modifications. Indeed, a tyr-o-sulfated form of leu-enkephalin has been isolated from brain that is devoid of opioid activity (119).

Receptor Selectivity

With the exception of leu-enkephalin, all opioid peptides derived from pro-enkephalin B have been shown to exhibit a pronounced selectivity for κ-opioid receptors (25, 28, 29, 81, 82, 120–123). In binding experiments, dynorphin A appears to have the highest affinity and highest selectivity for κ-binding sites, whereas its fragment dynorphin A (1–8) has a lower affinity and a somewhat lower selectivity for κ-sites in guinea-pig membranes (25). All these peptides are active in the rabbit vas deferens, a preparation that has been proposed to contain exclusively functional κ-receptors (26, 27, 81, 122, 124, 125).

Dynorphin A, α-neoendorphin, and dynorphin B are selective κ agonists in the guinea-pig ileum, a tissue containing μ- and κ-opioid receptors. Dynorphin A (1–8) and leumorphin appear to interact with κ- and μ-opioid receptors as assessed by differing sensitivities of the peptides to antagonism by naloxone (123). Similarly, in the mouse vas deferens, dynorphin A, dynorphin B, and leumorphin are selective κ agonists, whereas dynorphin A(1–8) and β-neoendorphin are distinctly less selective for κ-receptors and appear to interact also at δ-receptors as revealed in alkylation experiments (29) and in cross-tolerance studies (83). In the rat vas deferens, which contains a high abundance of ε-receptors, however, all proenkephalin B–derived peptides with the exception of leu-enkephalin are virtually inactive (85, 122).

The structural determinants for κ-selectivity appear to be an arginine residue at position 7 and another basic amino acid at position 10 or 11 (8). Dynorphin A, dynorphin B, and α-neoendorphin fulfill these criteria, but not dynorphin A(1–8) or β-neoendorphin, thus explaining their distinctly lower κ activity. Hence, if dynorphin A or α-neoendorphin were processed into dynorphin A(1–8) or β-neoendorphin, and further to leu-enkephalin, there would be a stepwise decrease in the selectivity for κ- and an increase in the selectivity for δ-opioid receptors.

In contrast to the POMC product β-endorphin and the majority of the proenkephalin A–derived peptides, the proenkephalin B–derived peptides have only weak analgesic properties, if any, when injected into the brain (34, 126). It is likely, however, that κ-opioid receptors are involved in mediating anti-nociception at the level of the spinal cord [reviewed in (82)].

In conclusion, the proteolysis of proenkephalin B generates a set of opioid peptides that exhibit selectivity for κ-opioid receptors. Dynorphin A is the most potent and selective peptide. Its further processing into dynorphin A(1–8) and further into leu-enkephalin occurs differentially in the various areas of the brain and this is associated with a change in the receptor selectivity towards δ-opioid receptors.

CONCLUDING REMARKS

This article reviews data evidence that posttranslational proteolysis of opioid peptide precursors occurs differently in various regions of the brain and pituitary and that the processing products can differ markedly in their selectivity for the various types of opioid receptors. In general, no simple allocation can be made between the opioid peptides of a precursor family and their preference for a certain class of receptors. Thus, processing of POMC yields peptides that interact with μ-, δ-, and ε-receptors; proenkephalin A–derived peptides interact with μ-, δ-, κ-, and ε-receptors; and the peptides derived from proenkephalin B interact preferentially with κ- and δ-opioid receptors. Some peptides exhibit a high selectivity for a certain receptor type, such as dynorphin A for κ-receptors or the enkephalins for the δ-receptors. Although some peptides have a prefer-ence for μ-receptors (β-endorphin and the peptides derived from peptide E), their selectivity is insufficient to accept them as prime candidates for the endogenous ligands of the μ-receptor. The only compound that has exclusive selectivity for the μ-type of receptors is thought to be of plant origin, namely morphine. Recent evidence suggests that such a compound is present in animals (127).

The formation from a single precursor of opioid peptides with presumably different biological activities offers a level at which physiological regulation may take place. Thus, specific processing enzymes may play a key role in regulating the biological activities of the opioid peptide system. It is important to remember that the opioid receptors are still poorly defined on the basis of relatively crude techniques and that the biological functions mediated by the various opioid receptor types are not understood. There is a clear need to define opioid receptors structurally, and it is likely that their structure, as well as the structures of the enzymes involved in opioid precursor processing, will be elucidated by recombinant DNA techniques in the near future. This will allow the regulation of the processing of the precursors and the interaction of the products with the opioid receptors to be studied at a molecular level. Finally, the design of specific inhibitors of the processing enzymes may provide further insight into the physiological role of opioid peptide processing and may offer a basis for the development of new opioids.

Literature Cited

1. Numa, S. 1984. Opioid peptide precursors and their genes. In *The Peptides,* ed. E. Gross, J. Meienhofer, Vol. 6. pp. 1–23. New York: Academic. 410 pp.
2. Eipper, B. A., Mains, R. E. 1980. Structure and biosynthesis of pro-adrenocorticotropin/endorphin and related peptides. *Endocrinol. Rev.* 1:1–27
3. Zakarian, S., Smyth, D. G. 1982. Distribution of β-endorphin-related peptides in rat pituitary and brain. *Biochem. J.* 202:561–71
4. Mains, R. E., Eipper, B. A., Glembotski, C. C., Dores, R. M. 1983. Strategies for the biosynthesis of bioactive peptides. *Trends Neurosci.* 6:229–35
5. Civelli, O., Douglass, J., Herbert, E. 1984. Pro-opiomelanocortin: A polyprotein at the interface of the endocrine and nervous systems. See Ref. 1, pp. 69–94
6. Lewis, R. V., Stern, A. S. 1983. Biosynthesis of the enkephalins and enkephalin-containing peptides. *Ann. Rev. Pharmacol. Toxicol.* 23:353–72
7. Udenfriend, S., Kilpatrick, D. L. 1984. Proenkephalin and the products of its processing: chemistry and biology. See Ref. 1, pp. 25–68
8. Goldstein, A. 1984. Biology and chemistry of the dynorphin peptides. See Ref. 1, pp. 95–145
9. Martin, W. R., Eades, C. G., Thompson, J. A., Huppler, R. E., Gilbert, P. E. 1976. The effects of morphine- and nalorphine-like drugs in the nondependent and morphine-dependent chronic spinal dog. *J. Pharmacol. Exp. Ther.* 197:517–22
10. Lord, J. A. H., Waterfield, A. A., Hughes, J., Kosterlitz, H. W. 1977. Endogenous opioid peptides: multiple agonists and receptors. *Nature* 267:495–99
11. Schulz, R., Wüster, M., Herz, A. 1981. Pharmacological characterization of the ε-opiate receptor. *J. Pharmacol. Exp. Ther.* 216:604–6
12. Paterson, S. J., Robson, L. E., Kosterlitz, H. W. 1984. Opioid receptors. See Ref. 1, pp. 147–89
13. Nakanishi, S., Inoue, A., Kita, T., Nakamura, M., Chang, A. C. Y., et al. 1979. Nucleotide sequence of cloned cDNA for bovine corticotropin-β-lipotropin precursor. *Nature* 278:423–27
14. Docherty, K., Steiner, D. F. 1982. Post-translational proteolysis in polypeptide

hormone biosynthesis. *Ann. Rev. Physiol.* 44:625–38

15. Gramsch, C., Kleber, G., Höllt, V., Pasi, A., Mehrain, P., Herz, A. 1980. Pro-opiocortin fragments in human and rat brain: β-endorphin and α-MSH are the predominant peptides *Brain Res.* 192:109–19

16. Kleber, G., Gramsch, C., Höllt, V., Mehrain, P., Pasi, A., Herz, A. 1980. Extrahypothalamic corticotropin and α-melanotropin in human brain. *Neuroendocrinology* 31:39–45

17. Weber, E., Evans, C. J., Barchas, J. D. 1981. Acetylated and non-acetylated forms of β-endorphin in rat brain and pituitary. *Biochem. Biophys. Res. Commun.* 103:982–89

18. Evans, C. J., Lorenz, R., Weber, E., Barchas, J. D. 1982. Variants of α-melanocyte stimulating hormone in rat brain and pituitary: Evidence that acetylated α-MSH exists only in the intermediate lobe of pituitary. *Biochem. Biophys. Res. Commun.* 106:910–19

19. O'Donohue, T. L., Handelman, G. E., Miller, R. L., Jacobowitz, D. M. 1982. N-acetylation regulates the behavioral activity of α-melanotropin in a multi-neurotransmitter neuron. *Science* 215:1125–27

20. Akil, H., Lin, H. L., Ueda, Y., Knobloch, M., Watson, S. J., Coy, D. 1983. Some of the α-NH$_2$-acetylated β-endorphin-like material in rat and monkey pituitary is acetylated α- and β-endorphin. *Life Sci.* 33(Suppl. 1):9–12

21. Dennis, M., Seidah, N. G., Chretien, M. 1983. Regional heterogeneity in the processing of pro-opiomelanocortin in rat brain. *Life Sci.* 33(Suppl. 1):49–52

22. Verhoef, J., Wiegant, V. M., De Wied, D. 1982. Regional distribution of α- and γ-type endorphins in rat brain. *Brain Res.* 231:454–60

23. Liotta, A. S., Advis, J. P., Krause, J. E., McKelvy, J. F., Krieger, D. T. 1984. Demonstration of in vivo synthesis of pro-opiomelanocortin, β-endorphin and α-melanotropin-like species in the adult rat brain. *J. Neurosci.* 4:956–65

24. Glembotski, C. C. 1981. Subcellular fractionation of proadrenocortin hormone/endorphin in rat intermediate pituitary. *J. Biol. Chem.* 256:7433–39

25. Kosterlitz, H. W., Paterson, S. J. 1985. Types of opioid receptors: relation to antinociception. *Philos. Trans. R. Soc. London Ser. B* 308:291–97

26. Oka, T., Negishi, K., Suda, M., Matsumiya, T., Inazu, T., Ueki, M. 1980. Rabbit vas deferens: a specific bioassay for opioid κ receptor agonists. *Eur. J. Pharmacol.* 73:235–36

27. Rezvani, A., Höllt, V., Way, E. L. 1983. κ-Receptor activities of the three opioid peptide families. *Life Sci.* 33(Suppl. 1):271–74

28. Höllt, V., Seizinger, B. R., Garzon, J., Loh, H. 1983. Receptor selectivities of the three opioid peptide families. In *Biochemical and Clinical Aspects of Neuropeptides: Synthesis, Processing and Gene Structure*, ed. G. Koch, D. Richter, pp. 59–72. New York: Academic. 250 pp.

29. Goldstein, A., James, I. F. 1984. Site-directed alkylation of multiple opioid receptors: Pharmacological selectivity. *Mol. Pharmacol.* 25:343–48

30. Law, P. Y., Loh, H. H., Li, C. H. 1979. Properties and localization of β-endorphin receptor in brain. *Proc. Natl. Acad. Sci. USA* 76:5455–59

31. Akil, H., Young, E., Watson, S. J., Coy, D. H. 1981. Opiate binding properties of naturally occurring N- and C-terminally modified β-endorphins. *Peptides* 2:289–92

32. Hammonds, R. G., Hammonds, A. S., Ling, N., Puett, D. 1982. β-Endorphin and deletion peptides. *J. Biol. Chem.* 257:2990–95

33a. Houghten, R. A., Johnson, N., Pasternak, G. W. 1984. [^{3}H]-β-Endorphin binding in rat brain. *J. Neurosci.* 10:2460–65

33b. McKnight, A. T., Corbett, A. D., Kosterlitz, H. W. 1983. Increase in potencies of opioid peptides after peptidase inhibition. *Eur. J. Pharmacol.* 86:393–402

34. Huidobro-Toro, J. P., Caturay, E. M., Ling, N., Lee, N. M., Loh, H. H., Way, E. L. 1982. Studies on the structural prerequisites for the activation of the β-endorphin receptor on the rat vas deferens. *J. Pharmacol. Exp. Ther.* 222:262–69

35. Höllt, V., Tulunay, F. C., Woo, S. K., Loh, H. H., Herz, A. 1982. Opioid peptides derived from proenkephalin A but not from proenkephalin B are substantial analgesics after administration into brain of mice. *Eur. J. Pharmacol.* 85:355–56

36. Hammonds, R. G., Nicolas, P., Li, C. H. 1984. β-Endorphin (1–27) is an antagonist of β-endorphin analgesia. *Proc. Natl. Acad. Sci. USA* 81:1389–90

37. Schweigerer, L., Bhakdi, S., Teschemacher, H. 1982. Specific non-opiate binding sites for human β-endorphin on the terminal complex of human complement. *Nature* 296:572–74

38. Hazum, E., Chang, K.-J., Cuatrecasas,

P. 1979. Specific non-opiate receptors for β-endorphins. *Science* 205:1033–35

39. Chang, K. J. 1984. Opioid peptides have actions on the immune system. *Trends Neurosci.* 7:234–35

40. Parish, D. C., Smyth, D. G., Norman-ton, J. R., Wolstencroft, J. H. 1983. Glycyl glutamine, an inhibitory neuropeptide derived from β-endorphin. *Nature* 306:267–70

41. Noda, M., Furutani, Y., Takahashi, H., Toyosato, M., Hirose, T., et al. 1982. Cloning and sequence analysis of cDNA for bovine adrenal preproenkephalin. *Nature* 295:202–6

42. Comb, M., Seeburg, P. H., Adelman, J., Eiden, L., Herbert, E. 1982. Primary structure of the human [Met]- and [Leu]-enkephalin precursor and its mRNA. *Nature* 295:663–66

43. Yoshikawa, K., Williams, C., Sabol, S. L. 1984. Rat brain preproenkephalin mRNA. *J. Biol. Chem.* 259:14301–8

44. Howells, R. D., Kilpatrick, D. L., Bhatt, R., Monohan, J. J., Poonian, M., Uden-friend, S. 1984. Molecular cloning and sequence determination of rat pre-proenkephalin cDNA: sensitive probe for studying transcriptional changes in rat tissues. *Proc. Natl. Acad. Sci. USA* 81:7651–55

45. Rosen, H., Douglas, J., Herbert, E. 1984. Isolation and characterization of the rat proenkephalin gene. *J. Biol. Chem.* 259:14309–13

46. Martens, G., Herbert, E. 1984. Polymorphism and absence of leu-enkephalin sequences in proenkephalin genes in *Xenopus laevis. Nature* 310:251–54

47. Patey, G., Liston, D., Rossier, J. 1984. Characterization of new enkephalin-containing peptides in the adrenal medulla by immunoblotting. *FEBS Lett.* 172: 303–8

48. Kilpatrick, D. L., Jones, B. N., Lewis, R. V., Stern, A. S., Kofima, J., et al. 1982. An 18,200 dalton adrenal protein that contains four [met]-enkephalin sequences. *Proc. Natl. Acad. Sci. USA* 79:3057–61

49. Jones, B. N. Shimely, J. E., Kilpatrick, D. L., Stern, A. S., Lewis, R. V., et al. 1982. Adrenal opioid proteins of 8,600 and 12,600 daltons: Intermediates in pro-enkephalin processing. *Proc. Natl. Acad. Sci. USA* 79:2096–2100

50. Stern, A. S., Jones, B. N., Shively, J. E., Stein, S., Udenfriend, S. 1980. Two adrenal opioid polypeptides: Proposed intermediates in the processing of pro-

enkephalin. *Proc. Natl. Acad. Sci. USA* 78:1962–66

51. Baird, A., Klepper, R., Ling, N. 1984. In vitro and in vivo evidence that the C-terminus of preproenkephalin-A circulates as an 8500-dalton molecule. *Proc. Soc. Exp. Biol. Med.* 175:304–8

52. Jones, B. N., Shively, J. E., Kilpatrick, D. L., Kojima, K., Udenfriend, S. 1982. Enkephalin biosynthetic pathway: a 5300 dalton adrenal polypeptide that terminates at its COOH end with the sequence [Met]enkephalin-arg-gly-leu-COOH. *Proc. Natl. Acad. Sci. USA* 79:1813–15

53. Jones, B. N., Stern, A. S., Lewis, R. V., Kimura, S., Stein, S., et al. 1978. Structure of two adrenal polypeptides containing multiple enkephalin sequences. *Arch. Biochem. Biophys.* 204:392–95

54. Seizinger, B. R., Liebisch, D. C., Gramsch, C., Herz, A., Weber, E., et al. 1985. Isolation and structure of a novel C-terminally amidated opioid peptide, amidorphin, from bovine adrenal medulla. *Nature* 313:57–59

55. Kilpatrick, D. L., Taniguchi, T., Jones, B. N., Stern, A. S., Shively, J. E., et al. 1981. A highly potent 3200 dalton adrenal opioid peptide that contains both a [Met]- and [Leu]enkephalin sequence. *Proc. Natl. Acad. Sci. USA* 78:3265–68

56. Mizuno, K., Minamino, N., Kangawa, K., Matsuo, H. 1980. A new family of endogenous "big" Met-enkephalins from bovine adrenal medulla: Purification and structure of Docosa-(BAM-22P) and Eicosapeptide (BAM-20P) with very potent opiate activity. *Biochem. Biophys. Res. Commun.* 97:1283–90

57. Evans, C. J., Erdelyi, E., Makk, G., Barchas, J. D. 1985. Identification of a novel proenkephalin derived opioid peptide in brain and adrenal. *Fed. Proc.* 44:422 (Abstr.)

58. Mizuno, K., Minamino, N., Kangawa, K., Matsuo, H. 1980. A new endogenous opioid peptide from bovine adrenal medulla: isolation and amino acid sequence of a dodecapeptide (BAM-12P). *Biochem. Biophys. Res. Commun.* 95: 1482–88

59. Weber, E., Esch, F. S., Böhlen, P., Paterson, S., Corbett, A. D., et al. 1983. Metorphamide: Isolation, structure and biologic activity of an amidated opioid octapeptide from bovine brain. *Proc. Natl. Acad. Sci. USA* 80:7362–66

60. Matsuo, H., Miyata, A., Mizuno, K. 1983. Novel C-terminally amidated opioid peptide in human phaeochromocytoma tumour. *Nature* 305:721–23

61. Bradbury, A. F., Finnie, M. D., Smyth, D. G. 1982. Mechanism of C-terminal amide formation by pituitary enzymes. *Nature* 298:686–88

62. Eipper, B. A., Mains, R. E., Glembotsky, C. C. 1983. Identification in pituitary tissue of a peptide α-amidation activity that acts on glycine-extended peptides and requires molecular oxygen, copper and ascorbic acid. *Proc. Natl. Acad. Sci. USA* 80:5144–48

63. Liston, D. R., Vanderhaeghen, J. J., Rossier, J. 1983. Presence in brain of synenkephalin, a proenkephalin-immuno-reactive protein which does not contain enkephalin. *Nature* 302:62–65

64. Rossier, J., Audigier, Y., Ling, N., Cros, J., Udenfriend, S. 1980. [Met]enkephalin-Arg^6-Phe^7, present in high amounts in brain of rat, cattle and man, is an opioid agonist. *Nature* 288:88–90

65. Giraud, A. S., Williams, R. G., Dockray, G. J. 1984. Evidence for different patterns of post-translational processing of pro-enkephalin in the bovine adrenal, colon and striatum indicated by radioimmunoassay using region-specific antisera to met-enk-arg^6-phe^7 and met-enk-arg^6-gly^7-leu^8. *Neurosci. Lett.* 46:223–28

66. Baird, A., Ling, N., Böhlen, P., Benoit, R., Klepper, R., Guillemin, R. 1982. Molecular forms of the putative enkephalin precursor BAM-12P in bovine adrenal, pituitary, and hypothalamus. *Proc. Natl. Acad. Sci. USA* 79:2023–25

67. Höllt, V., Haarmann, I., Grimm, C., Herz, A., Tulunay, F. C., Loh, H. H. 1982. Proenkephalin intermediates in bovine brain and adrenal medulla: Characterization of immunoreactive peptides related to BAM-22P and peptide F. *Life Sci.* 31:1883–86

68. Jingami, H., Nakanishi, S., Imura, H., Numa, S. 1984. Tissue distribution of messenger RNAs coding for opioid peptide precursors and related RNA. *Eur. J. Biochem.* 142:441–47

69. Pittius, C. W., Kley, N., Loeffler, J. P., Höllt, V. 1985. Quantitation of proenkephalin A messenger RNA in bovine brain, pituitary and adrenal medulla: Correlation between mRNA and peptide levels. *EMBO J.* 4:1257–60

70. Liston, D., Patey, G., Rossier, J., Verbanck, P., Vanderhaeghen, J. J. 1984. Processing of proenkephalin is tissue-specific. *Science* 225:734–37

71. Pittius, C. W., Seizinger, B. R., Pasi, A., Mehrain, P., Herz, A. 1984. Distribution and characterization of opioid peptides derived from proenkephalin A in human and rat central nervous system. *Brain Res.* 304:127–36

72. Beaumont, A., Metters, K. M., Rossier, J., Hughes, J. 1985. Identification of a proenkephalin precursor in striatal tissue. *J. Neurochem.* 44:934–40

73. Yang, H.-Y. T., Panula, P., Tang, J., Costa, E. 1983. Characterization and location of met^5-enkephalin-arg^6-phe^7 stored in various rat brain regions. *J. Neurochem.* 40:969–76

74. Lindberg, I., Yang, H.-Y. T. 1984. Distribution of met^5-enkephalin-arg^6-gly^7-leu^8-immunoreactive peptides in rat brain: Presence of multiple molecular forms. *Brain Res.* 299:73–78

75. Watson, S. J., Akil, H., Khachaturian, H., Young, E., Lewis, M. E. 1984. Opioid Systems: anatomical, physiological and clinical perspectives. In *Opioids Past Present and Future*, ed. J. Hughes, H. O. J. Collier, M. J. Rance, M. B. Tyers, pp. 145–78. London/Philadelphia: Taylor & Francis. 226 pp.

76. Giraud, A. S., Castanas, E., Patey, G., Oliver, C., Rossier J. 1983. Regional distribution of methionine-enkephalin-arg^6-phe^7 in the rat brain: Comparative study with the distribution of other opioid peptides. *J. Neurochem.* 41:154–60

77. Zamir, N., Palkovits, M., Weber, E., Mezey, E., Brownstein, M. J. 1984. A dynorphinergic pathway of leu-enkephalin production in rat substantia nigra. *Nature* 307:643–45

78. Miyata, A., Mizuno, K., Minamino, N., Matsuo, H. 1984. Regional distribution of adrenorphin in rat brain: comparative study with PH-8P. *Biochem. Biophys. Res. Commun.* 120:1030–36

79. Sonders, M., Barchas, J. D., Weber, E. 1984. Regional distribution of metorphamide in rat and guinea pig brain. *Biochem. Biophys. Res. Commun.* 122:892–98

80. Garzon, J., Jen, M. F., Sanchez-Blazquez, P., Höllt, V., Lee, N. M., Loh, H. H. 1983. Endogenous opioid peptides: comparative evaluation of their receptor affinities in the mouse brain. *Life Sci.* 33(Suppl. 1):291–94

81. Quirion, R., Weiss, A. S. 1983. Peptide E and other proenkephalin-derived peptides are potent κ-opiate receptor agonists. *Peptides* 4:445–49

82. Höllt, V., Sanchez-Blazquez, P., Garzon, J. 1985. Multiple opioid ligands and receptors in the control of nociception. *Philos. Trans. R. Soc. London Serv. B* 308:299–310

83. Wüster, M., Rubini, P., Schulz, R. 1981. The preference of putative pro-

enkephalins for different types of opiate receptors. *Life Sci.* 29:1219–27

84. Schulz, R., Wüster, M., Herz, A. 1982. Endogenous ligands for κ-opiate receptors. *Peptides* 3:973–76

85. Sanchez-Blazquez, P., Garzon, J., Lee, N. M., Höllt, V. 1984. Opiate activity of peptides derived from the three opioid peptide families on the rat vas deferens. *Neuropeptides* 5:181–84

86. Kakidani, H., Furutani, Y., Takahashi, H., Noda, M., Morimoto, Y., et al. 1982. Cloning and sequence analysis of cDNA for porcine β-neo-endorphin/dynorphin precursor. *Nature* 298:245–49

87. Minamino, N., Kangawa, K., Chino, N., Sakakibara, S., Matsuo, H. 1981. β-Neo-endorphin, a new hypothalamic "big" leu-enkephalin of porcine origin: Its purification and the complete amino acid sequence. *Biochem. Biophys. Res. Commun.* 99:864–70

88. Goldstein, A., Fischli, W., Lowney, L. I., Hunkapiller, M., Hood, L. 1981. Porcine pituitary dynorphin: Complete amino acid sequence of the biologically active heptadecapeptide. *Proc. Natl. Acad. Sci. USA* 78:7219–23

89. Tachibana, S., Araki, K., Ohya, S., Yoshida, S. 1982. Isolation and structure of dynorphin, an opioid peptide, from porcine duodenum. *Nature* 295:339–40

90. Nakao, K., Suda, M., Sakamoto, M., Yoshimasa, T., Morii, N., et al. 1983. Leumorphin is a novel endogenous opioid peptide derived from preproenkephalin B. *Biochem. Biophys. Res. Commun.* 117:695–701

91. Kangawa, K., Minamino, N., Chino, N., Sakakibara, S., Matsuo, H. 1981. The complete amino acid sequence of α-neoendorphin. *Biochem. Biophys. Res. Commun.* 98:871–88

92. Fischli, W., Goldstein, A., Hunkapiller, M. W., Hood, L. E. 1982. Isolation and amino acid sequence analysis of a 4000 dalton dynorphin from porcine pituitary. *Proc. Natl. Acad. Sci. USA* 79:5435–37

93. Kilpatrick, D. L., Wahlstrom, A., Lahm, H. W., Blacher, R., Udenfriend, S. 1982. Rimorphin, a unique, naturally occurring (leu)enkephalin-containing peptide found in association with dynorphin and α-neo-endorphin. *Proc. Natl. Acad. Sci. USA* 79:6480–83

94. Minamino, N., Kangawa, K., Fukuda, A., Matsuo, H., Iagaraski, M. 1980. A new opioid octapeptide related to dynorphin from porcine hypothalamus. *Biochem. Biophys. Res. Commun.* 95:1475–81

95. Seizinger, B. R., Höllt, V., Herz, A. 1981. Evidence for the occurrence of the opioid octapeptide dynorphin-(1–8) in the neurointermediate pituitary of rats. *Biochem. Biophys. Res. Commun.* 102:197–205

96. Weber, E., Evans, C., Barchas, J. D. 1982. Predominance of the aminoterminal octapeptide fragment of dynorphin in rat brain regions. *Nature* 299:77–79

97. Cone, R. I., Weber, E., Barchas, J. D., Goldstein, A. 1983. Regional distribution of dynorphin and neoendorphin peptides in rat brain, spinal cord and pituitary. *J. Neurosci.* 3:2146–52

98. Seizinger, B. R., Grimm, C., Höllt, V., Herz, A. 1984. Evidence for a selective processing of proenkephalin B into different opioid peptide forms in particular regions of rat brain and pituitary. *J. Neurochem.* 42:447–57

99. Seizinger, B. R., Höllt, V., Herz, A. 1981. Immunoreactive dynorphin in the rat adenohypophysis consists exclusively of 6000 dalton species. *Biochem. Biophys. Res. Commun.* 103:256–63

100. Maysinger, D., Höllt, V., Seizinger, B. R., Mehrain, P., Pasi, A., Herz, A. 1982. Parallel distribution of immunoreactive α-neo-endorphin and dynorphin in rat and human tissue. *Neuropeptides* 2:211–15

101. Seizinger, B. R., Hollt, V., Herz, A. 1984. Proenkephalin B (prodynorphin)-derived peptides: Evidence for a differential processing in lobes of the pituitary. *Endocrinology* 115:662–71

102. Watson, S. J., Akil, H., Ghazarossian, V. E., Goldstein, A. 1981. Dynorphin immunocytochemical localization in brain and peripheral nervous system: preliminary studies. *Proc. Natl. Acad. Sci. USA* 78:1260–63

103. Martin, R., Voight, K. H. 1981. Enkephalins co-exist with oxytocin and vasopressin in nerve terminals of rat neurophypophysis. *Nature* 289:502–4

104. Seizinger, B. R., Höllt, V., Herz, A. 1982. Dynorphin-related opioid peptides in the neurointermediate pituitary of rats are not α-N-acetylated. *J. Neurochem.* 39:143–48

105. Zamir, N., Zamir, D., Eiden, L., Palkovits, M., Brownstein, M. J., et al. 1985. Methionine and leucine enkephalin in rat neurohypophysis: Different responses to osmotic stimuli and T_2 toxin. *Science* 228:606–8

106. Höllt, V., Haarmann, I., Seizinger, B. R., Herz, A. 1981. Levels of dynorphin-(1–13) immunoreactivity in rat neurointermediate pituitaries are concommitantly altered with those of leucine

enkephalin and vasopressin in response to various endocrine manipulations. *Neuroendorinology* 33:333–39

107. Seizinger, B. R., Höllt, V., Herz, A. 1981. Evidence for an opiate-inactive N-acetylated derivative of leucine-enkephalin in the rat neurointermediate pituitary. *Biochem. Biophys. Res. Commun.* 101:289–97

108. Zamir, N., Weber, E., Palkovits, M., Brownstein, M. 1984. Differential processing of prodynorphin and pro-enkephalin in specific regions of the rat brain. *Proc. Natl. Acad. Sci. USA* 81:6886–89

109. Gramsch, C., Höllt, V., Pasi, A., Mehrain, P., Herz, A. 1982. Immunoreactive dynorphin in human brain and pituitary. *Brain Res.* 233:65–74

110. Suda, M., Nakao, K., Sakamoto, M., Yoshimasa, T., Morii, N., et al. 1984. Leumorphin is a novel endogenous-opioid peptide in man. *Biochem. Biophys. Res. Commun.* 123:148–155

111. Dores, R. M., Lewis, M. E., Khachaturian, H., Watson, S., Akil, H. 1985. Analysis of opioid and non-opioid end products of pro-dynorphin in the substantia nigra of the rat. *Neuropeptides* 5:501–4

112. Weber, E., Evans, C. J., Chang, J.-K., Barchas, J. D. 1982. Brain distributions of α-neo-endorphin and β-neo-endorphin: Evidence for regional processing differences. *Biochem. Biophys. Res. Commun.* 108:81–88

113. Zamir, N., Palkovits, M., Brownstein, M. J. 1984. Distribution of immunoreactive β-neo-endorphin in discrete areas of the rat brain and pituitary gland: Comparison with α-neo-endorphin. *J. Neurosci.* 4:1248–52

114. Hersh, L. P., McKelvy, J. F. 1979. Enzymes involved in the degradation of thyrotropin releasing hormone (TRH) and luteinizing hormone releasing hormone (LH-RH) in bovine brain. *Brain Res.* 168:553–64

115. Zhu, Y. X., Höllt, V., Loh, H. 1983. Immunoreactive peptides related to dynorphin B (=rimorphin) in the rat brain. *Peptides* 4:871–74

116. Vincent, S., Hökfelt, T., Christensen, I., Terenius, L. 1982. Immunohistochemical evidence for a dynorphin immunore

active striato nigral pathway. *Eur. J. Pharmacol.* 85:251–52

117. Palkovits, M., Brownstein, M. J., Zamir, N. 1984. On the origin of dynorphin A and α-neo-endorphin in the substantia nigra. *Neuropeptides* 4:193–99

118. Guthrie, J., Basbaum, A. I. 1984. Co-localization of immunoreactive pro-enkephalin and prodynorphin products in medullary neurons of the rat. *Neuropeptides* 4:437–45

119. Unsworth, C. D., Hughes, J., Morley, J. S. 1982. O-sulphated leu-enkephalin in brain. *Nature* 295:519–22

120. Huidobro-Toro, J. P., Yoshimura, K., Lee, N. M., Loh, H. H., Way, E. L. 1981. Dynorphin interaction at the κ-opiate site. *Eur. J. Pharmacol.* 72:265–66

121. Chavkin, C., Goldstein, A. 1981. Specific receptor for the opioid peptide dynorphin: Structure-activity relationships *Proc. Natl. Acad. Sci. USA* 78:6543–47

122. Corbett, A. D., Paterson, S. J., McKnight, A. T., Magnan, J., Kosterlitz, H. W. 1982. Dynorphin (1–8) and dynorphin (1–9) are ligands for the κ-subtype of opiate receptor. *Nature* 299:79–81

123. James, I. F., Fischli, W., Goldstein, A. 1984. Opioid receptor selectivity of dynorphin gene products. *J. Pharmacol. Exp. Ther.* 228:88–93

124. Oka, T., Negishi, K., Kajiwara, M., Watanabe, Y., Ishizuka, Y., Matsumiya, T. 1982. The choice of opiate receptor subtype by neoendorphins. *Eur. J. Pharmacol.* 79:301–5

125. Suda, M., Nakao, K., Yoshimasa, I., Ikeda, Y., Sakamoto, M., et al. 1983. A novel opioid peptide, leumorphin, acts as an agonist at the κ opiate receptors. *Life Sci.* 32:2769–75

126. Herman, B. H., Leslie, F., Goldstein, A. 1980. Behavioral effects and in vivo degradation of intraventricularly administered dynorphin-(1–13) and D-Ala²-dynorphin-(1–11) in rats. *Life Sci.* 27:883–92

127. Oka, K., Kantrowitz, J. D., Spector, S. 1984. Isolation of morphine from toad skin. *Proc. Natl. Acad. Sci. USA* 82:1852–54

Ann. Rev. Pharmacol. Toxicol. 1986. 26:79–99

DRUG OTOTOXICITY

Leonard P. Rybak

Departments of Surgery (Otolaryngololgy) and Pharmacology, Southern Illinois University, School of Medicine, Springfield, Illinois 62708

INTRODUCTION

Ototoxicity may be defined as the tendency of certain therapeutic agents and other chemical substances to cause functional impairment and cellular degeneration of the tissues of the inner ear, and especially of the end organs and neurons of the cochlear and vestibular divisions of the VIIIth cranial nerve (1). This is in contrast to neurotoxic drugs that may affect hearing or equilibrium by acting primarily on the brain-stem nuclei and central auditory or vestibular connections. Drug-induced hearing loss is one of several potential causes of iatrogenic deafness. The dangers of ototoxic agents such as quinine, arsenic, alcohol, aniline, and oil of chenopodium have long been recognized (2). Ototoxic agents in current clinical use include the aminoglycoside antibiotics, loop diuretics, nonsteroidal anti-inflammatory agents, chemotherapeutic agents and a variety of miscellaneous drugs. This review is limited to therapeutic agents most likely to cause hearing loss in humans.

ANATOMY AND PHYSIOLOGY OF THE AUDITORY PERIPHERY

The temporal bone is one of the complex bones of the cranial base. It contains the external auditory canal, tympanic membrane, middle and inner ear, vestibular apparatus, and the cochleovestibular and facial nerves. The inner ear or cochlea is a hollow, spirally wound tube, resembling a snail shell, which houses the auditory end organ. The cochlea is filled with fluids of distinct composition, endolymph and perilymph. The endolymph is contained within the central compartment or scala media, which also contains the basilar membrane and the organ of Corti, where the sensory cells (inner and outer hair cells) are suspended by supporting cells. The organ of Corti includes one row of inner hair cells and

79

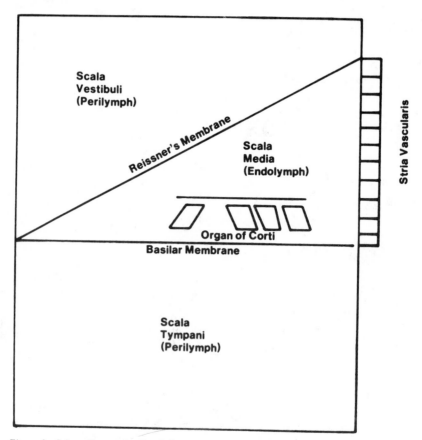

Figure 1   Schematic cross-sectional diagram of the cochlea.

three rows of outer hair cells; the supporting cells; the tunnel of Corti [a triangular space between the inner and outer hair cells (Figure 1)]; both efferent and afferent nerve endings; and the basilar and tectorial membranes. The primary auditory afferent dendrites convey impulses from the hair cell–eighth nerve synapse to the cell body in the medial wall—the spiral ganglion. The axons of the spiral ganglion leave the temporal bone via the internal auditory canal and travel intracranially to synapse in higher auditory centers in the brain stem. Space does not permit a complete description of current concepts of the physiology of hearing. The reader is referred to several recent publications for review (3–6).

Since its discovery in 1950, the resting endocochlear direct current (dc) potential (EP) has been studied by a number of investigators. The EP appears to consist of two components: a positive portion thought to be produced by an electrogenic sodium potassium pump, which can be inhibited by anoxia or ouabain; and a negative component unmasked by inhibitors such as anoxia or loop diuretics. The negative component is thought to result from potassium diffusion or a leakage of current from the cells of the organ of Corti (4). Fluid in the central compartment of the cochlea, endolymph, is very high in potassium but low in sodium content. On the other hand, perilymph (in the scala vestibuli and the scala tympani) is high in sodium and low in potassium. Perilymph is similar to the fluid that bathes the lateral surface of the receptor cells in the organ of Corti—the so-called cortilymph. Compartmental analysis strongly suggests that perilymph is an ultrafiltrate of plasma and that perilymph is the precursor of endolymph (7, 8).

The most thoroughly investigated sound-dependent potential is the cochlear microphonic (CM) potential. It can be recorded from various locations in and near the inner ear or even from the scalp. An electrode connecting the round window of an experimental animal to a suitable amplifier and loudspeaker will reproduce the voice of an individual who speaks into the ear of the animal. This potential most likely originates from the hair cells, and the recordings obtained from the round window reflect the activity of mainly the outer hair cells in the base of the cochlea. The summating potentials (SP) are dc potentials that can be most effectively recorded from the scala media inside the cochlea in response to a continuous tone. SP may consist of several components originating from different sources, such as the outer hair cells ($+SP$) and inner hair cells ($-SP$) (4).

The compound action potential (CAP or AP) is a sound-dependent potential reflecting excitation and synchronization of populations of auditory nerve fibers (3). The response is most prominent following transient stimuli such as clicks and the potential is composed of two negative peaks, named N_1 and N_2. The magnitude of the N_1 response is a function of both the stimulus intensity and the number of fibers firing synchronously. The N_1 amplitude and latency are thought to reflect the integrity of the cochlea and eighth nerve, whereas the N_2 component may originate from more central structures.

The auditory brain-stem response consists of a series of waves that can be recorded from the scalp. They may represent sequential activation of the auditory neuraxis in the brain stem. Single auditory nerve fibers can be studied with a microelectrode inserted into the nerve by an intracranial approach. These cells can be characterized by their spontaneous rate and pattern of firing and by the rate and pattern of firing with stimuli of known frequency and intensity. Both the receptor cells of the cochlea (inner hair cells) and the single neurons of the spiral ganglia and eighth nerve exhibit exquisite frequency selectivity, as demonstrated by the tuning curve. The tuning curve is a plot of neuron firing above threshold at various frequencies. The neural response at various frequencies is not the same, as one can see readily from the plot of the tuning curve. A turning curve consists of a low-frequency tail portion that indicates hearing response only to high-intensity sounds, and an extremely sharply tuned "tip" region. The latter is characterized by an extremely sudden transition from the high-threshold tail region to a narrow region where the nerves or receptor cells respond to their characteristic frequency. In this area, the neuron or receptor cell increases its firing rate abruptly at tones of low intensity near the characteristic frequency. At frequencies above the characteristic frequency, there is again an abrupt and rapid rise in the threshold of the neuron (3, 4). Auditory neurons also exhibit activity in the absence of sound (spontaneous activity) (4).

Spontaneous otoacoustic emissions and stimulated emissions (cochlear echoes) are interesting phenomena demonstrating that the reverse transmission of acoustic energy is in the cochlear partition. These may be generated by the so-called cochlear amplifier that may reside in the outer hair cells (5, 6).

Transduction of sound energy into electrical impulses transmitted to the brain is a complex process about which much is unknown. The shearing of the stereocilia of the hair cells relative to the tectorial membrane appears to elicit a receptor potential in the inner and outer hair cells. This presumably triggers the release of the excitatory afferent neurotransmitter that has not yet been fully characterized. Polyphosphoinositides, which appear to play a significant role in transduction in a variety of mammalian tissue cells (9), have been implicated in cochlear transduction recently (10) and may play a role in the ototoxicity of aminoglycosides.

OTOTOXIC ANTIBIOTICS

Aminoglycosides

The aminoglycoside antibiotics are a class of broad-spectrum antibiotics active against gram-positive and gram-negative organisms as well as mycobacteria. A large number of aminoglycoside antibiotics are in clinical use. Detailed descriptions of the chemistry and structure-activity relationships of aminoglycosides are available. The vestibulotoxic compounds such as streptomycin, gentamicin, and tobramycin tend to selectively destroy type I hair cells of the crista ampullaris (1). The cochleotoxic agents such as neomycin, kanamycin, amikacin, sisomycin, and lividomycin appear to cause a pattern of injury to the cochlea in experimental animals given ototoxic doses of these drugs similar to the injury pattern seen in human temporal bone studies (11).

Some comparative studies have been performed to rank aminoglycosides in order of their probability of auditory toxicity. Animal (12, 13) and clinical (14) studies suggest that netilmicin and dibekacin (15) may be considerably less ototoxic than other aminoglycosides currently in widespread use such as gentamicin, tobramycin, kanamycin, and amikacin. Comparisons of ototoxicity with antibacterial activity have shown that netilmicin has the highest therapeutic index. Tobramycin has been ranked next, followed by gentamicin C. Amikacin is said to have a therapeutic ratio less than 10% of netilmicin and 50% of that of tobramycin (16). Clinical studies show that the average incidence of cochlear toxicity was 13.9% for amikacin, 8.3% for gentamicin, 6.1% for tobramycin, and 2.4% for netilmicin (17).

MORPHOLOGIC CHANGES   The earliest cochlear lesions produced by amino-glycoside antibiotics in experimental animals and humans appear in the outer hair cells of the basal turn. The initial ultrastructural findings are fusion of stereocilia to form giant hairs (18). As the dosage and duration of administration of antibiotic is increased, the lesion extends apically, then to the inner hair cells (1, 19). The pattern of inner hair cell destruction varies, and may parallel or occur in the gradient opposite to that of the outer hair cells. This raises questions about the selectivity of aminoglycosides for the destruction of outer hair cells (20). Delayed degeneration of the afferent nerve endings after cessation of treatment can follow destruction of the inner hair cells (21). Damage to other cochlear structures lining the cochlear duct (including the spiral ligament, stria vascularis, vestibular membrane, spiral prominence, and pericapillary tissues of the outer sulcus) was described in animals treated with kanamycin (1). Hair cell damage and auditory dysfunction may be asymmetrical (11, 22).

PHARMACOKINETIC STUDIES   Because of the ease of obtaining pure samples, most studies of aminoglycoside pharmacokinetics have looked at the relationship of drug concentration in perilymph over time compared to simultaneous plasma concentration. It has been postulated that the slower rate of elimination of aminoglycosides from perilymph compared to plasma may be related to the aminoglycosides' cochleovestibular toxicity. Neomycin has the slowest elimination from the perilymph and also was the most ototoxic (23). Although earlier studies had suggested accumulation of aminoglycoside antibiotics in the perilymph of animals given large parenteral doses of aminoglycoside, gentamicin does not appear to accumulate in the perilymphatic compartment. Following prolonged infusion in animals, the perilymph-to-plasma ratios remained within a narrow range regardless of the plasma levels (24). This relatively constant ratio did not support the hypothesis of unlimited accumulation of aminoglycoside antibiotics in inner ear fluids, nor did it confirm the hypothesis of a "threshold" for entry into perilymph suggested by previous investigators (25). A review of the literature on the pharmacokinetics of aminoglycoside antibiotics in animals concluded that the vast majority of studies looked at concentrations of drugs in perilymph rather than endolymph, that their peak concentration in perilymph is reached later than the plasma peak, and that the half-lives of aminoglycoside in perilymph varied from 8 to 15 hours, which was much longer than the corresponding half-life in plasma (26).

Because of technical difficulties in obtaining pure endolymph, very few studies have been conducted on this fluid. Gentamicin enters this deep compartment extremely slowly. Following a constant infusion of gentamicin, the mean concentration of gentamicin achieved in endolymph by the end of the second day equaled that observed in a previous study after six days. This suggests that surrounding tissues have a large capacity to bind aminoglycosides or that a transport mechanism of the drug toward the endolymph became saturated (27).

PHYSIOLOGIC EFFECTS   Physiologic consequences of such damage include the shift and attenuation of the input-output (sound intensity versus amplitude of response) curves for the AP and CM. The resulting shifts in CM and N_1 thresholds have been observed, as well as elevation of threshold of single auditory fibers in the high-frequency range. Tuning curve tips appear to be blunted with hypersensitivity of the tails (21, 28) and a decreased rate of spontaneous activity (29).

POSSIBLE MECHANISMS OF OTOTOXICITY   Hypotheses have been proposed attempting to relate renal tubular transport of aminoglycosides to their nephrotoxic and ototoxic mechanisms. Aminoglycoside ototoxicity was originally thought to be caused by inhibition of protein synthesis in the organ of Corti (1). Although aminoglycosides can inhibit protein synthesis in mammalian liver mitochondria (30), this does not appear to be the mechanism for specific cellular destruction of the outer hair cells (31). It has been proposed that the aminoglycosides may inhibit carbohydrate uptake and/or metabolism and energy utilization in the outer hair cell. Kanamycin suppresses respiratory enzyme activity in the outer hair cell, with more pronounced effects on the basal turn (32). Biochemical studies suggest a selective inhibition of the Embden-Meyerhof pathway in the organ of Corti and in the kidney without alteration of the hexose monophosphate shunt (33). Neither pathway was found to be altered in the stria vascularis (33). This interference with carbohydrate metabolism may lead to inhibition of ATPase in the organ of Corti. There are reportedly fewer glycogen granules in normal outer hair cells of the basal turn of the cochlea, which is the area most susceptible to aminoglycoside damage, and these granules are depleted from the outer hair cells of animals treated with aminoglycosides (34). It has also been postulated that aminoglycosides may decrease the transport of glucose into the cochlea. Alloxan-diabetic rats were reportedly protected from kanamycin ototoxicity in proportion to the extent of hyperglycemia (35). The above concepts have been refuted by recent studies showing that gentamicin ototoxicity is not related to an effect on glucose uptake or utilization (36). On the other hand, diabetic rats were found to be protected from gentamicin-induced acute renal failure (37).

Phospholipids have been suggested as "receptors" for aminoglycoside antibiotic toxicity in both the membranes of the kidney and the inner ear (38). A series of experiments have led to the theory that ototoxicity caused by aminoglycoside antibiotics is related to phospholipid metabolism. Fractions of inner ear and kidney tissues each demonstrated high affinity for neomycin immobilized on glass beads (39). The components with this tendency to bind neomycin were two phospholipid fractions; namely, phosphatidylinositol phosphate and phosphatidylinositol diphosphate (39). Guinea pigs chronically treated with neomycin were found to have reduced labeling of phosphatidylinositol diphosphate in inner ear tissues when they were injected with radioactive phosphorus as a tracer to measure synthesis of these lipids (40). There appears to be a good correlation between effects of aminoglycoside drugs on cochlear microphonics and their interaction with polyphosphoinositide films in vitro (38, 41).

Some interesting recent studies of the lateral line organ of *Xenopus laevis* may explain all the biochemical findings discussed above and the clinical observations that, occasionally, the aminoglycoside antibiotics have reversible ototoxicity. Low concentrations of aminoglycoside antibiotics appear to have dual actions on sensory hair cells in the lateral line organ. The aminoglycosides appear to increase the spontaneous afferent nerve activity by altering the hair cell membrane. In addition, they markedly impair the mechano-electrical transduction process, perhaps by interfering with the motility of the sensory hairs (42). The gentamicin-induced loss of CM is reversed in the guinea pig with local perfusion of calcium (43). This also supports a two-step hypothesis for aminoglycoside ototoxicity: an initial membrane effect on phospholipids, antagonized by calcium; and a second step that is noncompetitive and leads to destruction of the hair cell. This hypothesis was further confirmed by double labeling experiments in which gentamicin was locally perfused into the ear and lipids were labeled by radioactive phosphate and radioactive glycerol. Uptake of radioactive phosphate into phospholipids was reduced in the organ of Corti, but labeled glycerol uptake into lipids was not altered in the ear treated with gentamicin. At the time that these effects were taking place, the CM were reduced but the ultrastructure of cochlear tissues was not altered. This may represent the reversible step that can be antagonized by calcium (43).

The aminoglycoside receptor in the cochlea may be a membrane-bound enzyme. Specific inhibition of proximal-tubule brush-border membrane phosphatidyl-specific phospholipase C in the kidney has been demonstrated (44). The binding of aminoglycosides to anionic phospholipids in the proximal-tubule cell membrane appears to be due to a charge interaction. This may allow sufficient aminoglycoside to enter the cell to allow an interaction with the above enzyme. By analogy, the receptor for aminoglycosides in the cochlea may be intracellular. Whether a similar enzyme exists in the cochlea needs to be explored.

Another explanation for the two-step hypothesis was briefly alluded to earlier. The initial step may be a charge interaction between the aminoglycoside and anionic phospholipids in the membrane of cells damaged by aminoglycosides. This interaction can be reversed by calcium. The second step may involve the inhibition of an important enzyme, such as phosphatidylinositol-specific phospholipase C, since the latter interaction is not altered by calcium in studies of the renal enzyme.

An alternative hypothesis was recently proposed to explain aminoglycoside ototoxicity, based on the finding that a radioprotectant compound WR 2721 [(3-aminopropylamino) ethyl phosphorothioate], which is thought to scavenge free radicals, protected guinea pigs against kanamycin ototoxicity as measured by behavioral and electrophysiological techniques (45). The onset of ototoxicity was delayed, its severity diminished, and its extent attenuated by pretreatment of animals with the radioprotectant compound. It was postulated that the mechanism of protection is mediated by scavenging of certain reactive species that may be generated by kanamycin in cochlear tissue (45). Another potential target for aminoglycoside ototoxicity is the protein melanin, suggested by the finding that albinos may be less vulnerable to aminoglycoside ototoxicity than are pigmented animals (46). Concomitant treatment of rats with fosfomycin appears to reduce both renal and inner ear damage caused by otherwise nephrotoxic and ototoxic doses of dibekacin (47). The mechanisms of this protective effect are unclear, but a chemical reaction between fosfomycin and dibekacin should be excluded.

Azthreonam is a new, completely synthetic monocyclic beta-lactam antibiotic that is active against aerobic gram-negative organisms and highly resistant to beta-lactamases (48). It is anticipated that azthreonam may replace aminoglycoside therapy in some patients. Preliminary studies show no evidence of ototoxicity in experimental animals (49).

Vancomycin

Vancomycin is a high-molecular-weight glycopeptide antibiotic that is structurally distinct from other currently used antibiotics. Recent advances in analytical techniques have permitted the complete elucidation of the structure of this unique antibiotic (50). Vancomycin and ristocetin are structurally related antibiotics that are both nephrotoxic and ototoxic and cause systemic reactions as well (51). The recent emergence of infections with methicillin-resistant strains of *Staphylococcus aureus* has resulted in a renewed interest in the use of vancomycin for such infections (52). Vancomycin is also used for enterococcal endocarditis in penicillin-sensitive individuals and is used orally for *Clostridium difficile* pseudomembranous colitis. Since some methicillin-resistant staphylococcal infections have failed to respond to vancomycin, rifampin or aminoglycosides may be added to the treatment regimen. An increased incidence of nephrotoxicity in humans and animals receiving vancomycin and aminoglycosides has been observed (53), suggesting the possibility of increased ototoxicity as well. Hearing loss in humans has been reported at blood levels exceeding 45 mg/liter (54) but has also been reported at blood levels of 30 mg/liter or lower (55, 56). Initial symptoms of cochlear damage may include tinnitus or deafness. Reversible tinnitus has been correlated to "peak" serum levels of 40–50 mg/liter (57). The risk of vancomycin ototoxicity appears to be greater in persons older than 65 years of age, in patients receiving other potentially ototoxic drugs, and in patients with reduced kidney function. A recent study has documented the reduced total systemic and renal clearances of vancomycin in the elderly even with normal renal function (58). Vancomycin pharmacokinetics have been more completely characterized with the modern techniques of high-pressure liquid chromatography (59) and radioimmunoassay (58, 60). Multicompartmental models have been proposed (58, 61). It is therefore important to know from which phase of the pharmacokinetic curve one is sampling before any meaningful statements can be made relating blood levels and ototoxicity (61). Also, infusion rate can drastically alter "peak" concentrations (61). Vancomycin has a significantly longer half-life and volume of distribution in premature than in full-term infants. For this reason, careful monitoring of vancomycin blood levels in premature infants has been strongly recommended (60). Significant oral absorption does not usually occur after oral administration of vancomycin (62).

Erythromycin

Initial animal testing for possible adverse effects of erythromycin on the inner ear consisted of vestibular screening. It was concluded that no eighth nerve cranial damage could be attributed to erythromycin (63). However, the importance of erythromycin in treating pneumonias caused by *Legionella pneumophila* and related pathogens has probably resulted in the increased utilization of intravenous erythromycin. At least 32 cases of bilateral, sensorineural hearing loss, which is typically uniform across frequencies, have been reported in association with high doses of intravenously or even orally administered erythromycin (64). Patients most likely to experience hearing loss are elderly females with hepatic or renal failure or Legionnaire's disease who receive 2 g or more of erythromycin daily (65). Symptoms include decreased hearing, "blowing" tinnitus, and occasionally, vertigo. Although none of 30 elderly patients receiving large doses of erythromycin stearate had any change in hearing despite renal or hepatic failure (66), the half-life of erythromycin is prolonged in patients with renal failure, and the serum levels may be three to five times as high as one would predict in a patient with normal renal function (67). Ototoxic blood levels were measured in two patients; one patient's level ranged from 63 to 78 mg/liter (68) and the other had a serum level of 100 mg/liter (67). Auditory changes observed after erythromycin have been shown to be reversible following cessation of therapy. Animal experiments are needed to define more clearly the mechanisms of erythromycin ototoxicity.

Chloramphenicol

Ototoxicity experiences related to chloramphenicol have been restricted to patients receiving extremely high doses (69). Animal studies have shown damage to the cochlea following topical application of chloramphenicol resulting in loss of succinic dehydrogenase activity in outer hair cells and nerve endings (70). A recent study has shown that combined otitis media, noise exposure, and chloramphenicol produced enhanced cochlear damage in rats (71). On the other hand, ethacrynic acid was found not to potentiate the ototoxicity of chloramphenicol, in contrast to the marked potentiation of kanamycin ototoxicity by ethacrynic acid (72).

LOOP DIURETICS

The "loop" or high-ceiling diuretics include a series of compounds that are very potent inhibitors of ion reabsorption in the loop of Henle. These compounds include ethacrynic acid, furosemide, bumetanide, piretanide, azosemide, ozolinone, and indacrinone (73). The last two of these compounds have optical isomers. The (−) isomer of ozolinone has diuretic activity (74) and is ototoxic (75); (−) indacrinone is more potent than its (+) isomer (76). Each of the active loop diuretics has been found to affect cochlear function adversely in experimental animals and most of them have been shown to be ototoxic in humans (usually reversible). The exact incidence of hearing loss associated with loop diuretics is unknown. Two patients of a series of 283 (0.7%) developed deafness while taking ethacrynic acid (77). Significant audiometric changes were found in 1.1% of patients treated with bumetanide, whereas 6.4% of patients receiving furosemide were found to have hearing loss (78). More detailed reviews of clinical ototoxicity of furosemide are discussed in recent publications (79, 80).

Morphological Studies

Morphological studies of loop diuretics ototoxicity have been reviewed in detail (1, 81, 82). Morphologic changes in the cochlea associated with loop diuretics occur in the stria vascularis, while sensory structures appear to be little affected except by large doses of ethacrynic acid (81), which appears to be more cytotoxic to outer hair cells of the basal turn of the cochlea. Animals (82) and humans (83) receiving ototoxic doses of loop diuretics were found to have edema, both between and within cells of the stria vascularis and most markedly in the basal turn. No changes were observed in the cochlear nerve fibers or ganglion cells.

Functional Changes

The EP is reduced in a dose-dependent manner by ethacrynic acid (19, 81), furosemide (84–86), bumetanide (87), and piretanide (88). Such changes are reversible, but the rate of recovery seems to be slowest for ethacrynic acid (89). The recovery of EP following furosemide injection correlates well with restoration of normal strial ultrastructure (90), in contrast with ethacrynic acid–treated animals (91). Permanent anoxia preceded by ethacrynic acid injection results in EP values that never reach the values usually obtained with anoxia alone (92). This may be caused by reduced permeability of the cochlear partition to potassium ions (93). CM is reduced after loop diuretics, especially ethacrynic acid, which has a greater effect on the outer hair cells (81). The reduction of the EP by loop diuretics appears to cause a reduction in the spontaneous firing rate of the eighth nerve, perhaps because of a reduction in the continuous release of neurotransmitter (94). Sound-evoked responses of the cochlea are also reduced, including AP (19, 75), evoked activity of single auditory nerve fibers (94, 95), auditory brain-stem response (96), and behavioral responses to sound (97). Furosemide appears to reduce the frequency selectivity of the cochlea, since significant blunting of the sharply tuned tip segment of the tuning curve can take place (94, 95). Loop diuretics abolish cochlear echoes (98). Impedance changes in the cochlear membranes following ethacrynic acid injection have been demonstrated (99) as well as an elevation of the effective resistance to the cochlear partition after furosemide injection (89). Piretanide may be less ototoxic than bumetanide or furosemide, but there may be species variations (75, 88).

Biochemical Effects

The concentration of potassium in endolymph is significantly reduced by ototoxic doses of loop diuretics (92, 100), with a reduction of chloride and elevation of sodium concentration (101).

Initially it was thought that ethacrynic acid inhibited Na,K-ATPase in the stria vascularis, but subsequent experiments have failed to confirm this (84). Adenylate cyclase is present in high concentrations in the stria vascularis and was thought to be a target for loop diuretics (84), but recently it has been shown that this cochlear enzyme is not altered by these agents (102, 103). Loop diuretics appear to block the potassium chloride cotransport system that moves these ions out of the stria vascularis into the endolymph (82, 104).

There have been extensive studies of ethacrynic acid metabolism in relation to ototoxicity. The drug itself (105) or its cysteine metabolite (106) may be the ototoxic species. A direct correlation has been found between the rate at which thiol conjugates of ethacrynic acid liberate free ethacrynic acid in vitro and their ototoxic potential in guinea pigs (107). Moreover, the diuretic efficacy of a series of thiol adducts of ethacrynic acid parallels their ototoxic potential (107). The ototoxic effects of furosemide may be mediated by a metabolite in premature infants (108). However, it is unclear whether this metabolite, CSA (2-amino-4-chloro-5-sulfamoyl anthranilic acid) is an artifact of the analytical procedure (109). The glucuronide metabolite has been found in both serum and perilymph of chinchillas receiving ototoxic doses of furosemide (86), but it is not known whether this metabolite is ototoxic. The different time course of appearance and disappearance of furosemide glucuronide in serum and perilymph (86) suggests the possibility that the cochlea is a drug-metabolizing organ.

The transfer of loop diuretics from the blood to the kidney lumen depends primarily on an active organic acid transport system in the proximal tubule (110). Similar anion carriers have been demonstrated in other tissues and a similar transport system may exist in the cochlea (111). Ethacrynic acid alters glutathione metabolism in the kidney, but the other loop diuretics do not (112) and it is not known whether glutathione is present in the inner ear.

Interactions

Various studies have demonstrated ototoxic potentiation between loop diuretics and aminoglycosides (19, 22).

The dose-ototoxic response curves for loop diuretics combined with a single dose of kanamycin were found to be parallel, but the relative ototoxic potential of bumetanide was less (113). Noise exposure has been shown to potentiate the damage to the inner ear caused by the aminoglycoside antibiotics, but not that caused by loop diuretics (114).

NONSTEROIDAL ANTI-INFLAMMATORY AND ANTIMALARIAL DRUGS

A hearing loss of 20–40 dB occurs across the audible frequency range in normal-hearing subjects and is preceded or accompanied by tinnitus with blood levels of salicylate in excess of 200–450 mg/liter (115). Auditory symptoms usually disappear within 24–72 hours after cessation of salicylates. Aspirin ototoxicity has been reported to occur in 11 per 1000 patients (77), but a much higher incidence has been reported after use of long-acting aspirin (116). Aspirin in large doses produces temporary changes in psychophysical measures of auditory function in normal human subjects, producing findings that mimicked those seen in subjects with permanent sensorineural deafness (117). Salicylates reach a maximum value in perilymph of 25–33% of the corresponding blood level about two hours after intraperitoneal injection (118, 119). Tritium-labelled salicylate was detected very quickly in the blood vessels of the stria vascularis and spiral ligament (120). Within an hour, the label was found around the outer hair cells and near the spiral ganglion cells, without accumulation in any specific structures (120). Direct perfusion of sodium salicylate reduces AP amplitude (121). Salicylates may inhibit cochlear transaminase and dehydrogenase systems (119) and/or acetylcholinesterase in efferent endings (120). ATP levels of Reissner's membrane of salicylate-intoxicated animals were significantly reduced (122). The ATP and phosphocreatine content of the cochlear nerve and stria vascularis were increased (122). Since nonsteroidal anti-inflammatory drugs are known to inhibit prostaglandin synthesis, depletion of these fatty acids may cause ototoxicity (19). Aspirin has been found to abolish spontaneous otoacoustic emissions in a reversible manner (123). The thresholds of single auditory nerve fibers were rapidly elevated following injection of large doses of sodium salicylate in cats. Fibers became less sharply tuned and there was an increase in spontaneous rate of neuron firing (124).

Because salicylates selectively reduced the AP in experimental animals (125), ultrastructural studies were carried out. No pathological changes of the auditory nerve were seen (126). Other ultrastructural studies of salicylate-intoxicated animals revealed normal cochlear structures (127). Humans with audiometrically documented salicylate-induced hearing loss were found in temporal bone studies to have no significant cellular alterations except those attributed to the age of the patient (128, 129). Salicylates may have a temporary metabolic effect that alters sensory receptor cells or neurons directly, or indirectly by decreased cochlear blood flow (1). Indomethacin-treated guinea pigs were found to have questionable distension of Reissner's membrane, but no ultrastructural abnormalities were detected (130). The auditory brain-stem response of guinea pigs chronically treated with ibuprofen was reported to be normal (131). Five patients were reported to suffer a hearing loss while receiving naproxen; only two recovered hearing after discontinuing the drug (132).

Abortifacient doses of quinine have resulted in deafness of the mother or of the infant when the pregnancy was not terminated (1). Animals given quinine in chronic doses of 50–100 mg/kg/day showed loss of hearing by behavioral testing (133). Histological study showed advanced degeneration of the cochlea, with the greatest injury in the base. Locally applied quinine resulted in reduced cochlear responses, and the outer hair cells and the stria vascularis were damaged (134). Transplacental ototoxicity resulting in deafness has been described in three children of a mother who had no toxic symptoms herself following chloroquine administration (135). Permanent and progressive ototoxicity in a teenager was reported (136). Ototoxicity may be reversed by cessation of chloroquine and the administration of corticosteroids (137). An autoradiographic study demonstrated accumulation of labelled chloroquine in melanin-containing tissues of the inner ear that persisted for nearly two weeks after injection; thus ototoxicity of chloroquine may be related to uptake by melanocytes in the stria vascularis (138).

Salicylates were found to exacerbate the temporary hearing loss induced by exposure to intense sound (139), but sulindac or diflunisal did not increase the sound-induced hearing loss in human subjects (140). Previous animal studies on the possible interactions of noise exposure and salicylates have produced conflicting results (114).

ANTINEOPLASTIC DRUGS

Cisplatinum is an inorganic platinum coordination complex with marked anti-neoplastic activity against solid tumors. The major organs affected by toxicity include kidney, bone marrow, gastrointestinal tract, and inner ear. The exact mechanism of cisplatinum-induced ototoxicity has not been defined, but it has been demonstrated that cisplatinum inhibits the activity of adenylate cyclase in cochlear tissues (141). There are morphologic similarities in the pattern of cochlear damage resulting from cisplatinum ototoxicity and due to aminogly-cosides. Animal studies have shown that the outer hair cells of the basal turn of the cochlea are damaged first, with eventual damage to more apical cells (142, 143). The first row of outer hair cells appears to suffer the greatest initial damage. Ultrastructural studies showed supporting cell damage, and irregular stereocilia of both inner and outer hair cells were observed (144). Marked degeneration of the stria vascularis has also been observed following cisplatinum injection (145). Recent studies of temporal bones from patients with cisplatinum-induced hearing loss have demonstrated large, fused stereocilia and damaged cuticular plate of the basal outer hair cells, with degeneration of spiral ganglion cells and cochlear neurons (146, 147).

It is difficult to define the exact incidence and severity of cisplatinum-induced auditory defects because of inconsistencies in previous studies and incomplete data from patients too ill to cooperate for hearing tests (148). The incidence of hearing loss following cisplatinum therapy has ranged from 9 to 91% (148). Symptoms that strongly suggest ototoxicity include otalgia, tinni-tus, and subjective deafness (149). Hearing loss is usually bilateral, but may be asymmetrical (150), and begins in the higher frequencies (6000 to 8000 Hz). Progression to lower frequencies (2000 and 4000 Hz) may occur with continued therapy (148). Some reversibility may be experienced but when the hearing loss is profound, it appears to be permanent. Higher frequency hearing loss may not be detected without audiometry. Speech understanding may be markedly re-duced (151). The critical cumulative ototoxic dose may be 3–4 mg/kg or 100 mg/m^2 (148). Ototoxicity can be more pronounced after bolus injection and may be minimized by using slow infusion and dividing the doses (152). Hearing loss prior to initiation of cisplatinum therapy may predispose to drug-induced hearing loss (148). Cochlear toxicity may be detected earlier with high-frequency audiometry than with conventional auditory testing (153). Children receiving high doses of cisplatinum (above 540 mg/m^2) have a high incidence of hearing loss (154) that appears to be accentuated by cranial irradiation (155). Animal studies have shown potentiation of cisplatinum-related loss of auditory function and damage to inner and outer hair cells by ethacrynic acid (156) or kanamycin (157).

Other antineoplastic agents have been reported to be ototoxic. Vinblastine destroys hair cells in the organ of Corti, without changing the cells or fibers of the spiral ganglion (158). Vincristine, on the other hand, was found to destroy not only the sensory cells but also the spiral ganglion cells and fibers (159).

Nitrogen mustard has also been reported to be ototoxic. Cats were found to have nearly total loss of hair cells and auditory function following injection of nitrogen mustard (160). The EP and CM were found to decrease rapidly after injection of nitrogen mustard, and then to recover gradually. However, a large ($-$) SP remained (161). The histological changes produced by nitrogen mustard resemble those produced by aminoglycosides.

ACKNOWLEDGMENTS

The preparation of this review was supported in part by grants from the Deafness Research Foundation and NIH Grants #R01-NS 22530 and #K07 NS 00705.

Literature Cited

1. Hawkins, J. E. Jr. 1976. Drug ototoxicity. In *Handbook of Sensory Physiology*, ed. W. D. Keidel, W. D. Neff, 5:707–48. New York: Springer

2. Stephens, S. D. 1982. Some historical aspects of ototoxicity. *Br. J. Audiol.* 16:76–80

3. Dallos, P. 1981. Cochlear physiology. *Ann. Rev. Psychol.* 32:153–90

4. Moller, A. R. 1983. *Auditory Physiology*, pp. 1–99. New York: Academic

5. McFadden, D., Wightman, F. L. 1983. Audition: some relations between normal and pathological hearing. *Ann. Rev. Psychol.* 34:95–128

6. Durrant, J. D., Lovrinic, J. H. 1984. *Bases of Hearing Science*. Baltimore: Williams & Wilkins. 276 pp. 2nd ed.

7. Sterkers, O., Ferrary, E., Amiel, C. 1984. Inter- and intracompartmental osmotic gradients within the rat cochlea. *Am. J. Physiol.* 247:F602–6.

8. Sterkers, O. 1984. La formation des li-

quides de l'oreille interne. *J. Fr. Oto-Rhino-Laryngol.* 33:239–50

9. Hirasawa, K., -G., Nishizuka, Y. 1985. Phosphatidylinositol turnover in receptor mechanism and signal transduction. *Ann. Rev. Pharmacol. Toxicol.* 25:147–70

10. Katsuki, Y., Horikoshi, T., Yanagisawa, K., Yoshioka, T. 1985. *Assoc. Res. Otolaryngol. Abstr.* 8:67 (Abstr)

11. Johnsson, L.-G., Hawkins, J. E. Jr., Kingsley, T. C., Black, F. O., Matz, G. J. 1981. Aminoglycoside-induced cochlear pathology in man. *Acta Oto-Laryngol.* 1981 (Suppl. 383):3–19

12. Parravicini, L., Forlani, A., Marzanatti, M., Arpini, A. 1983. Comparative ototoxicity of dibekacin and netilmicin in guinea pigs. *Acta Pharmacol. Toxicol.* 53:230–35

13. McCormick, G. C., Weinberg, E., Szot, R. J., Schwartz, E. 1985. Comparative ototoxicity of netilmicin, gentamicin and

tobramycin in cats. *Toxicol. Appl. Pharmacol.* 77:479–89

14. Lerner, A. M., Reyes, M. P., Cone, L. A., Blair, D. C., Jansen, W., et al. 1983. Randomized controlled trial of comparative efficacy, auditory toxicity and nephrotoxicity of tobramycin and netilmicin *Lancet* 1:1123–26

15. Aran, J. M., Erre, J. P., Guilhaume, A., Aurousseau, C. 1982. The comparative ototoxicities of gentamicin, tobramycin and dibekacin in the guinea pig. *Acta Oto–Laryngol.* 1982 (Suppl. 390):1–30

16. Brummett, R. E., Fox, K. E. 1982. Studies of aminoglycoside ototoxicity in animal models. In *The Aminoglycosides: Microbiology, Clinical Use and Toxicology*, ed. A. Whelton, H. C. Neu, pp. 419–52. New York: Dekker

17. Kahlmeter, G., Dahlager, J. I. 1984. Aminoglycoside toxicity—a review of clinical studies published between 1975 and 1982. *J. Antimicrob. Chemother.* 13 (Suppl. A):9–22

18. Theopold, H. M. 1977. Comparative surface studies of ototoxic effects of various aminoglycoside antibiotics on the organ of Corti in the guinea pig; a scanning electron microscopic study. *Acta Oto–Laryngol.* 84:57–64

19. Brown, R. D., Feldman, A. M. 1978. Pharmacology of hearing and ototoxicity. *Ann. Rev. Pharmacol. Toxicol.* 18:233–252

20. Browning, G. G., Northrop, R., Cortese, R. 1982. Selective destruction of outer hair cells in the chinchilla. *Clin. Otolaryngol.* 7:3–9

21. Kiang, N. Y. S., Liberman, M. C., Levine, R. A. 1976. Auditory-nerve activity in cats exposed to ototoxic drugs and high-intensity sounds. *Ann. Otol. Rhinol. Laryngol.* 85:752–68

22. Brummett, R. E. 1980. Drug-induced ototoxicity. *Drugs* 19:412–28

23. Voldrich, L. 1965. The kinetics of streptomycin, kanamycin and neomycin in the inner ear. *Acta Oto–Laryngol.* 60:243–48

24. Tran Ba Huy, P., Manuel, C., Meulemans, A. 1981. Kinetics of aminoglycoside antibiotics in perilymph and endolymph in animals. In *Aminoglycoside Ototoxicity*, ed. S. A. Lerner, G. J. Matz, J. E. Hawkins Jr., pp. 81–98. Boston: Little, Brown

25. Stupp, H. F., Kupper, K., Lagler, F., Sous, H., Quante, M. 1973. Inner ear concentrations and ototoxicity of different antibiotics in local and systemic application. *Audiology* 12:350–63

26. Tran Ba Huy, P., Manuel, C., Meulemans, A., Sterkers, O., Amiel, C. 1981. Pharmacokinetics of gentamicin in perilymph and endolymph of the rat as determined by radioimmunoassay. *J. Infect. Dis.* 143:476–86

27. Tran Ba Huy, P., Meulemans, A., Wassef, M., Manuel, C., Sterkers, O., et al. 1983. Gentamicin persistence in rat endolymph and perilymph after a two-day constant infusion. *Antimicrob. Agents Chemother.* 23:344–46

28. Robertson, D., Johnstone, B. M. 1979. Aberrant tonotopic organization in the inner ear damaged by kanamycin. *J. Acoust. Soc. Am.* 66:466–69

29. Kiang, N. Y.-S., Moxon, E. C., Levine, R. A. 1970. Auditory nerve activity in cats with normal and abnormal cochleas. In *Sensorineural Hearing Loss*, ed. G. E. W. Wolstenholme, J. Knight, pp. 241–68. London: Churchill, Livingstone

30. Buss, W. C., Piatt, M. K., Kauten, R. 1984. Inhibition of mammalian microsomal protein synthesis by aminoglycoside antibiotics. *J. Antimicrob. Chemother.* 14:231–41

31. Ylikoski, J., Wersäll, J., Björkroth, B. 1974. Degeneration of neural elements in the cochlea of the guinea pig after damage to the organ of Corti by ototoxic antibiotics. *Acta Oto–Laryngol.* 1974 (Suppl. 326):23–41

32. Kaku, Y., Farmer, J. C. Jr., Hudson, W. R. 1973. Ototoxic effects on cochlear histochemistry. *Arch. Otolaryngol.* 98:282–86

33. Tachibana, M., Mizukoshi, O., Kuriyama, L. 1976. Inhibitory effects of kanamycin on glycolysis in cochlea and kidney—possible involvement in the formation of oto- and nephrotoxicities. *Biochem. Pharmacol.* 25:2297–2301

34. Postma, D. S., Pecorak, J. B., Prazma, J., Logue, S. S., Fischer, N. D. 1976. Outer hair cell loss and alterations in glycogen due to tobramycin sulfate. *Arch. Otolaryngol.* 102:154–59

35. Guarcia-Quiroga, J., Norris, C. H., Glade, L., Bryant, G. M., Tachibana, M., et al. 1978. The relationship between kanamycin ototoxicity and glucose transport. *Res. Commun. Chem. Pathol. Pharmacol.* 22:535–47

36. Takada, A., Canlon, B., Schacht, J. 1983. Gentamicin ototoxicity dissociated from glucose uptake and utilization. *Res. Commun. Chem. Pathol. Pharmacol.* 42:203–12

37. Teixeira, R. B., Kelley, J., Alpert, H., Pardo, V., Vaamonde, C. A. 1982. Complete protection from gentamicin-

induced acute renal failure in the diabetes mellitus rat. *Kidney Int.* 21:600–12
38. Weiner, N. D., Schacht, J. 1981. See Ref. 24, pp. 113–21
39. Schacht, J. 1979. Isolation of an aminoglycoside receptor from guinea pig inner ear tissues and kidney. *Arch. Oto–Rhino–Laryngol.* 224:129–34
40. Orsulakova, A., Stockhorst, E., Schacht, J. 1976. Effect of neomycin on phosphoinositide labelling and calcium binding in guinea pig inner ear tissues in vivo and in vitro. *J. Neurochem.* 26:285–90
41. Wang, B. M., Weiner, N. D., Takada, A., Schacht, J. 1984. Characterization of aminoglycoside-lipid interactions and development of a refined model for ototoxicity testing. *Biochem. Pharmacol.* 33:3257–62
42. Kroese, A., Van den Bercken, J. 1982. Effects of ototoxic antibiotics on sensory cell functioning. *Hear. Res.* 6:183–97
43. Takada, A., Schacht, J. 1982. Calcium antagonism and reversibility of gentamicin-induced loss of cochlear microphonics in the guinea pig. *Hear. Res.* 8:179–86
44. Schwertz, D. W., Kreisberg, J. I., Venkatachalam, M. A. 1984. Effects of aminoglycosides on proximal tubule brush border membrane phosphatidylinositol-specific phospholipase C. *J. Pharmacol. Exp. Ther.* 231:48–55
45. Pierson, M. G., Moller, A. R. 1981. Prophylaxis of kanamycin-induced ototoxicity by a radioprotectant. *Hear. Res.* 4:79–87
46. Comis, S. D., Leng, G. 1980. Kanamycin ototoxicity and pigmentation in the guinea pig. *Hear. Res.* 3:249–51
47. Ohtsuki, K., Ohtani, I., Aikawa, T., Sato, Y., Anzai, T., et al. 1983. Protective effect of fosfomycin against aminoglycoside induced ototoxicity. *Nippon Jibi Inkoka Gakkai Kaiho* 86:1487–96
48. Sykes, R. B., Bonner, D. P., Bush, K., Georgopapadakou, N. H. 1982. Aztreonam (SQ 26,776), a synthetic monobactam specifically active against aerobic gram-negative bacteria. *Antimicrob. Agents Chemother.* 21:85–92
49. Myhre, J. L., DePaoli, A., Keim, G. R. 1985. Ototoxicity of subcutaneously administered aztreonam in neonatal rats. *Toxicol. Appl. Pharmacol.* 77:108–15
50. Perkins, H. R. 1982. Vancomycin and related antibiotics. *Pharmacol. Ther.* 16:181–97
51. Waisbren, B. A., Kleinerman, L., Skemp, J., Bratcher, G. 1960. Comparative clinical effectiveness and toxic-

ity of vancomycin, ristocetin and kanamycin. *Arch. Intern. Med.* 106:179–93
52. Watanakunakorn, C. 1982. Treatment of infections due to methicillin-resistant *Staphylococcus aureus*. *Ann. Intern. Med.* 97:376–78
53. Rybak, M. J., Boike, S. C. 1983. Additive toxicity in patients receiving vancomycin and aminoglycosides. *Clin. Pharm.* 2:508
54. Snavely, S. R., Hodges, G. R. 1984. The neurotoxicity of antibacterial agents. *Ann. Intern. Med.* 101:92–104
55. Traber, P. G., Levine, D. P. 1981. Vancomycin ototoxicity in a patient with normal renal function. *Ann. Intern. Med.* 95:458–59
56. Mellor, J. A., Kingdom, J., Cafferkey, M., Keane, C. 1984. Vancomycin ototoxicity in patients with normal renal function. *Br. J. Audiol.* 18:179–80
57. Alpert, G., Campos, J. M., Harris, M. C., Preblood, S. R., Plotkin, S. A. 1984. Vancomycin dosage in pediatrics reconsidered. *Am. J. Dis. Child.* 138:20–22
58. Cutler, N. R., Narang, P. K., Lesko, L. J., Ninos, M., Power, M. 1984. Vancomycin disposition: The importance of age. *Clin. Pharmacol. Ther.* 36:803–10
59. Hoagland, R. J., Sherwin, J. E., Phillips, J. M. Jr. 1984. Vancomycin: A rapid HPLC assay for a potent antibiotic. *J. Anal. Toxicol.* 8:75–77
60. Gross, J. R., Kaplan, S. L., Kramer, W. G., Mason, E. O. Jr. 1985. Vancomycin pharmacokinetics in premature infants. *Pediatr. Pharmacol.* 5:17–22
61. Banner, W. Jr., Ray, C. G. 1984. Vancomycin in perspective. *Am. J. Dis. Child.* 138:14–16
62. Kavanagh, K. T., McCabe, B. F. 1983. Ototoxicity of oral neomycin and vancomycin. *Laryngoscope* 93:649–53
63. Anderson, R. C., Harris, P. N., Chen, K. K. 1952. The toxicity and distribution of "Ilotycin". *J. Am. Pharm. Assoc.* (Sci. Ed.) 41:555–59
64. Schweitzer, V. G., Olson, N. R. 1984. Ototoxic effects of erythromycin therapy. *Arch. Otolaryngol.* 110:258–60
65. Haydon, R. C., Thelin, J. W., Davis, W. E. 1984. Erythromycin ototoxicity: analysis and conclusions based on 22 case reports. *Otolaryngol. Head Neck Surg.* 92:678–84
66. Hugues, F. C., Laccoureye, A., Lasserre, M. H., Toupet, M. 1984. Recherche d'une toxicité cochléaire de l'erythromycine chez le malade âgé. *Therapie* 39:591–94
67. Kroboth, P. D., McNeil, M. A., Kree-

ger, A., Dominguez, J., Rault, R. 1983. Hearing loss and erythromycin pharmacokinetics in a patient receiving hemodialysis. *Arch. Intern. Med.* 143:1263–65

68. Taylor, R., Schofield, I. S., Ramos, J. M., Bint, A. J., Ward, M. K. 1981. Ototoxicity of erythromycin in peritoneal dialysis patients. *Lancet* 2:935–36

69. Gargye, A. K., Dutta, D. V. 1959. Nerve deafness following chloramycetin therapy. *Indian J. Pediatr.* 26:265–66

70. Koide, Y., Hata, A., Hando, R. 1966. Vulnerability of the organ of Corti in poisoning. *Acta Oto–Laryngol.* 61:332–44

71. Henley, C. M., Brown, R. D., Penny, J. E., Kupetz, S. A., Hodges, K. B., et al. 1984. Impairment in cochlear function produced by chloramphenicol and noise. *Neuropharmacology* 23:197–202

72. Beaugard, M. E., Asakuma, S., Snow, J. B. Jr. 1981. Comparative ototoxicity of chloramphenicol and kanamycin with ethacrynic acid. *Arch. Otolaryngol.* 107:104–9

73. Jacobson, H. R., Kokko, J. P. 1976. Diuretics: Sites and mechanisms of action. *Ann. Rev. Pharmacol. Toxicol.* 16:201–14

74. Greven, J., Defrain, W., Glaser, K., Meywald, K., Heidenreich, O. 1980. Studies with the optically active isomers of the new diuretic drug ozolinone. I. Differences in stereoselectivity of the renal target structures of ozolinone. *Pfluegers Arch.* 384:57–60

75. Göttl, K. H., Roesch, A., Klinke, R. 1985. Quantitative evaluation of ototoxic effects of furosemide, piretanide, bumetanide, azosemide and ozolinone in the cat—a new approach to the problem of ototoxicity. *Naunyn-Schmiedeberg's Arch. Pharmacol.* In press

76. Blaine, E. H., Fanelli, G. M. Jr., Irvin, J. D., Tobert, J. A., Davies, R. O. 1982. Enantiomers of indacrinone: a new approach to producing an isouricemic diuretic. *Clin. Exp. Hypertension A* 4:161–76

77. Boston Collaborative Drug Surveillance Program. 1973. Drug-induced deafness. *J. Am. Med. Assoc.* 224:515–16

78. Tuzel, I. H. 1981. Comparison of adverse reactions to bumetanide and furosemide. *J. Clin. Pharmacol.* 21:615–19

79. Rybak, L. P. 1982. Pathophysiology of furosemide ototoxicity. *J. Otolaryngol.* 11:127–33

80. Rybak, L. P. 1985. Furosemide ototoxicity: clinical and experimental aspects. *Laryngoscope* 95(Suppl. 38):1–14

81. Matz, G. J. 1976. The ototoxic effects of ethacrynic acid in man and animals. *Laryngoscope* 86:1065–86

82. Santi, P. A., Lakhani, B. N. 1983. The effect of bumetanide on the stria vascularis: A stereological analysis of cell volume density. *Hear. Res.* 12:151–65

83. Arnold, W., Nadol, J. B. Jr., Weidauer, H. 1981. Ultrastructural histopathology in a case of human ototoxicity due to loop diuretics. *Acta Oto–Laryngol.* 91:399–414

84. Kusakari, J., Ise, I., Comegys, T. H., Thalmann, I., Thalmann, R. 1978. Effect of ethacrynic acid, furosemide, and ouabain upon the endolymphatic potential and upon high energy phosphates of the stria vascularis. *Laryngoscope* 88:12–37

85. Rybak, L. P., Green, T. P., Juhn, S. K., Morizono, T., Mirkin, B. L. 1979. Elimination kinetics of furosemide in perilymph and serum of the chinchilla. Neuropharmacologic correlates. *Acta Oto–Laryngol.* 88:382–87

86. Green, T. P., Rybak, L. P., Mirkin, B. L., Juhn, S. K., Morizono, T. 1981. Pharmacologic determinants of ototoxicity of furosemide in the chinchilla. *J. Pharmacol. Exp. Ther.* 216:537–42

87. Kusakari, J., Kambayashi, J., Ise, I., Kawamoto, K. 1978. Reduction of the endocochlear potential by the new "loop" diuretic, bumetanide. *Acta Oto–Laryngol.* 86:336–41

88. Rybak, L. P., Whitworth, C. 1985. Comparative ototoxicity of furosemide and piretanide. *Acta Oto–Laryngol.* In press

89. Asakuma, S., Snow, J. B. Jr. 1980. Effects of furosemide and ethacrynic acid on the endocochlear direct current potential in normal and kanamycin sulfate-treated guinea pigs. *Otolaryngol. Head Neck Surg.* 88:188–93

90. Pike, D. A., Bosher, S. K. 1980. The time course of the strial changes produced by intravenous furosemide. *Hear. Res.* 3:79–89

91. Brummett, R., Smith, C. A., Ueno, Y., Cameron, S., Richter, R. 1977. The delayed effects of ethacrynic acid on the stria vascularis of the guinea pig. *Acta Oto–Laryngol.* 83:98–112

92. Bosher, S. K. 1979. The nature of the negative endocochlear potentials produced by anoxia and ethacrynic acid in the rat and guinea pig. *J. Physiol.* 293:329–45

93. Bosher, S. K. 1980. The nature of the ototoxic actions of ethacrynic acid upon the mammalian endolymph system. I.

Functional aspects. *Acta Oto–Laryngol.* 89:407–18

94. Sewell, W. F. 1984. The relation between the endocochlear potential and spontaneous activity in the auditory nerve fibres in the cat. *J. Physiol.* 347:685–96

95. Evans, E. F., Klinke, R. 1982. The effects of intracochlear and systemic furosemide on the properties of single cochlear nerve fibres in the cat. *J. Physiol.* 331:409–27

96. Jung, W., Rosskopf, K. 1975. Evoked Response Audiometry (ERA) am Meerschweinchen vor und nach Lasix-induziertem Hörsturz. *Laryngol. Rhinol.* 54:411–18

97. Kameswaran, M., Visvanathan, M., Reddy, M. K., Bharathy, M., Kameswaran, S. 1977. Furosemide ototoxicity in guinea pigs. *Indian J. Otolaryngol.* 29:8

98. Anderson, S. D., Kemp, D. T. 1979. The evoked cochlear mechanical response in laboratory primates; a preliminary report. *Arch. Oto–Rhino–Laryngol.* 224:47–54

99. Himelfarb, M., Kroin, J., Strelioff, D. 1979. Evidence for intracochlear impedance changes following ethacrynic acid administration. *Otolaryngol. Head Neck Surg.* 87:880–87

100. Rybak, L. P., Morizono, T. 1982. Effect of furosemide upon endolymph potassium concentration. *Hear. Res.* 7:223–31

101. Brusilow, S. W. 1976. Propranolol antagonism to the effect of furosemide on the composition of endolymph in guinea pigs. *Can. J. Physiol. Pharmacol.* 54: 42–48

102. Marks, S. C., Schacht, J. 1981. Effects of ototoxic diuretics on cochlear Na^+-K^+-ATPase and adenylate cyclase. *Scand. Audiol.* 1981 (Suppl. 14):131–38

103. Thalmann, I., Kobayashi, T., Thalmann, R. 1982. Arguments against a mediating role of the adenylate cyclase-cyclic AMP system in the ototoxic action of loop diuretics. *Laryngoscope* 92:589–93

104. Marcus, D. C., Rokugo, M., Ge, X.-X., Thalmann, R. 1983. Response of cochlear potentials to presumed alterations of ionic conductance: Endolymphatic perfusion of barium, valinomycin and nystatin. *Hear. Res.* 12:17–30

105. Fox, K. E., Brummett, R. E. 1974. Protein binding of ethacrynic acid and its cysteine derivative in relation to depression of the cochlear potential in guinea pigs. *Fed. Proc.* 33:271

106. Brown, R. D. 1975. Comparison of the cochlear toxicity of sodium ethacrynate, furosemide, and the cysteine adduct of sodium ethacrynate in cats. *Toxicol. Appl. Pharmacol.* 31:270–82

107. Koechel, D. A. 1981. Ethacrynic acid and related diuretics: Relationship of structure to beneficial and detrimental actions. *Ann. Rev. Pharmacol. Toxicol.* 21:265–93

108. Aranda, J. V., Lambert, C., Perez, J., Turmen, T., Sitar, D. S. 1982. Metabolism and renal elimination of furosemide in the newborn infant. *J. Pediatr.* 101:777–81

109. Kerremans, A. L. M., Tan, Y., Van Ginneken, C. A. M., Gribnau, F. W. J. 1982. Specimen handling and high-performance liquid chromatographic determination of furosemide. *J. Chromatogr.* 229:129–39

110. Odlind, B. 1979. Relationship between renal tubular secretion and effects of five loop diuretics. *J. Pharmacol. Exp. Ther.* 211:238–44

111. Rybak, L. P., Green, T. P., Juhn, S. K., Morizono, T. 1984. Probenecid reduces cochlear effects and perilymph penetration of furosemide in chinchilla. *J. Pharmacol. Exp. Ther.* 230:706–9

112. Ahokas, J. T., Davies, C., Ravenscroft, P. J., Emmerson, B. T. 1984. Inhibition of soluble glutathione-s-transferase by diuretic drugs. *Biochem. Pharmacol.* 33: 1929–32

113. Brummett, R. E., Bendrick, T., Himes, D. 1981. Comparative ototoxicity of bumetanide and furosemide when used in combination with kanamycin. *J. Clin. Pharmacol.* 21:628–36

114. Humes, L. E. 1984. Noise-induced hearing loss as influenced by other agents and by some physical characteristics of the individual. *J. Acoust. Soc. Am.* 76:1318–29

115. Mongan, E., Kelly, P., Nies, K., Porter, W. W., Paulus, H. E. 1973. Tinnitus as an indication of therapeutic serum salicylate levels. *J. Am. Med. Assoc.* 226:142–45

116. Miller, R. 1978. Deafness due to plain and long-acting aspirin tablets. *J. Clin. Pharmacol.* 18:468–71

117. McFadden, D., Plattsmier, H. S., Pasanen, E. G. 1984. Aspirin-induced hearing loss as a model of sensorineural hearing loss. *Hear. Res.* 16:251–60

118. Juhn, S. K., Rybak, L. P., Jung, T. T. K. 1985. Transport characteristics of the blood-labyrinth barrier. In *Auditory Biochemistry*, ed. D. Drescher, pp. 488–99. Springfield, IL: Thomas

119. Silverstein, J., Bernstein, J., Davies, D. G. 1967. Salicylate ototoxicity; a biochemical and electrophysiological study. *Ann. Otol. Rhinol. Laryngol.* 76:118–28

120. Ishii, T., Bernstein, J. M., Balogh, K. Jr. 1967. Distribution of tritium-labelled

salicylate in the cochlea; an auto-radiographical study. *Ann. Otol. Rhinol. Laryngol.* 76:368–76

121. Bobbin, R. P., Thompson, M. H. 1978. Effects of putative transmitters on afferent cochlear transmission. *Ann. Otol. Rhinol. Laryngol.* 87:185–90

122. Krzanowski, J. J. Jr., Matschinsky, F. M. 1971. Phosphocreatine gradient opposite to that of glycogen in the organ of Corti and the effect of salicylate on adenosine triphosphate and P-creatine in cochlear structures. *J. Histochem.* 19:321–23

123. McFadden, D., Plattsmier, H. S. 1984. Aspirin abolishes spontaneous otoacoustic emissions. *J. Acoust. Soc. Am.* 76:443–48

124. Evans, E. F., Borerwe, T. A. 1982. Ototoxic effects of salicylates on the responses of single cochlear nerve fibres and on cochlear potentials. *Br. J. Audiol.* 16:101–8

125. Mitchell, C., Brummett, R., Himes, D., Vernon, J. 1973. Electrophysiological study of the effect of sodium salicylate upon the cochlea. *Arch. Otolaryngol.* 98:297–301

126. Falk, S. A. 1974. Sodium salicylate. *Arch. Otolaryngol.* 99:393

127. Deer, B. C., Hunter-Duvar, I. 1982. Salicylate ototoxicity in the chinchilla: a behavioral and electron microscope study. *J. Otolaryngol.* 11:260–64

128. Bernstein, J. M., Weiss, A. D. 1967. Further observation on salicylate ototoxicity. *J. Laryngol. Otol.* 81:915–25

129. DeMoura, L. F. P., Hayden, R. C. Jr. 1968. Salicylate ototoxicity; a human temporal bone report. *Arch. Otolaryngol.* 87:60–64

130. Morrison, M. D., Blakley, B. W. 1978. The effects of indomethacin on inner ear fluids and morphology. *J. Otolaryngol.* 7:149–57

131. Koopman, C. F. Jr., Glattke, T. A., Caffrey, J. D. 1982. Effect of ibuprofen upon hearing in the guinea pig. *Otolaryngol. Head Neck Surg.* 90:819–23

132. Chapman, P. 1982. Naproxen and sudden hearing loss. *J. Laryngol. Otol.* 96:163–66

133. Rüedi, L., Furrer, W., Lüthy, F., Nager, G., Tschirren, B. 1952. Further observations concerning the toxic effects of streptomycin and quinine on the auditory organ of guinea pigs. *Laryngoscope* 62:333–51

134. Hennebert, D., Fernandez, C. 1959. Ototoxicity of quinine in experimental animals. *Arch. Otolaryngol.* 70:321–33

135. Hart, C., Naunton, R. 1964. The ototoxicity of chloroquine phosphate. *Arch. Otolaryngol.* 80:407–12

136. Toone, E. C. Jr., Hayden, G. D., Ellman, H. M. 1965. Ototoxicity of chloroquine. *Arthritis Rheum.* 8:475–76

137. Mukherjee, D. K. 1979. Chloroquine ototoxicity—A reversible phenomenon? *J. Laryngol. Otol.* 93:809–15

138. Dencker, L., Lindquist, N. G. 1975. Distribution of labeled chloroquine in the inner ear. *Arch. Otolaryngol.* 101:185–88

139. McFadden, D., Plattsmier, H. S. 1983. Aspirin can potentiate temporary hearing loss induced by intense sounds. *Hear. Res.* 9:295–316

140. McFadden, D., Plattsmier, H. S., Pasanen, E. G. 1984. Temporary hearing loss induced by combinations of intense sounds and nonsteroidal anti-inflammatory drugs. *Am. J. Otolaryngol.* 5:235–41

141. Bagger-Sjoback, D., Filipek, C. S., Schacht, J. 1980. Characteristics and drug responses of cochlear and vestibular adenylate cyclase. *Arch. Oto–Rhino–Laryngol.* 228:217–22

142. Konishi, T., Gupta, B. N., Prazma, J. 1983. Ototoxicity of cis-dichlorodiammine platinum (II) in guinea pigs. *Am. J. Otolaryngol.* 4:18–26

143. Komune, S., Asakuma, S., Snow, J. B. Jr. 1981. Pathophysiology of the ototoxicity of cis-diamminedichloroplatinum. *Otolaryngol. Head Neck Surg.* 89:275–82

144. Estrem, S. A., Babin, R. W., Ryu, J. H., Moore, K. C. 1981. Cis-diamminedichloroplatinum (II) ototoxicity in the guinea pig. *Otolaryngol. Head Neck Surg.* 89:638–45

145. Tange, R. A., Vuzevski, V. D. 1984. Changes in the stria vascularis of the guinea pig due to cis-platinum. *Arch. Oto–Rhino–Laryngol.* 239:41–47

146. Wright, C. G., Schaefer, S. D. 1982. Inner ear histopathology in patients treated with cisplatinum. *Laryngoscope* 92:1408–13

147. Strauss, M., Towfighi, J., Lord, S., Lipton, A., Harvey, H. A., et al. 1983. Cisplatinum ototoxicity: clinical experience and temporal bone histopathology. *Laryngoscope* 93:1554–59

148. Moroso, M. J., Blair, R. L. 1983. A review of cis-platinum ototoxicity. *J. Otolaryngol.* 12:365–69

149. Reddel, R. R., Kefford, R. F., Grant, J. M., Coates, A. S., Fox, R. M., et al. 1982. Ototoxicity in patients receiving cisplatin: importance of dose and method

of drug administration. *Cancer Treat. Rep.* 66:19–23
150. Van Zeijl, L. G. P. M., Conijn, E. A. J. G., Rodenburg, M., Tange, R. A., Brocaar, M. P. 1984. Analysis of hearing loss due to cis-diamminedichloroplatinum—II. *Arch. Oto–Rhino–Laryngol.* 239:255–62
151. Rybak, L. P. 1981. Cis-platinum associated hearing loss. *J. Laryngol. Otol.* 95:745–47
152. Vermorken, J. B., Kapteijn, T. S., Hart, A. A. M., Pinedo, H. M. 1983. Ototoxicity of cis-diamminedichloroplatinum (II): Influence of dose, schedule and mode of administration. *Eur. J. Cancer Clin. Oncol.* 19:53–58
153. Fausti, S. A., Schechter, M. A., Rappaport, B. Z., Frey, R. H., Mass, R. E. 1984. Early detection of cisplatin ototoxicity. Selected case reports. *Cancer* 53:224–31
154. McHaney, V. A., Thibadoux, G., Hayes, F. A., Green, A. A. 1983. Hearing loss in children receiving cisplatin chemotherapy. *J. Pediatr.* 102:314–17
155. Granowetter, L., Rosenstock, J. G., Packer, R. J. 1983. Enhanced cis-platinum neurotoxicity in pediatric patients with brain tumors. *J. Neurooncol.* 1:293–97
156. Komune, S., Snow, J. B. Jr. 1981. Potentiating effects of cisplatin and ethacrynic acid in ototoxicity. *Arch. Otolaryngol.* 107:594–97
157. Schweitzer, V. G., Hawkins, J. E., Lilly, D. J., Litterst, C. J., Abrams, G., et al. 1984. Ototoxic and nephrotoxic effects of combined treatment with cis-diamminedichloroplatinum and kanamycin in the guinea pig. *Otolaryngol. Head Neck Surg.* 92:38–49
158. Serafy, A., Hashash, M., State, F. 1982. The effect of vinblastine sulfate on the neurological elements of the rabbit cochlea. *J. Laryngol. Otol.* 96:975–79
159. Serafy, A., Hashash, M. 1981. The effect of vincristine on the neurological elements of the rabbit cochlea. *J. Laryngol. Otol.* 95:49–54
160. Cummings, C. W. 1968. Experimental observations on the ototoxicity of nitrogen mustard. *Laryngoscope* 78:530–38
161. Asakuma, S., Snow, J. B. Jr. 1978. Bioelectric phenomena in the ototoxicity of nitrogen mustard. *Otolaryngology* 86:888–95

Ann. Rev. Pharmacol. Toxicol. 1986. 26:101–16

RENAL CALCIUM METABOLISM AND DIURETICS

Charles T. Stier, Jr. and Harold D. Itskovitz

Departments of Pharmacology and Medicine, New York Medical College, Valhalla, NY 10595

INTRODUCTION

The major purposes of diuretics are to enhance renal excretion of salt and water and to lower blood pressure. However, their effects are not limited to sodium and chloride; they may also influence the renal reabsorption and excretion of calcium, magnesium, potassium, and other ions. It is important to be aware of these effects in order to maintain appropriate body content of essential chemicals. The present review centers on the interactions of diuretic agents with calcium. Knowledge of these interactions may be useful in the appropriate application of diuretic agents for the maintenance of normal blood concentrations and body stores of calcium, especially during the chronic use of diuretic agents. Also, diuretic agents with differing effects on calcium metabolism may be indicated therapeutically in disorders of calcium metabolism. In the present review, we have taken into account the effects of diuretic agents on renal calcium metabolism relative to hormonal and nonhormonal factors and their direct actions within the nephron. Several excellent reviews of diuretics have been published in the past few years (1–3).

CALCIUM HANDLING BY THE KIDNEY

Filtration and Reabsorption

Calcium is present in plasma in three forms: free calcium, calcium anionic complexes, and calcium bound to protein. Filtration of calcium is limited owing to its binding to plasma proteins, and only free calcium and calcium anionic complexes can cross the glomerulus. Measurements of calcium concentrations

101

0362-1642/86/0415-0101$02.00

in the glomerular fluid of Bowman's space indicate that approximately 60% of plasma calcium may be filtered (4–6). This figure agrees in general with the reported ultrafilterability of calcium across artificial membranes (7). In tubular fluid of the proximal tubule the concentration of calcium is constant and is similar to or slightly exceeds the concentration of ultrafilterable calcium when measured in nondiuretic animals (4, 8–10). In fluid-expanded animals, active proximal tubular reabsorption of calcium has been demonstrated, because concentrations of tubular-fluid calcium lower than ultrafilterable glomerular calcium concentrations have been obtained (5, 8). Active calcium reabsorption in the proximal tubule has been postulated also on the basis of stop-flow microperfusion experiments in rats (11). The tubular basolateral membrane is thought to be the site of active transport of calcium since an appropriate electrochemical gradient for calcium entry into tubular cells exists on the luminal side (12). Two mechanisms of transport have been proposed. The first involves Ca^{2+}-ATPase: This enzyme has been found in the basolateral membrane of rat proximal tubular cells (13, 14). The second mechanism involves a sodium/calcium antiport, in which sodium enters the cell at the basolateral membrane in exchange for calcium. The latter mechanism is driven by the active pumping of intracellular sodium across the basolateral membrane. This explanation is supported by reports that ouabain and perfusion of peritubular capillaries with sodium-free solutions interfere with calcium reabsorption in the proximal tubule (11). Beyond the proximal tubule, reabsorption of calcium occurs in the pars recta and loop of Henle. Reabsorption in these zones accounts for 20–30% of the calcium that enters the tubular fluid at the glomerulus. At the hairpin turn of the loop of Henle, in the juxtamedullary nephron, tubular fluid/plasma concentrations of calcium are lower than those of sodium (15, 16), suggesting a dissociation of transport between these ions in either the pars recta or the descending limb of Henle's loop. This may relate to substantial reabsorption of calcium in segments of the straight proximal tubule (17) or perhaps to greater medullary recycling (entry into the descending limb) of sodium relative to calcium. Reabsorption of calcium has been demonstrated in isolated perfused segments of the thick ascending limb, both in its cortical (18, 19) and medullary (20) segments. Calcium reabsorption here has been found to be passive and is thought to be driven by a lumen-positive transepithelial potential generated in response to active chloride reabsorption (21). In contrast, other studies have reported active calcium reabsorption in perfused segments of cortical thick ascending limbs (20, 22, 23).

The reasons for these different findings are not clear. Studies in the early distal convoluted tubule indicate that the fractions of sodium and calcium reabsorbed are similar, and that they are equal at that point to approximately 85% of calcium filtered at the glomerulus (10, 24).

Hormonal Interactions

VITAMIN D   Vitamin D is converted in vivo to 1,25-dihydroxyvitamin D, which is its most active metabolic form. Parathyroid hormone (PTH) stimulates a final hydroxylation that occurs in the kidney. Thus, elevated levels of 1,25-dihydroxyvitamin D have been reported in some patients with hyperparathyroid disease. Vitamin D administration enhances calcium absorption in the intestine and increases plasma calcium concentrations. In parathyroidectomized animals, 1,25-dihydroxyvitamin D will increase urinary excretion of calcium (25). Vitamin D has been used in patients with deficient parathyroid function to raise plasma calcium levels and is usually associated with increased urinary calcium excretion. On the other hand, the renal reabsorption of calcium has been reported to increase after acute vitamin D administration (26). This may or may not be related to its effect of increasing blood calcium levels and secondarily increasing the filtration of calcium across the glomerulus. It has also been reported that administration of vitamin D can increase urinary calcium excretion without altering serum calcium or creatinine clearance (27). Preliminary micropuncture studies suggest possible distal nephron effects (28). The direct renal actions of vitamin D and its metabolites on various nephron segments remain to be fully investigated.

PARATHYROID HORMONE (PTH)   PTH plays an important regulatory role in body-calcium metabolism. PTH has extrarenal sites of action to increase bone resorption and intestinal calcium absorption and thus increase plasma calcium concentrations. In the kidney its hypocalciuric action further increases plasma calcium levels. Experimentally and clinically, parathyroidectomy or hypoparathyroidism is accompanied by an increase in urinary calcium excretion, whereas hyperparathyroid states are conversely manifested by reduced renal calcium clearance (29).

In contrast to its effects on calcium, PTH increases phosphate excretion by the kidney. Micropuncture and microperfusion studies have localized the principal sites of PTH actions to the distal nephron for increased calcium reabsorption and to the proximal tubule for its phosphaturic effect. After administration of PTH to intact or thyroparathyroidectomized dogs, delivery of calcium and sodium to the late proximal tubule is increased proportionately (30). However, in distal tubular fluid and the final urine the Ca/Na ratio is substantially decreased by PTH, supporting selective enhancement of calcium reabsorption at distal sites. In isolated perfused segments of cortical thick ascending tubules (20, 31–33) and in granular portions of the distal convoluted tubule and collecting duct (18, 32), PTH increases absorption of calcium when added to the bath. These nephron segments have been reported to possess

PTH-sensitive adenylate cyclase activity (32, 34). Analogs of cyclic AMP have been shown to mimic the effects of PTH on these nephron segments (31–33). In contrast, calcium absorption in perfused thick ascending medullary limbs (20) and cortical collecting tubules (18, 32, 33) is not affected by PTH. In these same areas, PTH-sensitive adenylate cyclase activity has been reported to be very low (32, 34).

CALCITONIN   Although calcitonin's extrarenal effects generally oppose those of PTH—it inhibits the reabsorption of bone calcium and decreases intestinal calcium absorption—its renal effects are similar to those of PTH in that it causes a hypocalciuric effect. Acute administration of calcitonin has been reported to exert a hypocalciuric action (35, 36) although in some studies calcium excretion was unchanged (37) or increased (38). Microperfusion studies in vivo have shown decreased urinary calcium excretion in association with increased calcium reabsorption in the loop of Henle, whereas calcitonin was observed to exert little effect on either proximal or distal tubular calcium absorption (39). In isolated perfused tubular preparations calcitonin increased calcium absorption and stimulated adenylate cyclase activity (40) in medullary thick ascending loops but had no effect on calcium absorption in cortical thick ascending limbs (41). Thus, calcitonin differs in its nephron sites of action from PTH, which stimulates calcium absorption in the cortical thick ascending limb but has no effect on medullary thick ascending loops. The hypocalciuric effect of calcitonin may depend also upon its ability to diminish plasma-calcium concentrations, since urinary calcium excretion is maintained when hypocalcemia is prevented by intravenous infusions of calcium chloride (39). Thus, the renal excretion of calcium after calcitonin is believed to be reduced relative both to its effects on the plasma calcium concentration and to its effects on the renal tubule.

Nonhormonal Interactions

Alterations in clearance of sodium are generally accompanied by similar alterations in the clearance of ultrafilterable calcium. This has led to the suggestion that the renal reabsorption of sodium and calcium are interdependent (29). Infusions of sodium chloride produce an increase in urinary calcium clearance that parallels the increase in sodium, even when the glomerular filtration of these ions is maintained below control levels (42). Micropuncture studies have shown proportionate reductions in proximal tubular reabsorption of sodium and calcium during saline volume expansion. On the other hand, a dissociation of sodium and calcium excretion occurs when sodium is infused with certain nonreabsorbable anions that complex with calcium. Thus, sodium sulfate infusions have been found to produce significantly greater increases in clearance of calcium than of sodium (29). However, when calcium is infused with other nonreabsorbable anions such as gluconate or lactate, the excretion of sodium is greater than that of calcium (43). In contrast, calcium chloride infusion markedly increases urinary calcium excretion, with little or no effect on sodium excretion (10). Even with a subsequent infusion of saline under this circumstance the dissociation persists and is believed to be related, in part, to suppression of PTH release (43).

During infusions of magnesium, the clearance of calcium greatly exceeds that of sodium. This dissociation relates in part to decreased PTH release secondary to hypermagnesemia. Magnesium also acts directly to diminish the tubular reabsorption of calcium to a greater extent than sodium reabsorption (44). In contrast to infusions of magnesium, those of phosphate decrease urinary calcium excretion (45) whereas phosphate depletion elevates urinary calcium.

Alterations in acid-base balance also influence the excretion of calcium. Chronic metabolic acidosis increases total urinary calcium excretion and the ratio of calcium-to-sodium clearance (46). The effects of acidosis do not appear to be due to lowering blood pH alone since respiratory acidosis has a delayed effect, increasing urinary calcium excretion only after several weeks when net acid excretion is increased. Alkalosis, resulting from bicarbonate administration, has an opposite effect and increases renal sodium excretion relative to that of calcium (46).

Nonionic substances, such as glucose or protein, which do not increase (but may decrease) sodium excretion, generally increase urinary calcium. The effects of glucose relate in part to increased insulin secretion. Hypercalciuria has also been reported after fasting which, in this case, has been related to the resultant ketoacidosis (43). Alterations in renal hemodynamics by vasodilator agents result in increases in fractional urinary calcium excretion that parallel that of sodium (47).

DIURETICS

By affecting one or another of the physiologic mechanisms that influence the renal handling of calcium, the different diuretics may either increase or decrease calcium excretion. Their final effects will be the result of many interrelated forces: direct renal actions and alterations in hormonal and nonhormonal factors. In the following discussion, we summarize the effects of diuretic agents on urinary calcium describing them in terms of the previously listed mechanisms.

Carbonic Anhydrase Inhibitors

Carbonic anhydrase inhibitors, typified by acetazolamide, exert their diuretic effects by blocking the generation of hydrogen ions. These ions have a major effect of enhancing the reabsorption of bicarbonate in the proximal tubule. Thus, carbonic anhydrase inhibitors produce a marked increase in urinary bicarbonate and phosphate excretion. Since phosphate anions are poorly reabsorbed beyond the proximal tubule, their excretion leads to an increased excretion of sodium and water. Generally, acetazolamide has been reported to produce an associated increase in calcium excretion (48–50), though it is less than that of sodium. In several studies calcium excretion was unaffected (51–53). The ability of acetazolamide to increase calcium excretion has been observed in thyroparathyroidectomized animals, suggesting that its calciuric effect is not related to changes in circulating PTH levels (50). Although administration both of PTH and of acetazolamide produces qualitatively similar results, no inhibitory effect of PTH or cyclic nucleotides on carbonic anhydrase activity has been reported. In stop-flow microperfusion studies of rat proximal tubules, acetazolamide did not influence active calcium transport, suggesting that its calciuric effect was passive (11). This is consistent with observations that acetazolamide does not inhibit microsomal calcium-activated ATPase from rat kidneys (52) or ATP-dependent calcium uptake by microsomes isolated from rat kidneys (54).

Micropuncture studies indicate that acetazolamide inhibits sodium and calcium reabsorption to parallel degrees in the proximal tubule of intact and parathyroidectomized animals (53). However, by the final urine, sodium excretion but not calcium excretion was increased, which was interpreted as indicating a greater distal reabsorption of calcium than of sodium. Also, during chronic acetazolamide administration the resultant metabolic acidosis may be associated with hypercalciuria. In studies using isolated canine kidneys perfused at constant pressure with autologous blood maintained in a nearly normal physiologic state, we observed significant increases in calcium excretion and comparable sodium clearance relative to calcium clearance following additions of acetazolamide (Figure 1). Our results support a direct action of acetazolamide on renal calcium metabolism, independent of changes in circulating hormones or systemic hemodynamics.

Loop Diuretics

The organomercurials, furosemide, and ethacrynic acid are diuretics that have the thick ascending loop of Henle as their main site of action. These agents act primarily to inhibit the $1 Na^+/1 K^+/2Cl^-$ cotransporter that is localized to the luminal membrane of the cortical and medullary portions of the thick ascending limb (55). The earliest effect of the loop diuretics (especially furosemide) is to increase urinary calcium excretion to a degree that parallels or most often is greater than their natriuretic effect. Few studies have tracked the long-term effects of loop diuretics on calcium balance. In isolated perfused rabbit cortical thick ascending limbs, furosemide inhibited calcium absorption in association

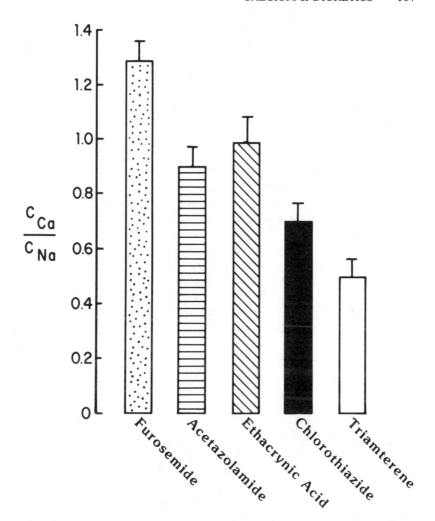

Figure 1 Ratio of calcium clearance to sodium clearance (C_{Ca}/C_{Na}) during peak natriuretic responses in isolated blood-perfused dog kidneys following bolus injections of diuretics. Furosemide (n = 9) > ethacrynic acid (n = 5) = acetazolamide (n = 8) ≥ chlorothiazide (n = 3) = triamterene (n = 11) by ANOVA.

with a reduction in the lumen-positive transepithelial voltage thought to drive passive calcium-ion transport in this segment (56). Furosemide causes slightly more calciuria than natriuresis (49, 50, 57–63). This dissociation appears to reside in the thick ascending limb of the loop of Henle. In vivo microperfusion studies in the rat have demonstrated relatively greater inhibition of calcium absorption than of sodium absorption in Henle's loop on intraluminal administration of furosemide, with little or no effect on the transport of these ions in the superficial distal tubule (64). Mercurial diuretics like furosemide have been reported to increase urinary calcium more than they do that of urinary sodium (65, 66). Ethacrynic acid, on the other hand, increases urinary calcium and sodium to similar degrees (48–50, 58, 59, 67). In our own studies using isolated, blood-perfused dog kidneys, we have shown that furosemide increases the clearance of calcium over that of sodium to a degree significantly greater than that caused by ethacrynic acid (Figures 1 and 2). Whereas furosemide consistently increased calcium clearance in excess of sodium clearance, ethacrynic acid affected calcium clearance to a similar (or slightly lesser) degree than sodium clearance on bolus administration (Figure 1) or infusion (Figure 2), respectively. We do not know the reason for this difference between furosemide and ethacrynic acid but have considered the possibility that it may relate to an additional effect ethacrynic acid has of enhancing calcium absorption relative to sodium absorption at an early distal site. This site is not shared by furosemide since other agents that act at distal sites beyond the loop of Henle (such as the thiazides and amiloride), tend to enhance the renal clearance of sodium relative to calcium in our isolated kidney preparation. When amiloride was infused during infusion of either furosemide or ethacrynic acid C_{Ca}/C_{Na} decreased (Figure 2). Chlorothiazide further decreased C_{Ca}/C_{Na} in kidneys infused with furosemide plus amiloride, but did not do so in kidneys that received ethacrynic acid plus amiloride. These results suggest that thiazides and ethacrynic acid share a distal site of action (perhaps the distal convoluted tubule) at which furosemide does not act.

Thiazide Diuretics

Thiazides and related diuretics, such as chlorthalidone, metolazone, and indapamide, have a primary effect at the early distal tubule diluting site. Agents acting at this site increase sodium excretion to a greater extent than excretion of chloride (in contradistinction to the loop diuretics) and cause a greater osmotic than water diuresis, which prevents the formation of a dilute urine. Acute administration of these agents produces a natriuresis and diuresis with little or no increase in calcium excretion (50, 59, 62, 65, 67). In some studies the clearance of calcium decreased (68, 69), resulting in a marked reduction in the calcium/sodium clearance ratio. Chronic thiazide administration causes an absolute reduction in calcium excretion (70–74) and this forms the basis for its therapeutic role of diminishing idiopathic hypercalciuria and preventing the formation of calcium-containing renal stones (75). Thiazides have also been used for treatment of bone demineralization states, such as osteoporosis. Different studies have suggested several different mechanisms for the hypocalciuric effects of thiazides. These effects include increasing calcium reabsorption by volume depletion and by increased plasma PTH levels as well as potentiation of the actions of PTH (73, 74). However, when administered

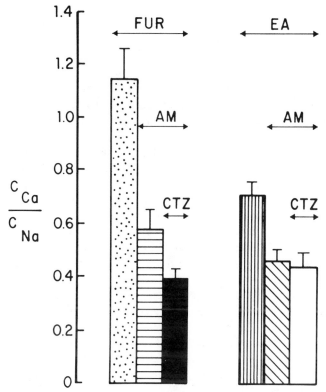

Figure 2   Ratio of calcium clearance to sodium clearance (C_{Ca}/C_{Na}) in isolated blood-perfused dog kidneys following a 1 mg bolus injection and continuous 0.2 mg/min infusion of furosemide (FUR) (n = 8) or ethacrynic acid (EA) (n = 5) and subsequent amiloride (AM) and chlorothiazide (CTZ) (n = 4) administration at the same dose level.

acutely to patients with hypoparathyroidism (76) or to thyroparathyroidectomized dogs (62, 77, 78), chlorothiazide has still been shown to reduce the calcium/sodium in the urine, indicating an effect independent of PTH. In our studies of isolated kidneys, where renal perfusion pressure and perfusate volume are constant, thiazides have been found to exert a direct effect on the kidney to diminish calcium excretion relative to sodium excretion (Figure 1). Microperfusion studies have localized the increase in calcium reabsorption in response to chlorothiazide to the distal convoluted tubule (79), predominantly to its early portion (80).

Potassium-Sparing Diuretics

Agents such as spironolactone (a competitive receptor antagonist of aldosterone) and triamterene or amiloride (which appear to block sodium channels) act at late distal tubular exchange sites to interfere with sodium potassium hydrogen ion exchange. As a result, urinary sodium and water excretion is increased while potassium- and hydrogen-ion excretion is diminished. In acute studies, triamterene has been found to cause an early increased urinary calcium excretion, followed by a reduction in urinary calcium after 6 hr (58). In other studies, water-loaded rats that received triamterene were shown to have significantly higher urine-sodium concentrations, while urinary calcium and magnesium were reduced (81). Still other studies in anesthetized dogs demonstrated that triamterene increased the clearance of sodium but had no consistent effect on that of calcium (78). Following administration of triamterene in isolated, blood-perfused dog kidneys, we observed an enhanced excretion of sodium relative to calcium (Figure 1). In a number of cases, calcium excretion was actually reduced. The effect of amiloride on calcium excretion was similar to that of triamterene. Microperfusion studies in rats and isolated segments of the rabbit nephron indicate that amiloride inhibits sodium reabsorption and potassium secretion and reverses the lumen-negative potential in the lumen of cortical collecting tubules, but has no effect in the cortical thick ascending limb (82, 83). Consistent with an action in the distal portion of the nephron, the direct intrarenal infusion of amiloride in clearance studies in dogs has been shown to produce a unilateral hypocalciuric effect (78). Recent microperfusion studies have localized enhancement of calcium absorption to the late segments of the distal tubule with little or no effect on the early distal convoluted tubule (84). Thus, the effects of amiloride on calcium can be observed even after administration of diuretics having earlier nephron sites of action. The hypocalciuric action of amiloride has been found to persist during furosemide diuresis in rats prepared for renal clearance studies (63) and in isolated blood-perfused dog kidneys (Figure 2). Maximally effective doses of amiloride and chlorothiazide have additive effects of reducing the ratio of calcium clearance/ sodium clearance (78). That this additivity is the result of different sites of action rather than different mechanisms of action is borne out by microperfusion studies indicating that the principal action of chlorothiazide is on the early distal convoluted tubule and that of amiloride is on the late distal convoluted tubule (80). It is unclear whether the increased calcium absorption of diuretics acting at the distal convoluted tubule and collecting duct is the result of loss of the lumen-negative transmembrane potential or whether it is the result of increased rates of sodium-calcium exchange. Although the increase in calcium absorption with amiloride is highly correlated with the decrease in sodium reabsorption, a similar quantitative relationship using chlorothiazide could not be established (80). Unlike thiazide diuretics, which markedly increase urinary potassium excretion, triamterene lowers urinary potassium, suggesting that the dissociation of sodium and calcium transport is not directly related to potassium in the distal tubule.

Spironolactone, like triamterene and amiloride, increases sodium excretion but decreases potassium excretion. In this case, the effects are dependent upon aldosterone blockade, since they are not observed in adrenalectomized animals. In intact dogs, adrenalectomy decreases the clearance of calcium relative to sodium. Subsequent administration of aldosterone increases the urinary calcium/sodium primarily by reducing the clearance of sodium (85). In rats on a low-calcium diet, mineralocorticoid administration increases calcium excretion, while sodium excretion is reduced (86). The effect of mineralocorticoids on urinary calcium excretion was thought to be due to extracellular fluid volume expansion subsequent to sodium retention, since an associated study in rats fed a diet low in sodium and calcium revealed no change in urinary calcium. In man, acute administration of aldosterone has resulted in inconsistent changes (87) or no change (88) in calcium excretion whereas spironolactone (Aldactone) has been found to increase both urinary calcium and sodium (89, 90). The latter results with calcium have been questioned subsequently, since substantial quantities of calcium were present in the spironolactone preparation administered (91), and the administration of vehicle alone produced the same degree of calciuria. It is likely that spironolactone may decrease the clearance of calcium relative to sodium clearance, as in the case of adrenalectomy. Taken together, these results indicate that aldosterone and the reversal of its effects exert only a modest influence on urinary calcium reabsorption in the distal nephron. The greater dissociation and hypocalciuria with triamterene and amiloride probably relate to a more complete inhibition of sodium reabsorption in terminal nephron segments by these agents.

CLINICAL USES OF DIURETICS WITH RESPECT TO CALCIUM

The differential actions of diuretic agents on calcium excretion have proved helpful in the clinical management of hypercalcemic and hypercalciuric states. In the former case, administration of furosemide and volume replacement with saline have been used to reduce plasma calcium concentrations acutely (92) and in the latter case of thiazides, to diminish urinary calcium levels. Although hypercalcemia usually does not result from thiazide treatment, an increased prevalence has been reported in patients with underlying disorders, such as primary hyperparathyroidism (93). In such cases hypercalcemia can be reversed by stopping thiazide treatment. Use of carbonic anhydrase inhibitors in the treatment of renal stone formation is limited to alkalinization of the urine. In patients forming calcium calculii, carbonic anhydrase inhibitors may increase urinary calcium excretion and promote calcium stone formation. Renal nephrolithiasis accounts for approximately 2–3% of hospital admissions (94). About 70% of kidney stones are composed of calcium oxalate and/or calcium phosphate. Normocalcemic hypercalciuria appears to predispose to calcium stone formation. Thiazide diuretics have been shown to reduce both calcium excretion and stone incidence in hypercalciuric patients (95). Combined use of thiazides and amiloride may be therapeutically advantageous since the hypocalciuric effects of these diuretics are additive while the hypokalemia produced by thiazides is prevented by amiloride (96, 97).

SUMMARY AND CONCLUSIONS

Diuretic agents have variable effects on calcium excretion as studied in vivo and in isolated kidneys and nephron segments. Generally, by increasing sodium and water excretion, diuretics will cause a concomitant increase in calcium excretion. As they diminish blood volume and alter renal hemodynamics, diuretics enhance calcium reabsorption in the proximal tubule, modulating their usual effects on calcium excretion. These general effects can be further modulated by additional metabolic actions. For instance, chronic administration of thiazide diuretics may diminish calcium excretion on the basis of altered levels of or responsiveness to PTH. Agents such as acetazolamide, which diminish bicarbonate reabsorption in the proximal tubule, will cause a modest calciuria, if any, because of reabsorption of the increased delivery of calcium, but not sodium, at the distal nephron. Agents acting in the loop of Henle that increase chloride excretion relative to sodium tend to cause greater calcium excretion. Finally, agents that act beyond the loop of Henle, which have their primary effects on cation excretion, tend to cause lesser degrees of calcium excretion, especially relative to sodium. These principles indicate that it may be appropriate to select a specific diuretic agent for different patients, depending upon the state of their calcium balance. It also may be possible to predict alterations in calcium balance, so that these may be anticipated and compensated for with patients on long-term therapy with various diuretic agents.

ACKNOWLEDGMENTS

The excellent secretarial assistance of Gail Price and Pam Blank is gratefully acknowledged. This work was supported in part by National Institute of Health Research Grant HL-28179.

Literature Cited

1. Baglin, A., Prinseau, J. 1981. Diurétiques et calcium. *Nephrologie* 2:189–96
2. Suki, W. N. 1982. Effects of diuretics on calcium metabolism. *Adv. Exp. Med. Biol.* 151:493–500
3. Sutton, R. A. L. 1985. Diuretics in calcium metabolism. *Am. J. Kidney Dis.* 5:4–9
4. Harris, C. A., Baer, P. G., Chirito, E., Dirks, J. H. 1974. Composition of mammalian glomerular filtrate. *Am. J. Physiol.* 227:972–76
5. Lassiter, W. E., Gottschalk, C. W., Mylle, M. 1963. Micropuncture study of renal tubular reabsorption of calcium in normal rodents. *Am. J. Physiol.* 204: 771–75

6. LeGrimellec, C., Poujeol, P., de-Rouffignac, C. 1975. ^{3}H-inulin and electrolyte concentrations in Bowman's capsule in rat kidney. *Pfluegers Arch.* 354:117–31

7. Toribara, T. Y., Terepka, A. R., Dewey, P. A. 1957. The ultrafiltrable calcium in human serum. I. Ultrafiltration methods and normal values. *J. Clin. Invest.* 36:738–48

8. Duarte, C. G., Watson, J. F. 1967. Calcium reabsorption in proximal tubule of the dog nephron. *Am. J. Physiol.* 212:1355–60

9. Agus, Z. S., Gardner, L. B., Beck, L. H., Goldberg, M. 1973. Effects of parathyroid hormone on renal tubular reabsorption of calcium, sodium and phosphate. *Am. J. Physiol.* 224:1143–48

10. Edwards, B. R., Sutton, R. A. L., Dirks, J. H. 1974. Effect of calcium infusion on renal tubular reabsorption in the dog. *Am. J. Physiol.* 227:13–18

11. Ullrich, K. J., Rumrich, G., Kloss, S. 1976. Active Ca^{2+} reabsorption in the proximal tubule of the rat kidney. Dependence on sodium and buffer transport. *Pfluegers Arch.* 364:223–28

12. Suki, W. N. 1979. Calcium transport in the nephron. *Am. J. Physiol.* 237:F1–F6

13. Kinne-Saffran, E., Kinne, R. 1974. Localization of a calcium-stimulated ATPase in the basal-lateral plasma membranes of the proximal tubule of the rat kidney cortex. *J. Membr. Biol.* 17:263–74

14. Doucet, A., Katz, A. I. 1982. High-affinity Ca-Mg-ATPase along the rabbit nephron. *Am. J. Physiol.* 242:F346–52

15. DeRouffignac, C., Morel, F., Moss, N., Roinel, N. 1973. Micropuncture study of water and electrolyte movements along the loop of Henle in *Psammomys* with special reference to magnesium, calcium and phosphorus. *Pfluegers Arch.* 344:309–26

16. Jamison, R. L., Frey, N. R., Lacy, F. B. 1974. Calcium reabsorption in the thin loop of Henle. *Am. J. Physiol.* 227:745–51

17. Rouse, D., Ng, R. C. K., Suki, W. N. 1980. Calcium transport in the pars recta and thin descending limb of Henle of the rabbit, perfused in vitro. *J. Clin. Invest.* 65:37–42

18. Shareghi, G. R., Stoner, L. C. 1978. Calcium transport across segments of the rabbit distal nephron in vitro. *Am. J. Physiol.* 235:F367–75

19. Bourdeau, J. E., Burg, M. B. 1979. Voltage dependence of calcium transport in the thick ascending limb of Henle's loop. *Am. J. Physiol.* 236:F357–64

20. Suki, W. N., Rouse, D., Ng, R. C. K., Kokko, J. P. 1980. Calcium transport in the thick ascending limb of Henle. Heterogeneity of function in the medullary and cortical segments. *J. Clin. Invest.* 66:1004–9

21. Burg, M. B. 1982. Thick ascending limb of Henle's loop. *Kidney Int.* 22:454–64

22. Rocha, A. S., Magaldi, J. B., Kokko, J. P. 1977. Calcium and phosphate transport in isolated segments of rabbit Henle's loop. *J. Clin. Invest.* 59:975–83

23. Imai, M. 1978. Calcium transport across the rabbit thick ascending limb of Henle's loop perfused in vitro. *Pfluegers Arch.* 374:255–63

24. Agus, Z. S., Chiu, P. J. S., Goldberg, M. 1977. Regulation of urinary calcium excretion in the rat. *Am. J. Physiol.* 232:F545–49

25. Rizzoli, R., Fleisch, H., Bonjour, J.-P. 1977. Effect of thyroparathyroidectomy on calcium metabolism in rats: role of 1,25-dihydroxyvitamin D_3. *Am. J. Physiol.* 233:E160–64

26. Puschett, J. B., Moranz, J., Kurnick, W. S. 1972. Evidence for a direct action of cholecalciferol and 25-hydroxycholecalciferol on the renal transport of phosphate, sodium, and calcium. *J. Clin. Invest.* 51:373–85

27. Alon, U., Wellons, M. D., Chan, J. C. M. 1983. Reversal of vitamin-D2-induced hypercalciuria by chlorothiazide. *Pediatr. Res.* 17:117–19

28. Sutton, R. A. L., Dirks, J. H. 1980. Renal handling of calcium, phosphate, and magnesium. In *The Kidney*, ed. B. M. Brenner, F. C. Rector Jr., pp. 551–618. Philadelphia: Saunders

29. Walser, M. 1961. Calcium clearance as a function of sodium clearance in the dog. *Am. J. Physiol.* 200:1099–1104

30. Sutton, R. A. L., Wong, N. L. M., Dirks, J. H. 1976. Effects of parathyroid hormone on sodium and calcium transport in the dog nephron. *Clin. Sci. Mol. Med.* 51:345–51

31. Bourdeau, J. E., Burg, M. B. 1980. Effect of PTH on calcium transport across the cortical thick ascending limb of Henle's loop. *Am. J. Physiol.* 239:F121–26

32. Imai, M. 1981. Effects of parathyroid hormone and N^6, $O^{2'}$-dibutyrl cyclic AMP on Ca^{2+} transport across the rabbit distal nephron segments perfused in vitro. *Pfluegers Arch.* 390:145–51

33. Shareghi, G. R., Agus, Z. S. 1982. Phosphate transport in the light segment of the

rabbit cortical collecting tubule. *Am. J. Physiol.* 242:F379–84

34. Chabardes, D., Imbert, M., Clique, A., Montegut, M., Morel, F. 1975. PTH sensitive adenyl cyclase activity in different segments of the rabbit nephron. *Pfluegers Arch.* 354:229–39

35. Sorensen, O. H., Hindberg, I. 1972. The acute and prolonged effect of porcine calcitonin on urine electrolyte excretion in intact and parathyroidectomized rats. *Acta Endocrinol.* 70:295–307

36. Rasmussen, H., Anast, C., Arnaud, C. 1967. Thyrocalcitonin, EGTA, and urinary electrolyte excretion. *J. Clin. Invest.* 46:746–52

37. Clark, J. D., Kenny, A. D. 1969. Hog thyrocalcitonin in the dog: urinary calcium, phosphorus, magnesium and sodium responses. *Endocrinology* 84:1199–1205

38. Aldred, J. P., Kleszynski, R. R., Bastian, J. W. 1970. Effects of acute administration of porcine and salmon calcitonin on urine electrolyte excretion in rats. *Proc. Soc. Exp. Biol. Med.* 134:1175–80

39. Quamme, G. A. 1980. Effect of calcitonin on calcium and magnesium transport in rat nephron. *Am. J. Physiol.* 238:E573–78

40. Chabardes, D., Imbert-Teboul, M., Montegut, M., Clique, A., Morel, F. 1976. Distribution of calcitonin-sensitive adenylate cyclase activity along the rabbit kidney tubule. *Proc. Natl. Acad. Sci. USA* 73:3608–12

41. Suki, W. N., Rouse, D. 1981. Hormonal regulation of calcium transport in thick ascending limb renal tubules. *Am. J. Physiol.* 241:F171–74

42. Blythe, W. B., Gitelman, H. J., Welt, L. G. 1968. Effect of expansion of the extracellular space on the rate of urinary excretion of calcium. *Am. J. Physiol.* 214:52–57

43. Goldberg, M., Agus, Z. S., Goldfarb, S. 1976. Renal handling of phosphate, calcium and magnesium. See Ref. 28, pp. 340–90

44. Massry, S. G., Ahumada, J. J., Coburn, J. W., Kleeman, C. R. 1970. Effect of MgCl₂ infusion on urinary Ca and Na during reduction in their filtered loads. *Am. J. Physiol.* 219:881–85

45. Lau, K., Goldfarb, S., Goldberg, M., Agus, Z. S. 1982. Effects of phosphate administration on tubular calcium transport. *J. Lab. Clin. Med.* 99:317–24

46. Sutton, R. A. L., Wong, N. L. M., Dirks, J. H. 1979. Effects of metabolic acidosis and alkalosis on sodium and

calcium transport in the dog kidney. *Kidney Int.* 15:520–33

47. Gonda, A., Wong, N., Seely, J. F., Dirks, J. H. 1969. The role of hemodynamic factors on urinary calcium and magnesium excretion. *Can. J. Physiol. Pharmacol.* 47:619–26

48. Barker, E. S., Elkinton, J. R., Clark, J. K. 1959. Studies of the renal excretion of magnesium in man. *J. Clin. Invest.* 38:1733–45

49. Sotornik, I., Schuck, O., Stribrna, J. 1969. Influence of diuretics on renal calcium excretion. *Experientia* 25:591–92

50. Eknoyan, G., Suki, W. N., Martinez-Maldonado, M. 1970. Effect of diuretics on urinary excretion of phosphate, calcium, and magnesium in thyroparathyroidectomized dogs. *J. Lab. Clin. Med.* 76:257–66

51. Besarab, A., Pomerantz, P., Swanson, J. W. 1982. Effect of exogenous adenosine 3′ : 5′-cyclic monophosphate, parathyroid hormone and acetazolamide on electrolyte excretion by the isolated perfused rat kidney. *Renal Physiol.* 5:124–35

52. Gemba, M., Nishimura, K. 1977. Effects of diuretics on calcium excretion and Ca⁺⁺-activated ATPase in rat kidney. *Jpn. J. Pharmacol.* 27:205–11

53. Beck, L. H., Goldberg, M. 1973. Effects of acetazolamide and parathyroidectomy on renal transport of sodium, calcium, and phosphate. *Am. J. Physiol.* 224:1136–42

54. Dan, T., Gemba, M. 1980. Effects of diuretics on calcium uptake and release in renal microsomes. *Biochem. Pharmacol.* 29:2339–43

55. Steinmetz, P. R., Koeppen, B. M. 1984. Cellular mechanisms of diuretic action along the nephron. *Hosp. Prac.* 19:125–34

56. Bourdeau, J. E., Buss, S. L., Vurek, G. G. 1982. Inhibition of calcium absorption in the cortical thick ascending limb of Henle's loop by furosemide. *J. Pharmacol. Exp. Ther.* 221:815–19

57. Antoniou, L. D., Eisner, G. M., Slotkoff, L. M., Lilienfield, L. S. 1967. Sodium and calcium transport in the kidney. *Clin. Res.* 15:476 (Abstr.)

58. Hanze, S., Seyberth, H. 1967. Effects of the diuretics furosemide and ethacrynic acid and triamterene on renal magnesium and calcium excretion. *Klin. Wochenschr.* 45:313–14

59. Duarte, C. G. 1968. Effects of ethacrynic acid and furosemide on urinary calcium, phosphate and magnesium. *Metabolism* 17:867–76

60. Antoniou, L. D., Eisner, G. M., Slot-

koff, L. M., Lilienfield, L. S. 1969. Relationship between sodium and calcium transport in the kidney. *J. Lab. Clin. Med.* 74:410–20

61. Tambyah, J. A., Lim, M. K. L. 1969. Effect of furosemide on calcium excretion. *Br. Med. J.* 1:751–52

62. Edwards, B. R., Baer, P. G., Sutton, R. A. L., Dirks, J. H. 1973. Micropuncture study of diuretic effects on sodium and calcium reabsorption in the dog nephron. *J. Clin. Invest.* 52:2418–27

63. Devane, J., Ryan, M. P. 1983. Dose-dependent reduction in renal magnesium clearance by amiloride during furosemide-induced diuresis in rats. *Br. J. Pharmacol.* 80:421–28

64. Quamme, G. A. 1981. Effect of furosemide on calcium and magnesium transport in the rat nephron. *Am. J. Physiol.* 241:F340–47

65. Parfitt, A. M. 1969. The acute effects of mersalyl, chlorothiazide and mannitol on the renal excretion of calcium and other ions in man. *Clin. Sci.* 36:267–82

66. Walser, M. 1971. Calcium-sodium interdependence in renal transport. In *Renal Pharmacology*, ed. J. W. Fischer, E. J. Cafruny, pp. 21–41. New York: Appleton-Century-Crofts.

67. Demartini, F. E., Briscoe, A. M., Ragan, C. 1967. Effect of ethacrynic acid on calcium and magnesium excretion. *Proc. Soc. Exp. Biol. Med.* 124:320–24

68. Duarte, C. G., Bland, J. H. 1965. Calcium, phosphorus and uric acid clearances after intravenous administration of chlorothiazide. *Metabolism* 14:211–19

69. Costanzo, L. S., Weiner, I. M. 1974. On the hypocalciuric action of chlorothiazide. *J. Clin. Invest.* 54:628–37

70. Lamberg, B. A., Kuhlback, B. 1959. Effect of chlorothiazide and hydrochlorothiazide on the excretion of calcium in urine. *Scand. J. Clin. Lab. Invest.* 11:351–57

71. Higgins, B. A., Nassim, J. R., Collins, J., Hilb, A. 1964. The effect of bendrofluazide on urine calcium excretion. *Clin. Sci.* 27:457–62

72. Seitz, H. Jaworski, Z. F. 1964. Effect of hydrochlorothiazide on serum and urinary calcium and urinary citrate. *Can. Med. Assoc. J.* 90:414–20

73. Brickman, A. S., Massry, S. C., Coburn, J. W. 1972. Changes in serum and urinary calcium during treatment with hydrochlorothiazide: Studies on mechanisms. *J. Clin. Invest.* 51:945–54

74. Parfitt, A. M. 1972. The interactions of thiazide diuretics with parathyroid hormone and vitamin D. Studies in patients with hypoparathyroidism. *J. Clin. Invest.* 51:1879–88

75. Yendt, E. R., Cohanim, M. 1978. Prevention of calcium stones with thiazides. *Kidney Int.* 13:397–409

76. Costanzo, L. S., Moses, A. M., Rao, K. J., Weiner, I. M. 1975. Dissociation of calcium and sodium clearances in patients with hypoparathyroidism by infusion of chlorothiazide. *Metabolism* 24:1367–73

77. Quamme, G. A., Wong, N. L. M., Sutton, R. A. L., Dirks, J. H. 1975. Interrelationship of chlorothiazide and parathyroid hormone: a micropuncture study. *Am. J. Physiol.* 229:200–5

78. Costanzo, L. S., Weiner, I. M. 1976. Relationship between clearances of Ca and Na: effect of distal diuretics and PTH. *Am. J. Physiol.* 230:67–73

79. Costanzo, L. S., Windhager, E. E. 1978. Calcium and sodium transport by the distal convoluted tubule of the rat. *Am. J. Physiol.* 235:F492–F506

80. Costanzo, L. S. 1985. Localization of diuretic action in microperfused rat distal tubules: Ca and Na transport. *Am. J. Physiol.* 248:F527–35

81. Ryan, M. P., Phillips, O. 1977. Diuretic-induced calcium and magnesium excretion in the rat. *Irish J. Med. Sci.* 146:303

82. Duarte, C. G., Chomety, F., Giebisch, G. 1971. Effect of amiloride, ouabain, and furosemide on distal tubular function in the rat. *Am. J. Physiol.* 221:632–39

83. Stoner, L. C., Burg, M. B., Orloff, J. 1974. Ion transport in cortical collecting tubule; effect of amiloride. *Am. J. Physiol.* 227:453–59

84. Costanzo, L. S. 1984. Comparison of calcium and sodium transport in early and late rat distal tubules; effect of amiloride. *Am. J. Physiol.* 246:F937–45

85. Massry, S. G., Coburn, J. W., Chapman, L. W., Kleeman, C. R. 1967. The acute effect of adrenal steroids on the interrelationship between the renal excretion of sodium, calcium and magnesium. *J. Lab. Clin. Med.* 70:563–70

86. Suki, W. N., Schwettmann, R. S., Rector, F. C., Seldin, D. W. 1968. Effect of chronic mineralocorticoid administration on calcium excretion in the rat. *Am. J. Physiol.* 215:71–74

87. Lamberg, B. A., Paloheimo, J., Torsti, P. 1964. Changes in the urinary excretion of calcium after intravenous injection of aldosterone. *Acta Med. Scand.* 179: (Suppl. 412):205–13

88. Lemann, J. Jr., Piering, W. F., Lennon, E. J. 1970. Studies of the acute effects of aldosterone and cortisol on the in-

terrelationship between renal sodium, calcium and magnesium excretion in normal man. *Nephron* 7:117–30

89. Wills, M. R., Gill, J. R., Bartter, F. C. 1969. The interrelationships of calcium and sodium excretions. *Clin. Sci.* 37:621–30

90. Ben-Ishai, D., Viskoper, R. J., Menczel, J. 1972. Effect of spironolactone on urinary calcium excretion. *Israel J. Med. Sci.* 8:495–501

91. Prati, R. C., Alfrey, A. C., Hull, A. R. 1972. Spironolactone-induced hypercalciuria. *J. Lab. Clin. Med.* 80:224–30

92. Suki, W. N., Yium, J. J., Von Minden, M., Saller-Hebert, C., Eknoyan, G., Martinez-Maldonado, M. 1970. Acute treatment of hypercalcemia with furosemide. *N. Engl. J. Med.* 283:836–40

93. Christensson, T., Hellstrom, K., Wengle, B. 1977. Hypercalcemia and primary hyperparathyroidism. *Arch. Int. Med.* 137:1138–42

94. Nordin, B. E. C., Hodgkinson, A., Peacock, M., Robertson, W. G. 1979. Urinary tract calculi. In *Nephrology*, ed. J. Hamburger, J. Crosnier, J. P. Grunsfeld, pp. 1090–1128. New York: Wiley

95. Cunningham, E., Oliveros, F. H., Nascimento, L. 1982. Metolazone therapy of active calcium nephrolithiasis. *Clin. Pharmacol. Ther.* 32:642–45

96. Leppla, D., Browne, R., Hill, K., Pak, C. Y. C. 1983. Effect of amiloride with or without hydrochlorothiazide on urinary calcium and saturation of calcium salts. *J. Clin. Endocrinol. Metab.* 57:920–24

97. Alon, U., Costanzo, L. S., Chan, J. C. M. 1984. Additive hypocalciuric effects of amiloride and hydrochlorothiazide in patients treated with calcitriol. *Min. Elec. Metab.* 10:379–86

Ann. Rev. Pharmacol. Toxicol. 1986 26:117–42
Copyright © 1986 by Annual Reviews Inc. All rights reserved

MARINE PHARMACOLOGY: BIOACTIVE MOLECULES FROM THE SEA

Pushkar N. Kaul and Pratibha Daftari

Department of Biology, Atlanta University, Atlanta, Georgia 30314

INTRODUCTION

Mankind has known for at least several thousand years that marine organisms contain substances capable of potent biological activity (1). Undoubtedly we are aware that most of the currently available therapeutic agents stem either directly or indirectly from naturally occurring organic molecules derived from terrestrial plants and/or animals. However, the abundant floras and faunas inhabiting the 70% of the Earth's surface covered by the ocean waters remain relatively unexplored. It is only in the past three decades that a significant research activity has suggested that the sea offers an enormous biomedical potential yet to be harnessed by man.

Attention to pharmacologically active substances in the sea in recent decades was first drawn by Emerson & Taft (2). Several subsequent reviews and monographs have dealt mostly with the pharmacology and toxicity of crude and semipurified extracts of marine organisms (3–13). More recent reviews, however, describe the pharmacology of some of the pure compounds of marine origin (14–17).

This review focuses on pharmacological activities of pure compounds isolated from marine organisms, as well as the pharmacologic activities of some highly potent substances broadly given the notorious name of marine toxins. Note that we take the same view of toxicity as Paracelsus—that at a given dosage level all compounds are toxic but that the right dose via the right route can make all the difference. Digitalis and tetrodotoxin (18) are but two examples among many that support this view.

117

CARDIOVASCULAR-ACTIVE SUBSTANCES

Marine Nucleosides

When subjected to chemical and pharmacological characterizations, an asystolic factor and a cardiotonic fraction from extracts of the sponge *Dasychalina cyathina* (19) led to the isolation of adenosine (20) and 2'-deoxyadenosine (21). Both these nucleosides showed negative inotropic and chronotropic activities on the isolated perfusing guinea-pig heart, leading to a heart block and a coronary vasodilation as would be expected of adenosine (particularly the heart block) (22). Spongosine, a methoxy derivative of adenosine (Figure 1), was obtained from the extract of the Caribbean sponge, *Cryptotethia crypta,* while being studied for the isolation of another asystolic activity (23). It should be pointed out here that it was the structural modification of an unusual arabinosylnucleoside obtained from *C. crypta* (24) that led to the development of cytosine arabinoside (ara C), a clinically effective antileukemic drug of choice available today (25). Doridosine, N^1-methylisoguanosine, was isolated from the nudibranch *Anisodoris nobilis* and found to be a prolonged hypotensive agent (26).

A comparative cardiovascular study (23) of various marine nucleosides in our laboratories shows that these compounds reduce both the rate and the force of contraction of the heart; their relative potencies are adenosine > doridosine > isoguanosine > spongosine. However, their potencies in increasing the coronary flow as a result of coronary dilation are adenosine > spongosine > isoguanosine > doridosine. Caffeine, a blocker of adenosinergic receptors, blocks these effects of marine nucleosides on the force as well as rate of myocardiac contractility, but somewhat less effectively on the coronary flow. Whether or not different types of purinergic receptors are involved in mediating the cardiac muscular and vascular effects remains an open question.

The hypotensive response in anesthetized rats and guinea pigs was most pronounced in the case of doridosine, followed by spongosine and isoguanosine. This may be attributable to the relatively longer half-life of the nucleosides in question, for in vitro incubation of these compounds with adenosine deaminase revealed virtually no disappearance with time of doridosine and less than 5% decrease of spongosine concentrations (P. Kaul, unpublished). On the other hand, adenosine disappeared rapidly while isoguanosine exhibited an intermediate rate of disappearance.

Intraperitoneal (i.p.) injections of the marine nucleosides (1–50 μg/kg) in mice as well as their injection into the lateral ventricles of conscious guinea pigs produced a dose-dependent fall in body temperature (27). The rate, magnitude, and duration of hypothermia were most profound in the case of doridosine, followed by spongosine and isoguanosine. This prolonged effect may be due to

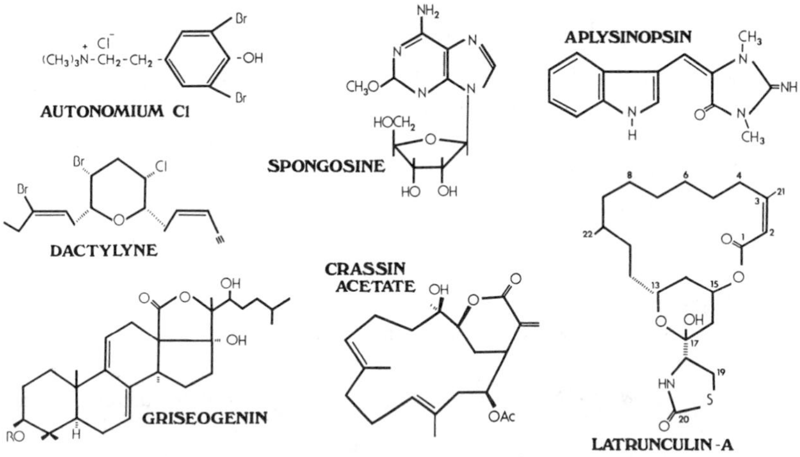

Figure 1   Various pharmacologically active molecules isolated from marine organisms.

a relatively slow disappearance of doridosine. The hypothermia was dose-dependently attenuated by pretreatment with theophylline (1–10 µg/kg i.p.). These prolonged hypotensive (26) and hypothermic (27) effects of doridosine make it an interesting candidate for further studies to determine its detailed pharmacological and toxicity profiles in order to assess its potential as a clinically useful agent.

Recently, pharmacology of two novel halogenated pyrrolopyrimidine derivatives of adenosine from marine organisms has been reported (28). 4-Amino-5-bromo-pyrrolo [2,3-d] pyrimidine from a sponge of genus *Echinodictyum* exhibited bronchodilatory activity similar to that of theophylline, but unlike theophylline it did not possess any central anti-adenosinergic activity. However, it has a potent inhibitory effect on adenosine reuptake and adenosine kinase in the brain tissue. The compound (10 or 30 mg/kg p.o.) had no significant effect on the heart rate or blood pressure of normotensive rats and only a small (about 5%) depressor effect in the desoxycorticosterone acetate (DOCA)/salt hypertensive rats.

The other nucleoside, 5'-deoxy-5-iodotubercidin, isolated from the red alga *Hypnea valentiae,* was found to be a muscle relaxant and hypothermic in mice. It was a very potent inhibitor of adenosine kinase of guinea-pig and rat brains and of rat liver. Interestingly, neither of the compounds was a substrate for or an inhibitor of adenosine deaminase. The iodotubercidin compound appears to be unique in that it is the first example of a naturally occurring 5'-deoxyribosyl nucleoside and an iodinated nucleoside (28). Because of its structural uniqueness and highly potent inhibitory activity on adenosine kinase, it may turn out to be an interesting research tool in physiology and pharmacology.

Marine Glycosides and Saponins

Terrestrial plants richly abound in glycosides and saponins, but in the animal kingdom only marine organisms have been found to contain these compounds, exclusively in the phylum *Echinodermata*. Of the five classes of this phylum, only *Holothuroidae* and *Asteroidae* contain appreciable quantities of saponins, generally referred to as holothurins and asterosaponins, respectively. The aglycones of the former are triterpenoids while those of the latter group are steroids analogous to the aglycones of digitalis glycosides. Holothurins in general appear to possess potent cardiotonic activity at low doses bordering on cardiotoxicity as observed on the isolated guinea pig heart (P. Kaul, B. Tursch, unpublished).

The well-known toxicity of starfishes is primarily due to the asterosaponins present in the starfish. These are lethal to fish (29–32) and toxic to annelids, molluscs, arthropods, and vertebrates (33, 34). Some of the purified saponins have been found, as would be expected, to cause hemolysis of fish and human erythrocytes blockable by cholesterol (31, 33). Asterosaponins from various marine organisms interfere in protein metabolism and possess cytolytic activity (35), anti-inflammatory, analgesic, and hypotensive actions (36), and neuro-muscular junction blocking activity as observed in phrenic nerve–diaphragm preparations (37).

Like asterosaponins, holothurins from sea cucumbers are also ichthyotoxic (35, 38). The general toxicity of dilute holothurin solution has been demonstrated with coelenterates, nematodes, annelids, molluscs, crustaceans, frogs, and protozoa (39). The LD_{50} of holothurin-A in mice was found to be 9 mg/kg intravenously (i.v.) and 10 mg/kg i.p. (40). This compound elicits convulsions, rigidity of limbs, and respiratory depression (41). It is extremely toxic to mammals by the systemic route, but is nontoxic via the oral route because it is destroyed by stomach acid.

The holothurins possess potent hemolytic action blockable by cholesterol (42). Rats infected by *Trypanosoma lewisi* and subsequently treated with holothurin showed elevated parasitemia, but a reduced parasitemia was observed in rats given holothurin either prior to or simultaneously with the infection (43, 44). This partial protection against the parasite only when holothurin was given prior to the infection may suggest a possible interaction between the glycoside and the rat immune system.

The antifungal activity of various holotoxins (desulfated holothurins) can be ranked as follows: Holotoxin A = holotoxin B > holotoxin C > all the nine plant saponins tested (45). Holothurins are less active than the holotoxins. The polyene antibiotics, which are specifically antifungal, act by disrupting the membrane and rendering the fungal cell wall leaky (cholesterol can prevent the disruption). The antifungal activity of holotoxins and holothurins is probably also due to their ability to complex with or displace cholesterol. However, it is questionable if this antifungal activity of the marine glycosides is specific, for these compounds also are potent cytolytic agents in general. A number of reports have appeared on the cytotoxic and antitumor activities of holothurins (35, 46–49).

Most of the neurotoxicity data on holothurins come from experiments on rat phrenic nerve–diaphragm and frog sciatic nerve–muscle preparations. Holthurin-A produced an irreversible block of both the neuromuscular junction and the muscle. However, both these responses were prevented by preincubating the preparations with dilute solutions (10^{-9} M) of anticholinesterases, e.g. physostigmine and neostigmine (37, 50–52). On the intact and internally perfused squid giant axon preparation, holothurin-A solution (10^{-4} M) increased Na^+ permeability, resulting in the nerve-membrane depolarization, apparently via the same general mechanism of action as the holothurins, i.e. complexation with the membrane cholesterol (53).

The effects of marine glycosides on Na^+-K^+ ATPase –dependent active transport have been studied more recently (54). Several triterpenoid glycosides, tested for their inhibitory activity on the rat brain Na^+-K^+ ATPase and Mg^{2+}-ATPase in vitro, showed a concentration-dependent inhibition of both the enzymes. The differences in the sugar moiety of the glycosides did not seem to matter, but the absence of sulfate groups appeared to enhance the Na^+-K^+ ATPase inhibition over that of the Mg^{2+}-ATPase. In general, the triterpenoid glycosides of sea cucumbers are more potent inhibitors of the ATPases than the steroidal glycosides from starfishes. All of the glycosides, however, lose their ATPase as well as other activities after pre-interaction with cholesterol (42, 54, 55).

In a bioassay-guided isolation of a CNS-depressant and hypothermic principle from *Holothuria floridana,* a saponin possessing potent and dose-dependent hypothermic and hemolytic activities was obtained that on hydrolysis yielded a known genin (16; P. Kaul and F. Schmitz, unpublished), griseogenin (Figure 1).

Peptides

ANTHOPLEURINS   One of the pharmacologically most interesting groups of marine peptides is the group of anthopleurins isolated from *Anthopleura xanthogrammica* (Brandt) and *A. elegantissima* (Brandt), which yield anthopleurins A and B from the former (56) and C from the latter coelenterate (57). Anthopleurins (AP) are homologous peptides of 47–49 amino acid residues. On sequencing, the presence of 49 amino acids was revealed in AP-A, with three intramolecular disulfide bridges (58). These can be distinguished from AP-C by their two additional residues, and different residues at four locations (Figure 2).

AP-A produces a strong positive inotropic effect in various animal species without any effect on heart rate, blood pressure, or Na^+-K^+ ATPase. The

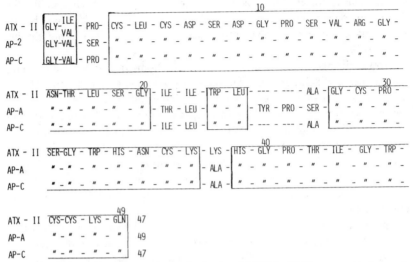

Figure 2   Amino acid sequences of anthopleurins A and C (AP-A, AP-C) compared to *Anemonia sulcata* toxin ATX-II. The boxed areas show common amino acids; the in-between areas show the differences in residues.

cardiotonic effect is unaffected by pretreatment with reserpine or α- and β-adrenergic blockers (59). In conscious dog, AP-A was found to be 35 times as cardiotonic as digoxin and nearly one third as toxic (60). Unlike digoxin, AP-A produced no ventricular extrasystole prior to the onset of ventricular fibrillation. At a single 2 μg/kg i.v. dose, AP-A increased the left ventricular pressure for over 2 hr in the conscious dog.

Conformational studies on AP-A with Laser-Raman and fluorescence spectroscopies reveal the molecule to be spherical with three pairs of CYS-CYS disulfide bridges (61). Correlation of structural modifications with cardiotonic activity revealed that the reduction of the disulfide bridges resulted in loss of activity and that most likely one or both of the lysine residues may be involved in mediating the response (62).

As a peptide of 5183 daltons, AP-A induces immune responses when given systemically to animals and loses activity when given orally (62). Obviously, systematic hydrolyses need to be carried out to explore the possibility of obtaining a smaller peptide that is either devoid of anaphylactic properties or is orally effective. This is analogous to the case of natural gastrin, which was replaced by an equally active pentapeptide, pentagastrin. The evidence that smaller peptides can be cardiotonic has come from another marine molecule, FMRFamide, a molluscan neurosecretory peptide. This tetrapeptide (Phe-Met-Arg-Phe-NH$_2$) stimulates cardiac as well as other excitable tissues (63). Further studies are clearly warranted to see if a tetra- or a pentapeptide can be obtained from AP-A, which retains the cardiotonic activity of the parent molecule.

CARDIOTOXIN-II   Biologically active polypeptides from sea anemones, resembling anthopleurins in both the amino acid sequence and cardiotonicity, have been studied extensively (64–70). Although seven peptides ranging from 2678 to 5630 daltons have been discovered (64), only anemonia toxin ATX-II has been studied at length.

A peptide of 47 amino acid residues (4770 daltons), ATX-II evoked a potent and dose-dependent cardiotonic response in various mammalian heart preparations. The changes in the steady-state cellular concentrations of Na^+, K^+, and Ca^{2+} affected by this peptide do not seem to account for its positive inotropic activity (65). Like AP-A, ATX-II also contains three pairs of cystein residues giving rise to three disulfide bridges and the resulting bifolded conformation (66). The primary difference between the amino acid sequences of ATX-II and AP-A lies in the charged center at residue 38, where second lysine of ATX-II is replaced by alanine in AP-A. This is 2–3 times as potent as the second lysine. This difference in the relative potencies has been attributed to this alanine/lysine variance, as well as to the considerably lower pKa value of the aspartate at residue 9 in ATX-II (69). Further structure-activity correlational studies have revealed that any modification of COOH in residue 9–aspartate or of arginine led to complete inactivation of ATX-II (70). It is conceivable that ionic dissociation, and thereby ionic and/or hydrogen bonding capability, of both these residues are involved in the interaction of ATX-II and the biological membrane receptors.

The cardiotonic effect of ATX-II is apparently not caused by a nonspecific membrane damage or by a direct action on the Na^+-K^+ ATPase, but by an indirect effect on the pump activity induced by increased Na^+ transport as a result of a delayed inactivation of fast sodium current (66). Thus, the sodium channels of the mammalian heart muscle cells appear to be the direct target for ATX-II. Further evidence in support of this sodium channel–specific action of this peptide has recently come from work on frog and mouse nerve–muscle preparations (68). The most characteristic action of ATX-II on the voltage-clamped denervated fast twitch muscle of the mouse is to slowly inactivate the Na^+ current. When this occurs, the rate constant of inactivation shows a reversed voltage dependence in the presence of the peptide. The significance of conformational disposition of these cardiotonic peptides from various sea anemones in relation to their activity was suggested originally for anthopleurins (57) but reemphasized recently for other peptides as well. The data obtained from comparative studies on AP-A and ATX-II, using circular dichroism and infrared spectroscopy and by application of modified Chou-Fasman method, suggest a similarity of the overall conformation of these peptides (71). This, coupled to their largely similar amino acid sequences, basicities, and three disulfide bridges, could explain their almost identical pharmacological activities. Similarity of cardiotonic activity of ATX-II to that of AP-A was emphatically pointed out years ago (64; L. Beress, personal communication).

OTHER PEPTIDES   Some of the less-studied peptides include a 147-residue peptide (20,000 daltons) from the sea anemone *Actinia equina*, which causes rapid hypotension, bradycardia, respiratory arrest in the intact rat, and pulmonary edema in preparations of the isolated rat lung (72); a 195-residue peptide (18,333 daltons) from the sea anemone *Condylactis gigantea*, which shows hemolytic action in rabbits blockable by sphingomyelin and is lethal to crayfish at nanogram doses (73); one of the smallest neurotoxic peptides (2000 daltons) from the sea anemone *Parasicyonis actinostoloides*, with an irreversible toxic action specific to crustacean neuronal tissue (74); several proteinase inhibitory, toxic, and hemolytic peptides ($\approx$6,000 daltons) from sea anemones of *Stoichactis* sp. (75, 76); a vasoactive and cardiotonic peptide (12,000 daltons) from a coral, *Goniopora* sp., which prolongs action potential in amphibian and mammalian atria caused by delayed inactivation of Na^+ current (77), analogous to the mechanism of action of ATX-II (66); and cytolasin A-III from the marine heteronemertine *Cerebratulus lacteus*, a highly basic protein (10,000 daltons) capable of binding to membrane macromolecules, with the help of its C-terminal region in an amphipathic helical conformation, and consequently able to release liposomal markers (78–80).

Autonomium

An unusual compound from *Verongia fistularis* (81) with an isosteric hybrid structure of epinephrine and acetylcholine, autonomium (Figure 1) exhibited not only α- and β-adrenergic activities blockable by the respective antagonists, but it also possessed cholinergic activity typical of acetylcholine. The distance between the quaternary nitrogen and the oxygen-bearing carbon in autonomium is 4.2 Å as compared with 4.1 Å for the same distance in acetylcholine (16). This interfunctional group distance may perhaps explain the cholinergic activity in autonomium. Likewise, the adrenergic activity may be gauged from the autonomium's β-phenethylamine structure typical of epinehrine. It is not uncommon to find biologic activities in compounds with structure and interatomic distances between functional sites similar to those of known naturally occurring bioactive compounds.

   Autonomium also shows CNS-stimulant effects in mice as gauged by a significant increase in spontaneous motor activity (81). The importance of such dual autonomically active compounds in marine environments is unknown, but it poses a question on the possibility of the occurrence of similar compounds in mammalians. Such compounds within CNS could conceivably play a role in regulating behavior, since much has been written on the balance between the cholinergic and the adrenergic systems within CNS required for normal behavior of both animals and man.

CYTOTOXIC/ANTICANCER COMPOUNDS

Perhaps hundreds of thousands of extracts, fractions, and compounds of marine origin have been screened by the NCI national testing program during the past three decades. Although the NCI's in vitro (KB) and in vivo (PS) tests have found as much as 10.9% of the tested samples from marine organisms to be active (82), only a few compounds have reached some degree of prominence and none other than cytosine arabinoside (ara C) is used clinically.

Cembranoids

Several dozens of 14-membered cyclic diterpenes (cembranoids) have been isolated from various species of soft corals and chemically characterized (82–85). Sinularin and its dihydro congener, both diterpene cembranoids with exocyclic lactones obtained from the soft coral *Sinularia flexibilis,* were found to be effective in the NCI's screens of potential anticancer agents (82). Crassin acetate (Figure 1) from the Caribbean gorgonian *Pseudoplexaura porosa* was found to possess no significant pharmacological activity in various mammalian systems and preparations but was cytotoxic (1–10 μg/ml) to mouse fibroblasts and human leukemic and HeLa cells in vitro (86). However, when this cembranoid was dissolved in dilute alkaline solutions in which the lactone opens up, the cytotoxic activity against cancer cells was lost several hundredfold. This observation should be a stimulus to medicinal chemists involved in structural design of drugs and structure-activity relational studies.

Some of the cembranoids have been found to deciliate protozoa (87) and larvae of a nudibranch (85). Of the five compounds tested, peunicin (5 ppm) was the most potent, paralyzing the larvae within 10 min of exposure. It is conceivable that some of these cembrane lactones or their structural modifications may be parasiticidal or spermicidal. These compounds clearly warrant further pharmacological investigations, since mammals tolerate the compounds relatively well (86).

Depsipeptides

Didemnins A, B, and C, cyclic depsipeptides from the Caribbean tunicate, *Trididemnum* sp., possess novel structural features (88). These compounds are potent inhibitors of L1210 leukemic cells in vitro, are active against P-388 leukemia and B-16 melanoma in vivo, and protect mice infected intravaginally with *Herpes simplex* type-2 virus (89). Clinical trials and other tests have revealed a high general toxicity of these compounds, but structural alterations and further testing should offer some hope in these novel compounds, particularly against *Herpes* infections.

Other Cytotoxic Agents

Antitumor and immunosuppressive effects of extracts and purified fractions of the sea squirt (tunicate) *Ecteinascidia turbinata* have been reported extensively since 1972, but to date no pure compound(s) with either of these activities has been isolated (90–93). An aqueous-alcoholic extract of the ascidian strongly inhibited the semiconservative DNA synthesis in human fibroblasts (93), which apparently is the primary mechanism of action for several antitumor compounds. However, in the ultraviolet-irradiated fibroblasts, only a weak inhibition of DNA excision repair was observed, which was also the case with arabinofuranosyl nucleosides, e.g. ara C and ara A (93). It should be interesting to witness the isolation of a pure molecular entity from *E. turbinata* possessing the claimed anticancer and immunomodulatory activities.

Of a series of 26-membered macrolides isolated from *Bugula neritina,* bryostatin and dolastatin have shown antileukemic activity in the NCI testing program (94). These macrolides are nearly twice the ring size of the anticancer cembranoids and represent a new class of potential anticancer molecules warranting further exploitation. A relatively new linear alcohol, triaconta-4,15,26-triene-1,12,18,29-tetrayne-3,14,17,28-tetraol, from a sponge of *Tetrosia* sp., has been found to inhibit mitosis in the sea urchin eggs at a concentration of 1 mg/ml (95). A number of similar polyacetylene alcohols have been isolated over the past several years, but their biological activity is yet to be determined.

An interesting observation has emerged more recently in the area of marine nucleosides, which had been found to occur only in sponges until a report appeared (96) that some of these nucleosides were isolated from the gorgonian *Eunicella cavolini*. Furthermore, the well-known antileukemic drug, ara A (9-B-D-arabinosyladenine), was originally developed as a semisynthetic modification of naturally occurring marine nucleosides, but now it has been found for the first time to exist in nature (96). Spongouridine, previously isolated from the sponge *Cryptotethia crypta* and found to possess antiviral activity, was also isolated from the coral *E. cavolini*.

A number of miscellaneous antitumor compounds and tumor promoters from marine prokaryotic organisms, especially the blue-green algae, have been described (97). A cyclic depsipeptide, majusculamide C from the alga *Lyngbya majuscula,* was found to partially inhibit X-5563 myeloma (0.5 mg/kg), but had no activity against P-388 leukemia, 6C3HED lymphoma, and 755 carcinoma in animal models. It is noteworthy that this compound resembles in structure the didemnins, which are also novel depsipeptides. However, didemnins have exhibited more potent and clear anticancer potential, though accompanied by extreme toxicity. Other carcinogenic-carcinostatic macromolecules from blue-green algae include aplysiatoxin, lingbyatoxin, teleocidins A and B, and oscillatoxins. Obviously, most of these potent macromolecules are far too toxic to be of practical clinical value as such. However, semisynthetic manipulations and structure-activity relationships should yield a viable avenue to the discovery of new anticancer agents.

Based on a good correlation observed for known anticancer agents between their potency and their ability to inhibit (a) microtubule assembly in the microtubule polymerization assay utilizing purified bovine brain microtubule proteins, and (b) synchronous cell division of the fertilized sea urchin eggs, 130 known and structurally defined marine organic compounds were screened by the two assays for potential anticancer activity (98). Nine compounds were found to inhibit the first division of the sea urchin embryo. Of these, elatol from *Laurencia elata* and its oxidation product, elatone, were found quite effective in the cell division assay, but only elatone was effective in the microtubule polymerization assay. This reflects some selectivity and specificity inherent in the latter assay. Subsequently, a polycyclic orthoquinone, stypoldione, from the brown seaweed *Stypodium zonale* was found to be a potent inactivator of soluble tubulin and thereby an inhibitor of the microtubule polymerization (99).

OTHER PHARMACOLOGIC ACTIVITIES

Enzyme Inhibitors

While pursuing the bioassay-guided isolation of a CNS-depressant activity in the crude extracts of sea hare, *Alysia dactylomela*, an unsaturated and halogenated cyclic ether, dactylyne (Figure 1), was isolated (100). This compound produced a dose-dependent prolongation of pentobarbital-induced hypnosis in animals but by itself did not have any other apparent effects. Detailed studies on its mechanism of action revealed that it inhibits the metabolism of pentobarbital (101). Other related halogenated cyclic ethers with exocyclic enine features also showed this pentobarbital potentiation, but dactylyne was the most potent of the compounds tested (102).

Since pentobarbital is eliminated largely by oxidation involving Cyt-P$_{450}$, we had proposed that through inhibition of this enzyme dactylyne might prove to be a general drug metabolism inhibitor of clinical value (103). Subsequent work has revealed that dactylyne does indeed reversibly bind to Cyt-P$_{450}$, as determined by spectral changes of the enzyme, and that it consequently inhibits the activity of the enzyme (P. Kaul and I. Schuster, unpublished). Enzyme inhibitors in molecular biology are becoming increasingly important in controlling cellular processes. The marine-derived enzyme inhibitors should be screened for activity against other enzymes of clinical significance. Furthermore, structural modifications for rigorous structure-activity studies may yield desired activities with specificity, the ultimate aim in designing restriction enzymes or enzyme inhibitors.

Anti-inflammatory and Antispasmodic Agents

Flexibilide, a diterpenoid cembrane from the soft coral *Sinularia flexibilis*, dendalone 3-hydroxybutyrate from the sponge *Phyllospongia dendyi*, and 6-*n*-tridecylsalicylic acid from the brown alga *Caulocystis cephalornithos* were found to be orally effective anti-inflammatory agents at 20–200 µmol/kg doses; the dendalone compound is the most potent but also most toxic (104). These marine compounds provide a different structural concept for anti-inflammatory activity from the usually accepted types of such pharmacologic agents.

Manoalide, a nonsteroidal anti-inflammatory compound isolated from the sponge *Luffariella variabilis*, is a rare molecular structure with analgesic activity and a selective anti-inflammatory profile, suggesting that it acts by directly inactivating phospholipase A_2 (105). This enzyme is a component of several neurotoxins and is also involved in prostaglandin synthesis in man. Manoalide, when pre-incubated with β-bungarotoxin, prevented the irreversible neurotoxicity of the toxin on the rat phrenic nerve–diaphragm preparation (105).

Marine indole derivatives, other than Tyrian purple known for 80 years, have been discovered only within the recent decade and are not yet extensively subjected to pharmacologic studies. Around 100 indoles, including many alkaloids, have been isolated from marine plants, acorn worms, gorgonians, sea anemones, sponges, and bryozoans (106). The indole alkaloids flustramine A and B, isolated from Swedish marine organism *Flustra foliacae* L. of the phylum Bryozoa (moss animals), were reported as muscle relaxants both in vitro and in vivo (107). These compounds weakened the grip of mice in the screen grip test and inhibited the contractions of isolated but electrically stimulated rat diaphragm and guinea-pig ileum. Contractions evoked by histamine were also inhibited by the two flustramines. Their mode of action, though unknown, appears to be different from other known relaxants.

Ionophore Antibiotics

Being experimentally the easiest of most bioassays, the antibiotic assays and therefore the antibiotic activities of marine-derived extracts, fractions, and pure compounds have been reported with the largest frequency and numbers (5, 6, 10, 12, 105–9). Despite such reports during the past three decades, no antibiotic of clinical significance has emerged. This is perhaps understandable in view of the fact that it is very difficult to surpass several broad-spectrum and specifically potent antibiotics available.

Recently, however, a novel polyether antibiotic, acanthifolicin, was isolated from the sponge *Pandaros acanthifolium* (110). In addition to being an interesting molecule structurally, it exhibits cytotoxic activity against certain cell lines but is lethal to mice at a 140 μg/kg i.v. dose. Another polyether cytotoxic compound, okadaic acid, has been isolated from two sponges of genus *Halichondria* (111). Also known as halichondrine-A, its LD_{50} in mice is 192 μg/kg i.v. It belongs to the group of compounds called ionophore polyethers capable of selectively carrying divalent ions such as Ca^{2+} across lipoidal membranes. However, in recent studies (112) okadaic acid caused contraction of various vascular smooth muscle preparations even in the absence of Ca^{2+}, a unique action indeed. This should reopen the question of mechanisms of smooth muscle contraction. Apparently, the role of okadaic acid–induced vascular contraction could not be explained by the Na^+K^+ pump involvement, since the acid has no effect on Na^+K^+ ATPase (112).

A group of unique boron-containing macrolide ionophores, aplasmomycins, has been isolated from the actinomycete *Streptomyces griseus,* probably of terrestrial origin, and found to be antimalarial against *Plasmodium berghei* (113). This may open inquiries into the development of new antimalarial drugs, as well as further exploration of marine microorganisms.

These types of polyether compounds have recently drawn much attention, but their toxicity appears to be relatively high. Whether or not any biomedically or clinically useful compounds will evolve out of these unique polyethers remains to be seen. There is no question, however, that these nearly linear macromolecules should be added to the list of other highly bioactive compounds from marine invertebrates that warrant investigation.

Latrunculins

Among scores of 14- and 16-membered macrocyclic diterpenes isolated from various corals and sponges, the most stimulating compounds perhaps are the latrunculins A (Figure 1) and B; these are isolated from a magnificent red-colored branching sponge, *Latruncula magnifica,* inhabiting the Red Sea at depths of 6–30 m (83, 114). The red juice expressed out of the fresh sponge into a fish aquarium agitates the fish within seconds and is lethal within 4–6 min apparently because of the latrunculin content of the juice.

Latrunculins at nanomolar concentrations induce profound changes in the microfilament organization without affecting the microtubules, an action strikingly similar to that of cytochalasins. In cultured mouse neuroblastoma clone NIE-115 and mouse fibroblasts, latrunculins (35 ng/ml) rapidly elicited morphological changes in the cells, which, however, were reversible upon removal of the marine compounds. Immunofluorescent studies revealed that the morphological changes resulted from the disruption of microfilaments at concentrations 1/10 to 1/100 that of cytochalasins. Also, unlike cytochalasins the latrunculins did not alter the rate of polymerization of the active filaments.

These differences have led to the belief that although the microfilament disruptive actions of the two classes of marine molecules are similar, their modes of action may be different (114).

Miscellaneous Activities

Aplysinopsin (Figure 1) from the yellow sponge *Verongia spengelii,* a tryptophan derivative, possesses cytotoxicity against KB, P-388, and L-1210 cell lines (115) as well as having an antidepressant profile in animals similar to that of imipramine (P. Kaul and S. Kulkarni, unpublished). When given orally, methylaplysinopsin from the sponge *Aplysinopsis reticulata* prevented the tetrabenazine-induced ptosis in mice and rats, inhibited MAO while simultaneously increasing brain serotonin concentration, reduced the neuronal reuptake of serotonin, and caused a generalized potentiation of serotonergic neurotransmission (116).

There are several dozens of compounds from marine invertebrates whose structures have been established, but on which only partial and preliminary pharmacological studies have been conducted. Some of these have shown hypotensive, antiarrhythmic, neuromuscular blocking, CNS depressant, and hypothermic activities (P. Kaul and F. Schmitz, unpublished).

MARINE TOXINS

It is beyond the scope of this review to include all of the marine toxins described as crude extracts, fractions, factors, amorphous mixtures, and structurally undefined molecules. Furthermore, it makes little sense to describe pharmacology of impure mixtures, because the pharmacology-toxicology and mode of action of pure toxins may eventually turn out to be quite different from parent crude materials. Therefore, this review is limited to only pure crystalline and structurally determined toxins, or those toxins whose homogeneity has been established prior to extensive studies. Even among these, only those toxins have been included that have either very potent activities or present an unusual mode of action.

Red-Tide Toxins

These toxins are produced by dinoflagellates that bloom periodically to produce both the toxins and the red carotenoid pigment, peridinin, believed to be responsible for the term "red tide." The main noxious species of this group of marine organisms include *Gonyaulax catenella, G. tamarensis,* and *Ptychodiscus brevis* (formerly known as *Gymnodinium breve*). The toxins accumulate in the shellfishes known to have a symbiotic relationship with the dinoflagellates; hence the name paralytic shellfish toxins.

The primary red-tide toxins isolated and studied at some length are saxitoxin (STX) produced by G. catenella, gonyautoxins (GTX$_{1-5}$) from G. tamarensis, and a number of lipid-soluble toxins from P. brevis (117). Like tetrodotoxin (TTX), the best-studied toxin, STX and GTXs are relatively polar heterocyclic molecules containing charged guanidinium groups.

SAXITOXIN AND GTXs   Also known as paralytic shellfish poisons, these toxins exhibit a pharmacological-toxicological profile similar to that of TTX. Mechanistically, these guanidinium-containing molecules bind specifically to the sodium channels on the outside of excitable membranes, allowing an influx of Na$^+$ in exchange for K$^+$ efflux within a few milliseconds, with the attendant membrane depolarization. Various aspects relative to the specificity and stoichiometry of binding of STX and TTX to sodium channel receptors have been thoroughly established (118–121). Although TTX and STX have no direct effect on the K$^+$ channel receptors, a natural analogue of TTX, chiriquitoxin, does affect K$^+$ channels in addition to resembling TTX in the rest of its electrophysiological effects (121).

BREVETOXIN   Within the past eight years, a large number of closely related toxins with varying and confusing nomenclature have been isolated from Ptychodiscus brevis and chemically characterized. This confusion has been somewhat cleared in a recent review (117), e.g. T$_{34}$ and GB-2 toxins claimed to be different by their respective discoverers have now been established as the same compound on the basis of comparative physicochemical data. In general, the lipid-soluble toxins produced by P. brevis have been classified into either hemolytic or neurotoxic groups. It is not clear how many toxins are produced by P. brevis grown in laboratory cultures, but the overall preponderance appears to be of the neurotoxins rather than the hemolytic components. At least several neurotoxins have been isolated either as crystalline or homogeneous materials.

The structure of brevetoxin-B (BTX-B) reveals a cyclic polyether nature of the molecule, with 11 fused oxygen-containing rings, an α, β-unsaturated lactone, and an aldehyde function (122, 123). Thus, unlike the paralytic shellfish poisons (TTX, STX, and GTX), the BTX-B does not contain any nitrogen. Earlier work with crystalline and homogeneous brevetoxin(s) with no defined structure showed the toxin to cause centrally mediated cardiovascular and respiratory failures (124), neuromuscular blockade via increased Na$^+$ permeability (125), a TTX-blockable release of amino acids and acetylcholine from mammalian cortical synaptosomes (126), bronchoconstriction apparently mediated by ACh release (127), and a muscarinic crisis (128). Studies on the structurally defined BTX-B have revealed that it possesses positive inotropic and arrythmogenic activities on rat and guinea-pig hearts accompanied by A-V block (129), ability to depolarize nerve membranes and terminals by activating the Na^+ channels at sites other than those specific for TTX and/or AP-A (130), and neuromuscular blocking activity resulting from persistent depolarization of the nerve terminal (131).

Specific polyclonal antibodies have been prepared against brevetoxins for trace detection of the toxins in the food chain (shellfish) prior to consumption, but attempts have failed to prevent the BTX-induced toxicological symptoms in fish by the use of these antibodies (132).

From the cyclic polyether structural information of at least one of the brevetoxins (BTX-B) it appears that there might be some similarities, in the yet to be uncovered biological activities, between the so-called ionophore polyethers and brevetoxins. For the present, these novel marine molecules are clearly bound to stimulate a lot of pharmacological and biochemical investigations.

Ciguatoxin

Although not directly related to the red tide, ciguatera poisoning in tropical and subtropical waters also results from periodic outbursts of dinoflagellates and is carried to man not through shellfish but through the consumption of some types of reef fishes. Ciguatera poisoning is characterized by neurological, gastrointestinal, and cardiovascular syndromes developing within 2 to 24 hours of eating the contaminated fish. The factor responsible for the toxicity was isolated from Pacific red snapper and termed ciguatoxin (CTX). It appears to be a complex lipid (133), and has recently been thought to originate from the dinoflagellate *Gambierdiscus toxicus* (134). Preliminary data have revealed the presence of one oxygen atom to every three carbons (117), suggesting that the CTX molecule is similar to the polyether toxins, e.g. BTX-B. Since pure crystalline CTX as a single molecular moiety was only recently obtained (135), its X-ray crystal structure should be forthcoming shortly, if it has not already been published before this review appears.

In anesthetized cats and rats, CTX at low doses (5–30 μg/kg, i.v.) elicited respiratory stimulation and bradycardia, while at higher but sublethal doses (40–80 μg/kg) respiratory depression as well as marked bradycardia and hypertension developed (136). At low concentrations in the perfusion fluid (100 pg/ml), CTX was found strongly cardiotonic (137), but this observation has been attributed to variabilities in tissue sensitivity and toxin purity (138). It also induces a marked release of norepinephrine (NE) from the presynaptic sites in the neuromuscular junction of guinea-pig vas deferens and causes supersensitivity at the postsynaptic sites due to an increase in the permeability of TTX-sensitive Na^+ channels in the smooth muscle membrane (139). However, the site of interaction for CTX is entirely different from that of any other site, making it a new type of Na^+ channel toxin among a total of six different groups of toxins affecting Na^+ permeability, each by interacting with a specific site (140).

Palytoxin

One of the most interesting vasoactive molecules is palytoxin (PTX) isolated from various *Palythoa* species inhabiting the Caribbean (141) and Pacific (142) oceans. The structure of PTX has been elucidated (143) as a polyhydroxy, long chain macromolecule (Figure 3). It is the most potent marine toxin (144) and also the most potent coronary vasoconstrictor substance (16) known. As few as 1.6×10^{-17} moles can produce a nearly total constriction of the coronary artery in an isolated guinea-pig heart (145). Although this potent coronary vasoconstriction has been tentatively postulated as the mechanism of PTX toxicity (16), the toxin also has direct effects on a number of other muscle and nerve tissues (144–148).

The data on the action of PTX on nerve membranes indicate that the mechanism of action of PTX on the nerve tissues is clearly different from that of TTX. These data were obtained by intracellular and extracellular microelectrode recordings of neuronal activity in the coupled Retzius cells of horse leech ganglia. In these ganglia the membrane resistance as well as resting potential are unaffected by PTX (16). In both the nerve and the conducting system of the heart muscle, PTX appears to simulate the effects of large doses of extracellular

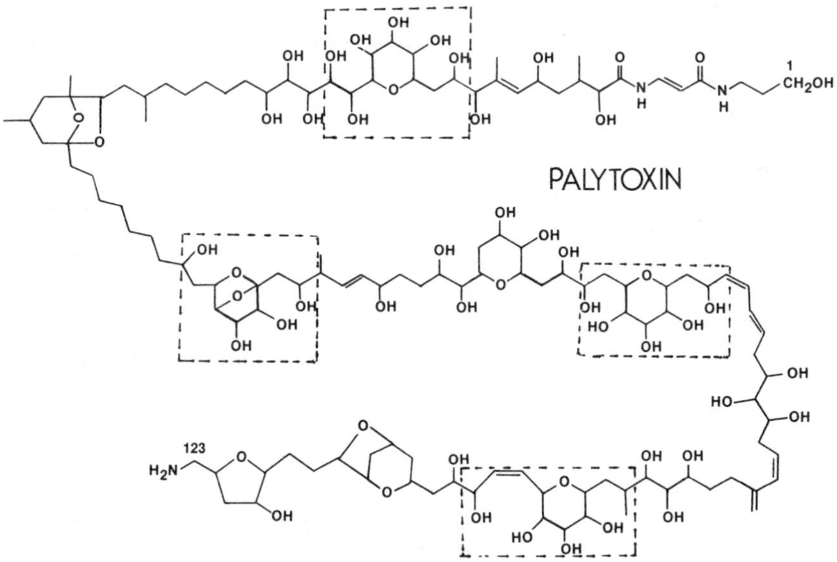

Figure 3   Structure of palytoxin (PTX). Boxed areas in dotted lines show possible chelation sites.

K^+ (16, 149, 150). In contrast to these observations, a decrease in the membrane resting potential in rabbit papillary muscle was noted in one study (151). However, it is questionable if this was really an effect of PTX, since a partially purified fraction of *Palythoa,* and not pure PTX, was used in this study. A biphasic contractile action of PTX observed on vas deferens has been attributed to a direct effect on the smooth muscle (first phase) and the release of NE from the adrenergic nerve terminals (second phase), since the second phase could be markedly inhibited by pretreatment with phentolamine or by predepletion of NE by reserpine (152).

An interesting effect of PTX is on the EKG of the rat, the dog, and the guinea pig, in which it elevates T-wave and S-T segment (16, 149) in a manner similar to that observed in patients suffering from variant or Prinzmetal angina (153). It is conceivable that PTX induces a coronary vascular spasm analogous to the spasm experienced in the variant angina. Thus, PTX may serve as a physiological tool to study animal models of this disease. Another very interesting observation is the potent inhibition of sperm motility induced by PTX (10^{-13} M) acting on the outer surface of the sperm membrane (154). Based on these studies, the use of sperm has been suggested for determining the mechanism of action of PTX.

The structure of PTX deserves an in-depth look, for it is one of the most unusual macromolecules in nature. There are several polyhydroxy and cyclic ether clusters (see dotted, boxed-in areas in its structural formula in Figure 3) suggestive of chelation sites. The molecule in general shows a high capability for both intra- and inter-molecular hydrogen bonding. It should also show a high binding capacity to biological macromolecules.

Other Marine Toxins

Halitoxin (HTX) from *Haliclona rubens,* the red "fire sponge", is a mixture of chemically defined heterocyclic molecules containing quaternary charged nitrogens as pyridinium moieties (155), analogous to curare alkaloids. It is a potent neuromuscular blocker and kills mice and rats by respiratory paralysis preceding cardiac arrest (P. Kaul, unpublished). Lophotoxin (LTX) from the sea whip coral (*Lophogorgia rigida*) is a cembranoid with two epoxides, an aldehyde, and an exocyclic lactone as its main chemical features (156). It has been claimed to be a new type of neuromuscular blocker acting on neuromuscular junction but on sites other than cholinoceptive receptors (157).

Maitotoxin (MTX) from the dinoflagellate *Gambierdiscus toxicus,* extensively studied though not yet chemically characterized, is a Ca^{2+} channel activator erroneously claimed (158) to be the most potent marine toxin known (See Table 1). It stimulates Ca^{2+} channels in insect skeletal muscles (159) and increases Ca^{2+} uptake in cultured NG108-15 neuroblastoma × glioma cells (160) by altering the voltage dependence of calcium channel activation.

Table 1 Relative toxicity of some of the marine toxins

Toxin	Organism	LD$_{50}$/kg (i.p.)	Species
Palytoxin	*Palythoa mammilosa*	50–100 ng	mice
Maitotoxin	*Gambierdiscus toxicus*	170 ng[a]	mice
Ciguatoxin	*G. toxicus*	450 ng	mice
Saxitoxin	*Saxidomus giganteus*	10 μg	mice
Tetrodotoxin	*Tapes semidecussata*	8–20 μg	mice
Laticatoxin	*Laticauda semifasciata*	130 μg	mice
Brevetoxin	*Ptychodiscus brevis*	250 μg	mice
Cephalotoxin	*Octopus vulgaris*	150–300 μg[b]	dogs
Lophotoxin	*Lophogorgia* sp.	8 mg	mice
Holotoxin	*Holothuria tubulosa*	5–15 mg[c]	mice
Nereistoxin	*Lumbriconeresis heteropoda*	33 mg[c]	mice
Halitoxin	*Haliclona viridis*	2.5 mg[c]	mice

[a]Minimum lethal dose.
[b]Subcutaneous.
[c]Intravenous.

Neosurugatoxin (NSTX) from the Japanese ivory mollusc, *Babylonia japonica,* is a potent blocker of sympathetic ganglia and a specific antagonist of nicotinic ACh receptors, as revealed by experiments on isolated guinea-pig ileum and radioligand binding studies with rat forebrain membranes (161). It is a nitrogenous heterocyclic compound with strong conjugation in a fused multi-ring system and contains sugar moieties.

BIOMEDICAL POTENTIAL AND BIOTECHNOLOGY

The biomedical potential of the sea has been emphasized repeatedly in recent decades (2, 6, 12, 14–17, 162). Clearly, a large number of unique organic molecules have been discovered and some of these have been found to possess either novel or potent pharmacologic activities. Of over 1000 structurally defined compounds of marine origin, only a score or two have been studied pharmacologically and only partially at that. This is so because in contrast to a relatively much larger number of dedicated marine natural-product chemists globally engaged in this field, only a handful of pharmacologists/biologists have been involved. Considering the usual ratio of one chemist to 4–6 biologists prevalent in industrial drug research, it is impossible to make serious progress in marine pharmacology/biomedicine unless many pharmacologists move toward the scientific novelties the sea has to offer. It is encouraging that ASPET in recent years has given some endorsement to marine pharmacology by including a few symposia on the subject, but, for a meaningful advance to occur in marine biomedicine, there will have to be a more substantial push from the industry and from federal funding agencies to catalyze the involvement of more and competent chemists and pharmacologists.

Biotechnology, of course, has become the key word in every field, including electronics. It certainly has a realistic potential in marine pharmacology. It was quite an appropriate step, therefore, for the MIT Sea Grant Program to host a key lecture series on biotechnology interfacing with marine sciences (162). Application of genetic engineering to mariculture has already begun to demonstrate the potential of biotechnology in the marine sciences. It is a logical step to apply recombinant DNA technology to the production of reasonable amounts of otherwise oligopeptides and other potent bioactive molecules present in trace amounts in marine organisms. In fact, some investigators may already have begun in this direction. Approaches such as these will allow for new drug development at a rate commensurate with other advances both on Earth and in space.

CONCLUSION

The claims by skeptics that no new drugs have emerged from the sea despite the noise made by some of us fanatical marine pharmacologists and chemists must be viewed realistically. Firstly, not much effort is going on in the field compared to what has been and is now going into synthetic and terrestrial natural-products research—tens of thousands of chemists and biologists globally having spent hundreds of billions of dollars over the past 80 years. Secondly, at least several decades lapse between the first discovery of pharmacological activity of a compound and its final use as a drug. Thirdly, man has always gone to nature for a structural lead in just about every class of therapeutic agents. These facts, coupled with the evidence presented in this review of highly active and novel marine molecules, offer a challenge full of hope, which we can meet only by an aggressive and determined dip into the sea. We have no doubt whatsoever that the new drugs in the space-age of the twenty-first century will emerge from the oceans.

ACKNOWLEDGMENTS

One of the authors (PNK) is grateful to Dr. Leon Ciereszko for his initial encouragement and knowledgable guidance during 17 years of involvement in pharmacologic studies on marine natural products. It has been a pleasure working collaboratively with him and the other members of the Oklahoma marine research group, Drs. Francis Schmitz and Alfred Weinheimer (now at University of Houston). This author is indebted to Dr. Dave Attaway of the National Sea Grant Program for his professional courtesies and advice, and to the Sea Grant Office, USDC-NOAA, for continuous support of our work that led to this review.

Literature Cited

1. Halstead, B. W. 1965. *Poisonous and Venomous Marine Animals of the World,* Vol. 1, pp. 1–29. Washington, DC: US GPO. 994 pp.
2. Emerson, G. A., Taft, C. H. 1945. Pharmacologically active agents from the sea. *Toxicol. Rep. Biol. Med.* 3:302–38
3. Nigrelli, R. F., ed. 1960. *Biochemistry and Pharmacology of Compounds Derived from Marine Organisms,* pp. 615–950. New York: Ann. NY Acad. Sci.
4. Freudenthal, H. D., ed. 1968. *Drugs From the Sea.* Washington, DC: Marine Technol. Soc. 297 pp.
5. Der Marderosian, A. 1969. Marine pharmaceuticals. *J. Pharm. Sci.* 58:1–33
6. Baslow, M. H. 1969. *Marine Pharmacology.* Baltimore: Williams & Wilkins. 286 pp.
7. Youngken, H. W., ed. 1969. *Food Drugs from the Sea Proceedings.* Washington, DC: Marine Technol. Soc. 396 pp.
8. Russel, F. E. 1971. Pharmacology of toxins of marine organisms. In *International Encyclopedia of Pharmacology and Therapeutics,* 2:3–114. New York: Pergamon
9. Worthen, L. R., ed. 1972. *Food Drugs from the Sea Proceedings.* Washington, DC: Marine Technol. Soc. 396 pp.
10. Martin, D., Padilla, G., eds. 1973. *Marine Pharmacognosy.* New York: Academic
11. Webber, H. H., Ruggieri G. D., eds. 1976. *Food Drugs from the Sea Proceedings.* Washington, DC: Marine Technol. Soc. 509 pp.
12. Ruggieri, G. D. 1976. Drugs from the sea. *Science* 194:491–96
13. Hashimoto, Y. 1979. *Marine Toxins and Other Bioactive Marine Metabolites.* Tokyo: Japan Sci. Soc.
14. Kaul, P. N., Sindermann, C. J., eds. 1978. *Drugs and Food from the Sea— Myth or Reality,* pp. 37–150. Norman: Oklahoma Univ. Printing. 448 pp.
15. Kaul, P. N. 1979. The Sea's biomedical potential. *Impact Sci. on Soc.* 29:123–34
16. Kaul, P. N. 1981. Compounds from the sea with actions on the cardiovascular and central nervous systems. *Fed. Proc.* 40:10–14
17. Kaul, P. N. 1982. Biomedical potential of the sea. *Pure Appl. Chem.* 54:1963–72
18. Ogura, Y., Mori, Y. 1968. Mechanism of local anesthetic activity of crystalline tetrodotoxin and its derivatives. *Eur. J. Pharmacol.* 3:58–67
19. Zelenski, S. G., Weinheimer, A. J.,

Kaul, P. N. 1976. A cardioactive compound isolated from the sponge, *Dasychalina cyathina.* See Ref. 11, pp. 288–96
20. Chang, C. W. J., Weinheimer, A. J., Matson, J. A., Kaul, P. N. 1978. Adenosine as the causative asystolic factor from a marine sponge. See Ref. 14, pp. 89–95
21. Weinheimer, A. J., Chang, C. W. J., Matson, J. A., Kaul, P. N. 1978. Marine cardioactive agents. Adenosine and 2'-doxy-adenosine from *Dasychalina cyathina. Lloydia* 41:488–90
22. Rand, M., Stafford, A., Thorp, R. H. 1955. The effect of cardiac glycosides on the heart block produced in the guinea pig by adenosine and its derivatives. *Aust. J. Exp. Biol.* 33:663–70
23. Kaul, P. N. 1982. Biomedical potential of the sea. *Pure Appl. Chem.* 54:1966
24. Bergmann, W., Burke, D. C. 1955. Contributions to the study of marine products. XXIX. The nucleosides of sponges III. Spongothymidine and Spongouridine. *J. Org. Chem.* 20:1501–7
25. Cohen, S. S. 1977. The mechanisms of lethal action of arabinosyl cytosine (ara C) and aradinosyl adenine (ara A). *Cancer* 40:509–18
26. Fuhrman, F. A., Fuhrman, G. J., Kim, Y. H., Pavelka, L. A., Mosher, H. S. 1980. Doridosine: A new hypotensive *N*-methylpurine riboside from the nudibranch *Anisodoris nobbilis. Science* 207:193–95
27. Kaul, P. N. 1984. *Future drugs from the sea.* Presented at Romanian Natl. Pharm. Congr., 8th, Bucharest
28. Davis, L. P., Jamieson, D. D., Baird-Lambert, J. A., Kazlauskas, R. 1984. Halogenated pyrrolopyrimidine analogues of adenosine from marine organisms. Pharmacological activities and potent inhibition of adenosine kinase. *Biochem. Pharmacol.* 33:347–55
29. Parker, C. A. 1881. Poisonous qualities of the starfish. *Zoologist* 5:214–15
30. Rio, G. J., Stampien, M. F., Nigrelli, R. F., Ruggieri, G. D. 1965. Echinoderm toxins: 1. Some biochemical and physiological properties of toxins from several species of *Asteroidea. Toxicon* 3:147–55
31. Ruggieri, G. D., Nigrelli, R. F. 1964. Jelly-precipitating reactions in sea urchin eggs by antibiotic substances from sponges. *Am. Zool.* 4:431 (Abstr.)
32. Mackie, A. M., Singh, H. T., Owen, J. M. 1977. Studies on the distribution, biosynthesis and function of steroidal

saponins in echinoderms. *Comp. Biochem. Physiol. B* 56:9–14

33. Owellen, R. J., Owellen, R. G., Gorog, M. A., Klein, D. 1973. Crytolytic saponin fraction from *Asterias vulgaris*. *Toxicon* 11:319–23

34. Patterson, M. J., Bland, J., Lindgren, E. W. 1978. Physiological response of symbiotic polychaetes to host saponins. *J. Exp. Mar. Biol. Ecol.* 33:51–56

35. Ruggieri, G. D., Nigrelli, R. F. 1974. Physiologically active substances from echinoderms. In *Bioactive Compounds from the Sea*, ed., H. Humm, C. Lane, pp. 183–95. New York: Dekker. 251 pp.

36. Goldsmith, L. A., Carlson, G. P. 1976. Pharmacological evaluation of an asterosaponin from *Asterias forbesi*. See Ref. 11, pp. 366–74

37. Friess, S. L. 1972. Mode of action of marine saponins on neuromuscular tissues. *Fed. Proc.* 31:1146–49

38. Bakus, G. J., Green, G. 1974. Toxicity in sponges and holothurians. *Science* 185:951–53

39. Burnell, D. J., ApSimon, J. W. 1983. Echinoderm saponins. In *Marine Natural Products*, ed. P. J. Scheuer, 5:365–69. New York/London: Academic. 442 pp.

40. Sullivan, T. D., Ladue, K. T., Nigrelli, R. F. 1955. The effect of holothurin, a steroid saponin of animal origin, on Krebs-2 ascites tumors in swiss mice. *Zoologica* 40:49–52

41. Friess, S. L., Durant, R. C., Chanley, J. D., Fash, F. J. 1967. Role of sulphate charge center in irreversible interactions of holothurin-A with chemoreceptors. *Biochem. Pharmacol.* 16:1617–25

42. Nigrelli, R. F., Jakowska, S. 1960. Effects of holothurin, a steroidal saponin from Bahamian sea cucumber, *Actinopyga agassizi*, on various biological systems. *Ann. NY Acad. Sci.* 90:884–92

43. Styles, T. J. 1970. Effect of holothurin on *Trypanosoma lewisi* infections in rats. *J. Protozool.* 17:196–98

44. Sen, D. K., Lin, V. K. 1977. Effect of holothurin on *Trypanosoma duttoni* in mice: Response of trypanosomes to biotoxin. *Va. J. Sci.* 28:9–12

45. Kitagawa, I., Sugawara, T., Yosioka, I., Kuriyama, K. 1976. Saponin and Sapogenol. 14. Antifungal glycosides from the sea cucumber *Stichopus japonicus*, Selenka. 1. Structure of stichopogenin A_4, the genuine aglycone of holotoxin-A. *Chem. Pharm. Bull.* 24:266–74

46. Anisimov, M. M., Prokofieva, N. G., Korotkikh, L. Y., Kapustina, I. I., Stonik, V. A. 1980. Comparative study of

cytotoxic activity of triterpene glycosides from marine organisms. *Toxicon* 18:221–23

47. Nigrelli, R. F., Zahl, P. A. 1952. Some biological characteristics of holothurin. *Proc. Soc. Exp. Biol. Med.* 81:379–80

48. Pettit, G. R., Herald, C. L., Herald, D. L. 1976. Antineoplastic sea agents XLV: Sea cucumber cytotoxic saponins. *J. Pharm. Sci.* 65:1558–59

49. Sullivan, T. D., Nigrelli, R. F. 1956. The antitumorous action of biologics of marine origin. 1. Survival of Swiss mice inoculated with Krebs-2 ascites tumor and treated with holothurin, a steroid saponin from the sea cucumber, *Actinopyga agassizi*. *Proc. Am. Assoc. Cancer Res.* 2:151 (Abstr.)

50. Friess, S. L., Durant, R. C. 1965. Blockade phenomena at the mammalian neuromuscular synapse. Competition between reversible anticholinesterases and an irreversible toxin. *Toxicol. Appl. Pharmacol.* 7:373–81

51. Thron, C. D. 1964. Hemolysis by holothurin-A, digitonin, and quillaia saponin: estimates of the required cellular lysin uptakes and free lysin concentrations. *J. Pharmacol. Exp. Ther.* 145:194–202

52. Friess, S. L., Durant, R. C., Chanley, J. D., Mezzetti, T. 1965. Some structural requirements underlying holothurin-A interactions with synaptic chemoreceptors. *Biochem. Pharmacol.* 14:1237–47

53. DeGroof, R. C., Narahashi, T. 1976. The effects of holothurin-A on the resting membrane potential and conduction of squid axon. *Eur. J. Pharmacol.* 36:337–46

54. Gorshkov, B. A., Gorshkov, I. A., Stonik, V. A., Elyakov, G. B. 1982. Effect of marine glycosides on adenosinetriphosphatase activity. *Toxicon* 20:655–58

55. Anisimov, M. M., Popov, A. M., Dizizenko, S. N. 1979. The effect of light lipids from sea urchin embryos on cytotoxic activity of certain triperpene glycosides. *Toxicon* 17:319–21

56. Norton, T. R., Shibata, S., Kashiwagi, M., Bentley, J. 1976. Isolation and characterization of the cardiotonic polypeptide anthopleurin-A from the sea anemone *Anthopleura xanthogrammica*. *J. Pharm. Sci.* 65:1368–74

57. Norton, T. R., Kashiwagi, M., Shibata, S. 1978. Anthopleurin A, B and C, cardiotonic polypeptides from the sea anemones *Anthopleura xanthogrammica* (Brandt) and *A. elegantissima* (Brandt). See Ref. 14, pp. 37–50

58. Tanaka, M., Haniu, M., Yasunobu, K. T., Norton, T. R. 1977. Amino acid sequence of the *Anthopleura xanthogrammica* heart stimulant, anthopleurin-A. *Biochemistry* 16:204–8

59. Shibata, S., Norton, T. R., Izumi, T., Matsuo, T., Katsumi, S. 1976. A polypeptide (AP-A) from sea anemone *(Anthopleura xanthogrammica)* with potent positive inotropic action. *J. Pharmacol. Exp. Ther.* 199:298–309

60. Scriabine, A., van Arman, C. G., Morris, A. A., Morgan, G., Bennett, C. D. 1977. Cardiotonic activity of anthopleurine-A (AP-A), a polypeptide from sea anemone *(Anthopleura xanthogrammica)* in dogs. *Fed. Proc.* 36:973 (Abstr.)

61. Ishizaki, H., McKay, R. H., Norton, T. R., Yasunobu, K. T., Lee, J., et al. 1979. Conformational studies of peptide heart stimulant anthopleurin-A: Laser-Raman, circular dichroism, fluorescence spectral studies and Chou-Fasman calculations. *J. Biol. Chem.* 254:9651–56

62. Norton, T. R. 1981. Cardiotonic polypeptides from *Anthopleura xanthogrammica* (Brandt) and *A. elegantissima* (Brandt). *Fed. Proc.* 40:21–25

63. Greenberg, M. J., Painter, S. D., Doble, K. E., Nagle, G. T., Price, D. A., et al. 1983. The molluscan neurosecretory peptide FMRFamide: comparative pharmacology and relationship to the enkephalins. *Fed. Proc.* 42:82–86

64. Beress, L. 1978. Biologically active polypeptides, toxins and proteinase inhibitors from the sea anemones *Anemonia sulcata* and *Condylactis aurantiaca*. See Ref. 14, pp. 59–72

65. Alsen, C., Peters, T., Scheufler, E. 1982. Studies on the mechanism of the positive inotropic effect of ATX-II *(Anemonia sulcata)* on isolated guinea pig atria. *J. Cardiovasc. Pharmacol.* 4:63–69

66. Alsen, C. 1983. Biological significance of peptides from *Anemonia sulcata*. *Fed. Proc.* 42:101–8

67. Rack, M., Meves, H., Beress, L., Grünhagen, H. H. 1983. Preparation and properties of fluorescence labeled neuro- and cardiotoxin II from the sea anemone *(Anemonia sulcata)*. *Toxicon* 21:231–37

68. Erxleben, C., Rathmayer, W. 1984. Effects of the sea anemone *Anemonia sulcata* toxin II on skeletal muscle and on neuromuscular transmission. *Toxicon* 22:387–99

69. Norton, R. S., Zwick, J., Beress, L. 1980. Natural abundance of ^{13}C nuclear-magnetic-resonance study of toxin II from *Anemonia sulcata*. *Eur. J. Biochem.* 113:75–83

70. Barhanin, J., Hugues, M., Schweitz, H., Vincent, J. P., Lazdunski, M. 1982. Structure-function relationships of sea anemone toxin II from *Anemonia sulcata*. *Toxicon* 20:59 (Abstr.)

71. Nabiullin, A. A., Odinokov, S. E., Kozlovskaya, E. P., Elyakov, G. B. 1982. Secondary structure of sea anemone toxins: circular dichroism, infrared spectroscopy and Chou-Fasman calculations. *FEBS Lett.* 141:124–27

72. Lafranconi, W. M., Ferlan, I., Russell, F. E., Huxtable, R. J. 1984. The action of equinatoxin, a peptide from the venom of sea anemone, *Actinia equina*, on the isolated lung. *Toxicon* 22:347–52

73. Bernheimer, A. W., Avigad, L. S., Lai, C. Y. 1982. Purification and properties of a toxin from the sea anemone *Condylactis gigantea*. *Arch. Biochem. Biophys.* 214:840–45

74. Fujita, S., Warashina, A. 1980. Parasicyonis toxin: Effect on crayfish giant axon. *Comp. Biochem. Physiol.* 67:71–74

75. Mebs, D., Gebauer, E. L. 1980. Isolation of proteinase inhibitory, toxic and hemolytic polypeptides from a sea anemone, *Stoichactis* sp. *Toxicon* 18:97–106

76. Mebs, D., Liebrich, M., Reul, A., Samejima, Y. 1983. Hemolysins and proteinase inhibitors from sea anemones of the Gulf of Aqaba. *Toxicon* 21:257–64

77. Noda, M., Muramatsu, I., Fujiwara, M. 1984. Effects of Goniopora toxin on the membrane currents of bullfrog atrial muscle. *Naunyn-Schmiedeberg's Arch. Pharmacol.* 327:75–80

78. Blumenthal, K. M. 1984. Release of liposomal markers by *Cerebratulus* toxin A-III. *Biochem. Biophys. Res. Commun.* 121:14–18

79. Blumenthal, K. M. 1985. Binding of *Cerebratulus* cytolysin A-III to human erythrocyte membranes. *Biochem. Biophys. Acta* 812:127–32

80. Dumont, J. A., Blumenthal, K. M. 1985. Structure and action of heteronemertine polypeptide toxins: Importance of amphipathic helix for activity of *Cerebratulus lacteus* toxin A-III. *Arch. Biochem. Biophys.* 236:167–75

81. Hollenbeak, K. H., Schmitz, F. J., Kaul, P. N., Kulkarni, S. K. 1978. A dual adrenergic compound from the sponge *Verongia fistularis*. See Ref. 14, pp. 81–87

82. Weinheimer, A. J., Matson, J. A., Karms, T. K. B., Hossain, M. B., van

der Helm, D. 1978. Some new marine anticancer agents. See Ref. 14, pp. 117–21

83. Kashman, Y., Groweiss, A., Carmely, S., Kinamoni, Z., Czarkie, D., et al. 1982. Recent research in marine natural products from the Red Sea. *Pure Appl. Chem.* 54:1995–2010

84. Tursch, B., Braekman, J. C., Daloze, D., Kaisin, M. 1978. Terpenoids from coelenterates. In *Marine Natural Products*, ed. P. J. Scheuer, 2:247–96. New York/London: Academic. 392 pp.

85. Hadfield, M. G., Ciereszko, L. S. 1978. Action of cembranolides derived from octocorals on larvae of the nudibranch *Phastilla sibogae*. See Ref. 14, pp. 145–50

86. Kaul, P. N. 1972. Pharmacologically active substances of marine origin. See Ref. 9, pp. 299–307

87. Perkins, D. L., Ciereszko, L. S. 1973. The environmental toxicity of crassin acetate using *Tetrahymena pyriformis* as a model. *Hydrobiologia* 42:77–84

88. Rinehart, K. L., Gloer, J. B., Cook, J. C., Mizsak, S. A., Scahill, T. A. 1981. Structures of the didemnins, antiviral and cytotoxic depsipeptides from a Caribbean tunicate. *J. Am. Chem. Soc.* 103:1857–59

89. Rinehart, K. L., Gloer, J. B., Wilson, G. R., Hughes, R. G., Li, H. L., et al. 1983. Antiviral and antitumor compounds from tunicates. *Fed. Proc.* 42:87–90

90. Lichter, W., Wellham, L. L., van der Werf, B. A., Middlebrook, R. E., Sigel, M. M., et al. 1972. Biological activities exerted by extract of *Ecteinascidia turbinata*. See Ref. 9, pp. 117–27

91. Lichter, W., Ghaffar, A., Wellham, L. L., Sigel, M. M. 1978. Immunomodulation by extract of *Ecteinascidia turbinata*. See Ref. 14, pp. 137–44

92. Sigel, M. M., Lichter, W., Ghaffar, A., Wellham, L. L., Weinheimer, A. J. 1979. Substances from marine organisms influencing tumor growth and immune responses. *Adv. Exp. Med. Biol.a.* 121:577–88

93. Dunn, W. C., Carrier, W. L., Regan, J. D. 1982. Effects of an extract from the sea squirt *Ecteinascidia turbinata* on DNA synthesis and excision repair in human fibroblasts. *Toxicon* 20:703–8

94. Pettit, G. R., Herald, C. L., Doubej, D. L., Herald, D. L. 1982. Isolation and structure of bryostatin 1. *J. Am. Chem. Soc.* 104:6846–48

95. Fusetani, M., Kato, Y., Matsumaga, S., Hashimoto, K. 1983. Bioactive marine metabolites. 3. A novel polyacetylene

alcohol, inhibitor of cell division in fertilized sea urchin egg, from the sponge *Tetrosia* sp. *Tetrahedron Lett.* 24:2771–74

96. Cimino, G., DeRosa, S., De Stefano, S. 1984. Antiviral compounds from a gorgonian, *Eunicella cavolini*. *Experientia* 40:339–40

97. Moore, R. E. 1982. Toxins, anticancer agents, and tumor promoters from marine prokaryotes. *Pure Appl. Chem.* 54:1919–34

98. Jacobs, R. S., White, S., Wilson, L. 1981. Selective compounds derived from marine organisms: effect on cell division in fertilized sea urchin eggs. *Fed. Proc.* 40:26–29

99. O'Brien, E. T., Jacobs, R. S., Wilson, L. 1983. Inhibition of bovine brain microtubule assembly in vitro by stypoldione. *Mol. Pharmacol.* 24:493–99

100. Schmitz, F. J., Campbell, D. C., Hollenbeak, K. H., Vanderah, D. J., Ciereszko, L. S., et al. 1977. The search for drugs from the sea. Chemistry related to the search for drugs from the sea. In *Marine Natural Products Chemistry*, ed. D. J. Faukner, W. H. Fenical, IV-1:293–310. New York/London: Plenum. 433 pp.

101. Kaul, P. N., Kulkarni, S. K. 1978. New drug metabolism inhibitors of marine origin. *J. Pharm. Sci.* 67:1293–96

102. Kaul, P. N., Kulkarni, S. K., Kurosawa, E. 1978. Novel substances of marine origin as drug metabolism inhibitors. *J. Pharm. Pharmacol.* 30:589–90

103. Kaul, P. N., Kulkarni, S. K., Schmitz, F. J., Hollenbeak, K. H. 1978. Pharmacologically active substances from the sea. 3: A marine derived inhibitor of drug metabolism. See Ref. 14, pp. 99–106

104. Buckle, P. J., Blado, B. A., Taylor, K. M. 1980. The anti-inflammatory activity of marine natural products—6-*n*-tridecylsalicylic acid, flexibilide and dendalone, 3-hydroxybutyrate. *Agents Actions* 10:361–67

105. de Freitas, J. C., Blankemeier, L. A., Jacobs, R. S. 1984. *In vitro* inactivation of the neurotoxic action of β-bungarotoxin by the marine natural product, manoalide. *Experientia* 40:864–66

106. Christophersen, C. 1983. Marine indoles. See Ref. 39, pp. 259–85

107. Sjoblom, T., Bohlin, L., Christopheren, C. 1983. Studies of Swedish marine organisms. 2. Muscle relaxant alkaloids from marine bryozoan *Flustra foliacea*. *Acta Pharm. Suec.* 20:415–19

108. Scheuer, P. J. 1973. *Chemistry of Marine Natural Products*. New York: Academic. 214 pp.

109. Baker, J., Murphy, V. 1976. *Handbook*

of Marine Sciences. Cleveland: CRC Press 226 pp.

110. Schmitz, F. J., Gropichand, Y., Michaud, D., Prasad, R. S., Ramaley, S., et al. 1981. Recent developments in research on metabolites from Caribbean marine invertebrates. Pure Appl. Chem. 53:853–65

111. Tachibana, K., Sheuer, P. J., Tsukitani, Y., Kiruchi, H., van Engen, D., et al. 1981. Okadaic acid, a cytotoxic polyether from two marine sponges of genus Halichondria. J. Am. Chem. Soc. 103:2469–71

112. Shibata, S., Ishida, Y., Kitano, H., Ohizumi, Y., Habon, J., et al. 1982. Contractile effects of okadaic acid, a novel ionophore-like substance from black sponge, on isolated smooth muscle under the condition of Ca^{++} deficiency. J. Pharmacol. Exp. Ther. 223:135–43

113. Okami, Y. 1982. Potential use of marine micro-organisms for antibiotic and enzyme production. Pure Appl. Chem. 54:1951–62

114. Spector, I., Schochet, N. R., Kashman, Y., Groweiss, A. 1983. Latrunculins: novel marine toxins that disrupt microfilament organization in cultured cells. Science 219:493–95

115. Hollenbeak, K. H., Schmitz, F. J. 1977. Aplysinopsin: antineoplastic tryptophan derivative from the marine sponge Verongia spengelii. Lloydia 40:479–81

116. Taylor, K. M., Baird-Lambert, J. A., Davis, P. A., Spence, I. 1981. Methylaphysinopsin and other marine natural products affecting neurotransmission. Fed. Proc. 40:15–20

117. Baden, D. G. 1983. Marine food-borne dinoflagellate toxins. Int. Rev. Cytology 82:99–150

118. Kao, C. Y. 1966. Tetrodotoxin, saxitoxin and their significance in the study of excitation phenomena. Pharmacol. Rev. 18:997–1049

119. Narahashi, T. 1974. Chemicals as tools in the study of excitable membranes. Physiol. Rev. 54:813–89

120. Ritchie, J. M., Rogart, R. B. 1977. The binding of saxitoxin and tetrodotoxin to excitable tissues. Rev. Physiol. Biochem. Pharmacol. 79:2–50

121. Kao, C. Y. 1981. Tetrodotoxin, saxitoxin and chiriquitoxin: new perspectives on ionic channels. Fed. Proc. 40:30–35

122. Lin, Y. Y., Risk, M., Ray, S. M., Engen, D. V., Clardy, J., et al. 1981. Isolation and structure of brevetoxin-B from the "red tide" dinoflagellate Ptychodiscus brevis (Gymnodinium breve). J. Am. Chem. Soc. 103:6773–75

123. Schmizu, Y. 1982. Recent progress in marine toxin research. Pure Appl. Chem. 54:1973–80

124. Borison, H. L., Ellis, S., McCarthy, L. E. 1980. Central respiratory and circulatory effects of Gymnodinium breve toxin in anesthetized rats. Br. J. Pharmacol. 70:249–56

125. Shinnick-Gallagher, P. 1980. Possible mechanism of action of Gymnodinium breve toxin at the mammalian neuromuscular junction. Br. J. Pharmacol. 69:373–78

126. Risk, M., Norris, P. I., Coutinho-Netto, J., Bradford, H. F. 1982. Action of Ptychodiscus brevis red tide toxin on metabolic and transmitter-releasing properties of synaptosomes. J. Neurochem. 39:1485–88

127. Baden, D. G., Mende, T. J., Bikhazi, G., Leung, I. 1982. Bronchoconstriction caused by Florida red tide toxins. Toxicon 20:929–32

128. Baden, D. G., Mende, T. J. 1981. Toxicity of two toxins from the Florida red tide marine dinoflagellate, Ptychodiscus brevis. Toxicon 20:457–61

129. Rodgers, R. L., Chou, H. N., Temma, K., Akera, T., Shimizu, Y. 1984. Positive inotropic and toxic effects of brevetoxin-B on rat and guinea pig heart. Toxicol. Appl. Pharmacol. 76:296–305

130. Huang, J. M. C., Wu, C. H., Baden, D. G. 1984. Depolarizing action of a red-tide dinoflagellate brevetoxin on axonal membranes. J. Pharmacol. Exp. Ther. 229:615–21

131. Baden, D. G., Bikenazi, G., Decker, S. J., Foldes, F. F., Leung, I. 1984. Neuromuscular blocking action of two brevetoxins from the Florida red tide organism Ptychodiscus brevis. Toxicon 22:75–84

132. Baden, D. G., Mende, T. J., Walling, J., Schultz, D. R. 1984. Specific antibodies directed against toxins of Ptychodiscus brevis (Florida's red tide dinoflagellate). Toxicon 22:783–89

133. Scheuer, P. J., Takahashi, W., Tsutsumi, J., Yoshida, T. 1967. Ciguatoxin: Isolation and chemical nature. Science 155:1267–68

134. Adachi, R., Fukuyo, T. 1979. The thecal structure of a marine toxic dinoflagellate Gambierdiscus toxicus gen. et sp.-nov. collected in a ciguatera-endemic area. Bull. Jpn. Soc. Sci. Fish. 45:67–71

135. Nukina, M., Koyanagi, L. K., Scheuer, P. J. 1984. Two interchangeable forms of ciguatoxin. Toxicon 22:169–76

136. Legrand, A. M., Galonnier, M., Bagnis, R. 1982. Studies on the mode of action of ciguateric toxins. Toxicon 20:311–15

137. Miyahara, J. T., Akau, C. K., Yasumoto, T. 1979. Effect of ciguatoxin and maitotoxin on the isolated guinea pig atria. *Res. Commun. Chem. Pathol. Pharmacol.* 25:177–80

138. Legrand, A. M., Bagnis, R. 1984. Effect of ciguatoxin and maitotoxin on isolated rat atria and rabbit duodenum *Toxicon* 22:471–75

139. Ohizumi, Y., Ishida, Y., Shibata, S. 1982. Mode of the ciguatoxin-induced supersensitivity in the guinea pig vas deferens. *Pharmacol. Exp. Ther.* 221:748–52

140. Bidard, J. N., Vijverberg, H. P. M., Frelin, C., Chungue, E., Legrand, A. M., et al. 1984. Ciguatoxin is a novel type of Na⁺ channel toxin. *J. Biol. Chem.* 259:8353–57

141. Attaway, D. H., Ciereszko, L. S. 1974. Isolation and partial characterization of Caribbean palytoxin. *Proc. Soc. Int. Coral Reef Sym.* 7:497–504

142. Moore, R. E., Scheuer, P. J. 1971. A new marine toxin from coelenterate. *Science* 172:495–97

143. Moore, R. E., Bartolini, G. 1981. Structure of palytoxin. *J. Am. Chem. Soc.* 103:2491–94

144. Kaul, P. N., Farmer, M. R., Ciereszko, L. S. 1974. Pharmacology of palytoxin—the most potent marine toxin known. *Proc. West. Pharmacol. Soc.* 17:294–301

145. Kaul, P. N. 1976. A new physiological tool. *Science* 194:311–23

146. Wiles, J. S., Vick, J. A., Christensen, M. K. 1974. Toxicological evaluation of palytoxin in several animal species. *Toxicon* 12:427–33

147. Deguchi, T., Urukawa, N., Takamatsu, S. 1976. Some pharmacological properties of palythoatoxin isolated from the zoanthid, *Palythoa tuberculosa*. In *Animal, Plant and Microbial Toxins*, ed. A. Ohsaka, K. Hayashi, Y. Sawai, 2:379–94. New York/London: Plenum

148. Beress, L. 1982. Biologically active compounds from coelenterates. *Pure Appl. Chem.* 54:1981–94

149. Kulkarni, S. K., Kirlin, W. G., Kaul, P. N. 1978. Mechanism of cardiovascular effects of palytoxin. See Ref. 14, pp. 73–80

150. Ito, K., Karaki, H., Urukawa, N. 1977. The mode of contractile action of palytoxin on smooth muscle. *Eur. J. Pharmacol.* 46:9–14

151. Weidmann, S. 1977. Effect of palytoxin on the electrical activity of dog and rabbit heart. *Experientia* 33:1487–88

152. Ohizumi, Y., Shibata, S. 1980. Mechanism of the excitatory action of palytoxin and N-acetylpalytoxin in the isolated guinea pig vas deferens. *J. Pharmacol. Exp. Ther.* 214:209–12

153. Selzer, A., Langston, M., Ruggeroli, L., Cohen, K. 1976. Clinical syndrome of variant angina with normal coronary arteriogram. *N. Engl. J. Med.* 295:1343–47

154. Morton, B. E., Fraser, C. F., Thenawidjaja, M., Albagli, L., Rayner, M. D. 1982. Potent inhibition of sperm motility by palytoxin. *Exp. Cell Res.* 140:261–65

155. Schmitz, F. J., Hollenbeak, K. H., Campbell, D. C. 1978. Marine natural products: Halitoxin, toxic complex of several marine sponges of genus *Haliclona. J. Org. Chem.* 43:3916–22

156. Fenical, W., Okuda, R. K., Bandurraga, M. M., Culver, P., Jacobs, R. J. 1981. Lophotoxin: a novel neuromuscular toxin from Pacific sea whips of the genus *Lophogorgia. Science* 212:1512–14

157. Langdon, R. B., Jacobs, R. S. 1983. Quantal analysis indicates an α-toxin-like block by lophotoxin, a non-ionic marine natural product. *Life Sci.* 32:1223–28

158. Takahashi, M., Tatsumi, M., Ohizumi, Y. 1983. Ca⁺⁺ channel activating function of maitotoxin, the most potent marine toxin known, in clonal rat pheochromocytoma cells. *J. Biol. Chem.* 258:10944–49

159. Miyamoto, T., Ohizumi, Y., Washio, H., Yasumoto, Y. 1984. Potent excitatory effect of maitotoxin on Ca⁺⁺ channels in the insect skeletal muscle. *Pfleugers Arch.* 400:439–41

160. Freedman, S. B., Miller, R. J., Miller, D. M., Tindall, D. R. 1984. Interactions of maitotoxin with voltage-sensitive calcium channels in cultured neuronal cells. *Proc. Natl. Acad. Sci. USA* 81:4582–85

161. Hayashi, E., Ingai, M., Kagaria, K., Takayanagi, N., Yamada, S., 1984. Neosurugatoxin, a specific antagonist of nicotinic acetylcholine reception. *J. Neurochem.* 42:1491–94

162. Colwell, R. R., Pariser, E. R., Sinskey, A. J., eds. 1984. *Biotechnology in the Marine Sciences.* New York: Wiley. 293 pp.

Ann. Rev. Pharmacol. Toxicol. 1986. 26:143–60

THE PHARMACOLOGY OF INTRAVASCULAR RADIOCONTRAST MEDIA

Thomas W. Morris[1] and Harry W. Fischer[2]

Departments of Radiology and Physiology[1] and Radiology[2], University of Rochester, Rochester, New York 14642

INTRODUCTION

Radiopaque contrast media are used for many diagnostic procedures that require X-ray opacification of blood vessels or tissue. Contrast media are injected both intravenously and intra-arterially to achieve this purpose. An ideal contrast media would exert no effect on the physiologic state while achieving the desired opacification in the selected organ or vessel. As with all drugs the ideal has not yet been achieved; however, the current generation of contrast media are considerably less toxic than the original commercial agents. There are several thorough reviews of the development, utilization, and pharmacology of contrast media, therefore the emphasis in this review is on general characteristics and current or new contrast media molecules (1–6).

STRUCTURE

All the currently used intravascular contrast media are derivatives of tri-iodinated benzoic acids (7, 8). The iodine molecule is an effective X-ray absorber in the energy range where most clinical systems operate (9, 10). Figure 1 illustrates examples of the different contrast media molecules currently available. The anion diatrizoate is the most commonly used contrast media in the United States and is supplied as either a meglumine or sodium salt. Not shown in the figure are iothalamate and metrizoate, two similar ionic monomers. Metrizamide, iopamidol, and iohexol are nonionic molecules with an organic side chain replacing the carboxyl group. Ioxaglate is a "mono-acidic

143

0362-1642/86/0415-0143$02.00

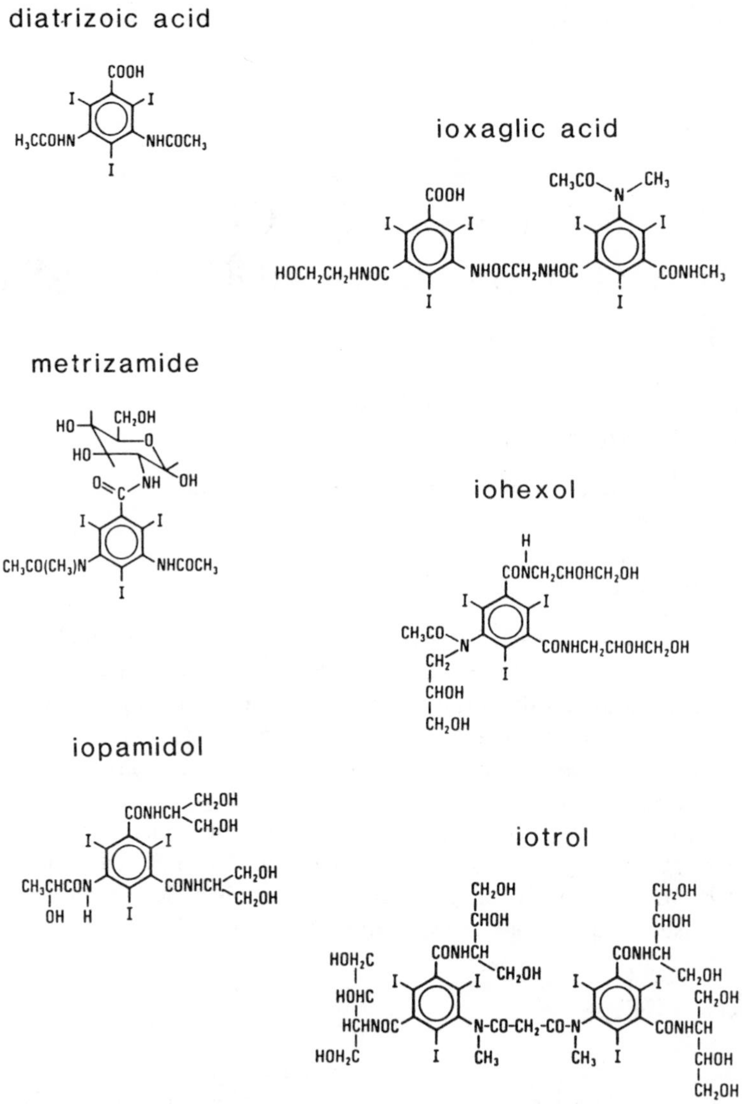

Figure 1 The structure of six different molecules currently in use in Europe or the United States illustrates the four classes of media available. All of the intravascular contrast media are derived from tri-iodinated benzoic acid precursors.

dimer" in which two of the "monomer" molecules have been linked to form a monovalent anion while iotrol is a nonionic "dimer." Iohexol, ioxaglate, and iopamidol contrast media are available for intravascular use in Europe and their approvals are currently pending in the United States. Intravascular injections of iohexol, iopamidol, and ioxaglate have been shown in numerous animal and clinical studies to be less toxic than the currently used anion "monomers" (11–13). Metrizamide is currently approved in the United States for intrathecal use while iohexol, iopamidol, and iotrol approvals are pending for that route of administration.

As shown by the intravascular LD_{50} data in Table 1, contrast media are among the most inert compounds biologically and most of their physiologic and pharmacologic effects are related to their high concentration and, more specifically, to their high osmolality. The different media are often grouped according to the number of iodine molecules divided by the number of particles in an ideal solution. Thus the ionic monomers yield a ratio of 1.5 iodine molecules for each particle in an ideal solution; the nonionics and mono-acidic dimer have ratios of 3 to 1.

CONCENTRATION AND COLLIGATIVE PROPERTIES

Most intravascular drugs achieve their primary function at doses in the $\mu g/kg$ range. Contrast media must absorb X rays to perform their function and are therefore generally used in dose ranges measured in g/kg and in concentrations as high as 1.5 Molal, or 10 times higher than the concentration of body fluids. At these high concentrations the colligative properties of these contrast media solutions are very important. Osmolality and viscosity are shown as a function of concentration (in mgI/ml) in Figure 2 and 3 for three types of contrast media. The osmolalities of contrast media solutions are considerably lower than expected for ideal solutions. Thus a 1.5 Molal solution of diatrizoate has an osmolality of only 1.7 rather than 3.0 Osmoles/kg. The viscosity of the concentrated solutions is higher than that of blood and plasma, and contrast media can produce alterations in local blood flow.

DIAGNOSTIC UTILIZATION

There are three general modes of utilizing intravascular radiopaque contrast media in clinical practice. The first is the direct injection of the media into a vascular structure to provide opacification of the vascular lumen. This procedure is performed at injection rates sufficient to replace blood flow through the structure. If the X-ray images are being recorded directly on film, concentrations from 280 to 370 mgI/ml are used. More recently the development of computerized tomography (CT) and digital subtraction angiography (DSA) have made it possible to visualize vascular structures with concentrations as low as 2 to 8 mgI/ml.

A second mode of using contrast media is to visualize and monitor their distribution in body fluid compartments. This is primarily used in contrast-enhanced CT studies. The X-ray absorbance of soft tissues is low and only small differences are observed in normal and pathologic tissue. The use of

Table 1 Comparisons of several parameters for six different contrast media molecules

Contrast media	Molecular weight	Moles of iodine per mole particles in solution	Type of Molecule	Acute LD_{50}[a] in mice (gI/kg)	Half time[b] in man (min)
Diatrizoate	636	1.5	ionic, monomer	7.5 (14)	101 (15a)
Ioxaglate	1269	3.0	ionic, dimer	13.4 (14)	92[c]
Metrizamide	789	3.0	nonionic, monomer	18.6 (14)	75 (15b)
Iohexol	821	3.0	nonionic, monomer	24.2 (14)	121 (15b)
Iopamidol	777	3.0	nonionic, monomer	22.1 (14)	128 (15c)
Iotrol	1626	6.0	nonionic, dimer	26.0 (15)	—

[a]Acute lethal dose 50 following intravenous administration in units of grams of iodine per kilogram body weight. Numbers in parentheses are references.
[b]This time is calculated from a 2-exponential model and represents the half time of the slow excretion component.
[c]Half time supplied by Guerbet Laboratories.

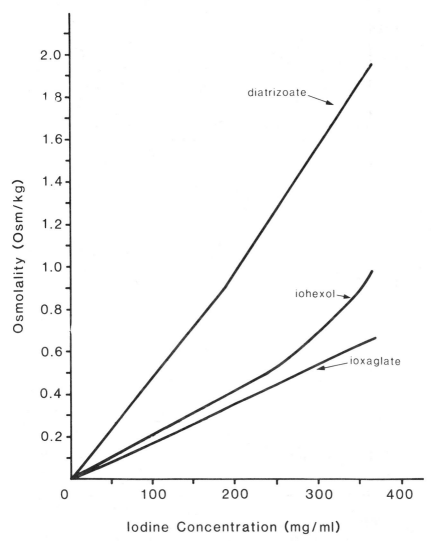

Figure 2   Osmolality in units of osmoles/kilogram (Osm/kg) water is shown as a function of iodine concentration for contrast media representing three types of media: ionic monomers (diatrizoate), monovalent ionic dimers (ioxaglate), and nonionic (iohexol). An iodine concentration of 190 mgI/ml would be 0.5 molar for diatrizoate or iohexol and 0.25 molar for ioxaglate. As the concentration increases, the solute volume of the solutions becomes substantial. For example, at 370 mgI/ml one ml of a diatrizoate solution contains 0.66 ml of H_2O and 0.34 ml of solute. This large solute volume is responsible for the upward curvature of these plots.

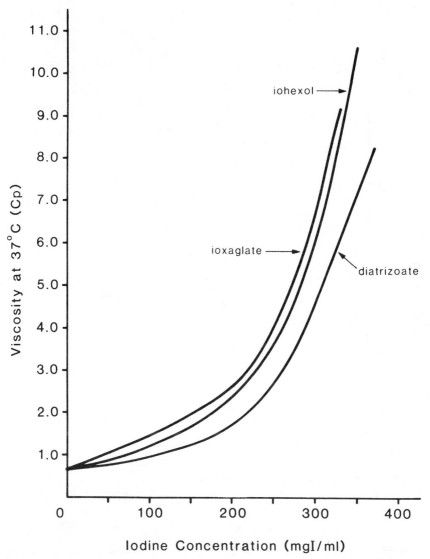

Figure 3   Viscosity in units of centipoise (Cp) is shown as a function of iodine concentration for the same three contrast media. At the higher concentrations solute-solute interactions and viscosity increase rapidly. The most commonly used radiocontrast media concentrations of 370 and 300 mgI/ml have viscosities several times greater than the viscosity of plasma.

contrast agents can enhance the difference in the absorbance of soft tissue because of the difference in the distribution of the contrast media molecules (9, 10). For example, some brain tumors lack a blood-brain barrier and contrast media will diffuse into them while they will not diffuse into areas retaining a normal blood-brain barrier (16). The distribution volume of contrast media is often used to quantify these studies. The distribution volume is calculated as 100 times the ratio of tissue concentration divided by plasma concentration and can be obtained directly from CT data and the blood hematocrit ratio.

A third mode of using contrast media is to visualize their route of excretion from the body. Most of the current molecules for intravascular use are excreted primarily by the kidney (17). As these molecules are cleared by the kidney they will opacify the renal parenchyma, then the tubular structures, the renal calyces and pelvis, and finally the ureter and bladder. These agents are concentrated by the kidney and thus provide excellent visualization of the entire renal system. In patients with renal failure there is a much slower vicarious excretion of contrast media through the biliary system and bowel. There is an additional class of intravascular contrast media that are excreted primarily into the biliary system by the hepatocytes (18). These media, such as iodipamide, are not frequently used today because of their higher toxicity and because of the increased use of CT and ultrasound to examine the liver and biliary system.

The dose of contrast media used varies considerably depending on the procedures to be performed. For example, peripheral intra-arterial DSA procedures may require less than 0.15 gI/kg while a complete conventional cardiac study can require as much as 1.5 gI/kg. The procedures requiring the highest doses usually involve multiple injections, often at different vascular sites.

DISTRIBUTION

All of the contrast media molecules available have molecular weights ranging from 600 to 1700 and have low lipid solubility (this is excluding the biliary agents). These molecules distribute in body fluids in much the same way as extracellular markers such as sucrose, Cr-EDTA, Tc^{99m} DTPA, or inulin. The molecules do not enter normal cells in significant amounts although very small intracellular concentrations have been reported (19). The molecules enter the interstitial space quickly in most tissue (20, 21) but they do not appear to cross the blood-brain barrier. The molecules do enter cerebrospinal fluid through fenestrated areas such as the choroid plexus (16).

Diagnostic procedures take advantage of the differential distribution space and kinetics of normal and abnormal tissue. Figure 4 illustrates the CT attenuation of blood and different tissues in a series of patients (22). The CT attenuation at equilibrium depends on the dose given and the extracellular space or distribution volume of tissue, which does vary with tissue type. The kinetics of

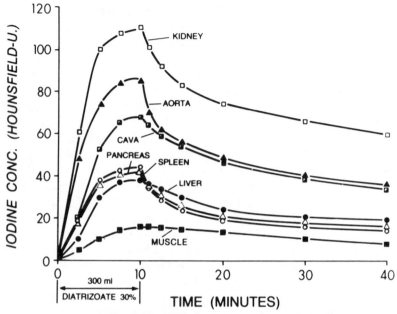

Figure 4 Iodine concentrations derived from CT measurements and presented as Hounsfield units are shown as a function of time in patient blood and tissues. (25 Hounsfield units are equivalent to 1 mgI/ml.) The greatest differences in iodine concentrations among the tissues occur during the infusion of contrast media and are related to distribution kinetics (22). (Reprinted with permission from the authors and *Am. J. Roentgenol.*)

contrast media distribution vary considerably more than the extracellular space and depend on blood flow, capillary density, capillary permeability, interstitial diffusion distances, and the diffusivity of the interstitial matrix. All of these factors can be altered in different types of abnormal tissue. By obtaining CT images at different times after intravascular injection, one can take advantage of the differences in tissue contrast media accumulation. As illustrated in Figure 4, this is most effective during or immediately after the contrast media infusion. The distribution kinetics of the new low osmolality contrast media appear to be very similar to the distribution kinetics of the conventional ionic monomers (23).

CLEARANCE

The contrast media molecules are excreted primarily by filtration at the renal glomerulus. They are not significantly secreted or reabsorbed in the tubules at clinical doses and are essentially equivalent to the standard marker for glomerular filtration, inulin (17, 24). The half times for excretion calculated from two compartment models are given in Table 1 for several different contrast media molecules.

During renal artery injections, small differences in clearance rates for different molecules have been observed and may relate to their osmolality. During intra-arterial injections the higher osmolality ionic monomer contrast media cause greater shrinkage of glomerular endothelial cells that may lead to increased filtration. In isolated perfused canine kidneys we observed that the renal vein concentration of ioxaglate was highest, nonionic monomers were intermediate, and and the ionic monomers were the lowest (25).

Although the total excretion is similar for all contrast media following i.v. injections, the urine concentration depends on the type of molecule. The low osmolality nonionic and mono-acidic dimer contrast media are more highly concentrated in the urine than the more hypertonic ionic monomer contrast media (26–28). The ionic monomer contrast media cause higher water flux into the tubules and a greater diuresis. The larger fluid volume causes greater distention of the pelvic structures. The higher urine concentrations of the low osmolality contrast media produce greater visualization of small structures and boundaries. A smaller difference in urine concentration has been noted between meglumine and sodium salts of the ionic monomers (29). The sodium salts are believed to reach higher concentrations because of sodium reabsorption.

LOCAL EFFECTS

The direct injection of radiopaque contrast media into arteries causes alterations in fluid and electrolyte balance, hemodynamics, and vascular resistance. These changes are caused primarily by the high osmolality and viscosity of the media. During and immediately following an intra-arterial injection, the contrast media viscosity raises the vascular resistance in the downstream vascular bed (30). This effect is apparent only for the brief period during which the media is located in the resistance vessels or arterioles (30). The high osmolality of the contrast media causes a rapid loss in water by red cells, endothelium, and tissue extravascular space (25, 31, 32). Figure 5 illustrates the relationship between red cell volume and solution osmolality that we have observed with contrast media. A similar loss of water by endothelial cells can result in shrinkage of the endothelial cells and the opening of tight junctions such as those in the blood-brain barrier (16). Recent studies of the endothelium have demonstrated that the molecular structure of the contrast media also plays a role in producing endothelial damage (33).

The shift of water from tissue parenchyma is biphasic with an initial loss followed by a later gain (25). This response appears to result because the bolus of blood and contrast media first passing through the tissue capillaries removes tissue water and raises tissue osmolality. As this mixture is washed through the

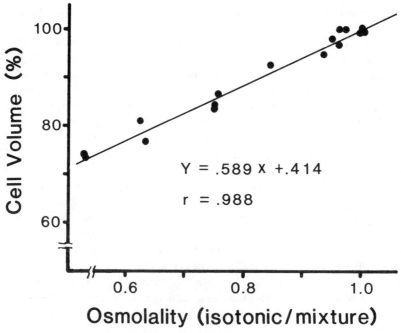

Figure 5   Red blood cell volume, presented as a percentage of the isotonic volume, is shown as a function of the ratio of isotonic and test solution osmolalities. The test solutions were made hypertonic by adding sodium diatrizoate. Red cell volumes were measured using both isotope and microcapillary hematocrit techniques and are corrected for dilutions.

capillaries it is replaced by blood of normal osmolality and water is then lost to the tissue. The return of fluid to tissues is enhanced by the increased solute concentration caused by the movement of contrast media molecules from capillaries to the interstitial space. The loss of tissue water and increase in tissue osmolality are the most likely causes of the vasodilation observed in most vascular beds following intra-arterial contrast media injections (34, 35). Figure 6 illustrates the changes we have observed in femoral blood flow with 5-sec injections of different contrast media solutions (36). When the solutions were isotonic there was no difference between the maximum flow observed for contrast media and blood, while hypertonic solutions caused large increases in flow.

The high osmolality of contrast media has also been associated with pain during selective arteriography in many sites (37). It has been shown in several clinical studies that the new low osmolality contrast media produce significantly less pain (38–42).

The injection of contrast media into coronary arteries can cause effects on myocardial electrical and mechanical function (43, 44). The hypertonic ionic

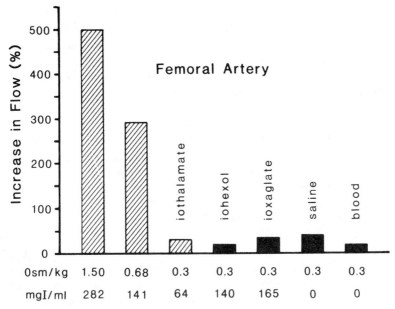

Figure 6   The maximum increase in femoral artery flow (at constant arterial pressure) is shown from a single canine experiment. The injection was for 5 seconds at 0.5 ml/second and maximum flow occurred between 5 and 60 seconds after the start of the injection. The isotonic solutions produce similar maximum flows that are much smaller than those for hypertonic iothalamate solutions.

solutions have been shown to cause both bradycardia and significant decreases in contractile function, while hypertonic nonionic solutions have been shown to cause an increase in contractile force (43, 45, 46). During prolonged exposures of the myocardium to contrast media the importance of electrolyte composition is also apparent. In dog experiments it has been shown that both calcium chelators and the lack of sodium increase the risk of ventricular arrhythmias and fibrillation (47–50). These electrolyte effects appear to be related to decreases caused in conduction velocities and cell repolarization (51). The importance of electrolyte composition in clinical practice is less well established, but there is some agreement with animal studies (52–54).

Renal artery injections of contrast media produce hemodynamic changes different from those observed in other vascular beds. In the kidney there is an initial vasodilation followed by a later, more prolonged increase in vascular resistance (55). This increase in vascular resistance coincides with the period during which the kidney tissue is regaining water from blood (25). There has been much debate over the mechanism for this increase in resistance (56–58). The bulk of the existing evidence seems to indicate that the increased resistance can be explained by an increase in tubular pressure and a subsequent decrease in filtration fraction, and glomerular filtration plus compression of glomerular capillaries (57). The increased tubular pressure might also tend to cause compression of post-glomerular vessels. Many vasoconstrictor substances have also been suggested and may play some role. The injection of contrast media into the renal artery has also been shown to cause a transient proteinuria (59), presumably from osmotic disruption of the glomerular endothelial cells. Both the hemodynamic effects and the proteinuria are significantly reduced with the use of the new low osmolality contrast media (60, 61).

Since the kidney is the primary organ for excretion of contrast media all arterial and venous injections of contrast media result in high renal concentrations of contrast media. Thus the hemodynamic alterations observed with renal artery injections can also be observed with all contrast media injections, but they are delayed and of lesser magnitude (62).

Rapid intravenous injections such as those used in angiocardiography, dynamic CT scanning, and i.v. DSA produce effects in the lungs very similar to the effects of intra-arterial injections in other tissues. The large bolus (typically 20 to 40 ml) is delivered in less than two seconds and results in a high osmolality mixture of blood and contrast media entering the pulmonary vascular system. Thus the same fluid shifts that occur in other tissues occur in the lungs (63). A large increase in pulmonary water content has been documented using a combination of thermal and dye tracers with an indicator dilution analysis (64). The mechanism is believed to be a leakage of serum proteins as well as contrast media into the pulmonary interstitium following the osmotic shrinkage of endothelial cells. As would be expected, there is less of an increase in lung water with the new low osmolality contrast media (65).

In a clinical study it was observed that all patients receiving intravenous contrast media had a mild but measurable bronchospasm (66). The bronchospasm could be related to water shifts or to the release of a substance such as histamine. The intravenous injection of contrast also causes an increase in pulmonary artery pressure that may be related to the shrinkage and decreased deformability of red blood cells (67). This increase in pulmonary artery pressure has been shown to be reduced with the new low osmolality contrast media (68).

A recent study has demonstrated a local effect of intravenous contrast media on the production of cerebrospinal fluid (69). This decrease was significant even at clinical doses and did not appear to be related to hypertonicity. The mechanism may be related to the specific structure of the contrast media molecules.

SYSTEMIC EFFECTS

Both intravenous and selective intra-arterial injections can cause systemic responses and reactions. Selective intra-arterial injections in the carotid and vertebral arteries are known to produce bradycardia and systemic vasodilation that are mediated by the autonomic nervous system (70–72). The mechanism is believed to be initiated by carotid chemoreceptors and other receptors in the cerebral vasculature (71). Coronary artery injections of contrast media cause changes in cardiac output because of their effects on both heart electrophysiologic and contractile function (44).

Intravenous contrast media injections have been shown to cause hypotension and bradycardia in both animal and patient studies (73–75). Based on the animal studies these effects seem to be dose dependent (73) and to be reduced with the new low osmolality contrast media (74). In a study of 97 patients, 51 were observed to respond with a measurable decrease in arterial pressure and 6 had mean arterial pressures drop below 60 mm Hg (75). In animal studies this effect has been shown to be markedly potentiated by a preexisting dehydration (76).

ADVERSE REACTIONS

Adverse reactions to contrast media are classified as minor, intermediate, or severe (77). Minor reactions include all reactions such as nausea, vomiting, mild rash or urticaria, and mild dyspnea that require no treatment. Intermediate reactions are those that require treatment (but not hospitalization) and include bronchospasm, mild laryngeal and facial edema, dyspnea, hypotension, extensive urticaria, and mild chest pain. Severe reactions that are life threatening and require hospitalization include laryngeal and pulmonary edema, circulatory collapse with refractory hypotension, angina, cardiac arrhythmias, and cardiac or respiratory arrest. The incidence of these 3 types of reactions is not precisely known (77–79) but they are relatively infrequent. Conservative estimates for the ionic monomer contrast media are that minor reactions occur in 1 out of 20 patients, intermediate reactions in 1 out of 100, and severe reactions in 1 out of 2000 (80). The mortality rate reported in the literature is quite variable, ranging from 1 in 14,000 to 1 in 117,000 patients (81). Sample size limitations and patient population characteristics make it difficult to assess this rate more precisely; however, the figure most generally quoted is 1 in 40,000 patients. The risk of having a severe reaction to contrast media appears to increase with some predisposing risk factors (80). These factors include a previous reaction, a history of allergy, asthma, dehydration, cardiac disease, and advanced age. The incidence of these reactions seems to be lower with the new low osmolality contrast media (82–84), but the number of patients studied is too small for a statistical assessment.

The development of CT and DSA technology has led to a general increase in the total number of contrast media studies and to an increase in the number of contrast media studies performed in elderly patients and in patients with renal impairment. Coincident with this, there has been an increase in the number of reported cases of acute renal failure (85–87). Many renal specialists believe that it is the presence of preexisting risk factors and acute stresses that potentiate these renal responses to contrast media (85, 88). The new lower osmolality media will substantially reduce the osmotic load on the kidneys and should reduce the incidence of acute renal failure.

Several hypotheses have been developed to explain the occurrence of adverse reactions to radiopaque contrast media (89–93). Many of the reactions appear similar to anaphylactic reactions and some researchers believe there is an antigen-antibody response (91). Other researchers in the field, however, believe that the reactions are more properly termed anaphylactoid and that they are induced by other mechanisms that may involve some of the same reaction "pathways" (93). These hypotheses are based on the premise that the hypertonic contrast media cause endothelial disruptions and the release of active chemical substances or transmitters. It has also been suggested that the contrast media enter areas of the CNS having fenestrated capillaries and then cause autonomic responses that produce the reactions (93). All of these mechanisms are possible but it is difficult for one hypothesis to explain all the observed reactions. The literature appears to indicate that the mechanisms for adverse reactions are multifaceted and complex. We do know, however, that preexisting factors play a role (80). The accumulation of clinical data for the new low osmolality contrast media should test the hypothesis that the initiating mechanism is related to hypertonicity.

CONCLUDING REMARKS

Radiopaque contrast media are an extremely important diagnostic tool. They are among the least toxic of intravascular agents but they commonly must be used in high concentrations and doses to achieve their X-ray absorbing function. These high concentrations and doses will always produce transient physiologic and pharmacologic alterations. These responses are generally small and of little clinical concern. Adverse reactions requiring medical treatment are infrequent with conventional ionic monomer molecules, but they are still of medical concern. New low osmolality contrast media molecules will soon be available in the United States that have been shown to produce significantly smaller physiologic and pharmacologic responses. It is believed that these new molecules will also reduce the incidence of adverse reactions significantly, but the patient data available is still incomplete.

ACKNOWLEDGMENTS

The authors wish to thank Ms. Suzanne Ayers and Mr. John Groves for their help with this manuscript.

Literature Cited

1. Knoefel, P. K., ed. 1971. *Radiocontrast Agents*, Vol. 2. Oxford: Pergamon. 691 pp.
2. Miller, R. E., Skucas, J. 1977. *Radiographic Contrast Agents*. Baltimore: Univ. Park Press. 515 pp.
3. Amiel, M., ed. 1982. *Contrast Media in Radiology*. New York: Springer. 353 pp.
4. Taenzer, V., Zeitler, E., eds. 1983. *Contrast Media in Urography, Angiography and Computerized Tomography*. New York: Thieme Verlag. 173 pp.
5. Sovak, M., ed. 1984. *Radiocontrast Agents*. Berlin/New York: Springer-Verlag. 609 pp.
6. Granger, R. G. 1982. Intravascular contrast media—the past, the present and the future. *Br. J. Radiol.* 55:1–18
7. Hoey, G. B., Smith, K. R. 1984. Chemistry of X-ray contrast media. See Ref. 5, pp. 23–125
8. Speck, U., Muetzel, W., Weinmann, H-J. 1983. Chemistry, physiochemistry and pharmacology of known and new contrast media for angiography, urography and CT enhancement. See Ref. 4, pp. 2–10
9. Plewes, D. B., Violante, M. R., Morris, T. W. 1980. Intravenous contrast material and tissue enhancement in CT. In *Medical Physics and Ultrasound*, ed. G. D. Gullerton, J. A. Zagzebski, pp. 176–220. New York: Am. Inst. Physics
10. Dean, P. B., Plewes, D. B. 1984. Contrast media in computed tomography. See Ref. 5, pp. 419–23
11. Potts, D. G., Higgins, C. B., ed. 1985. A worldwide clinical assessment of a new nonionic contrast medium: iohexol. *Invest. Radiol.* 20(1): S1–S121. (Suppl.)
12. McClennan, B. L., ed. 1984. Ioxaglic acid: a new low osmolality contrast medium. *Invest. Radiol.* 19(6): S289–S392 (Suppl.)
13. Drayer, B. P., ed. 1984. Iopamidol: intravascular and intrathecal applications. *Invest. Radiol.* 19(5): S161–S287 (Suppl.)
14. Shaw, D. D., Potts, D. G. 1984. Toxicology of iohexol. *Invest. Radiol.* 20(1):S10–S13 (Suppl.)
15. Sovak, M. 1984. Introduction: state of the art and design principles of contrast media. See Ref. 5, pp. 1–22
15a. Nagel, R., Leistenschneider, W., Speck, U., Clauss, W. 1978. Pharmacokinetics and clinical studies of ioglicinate, a new contrast medium for intravenous urography. *Int. J. Clin. Pharmacol. Ther. Toxicol.* 16:49–53

15b. Olsson, B., Aulie, A. S. E., Sven, K., Andrew, E. 1983. Human pharmacokinetics of iohexol a new nonionic contrast medium. *Invest. Radiol.* 18:177–82
15c. McKinstry, D. N., Rommel, A. J., Sugerman, A. 1984. Pharmacokinetics, metabolism, and excretion of iopamidol in healthy subjects. *Invest. Radiol.* 19:S171–174 (Suppl.)
16. Sage, M. R. 1983. Kinetics of water soluble contrast media in the central nervous system. *Am. J. Roentgenol.* 141: 815–24
17. Donaldson, M. L. 1968. Comparison of the renal clearance of inulin and radioactive diatrizoate as measures of glomerular filtration rate in man. *Clin. Sci.* 35:513–24
18. Barnhart, J. L. 1984. Hepatic disposition and elimination of biliary contrast media. See Ref. 5, pp. 367–418
19. Guidolet, J., Barbe, R., Borsson, F., Gateau, O., Amiel, M., Louisot, P. 1980. Subcellular localization of uroangio-graphic contrast by I-125-labelled media. *Invest. Radiol.* 15(6): S215–S19 (Suppl.)
20. Dean, P. B., Kivisaari, L., Kormano, M. 1978. The diagnostic potential of contrast enhancement pharmacokinetics. *Invest. Radiol.* 13:533–40
21. Newhouse, J. H., 1977. Fluid compartment distribution of intravenous iothalamate in the dog. *Invest. Radiol.* 12:364–67
22. Burgener, F. A., Hamlin, D. J. 1981. Contrast enhancement in abdominal CT: bolus vs. infusion. *Am. J. Roentgenol.* 137:351–58
23. Dean, P. B., Kivisaari, L., Kormano, M. 1983. Contrast enhancement pharmacokinetics of six ionic and nonionic contrast media. *Invest. Radiol.* 18(4):368–74
24. Morris, A. M., Elwood, C., Sigman, E. M., Cotanzaro, A. 1965. The renal clearance of I-131 labelled meglumine diatrizoate in man. *J. Nucl. Med.* 6:183–91
25. Morris, T. W., Harnish, P. P., Reece, K., Katzberg, R. W. 1983. Tissue fluid shifts during renal arteriography with conventional and low osmolality agents. *Invest. Radiol.* 18:335–40
26. Spataro, R. F. 1984. Newer contrast media for urography. *Radiol. Clin. North Am.* 22(2):365–80
27. Spataro, R. F., Fischer, H. W., Boylan, L. 1982. Urography with low osmolality contrast media. Comparative urinary excretion of iopamidol, hexabrix and diatrizoate. *Invest. Radiol.* 17:494–500

28. Sjoberg, S., Almen, T., Golman, K. 1980. Excretion of urographic contrast media. I. Iohexol and other media during free urine flow in the rabbit. *Acta Radiol. Suppl.* 362:93–98

29. Benness, G. T. 1970. Urographic contrast agents. A comparison of sodium and methylglucamine salts. *Clin. Radiol.* 21:150–56

30. Morris, T. W., Kern, M. A., Katzberg, R. W. 1982. The effects of media viscosity on hemodynamics in selective arteriography. *Invest. Radiol.* 17(1):70–76

31. Laurum, F. 1984. Injurious effects of contrast media on human vascular endothelium. *Invest. Radiol.* 20(1):S98–S99 (Suppl.)

32. Nyman, U., Almen, T. 1980. Effects of contrast media on aortic endothelium. Experiments in the rat with nonionic and ionic monomer and monoacidic dimeric contrast media. *Acta Radiol. Suppl.* 362:65–72

33. Gospos, C., Freudenberg, N., Staubesand, J., Mathias, K., Papacharlampos, X. 1983. The effect of contrast media on the aortic endothelium of rats. *Radiology* 147:685–88

34. Hilal, S. 1966. Hemodynamic changes associated with intra-arterial injection of contrast media. *Radiology* 86:615–33

35. Morris, T. W., Francis, M., Fischer, H. W. 1979. A comparison of the cardiovascular responses to carotid injections of ionic and nonionic contrast media. *Invest. Radiol.* 14(3):217–23

36. Morris, T. W. 1984. Contrast media for digital subtraction angiography. *Invest. Radiol.* 19:S114–15 (Suppl.)

37. Hagen, B., Klink, G. 1983. Contrast media and pain: hypothesis on the genesis of pain occurring on intra-arterial administration of contrast media. See Ref. 4, pp. 50–56

38. Wolf, K. J., Steidle, B., Banzer, D., Seyferth, W., Keysser, R. 1983. Comparative evaluation of low osmolar contrast media in femoral arteriography. See Ref. 4, pp. 102–6

39. Stuart, C., Foresti, M., Gambaccini, P., Tenti, L., Toti, A., et al. 1982. A double blind multicenter study of Iopamiro 370 versus sodium-methylglucamine diatrizoate 76% in aortography and selective arteriography. *Rays* 7:49–60 (Suppl.)

40. Sacks, B. A., Ellison, H. P., Bartek, S., Vine, H. S., Palestrant, A. M. 1984. A comparison of Hexabrix and Renografin-60 in peripheral arteriography. *Invest. Radiol.* 19:S320–22 (Suppl.)

41. Reidy, J. F. 1984. Iopamidol in peripheral angiography. *Invest. Radiol.* 19:S206–9 (Suppl.)

42. Wolf, G. L. 1984. Adult peripheral angiography. Results from four North American randomized clinical trials of ionic media vs. iohexol. *Invest. Radiol.* 20:S108–11 (Suppl.)

43. Higgins, C. B. 1984. Contrast media in the cardiovascular system. See Ref. 5, pp. 193–251

44. Fischer, H. W., Thomson, K. B. 1978. Contrast media in coronary arteriography: a review. *Invest. Radiol.* 13(5):450–59

45. Higgins, C. B. 1977. Effects of contrast media on the conducting system of the heart. *Radiology* 124:599–606

46. Higgins, C. B., Schmidt, W. 1978. Direct and reflex myocardial effects of intracoronary administered contrast materials in the anesthetized and conscious dog: Comparison of standard and newer contrast materials. *Invest. Radiol.* 13:205–16

47. Thomson, K. R., Violante, M. R., Kenyon, T. 1978. Reduction in ventricular fibrillation using calcium enriched Renografin 76. *Invest. Radiol.* 13:238–40

48. Morris, T. W., Sahler, L. G., Whynot, L. K., Hayakawa, K. 1984. Contrast media induced fibrillation with Angiovist-370 and Renografin-76. *Radiology* 152:203–4

49. Morris, T. W., Hayakawa, K., Sahler, L. G., Ekholm, S. 1985. Incidence of fibrillation with isotonic contrast media for intra-arterial coronary digital subtraction angiography. *Diagn. Imaging Clin. Med.* In press

50. Snyder, C. F., Formanek, A., Frech, R. S., Amplatz, K. 1971. The role of sodium in promoting ventricular arrhythmia during selective coronary arteriography. *Am. J. Roentgenol.* 113:567–71

51. Miller, D., Lohse, J., Wolf, G. 1976. Slow response induced in canine purkinje fibers by contrast medium. *Invest. Radiol.* 11:577–87

52. Zipfel, J., Baller, D., Blanke, H. 1980. Decrease in cardiotoxicity of contrast media in coronary arteriography by added calcium. *Ann. Radiol.* 23:382–83

53. Wolf, G. L., Hirshfeld, J. W. 1983. Changes in QT_c interval induced with Renografin-76 and Hypaque-76 during coronary arteriography. *J. Am. Coll. Cardiol.* 1:1489–92

54. Hildner, F. J., Scherlag, B., Samet, P. 1971. Evaluations of Renografin-M76 as a contrast agent for angiocardiography. *Radiology* 100:329–34

55. Katzberg, R. W., Morris, T. W., Burgener, F. A., Kamm, D. E., Fischer, H. W. 1977. Renal renin and hemodynamic responses to selective renal artery catheterization and angiography. *Invest. Radiol.* 5:381–88

56. Bakris, G. L., Burnett, J. C. 1985. A role for calcium in radiocontrast induced reductions in renal hemodynamics. *Kidney Int.* 27:465–68

57. Katzberg, R. W., Schulman, G., Meggs, L. G., Caldicott, W. J. H., Damiano, M. M., Hollenberg, N. K. 1983. Mechanism of renal response to contrast medium in dogs: decrease due to hypertonicity. *Invest. Radiol.* 18:74–80

58. Larson, T. S., Hudson, K., Merty, J. I., Romero, J. C., Knox, F. G. 1983. Renal vasoconstrictive response to contrast medium. *J. Lab. Clin. Med.* 101:385–91

59. Tejler, L., Almen, T., Holtas, S. 1977. Proteinuria following nephroangiography. 1. Clinical experiences. *Acta Radiol. Diagn.* 18:634–40

60. Morris, T. W., Katzberg, R. W., Fischer, H. W. 1978. A comparison of the hemodynamic resposes to metrizamide and meglumine/sodium diatrizoate in canine renal angiography. *Invest. Radiol.* 13:74–78

61. Tornquist, C., Almen, T., Golman, K., Holtas, S. 1980. Proteinuria following nephroangiography. 3. Comparison between ionic monomeric, monoacidic dimeric and nonionic contrast media in the dog. *Acta Radiol. Suppl.* 362:49–52

62. Katzberg, R. W., Morris, T. W., Schulman, G. 1983. Reaction to intravenous contrast media. Part 2. Acute renal response in euvolemic and dehydrated dogs. *Radiology* 147:331–34

63. Morris, T. W., Hayakawa, K., Sahler, L. G. 1984. Evaluation of IV-DSA protocols to increase aortic opacification. *Invest. Radiol.* 19(5):S32 (Abstr.)

64. Slutsky, R. A., Brown, J. J., Strich, G. 1984. Extravascular lung water: effects of using ionic contrast media at varying levels of left atrial pressure and during myocardial ischemia. *Radiology* 152:575–78

65. Slutsky, R. A., Hackney, D. B., Peck, W. W., Higgins, C. B. 1983. Extravascular lung water: effects of ionic and nonionic contrast media. *Radiology* 149:375–78

66. Littner, M. R., Rosenfield, A. T., Ulreich, S., Putman, C. E. 1977. Evaluation of bronchospasm during excretory urography. *Radiology* 124:17–21

67. Read, R. C., Vick, J. A., Meyer, M. W. 1959. Influence of perfusate characteris-

tics on the pulmonary vascular effects of hypertonic solutions. *Fed. Proc.* 18: 1240–46

68. Almen, T., Aspelin, P. 1975. Cardiovascular effects of ionic monomeric, ionic dimeric and nonionic contrast media. *Invest. Radiol.* 10:557–63

69. Harnish, P. P., DiStefano, V. 1984. Decreased cerebrospinal fluid production by intravenous sodium diatrizoate. *Invest. Radiol.* 19:318–23

70. Morris, T. W., Francis, M., Fischer, H. W. 1979. A comparison of the cardiovascular responses to carotid injections of ionic and nonionic contrast media. *Invest. Radiol.* 14:217–23

71. Higgins, C. B., Schmidt, W. S. 1979. Identification and evaluation of the contribution of the chemoreflex in the hemodynamic response to intracarotid administration of contrast materials in the conscious dog: Comparison to nicotine. *Invest. Radiol.* 14:438–46

72. Hayakawa, K., Morris, T. W., Katzberg, R. W., Fischer, H. W. 1985. Cardiovascular response to the intervertebral injection of hypertonic contrast media in the dog. *Invest. Radiol.* 20:217–21

73. Fischer, H. W., Morris, T. W. 1980. Possible factors in intravascular contrast media toxicity. *Invest. Radiol.* 15:S232–S238 (Suppl.)

74. Higgins, C. B., Gerber, K. H., Mattrey, R. F., Slutsky, R. A. 1982. Evaluation of hemodynamic effects of intravenous administration of ionic and nonionic contrast materials. *Radiology* 142:681–86

75. Fischer, H. W., Katzberg, R. W., Morris, T. W., Spataro, R. F. 1984. Systemic response to excretory urography. *Radiology* 151:31–33

76. Katzberg, R. W., Morris, T. W., Schulman, G., Faillace, R. T., Boylan, L. M., et al. 1983. Intravenous contrast media: severe and fatal reactions in a canine dehydration model. *Radiology* 147:327–30

77. Ansell, G. 1970. Adverse reactions to contrast agents. Scope of problem. *Invest. Radiol.* 5:374–84

78. Hobbs, B. B. 1981. Adverse reactions to intravenous contrast agents in Ontario. *J. Can. Assoc. Radiol.* 31:8–10

79. Lalli, A. F. 1980. Contrast media reactions: data analysis and hypothesis. *Radiology* 134:1–12

80. Ansell, G., Tweedie, M. C. K., West, C. R., Evans, P., Couch, L. 1980. The current status of reactions to intravenous contrast media. *Invest. Radiol.* 15:S32–S39 (Suppl.)

81. Hartman, G. W., Hattery, R. R., Witten, D. M., Williamson, B. 1982. Mortality

during excretory urography: Mayo Clinic experience. *Am. J. Roentgenol.* 139: 919–22

82. Dahlstrom, K., Shaw, D. D., Clauss, W., Andrew, E., Sveen, K. 1985. Summary of US and European intravascular experience with iohexol based on the clinical trial program. *Invest. Radiol.* 20:S117–21 (Suppl.)

83. Holtas, S. 1984. Iohexol in patients with previous adverse reactions to contrast media. *Invest. Radiol.* 19:563–65

84. Rapaport, S., Bookstein, J. J., Higgins, C. B., Carey, P. H., Sovak, M., Lasser, E. C. 1982. Experience with metrizamide in patients with previous severe anaphylactoid reactions to ionic contrast agents. *Radiology* 143:321–25

85. Berkseth, R. O., Kjellstrand, C. M. 1984. Radiologic contrast-induced nephropathy. *Med. Clin. North Am.* 68: 351–70

86. Byrd, L., Sherman, R. L. 1979. Radiocontrast-induced acute renal failure: a clinical and pathophysiologic review. *Medicine* 58:270–79

87. Mudge, G. H. 1980. Nephrotoxicity of urographic radiocontrast drugs. *Kidney Int.* 18:540–52

88. Rasmussen, H. H., Ibels, L. S. 1982. Acute renal failure. *Am. J. Med.* 73:211–18

89. Ekholm, S. E. 1985. Adverse reactions to intravascular and intrathecal contrast media. Iatrogenic diseases, *Crit. Rev. in Diagn. Imaging.* In press

90. Goldberg, M. 1984. Systemic reactions to intravascular contrast media: a guide for the anesthesiologist. *Anesthesiology* 60:46–56

91. Brasch, R. C. 1980. Allergic reactions to contrast media: accumulated evidence. *Am. J. Roentgenol.* 134:797–801

92. Lasser, E. C., Lang, J. H., Hamblin, A. E., Lyon, S. G., Howard, M. 1980. Activation systems in contrast idiocyncrasy. *Invest. Radiol.* 15:S52–S55 (Suppl.)

93. Lalli, A. F., Greenstreet, R. 1981. Reactions to contrast media: testing the CNS hypothesis. *Radiology* 138:47–49

Ann. Rev. Pharmacol. Toxicol. 1986. 26:161–81

POTENTIAL ANIMAL MODELS FOR SENILE DEMENTIA OF ALZHEIMER'S TYPE, WITH EMPHASIS ON AF64A-INDUCED CHOLINOTOXICITY

Abraham Fisher

Israel Institute for Biological Research, Ness-Ziona, 70450, Israel

Israel Hanin

Department of Psychiatry, Western Psychiatric Institute and Clinic, University of Pittsburgh School of Medicine, Pittsburgh, Pennsylvania 15213

INTRODUCTION

A number of excellent reviews have been published over the past decade, dealing with neurotoxic substances specific for neurotransmitter systems (1–12). Application of a few such agents has provided new animal models for various neuropsychiatric disease states, including Parkinson's disease, Huntington's disease, Senile Dementia of Alzheimer's Type (SDAT), epilepsy, and some ataxias.

These all serve as background for the subject of this review, which focuses on literature pertaining to ethylcholine aziridinium ion (AF64A) (e.g. 13–45). We have recently proposed this agent as a potential tool in developing an animal model for SDAT (13, 20, 26), a disease in which a central cholinergic hypofunction has been implicated (46–55).

In this review, the clinical, neuropathological, and behavioral features of SDAT will first be described briefly, to enable us to evaluate the relevance of AF64A-induced cholinotoxicity in vivo as a potential animal model for SDAT. We then compare the AF64A model with other experimental models of SDAT.

161

0362-1642/86/0415-0161$02.00

We provide an overview of research conducted with the AF64A-treated animal, based on published reports in the literature. Finally, we discuss the potential of the AF64A-treated animal as a model of SDAT, in light of AF64A's biological effects in vivo.

THE CHOLINERGIC HYPOFUNCTION IN SDAT

The neurological disorder SDAT is highly prevalent today. Yet, to date there is no effective therapy for this disease state (46, 47). The term SDAT is now generally applied to cases of presenile dementia in which onset occurs in the fifth decade, as well as to cases of senile dementia in which patients are 60–65 years or older. SDAT is characterized by a progressive, chronic cognitive dysfunction, with severe impairment of memory of recent events, while memory for the more distant past remains relatively intact (46).

Histopathological studies on brains taken at autopsy from patients with SDAT show characteristic abnormalities such as plaques, consisting of abnormal neurites and having a central core of amyloid surrounded by argentophilic granules and filaments; neurofibrillary tangles, which are composed of bundles of paired helical filaments that accumulate within the cell bodies of neurons; and granulovacuolar degeneration. These abnormalities are most prominent in the cerebral cortex and hippocampal formation (46, 47).

A loss of specific populations of nerve cells from SDAT patients' brains taken at autopsy has been reported in the frontal and temporal cortexes, the medial septum, diagonal band of Broca (dbB), and the nucleus basalis of Meynert (nbM), a basal forebrain cholinergic network that projects directly to the hippocampus and neocortex (reviewed in 46, 47). It is therefore important to note that, over the past few years, neurochemical studies have also demonstrated that presynaptic cholinergic markers[1] are significantly reduced in the cerebral cortices and hippocampi of affected individuals (55), as well as in their medial septa, dbBs, and nbMs (46–69).

These changes are paralleled by increasing morphological alterations, probably due to nerve terminal degeneration, which in turn correlate with increasing dementia scores (46, 49). Such observations, coupled with pharmacological investigations in humans and animals indicating a major role of the cholinergic system in learning and memory (52–56), are consistent with a hypothesis of a cholinergic dysfunction in SDAT. In fact, SDAT appears to be caused primarily by a cholinergic hypofunction in selected brain areas, while other neurotransmitter systems appear to be affected less or later in the course of the disease (46, 47, 51, 53–57, 65).

---

[1]Presynaptic cholinergic markers include choline acetyltransferase (ChAT) and acetylcholinesterase (AChE) activities; high-affinity transport of choline (HAChT); acetylcholine (ACh) synthesis; and muscarinic receptor (mAChR) binding.

Clinical trials have been conducted in which lecithin or physostigmine have been administered to SDAT patients, because of the presumed ability of these agents to elevate and thus restore cholinergic activity in the central nervous system (66, 67, 69). Unfortunately, results to date have not been conclusive, and clinicians do not agree about the efficacy of treating SDAT with such drugs. Recently, however, a marked improvement in SDAT patients was reported following the intracerebroventricular infusion of bethanechol, lending further credence to the cholinergic hypothesis of SDAT (68).

RELEVANT ANIMAL MODELS OF SDAT

A major problem in the basic research and drug development for SDAT is the lack of adequate animal models that can mimic all aspects of this disease. Generally, an animal model should allow for a more detailed evaluation of the neurochemical, neuropathological, and behavioral sequelae of the primary cholinergic hypofunction suggested in this disorder. Such a model would be instrumental in testing a wide variety of drugs, to determine whether they correct the cholinergic hypofunction and restore cognitive functions to normal. An animal model would obviously provide information in studies that cannot readily be performed in humans (e.g. analysis of neurotransmitter levels and metabolism in brain areas in vivo). Finally, an animal model that reproduces the specific neuronal deficits and cognitive dysfunction of SDAT may offer some clues about the underlying deficits of this disease state.

The ideal model would be one that exhibits the same biochemical, behavioral, and histopathologic abnormalities as the human disease state. However, there is at present no homologous animal for SDAT, since the etiology of this disorder is still unknown. Partial success could therefore be achieved at this stage only with *isomorphic models;* that is, despite parallelism between the model and the human conditions, the cause of the condition in the animal may be quite different from the cause in man.

A number of experimental approaches or paradigms have been used that mimic different aspects of this progressive neurological disorder. These include:

1. aged rodents and aged monkeys;
2. anoxic/hypoxic rodents;
3. scopolamine- or hemicholinium-treated experimental animals;
4. aluminum-treated experimental animals;
5. excitotoxin-lesioned rats or monkeys; and
6. AF64A-lesioned rodents.

The following is an overview and critique of each of these specific experimental models. Available space precludes an extensive evaluation of each of these models since the primary emphasis of the review is on the AF64A-treated animal. The reader is therefore urged to refer to the pertinent publications listed in the discussion of each of the other individual models for further specific information.

Aged Rodents and Aged Monkeys

Learning and memory deficits are recognized as severe and consistent behavioral impairments in the elderly. Since SDAT is a neurological disorder associated with aging, aged animals have been evaluated in many studies as possible animal models for age-related memory deficits and for SDAT (56).

Aged rodents (mice and rats) were shown, for example, to suffer deficits of retention of a single-trial passive-avoidance task. This deficit is conceptually similar to the severe memory loss reported in aged monkeys and humans (56). Control studies have indicated that a major source of this impairment is loss of memory for the learned event.

Drugs known to produce subtle improvements in SDAT patients also improved the performance of aged rodents in a task sensitive to age-related loss of memory (56). Thus, such experimental animals can be useful in evaluating drugs for the treatment of SDAT. Similarly, old monkeys showed reduced memory for recent events, increased perseveration in a reversal learning task, and hypersensitivity to interference. Drug effects on memory in the aged monkey also appeared to resemble those in humans (56).

Neuritic plaques occur in aging human brain and are more numerous in SDAT. Furthermore, in SDAT they correlate with the severity of dementia and magnitude of cortical cholinergic deficits (49). Neuritic plaques have also been found in aged (23–31 years) rhesus monkeys (70). In this regard, therefore, these aged nonhuman primates are an important model for testing hypotheses about the evolution and significance of these plaques.

Thus, the aged rodent or monkey does have value as an experimental animal in modelling SDAT. This model also has a few disadvantages:

1. Since SDAT is a neurological progressive disease distinct from normal aging (46, 48, 49, 71–73), aged rodents or monkeys are not ideal animal models for this disorder (74). Moreover, aged rodents mimic to a certain degree the neurochemical changes associated with normal aging, but not those presynaptic cholinergic dysfunctions (e.g. decreased ChAT activity) reported in SDAT (54).

2. The high cost of old monkeys and even old rats in drug screening also severely restricts the practical use of these animals for research purposes.

3. Poor health of aging animals and individual pharmacokinetic variabilities in drug absorption, metabolism, and distribution may sometimes yield statistically inconclusive data.

Anoxic or Hypoxic Rodents

The brains of many aged mammals differ from those of young mammals in energy-dependent biochemical functions (56). By depriving young rodents of oxygen, an energy-deficient state is induced that resembles the functional characteristics of the aging brain. Anoxia may be analogous to aging because both aging and anoxia impair oxidative metabolism and lead to similar behavioral deficits.

The anoxic model is produced by training animals in a single-trial passive-avoidance task and then exposing them immediately to an oxygen-deficient environment. The anoxic situation causes a retrograde retention deficit for the training trial (56). Hypoxia as a model for aging is analogous in many aspects to the anoxia-induced experimental model (74).

The anoxia/hypoxia experimental model generally resembles the aged rodent both neurochemically and behaviorally, thus allowing evaluation of drugs to be used for experiments in and treatment of geriatric memory and learning deficits. In fact, drugs shown to have some marginal beneficial effects in SDAT are effective in this test as well (56). This simple and inexpensive model can therefore be used for preliminary screening in developing drugs for memory disorders.

On the other hand, anoxic or hypoxic animals do not selectively exhibit those brain-area specific cholinergic deficits generally reported in this disorder. In fact, the key disadvantage in this model is that the anoxic/hypoxic animals mimic a generalized neuropathology associated with various neurotransmitters, including the cholinergic system. Another disadvantage of this model is its lack of histopathological characteristics similar to those of SDAT brains.

Scopolamine- or Hemicholinium-Treated Experimental Animals

The primary pharmacological support for the theory that the cholinergic system plays an important role in cognitive function is the finding that blockade of central $mAChR$ binding induces a cognitive deficit in young volunteers. The deficit is qualitatively similar to that occurring naturally in aged subjects. Scopolamine administration induced cognitive deficits similar to those found naturally in aged subjects tested on the same clinical battery (reviewed in 54). One such deficit was loss of memory in young subjects for recent (but not immediate) events. Similarly, scopolamine injected into young monkeys caused memory deficits similar to those occurring naturally in aged monkeys (54).

Although the scopolamine-treated animal provides a good model for evaluating the cognitive effects of pharmacological disruption of cholinergic function, it lacks certain features necessary for studying the pathophysiology of SDAT: (a) SDAT is a progressive, irreversible, neurological disease whereas the effects induced by scopolamine in animals (or humans) are reversible. (b) In

SDAT the cholinergic system is irreversibly compromised as a result of pre-synaptic degeneration of cholinergic neurons, without a significant decrease in postsynaptic $mAChR$ (54, 60, 62–64; but see also 61); therefore scopolamine, which causes mainly reversible blockade of postsynaptic $mAChR$, mimics only some features of SDAT (75).

Hemicholinium-3 injected intracerebroventricularly (i.c.v.) in mice, rats, or marmosets has also been shown to impair certain cognitive functions (75, 76). Hemicholinium-3 induces a state of presynaptic cholinergic hypofunction by blocking HAChT. However, although this model may mimic some aspects of the memory disorder in SDAT it, again, is not the ideal model for this disease state since it only partially mimics the central cholinergic hypofunction. Moreover, the effect is reversible, whereas SDAT is a chronic and progressive disorder.

Aluminum-Treated Experimental Animals

Aluminum has been implicated as being involved with SDAT. Perl & Brody (77) have reported the presence of aluminum in the nuclear region of neurofi-brillary tangles containing neuronal cells from Alzheimer's patients. Alumi-num injected into rabbit brains also causes formation of neurofibrillary tangles (78). Additionally, following aluminum administration into cat brains, some memory loss and abnormal behavior have been observed (79). Also, recently, intracranial administration of aluminum was shown to produce avoidance-learning deficits in immature rabbits (80).

The morphology of the neurofibrillary tangles induced by aluminum, howev-er, differs significantly from that of human SDAT-type tangles (46, 79, 80). Central cholinergic activity (which is markedly reduced in SDAT) is, moreov-er, normal in rabbits with aluminum-induced neurofibrillary changes, and the direct activity of aluminum on cholinergic markers such as ChAT is minimal (81). Also, the brain areas affected by aluminum in animals are significantly different from those areas affected in SDAT (81). In addition, McDermott et al (82) showed that there was no difference in aluminum accumulation between SDAT and age-matched controls. Furthermore, they found an increase in brain aluminum content associated with aging.

Based on the above-mentioned data it appears that the induction by alumi-num of neurofibrillary tangles in experimental animals, while an intriguing phenomenon definitely worth further exploration, is not a perfectly matching animal model for SDAT. Moreover, its relevance to the etiology of this disorder is still an unsettled issue.

Excitotoxin-Lesioned Rats and Monkeys

The magnocellular system of the basal forebrain consists of clusters of large neurons located in the septum, dbB, and nbM. This system has been shown to be cholinergic (48, 83). In SDAT the cholinergic deficiency in the cortex and hippocampus appears to be due to a loss of neurons from this magnocellular cholinergic system. In concordance with this observation, electrolytic or excitotoxin-induced lesions of the ventromedial corner of the rat globus pallidus (equivalent to the nbM in humans and nonhuman primates) reduce ChAT activity, ACh levels, and Ch uptake in different parts of the cortex (48, 72, 83).

Electrolytic lesions are nonspecific, however, and result in axonal destruction and anterograde and retrograde neuronal degeneration. Intracerebrally injected excitotoxins, including kainic acid, ibotenic acid, N-methyl aspartate, and quinolinic acid do, on the other hand, produce a selective pattern of neuronal degeneration. This effect is focussed at neuronal perikarya near the injection site; axons of passage or of termination are essentially spared from destruction (72, 84–86).

Some of the excitotoxins listed above have been used for lesioning the nbM, in order to induce in experimental animals (rats or monkeys) cortical cholinergic lesions similar to those reported in SDAT. A wealth of information regarding these types of lesions in the nbM has been accumulated in the last few years, including neurochemical, histochemical, behavioral, and pharmacological observations. Some representative examples follow.

Neurochemical studies with kainic acid–induced lesions in the rat nbM have demonstrated a 45–50% loss of cortical ChAT (72, 87). This decrease in cortical ChAT has been paralleled by a decrease in ACh levels and in HAChT and AChE activity, but with no significant change in cortical GABA-ergic, noradrenergic, serotonergic, or histaminergic presynaptic markers (72). Behaviorally, this kind of lesion with kainic acid induces a marked retention deficit, 24 hr after the initial training trial, in a step-through passive-avoidance task (87). Thus, this lesion with kainic acid may be capable of producing a potential animal model for SDAT (72, 87).

However, kainic acid, as a potent convulsant, can produce distant damage (88, 89). Therefore ibotenic acid is presently preferred in a large number of laboratories (72, 84, 90–100).

Ibotenic acid–induced lesion of the nbM reduces ChAT activity in different parts of the cortex; the decrease is generally smaller than that reported with kainic acid (but see also 72, 84). Behaviorally, rats with ibotenic acid–nbM lesions show deficits in the retention of a step-through passive-avoidance response; an impairment of spatial-reference memory in a 16-arm radial maze; and recent-memory deficits (in an 8-arm radial maze), analogous to those seen in SDAT patients (84, 99). On the other hand, working memory is not disrupted by such lesions (84). Lesions of the nbM and medial septal areas of rats with ibotenic acid also impair spatial "working" memory in a T-maze task (98).

A few pharmacologically oriented studies have already been initiated in which attempts have been made to reverse learning and memory deficits caused by nbM lesions induced by ibotenic acid. Such deficits can be reversed by treatment with the cholinesterase inhibitor physostigmine (84, 95), but not with the direct muscarinic agonist oxotremorine (99). Monkeys injected with ibotenic acid into the nbM can still perform normally in a recognition memory task, but their performance is more easily disrupted than that of normal animals when challenged with the muscarinic antagonist scopolamine (93).

All these results, when combined, lend support to the view that excitotoxin-induced lesions can be useful in production of animal models of the cortical cholinergic deficiency in SDAT. However, several deficiencies in these models should be pointed out. Specifically, these are the following.

1. The excitotoxin-induced lesions do not produce the histopathological features characteristic of SDAT such as neuritic plaques and neurofibrillary tangles. Nor do they cause deficits in somatostatin, which is also affected in SDAT (46, 51, 96).
2. Since these excitotoxins generally affect all neuronal perikarya regardless of neurotransmitter used, these lesions provide only limited information on the specific role of the cholinergic system in memory and learning deficits.
3. Another deficiency with these excitotoxin lesions is that they damage contiguous noncholinergic neurons at the injection site (72). Thus, rats with ibotenic lesions in the dorsolateral globus pallidus exhibited passive-avoidance deficits even though their cortical ChAT activity was not decreased (90). This limitation might be avoided through the use of AF64A (see below).
4. Finally, excitotoxin-induced lesion of the nbM mimics only the cortical presynaptic cholinergic deficit in SDAT; ChAT activity in the hippocampus is not affected in these excitotoxin-lesioned animals.

AF64A-Lesioned Rodents

Progress in the amelioration of SDAT could be hastened considerably if an animal model could be found that *directly* mimics the cholinergic abnormality reported in SDAT (13). Steps in this direction have been taken, based on our current understanding of factors regulating cholinergic function in vivo.

Although cholinergic neurons do not take up their neurotransmitter ACh, they possess an avid, high-affinity transport mechanism for its precursor choline, the HAChT, which appears to be restricted to, or at least highly concentrated on, cholinergic neurons, and tightly linked to ACh synthesis. It can be distinguished from a nonspecific transport process for choline, found in most cells that have a much lower affinity for choline transport (LAChT) (13, 101). A chemical analog of choline was therefore sought, which would be selectively targeted toward the HAChT system because of its structural similarity to choline, but which, at the same time, would be cytotoxic at the site of its accumulation in vivo.

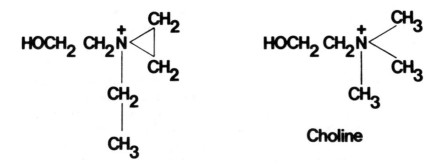

AF64A

Figure 1   Structural representation of AF64A and choline. Note the close similarity in chemical structure of these two molecules.

Such a cholinotoxin, ethylcholine aziridinium, (AF64A) (Figure 1) fulfills that requirement. It induces in vivo a persistent central cholinergic hypofunction of presynaptic origin. To date, we and others have conducted extensive neurochemical, electrophysiological, behavioral, and histochemical studies to evaluate the AF64A-treated animal as a potential animal model for SDAT.

The following is an overview of some key reports on the biological effects of AF64A in vivo. Because the data are pertinent vis-à-vis animal models of SDAT, and selectivity of action of the neurotoxin, we focus in this section on results from studies conducted with rats, with particular emphasis on neurochemical findings as well as on behavioral consequences of AF64A administration.

INTRAHIPPOCAMPAL ADMINISTRATION OF AF64A   In early studies performed in vitro on rat hippocampal tissue, we were able to show that AF64A is a very specific inhibitor of HAChT (IC_{50} = 3.4 μM). Its effect on HAChT was 17, 1209, 1494, 1735, and at least 10,000 times more potent than on the LAChT, $mAChR$, ChAT, or AChE activity, or on serotonin uptake, respectively. Thus, at low concentrations in vitro, AF64A interacts only with the HAChT system (25). These findings are in concordance with the in vitro studies of Rylett & Colhoun (19), in which they demonstrated irreversible inhibition of HAChT in rat forebrain synaptosomes, using ethylcholine aziridinium.

We have expanded these data in rats, in vivo. When 2 nmol (in 2μl) AF64A were injected intracerebrally (i.c.) into the dorsal hippocampal area of rats, ACh levels in this tissue were significantly lowered (-57%) within 5 days. This was paralleled by a significant decrease in the activity of HAChT (-77%), and ChAT (-58%), while choline levels and $mAChR$ were unchanged in the same brain area. Moreover the LAChT (found on many cell types), serotonin uptake, and norepinephrine levels were also unchanged (25).

In a longitudinal study 5 days, 3 weeks, and 6 weeks following i.c. injection of AF64A (6 nmol/side into the dorsal hippocampus), HAChT and AChE activity were greatly reduced (-60–70%), and AChE staining was markedly decreased (23).

INTRASTRIATAL ADMINISTRATION OF AF64A   Striatal lesions induced in rats by AF64A (8 nmol bilaterally) resulted in significant impairments in the acquisition and retention of a step-down passive-avoidance task. No significant differences between the same control and AF64A-injected rats were found in sensitivity to electric shock or in various measures of spontaneous locomotor activity. Striatal ChAT activity was significantly decreased (-25%) in these AF64A-treated rats when compared with controls, whereas glutamic acid decarboxylase activity was not affected in the same brain area. Furthermore, there were no significant differences between the two groups in activities of ChAT and glutamic acid decarboxylase, in either the cortex or the hippocampus, thus supporting the specificity of the lesion to the striatum (33).

The above study concurs with a previous series of experiments employing similar conditions, where it was shown that AF64A acted specifically on striatal cholinergic neurons, inducing a long-lasting cholinergic underactivity (lasting at least up to 3 months), while sparing neurons containing norepinephrine, dopamine, serotonin, and GABA (31). Interestingly, under similar experimental conditions AF64A increased spontaneous nocturnal locomotor activity in rats (35). The hyperactivity found in these rats after intrastriatal injection of AF64A was interpreted as evidence that the striatal cholinergic system plays a role in locomotor behavior.

INJECTION OF AF64A INTO THE nbM   Very low concentrations of AF64A (0.02 nmol/μl or 10 μl), unilaterally administered directly into the rat nbM, decreased AChE staining in the nbM when the brain region was analyzed 7 or 14 days after injection. This reduction was paralleled by a significant decrease in cortical activity of ChAT (-17%); cortical levels of dopamine and serotonin were not affected in the same tissue (41).

On the other hand, in another study doses above 0.5 nmol of the cytotoxin, when administered into the striatum and nbM, produced appreciable nonselective damage in both the caudate putamen complex and nucleus basalis. More selective effects were seen, however, in the range of 0.1–0.5 nmol, and these were accompanied by minimal effects on cholinergic neurons (42).

The consequences of AF64A administration into the nbM thus remain equivocal, and are subject to establishing the optimal dose of the substance that should be used in future studies.

INTRACEREBROVENTRICULAR ADMINISTRATION OF AF64A   A considerable amount of information has been generated recently as a result of the i.c.v. administration of AF64A in rats. A variety of neurochemical parameters, as well as behavioral correlates of administration of various concentrations of this substance, have been measured in different brain areas. The following summarizes some of the findings obtained so far.

In the studies of Walsh and coworkers (38), rats were infused i.c.v., bilaterally, with either 7.5 or 15 nmol of AF64A (i.e. 15 and 30 nmol per brain). The results obtained in this set of experiments were as follows:

Retention of step-through passive-avoidance task, assessed 35 days after dosing, was impaired in both the 7.5- and 15-nmol groups.

Radial-arm maze performance, measured 60–80 days following treatment, was markedly impaired in the treated groups. Animals treated with AF64A made fewer correct responses in their first eight choices, required more total selections to complete the task, and had an altered pattern of spatial responding in the maze. It appears that the "working memory" rather than the "reference memory" was impaired in this test.

In these same rats neurochemical changes were evaluated 120 days later (following an extensive behavioral evaluation). Significant decreases in ACh levels in both the hippocampus (-44 to -62% in the 7.5- and 15-nmol groups) and the frontal cortex (-63% in the 15-nmol group) were observed, whereas ACh levels in the striatum were unchanged when compared with the control group. The concentrations of catecholamines, indoleamines, their metabolites, and of choline in these brain regions were not affected by AF64A treatment (38). Thus, AF64A caused a persistent decrease in ACh levels in selected brain areas reminiscent of the data obtained in mice (17).

In a similar behavioral study, smaller doses of AF64A (3 and 6 nmol) were injected i.c.v. into rats, and performance in an 8-arm radial maze was evaluated 21 days following treatment (30). "Working memory" function in the radial maze was impaired on both "place" and "cue" tasks, while "reference memory" performance was disrupted only on the "place" task. Treatment of rats i.c.v. with 3 nmol AF64A induced, after one week, a large reduction of ACh levels in the hippocampus and striatum without affecting norepinephrine or dopamine levels in the hippocampus and striatum, respectively. The authors claimed that this behavioral pattern is similar to the behavior exhibited following lesions of the fimbria-fornix. However, they also indicated that, under their experimental conditions, it was not clear whether the behavioral and neurochemical effects of AF64A were due to cholinergic specificity of this agent, or whether they resulted from a nonspecific lesion of the fimbria-fornix.

Comparable behavioral observations were also made with AF64A (3 and 5 nmol/side, icv) (44), using the one-trial passive-avoidance test. Interestingly, this AF64A-induced memory impairment could be reversed by intraperitoneal (i.p.) pretreatment of animals with physostigmine (0.06 mg/kg), thus emphasizing the potential use of this animal model for SDAT in evaluating new drugs for the disorder (44).

When rats were injected bilaterally with AF64A (3 nmol/3 µl/side) and analyzed for various cholinergic parameters 7 and 21 days after injection (45), hippocampal ChAT was found to be reduced to 42% of control level both 7 and 21 days after AF64A treatment; HAChT was reduced to 33% and 48% of control respectively; AChE was reduced to 40% and 30% of control, respectively; and K^+-stimulated ACh release was reduced to 24% or 35% of control, respectively. Meanwhile $mAChR$ binding ([^{3}H]QNB binding) was either unchanged (at 7 days), or slightly decreased (-11%, by 21 days). Neither HAChT nor [^{3}H]QNB binding in striatum and cortex were altered by AF64A treatment. Interestingly, under the specific conditions of this study, the effect of AF64A appeared to be selective for the hippocampus. These data, using a low dose of i.c.v. AF64A, further emphasize the value of using AF64A as a selective tool for inducing a persistent cholinergic hypofunction in vivo.

In yet another study (36) AF64A was administered i.c.v. (20 nmol/5µl) to 3–4-month-old rats, and a variety of tests were performed three months later with the following results:

Locomotor activity was markedly increased (which is also seen with anticholinergics). Habituation was not influenced by AF64A treatment. REM sleep was reduced, and REM latency increased. The latter was also found to be the case in old rats (>30 months) that were compared with the AF64A-treated rats. Finally, postsynaptic excitability of hippocampal pyramidal cells was not changed, while a presynaptic cholinotoxic site of action of AF64A was indicated. In some respects the changes observed were also found in old animals.

Thus, AF64A mimics, at least qualitatively, the profound reduction of presynaptic cholinergic markers observed in most regions of the forebrain, and particularly the hippocampus and cortex, of SDAT patients (46, 48).

In addition, the persistent cholinergic deficiencies in hippocampus and cortex induced by AF64A (administered to rats) are paralleled by a long-term impairment of cognitive function in the affected animals. In SDAT a decrease of presynaptic cholinergic markers is paralleled by chronic cognitive dysfunction (46, 49, 51).

The cognitive deficit in SDAT is severe for memory of recent events (short-term memory) whereas memory for the past remains relatively intact. A similar behavior pattern was observed in the 8-arm radial maze, as a result of AF64A-induced cholinotoxicity following i.c.v. injection in rats (38, 44).

Finally, AF64A administration is superior to the excitotoxin-lesioning approach of developing animal models for SDAT since the excitotoxins, because of their postulated cytotoxic mechanism, must be injected very close to the cell bodies rather than in the terminal field, where they are inactive.

However, the AF64A-animal model also has its deficiencies:

1. We have not shown yet that it can mimic the histological characteristic found in SDAT (that is, plaques and tangles). This limitation is inherent in the excitotoxin-induced lesions as well (72).

2. This animal model mimics the cholinergic hypofunction reported in SDAT. However, we do not yet know if it can reproduce deficits in somatostatin that have been reported to be reduced in SDAT (46, 50).

3. Still to be established, using conventional cholinergic drugs such as arecoline or oxotremorine, is whether such agents are capable of alleviating memory disorders induced by AF64A. In this regard the beneficial effect of physostigmine in this animal model (44) holds great promise for the future.

4. It still is important to evaluate the effect of nootropic drugs (54) on this animal model.

POSSIBLE MECHANISMS OF AF64A-INDUCED CHOLINOTOXICITY

From the literature to date we can deduce that AF64A, when used at appropriate concentrations, is a unique, selective, and specific presynaptic cholinotoxin capable of inducing a long-term or even persistent cholinergic hypofunction in vivo. How AF64A actually induces such a state of diminished cholinergic activity, while sparing other neurotransmitter systems such as the catecholaminergic, serotonergic, or GABA-ergic systems, remains to be answered.

At this stage, we have some clues regarding the chain of events leading to a long-term presynaptic cholinotoxicity and eventual cytotoxicity of cholinergic neurons following AF64A administration:

The specificity of AF64A to cholinergic neurons originates from its very close structural similarity to choline; the volume of the cationic head in AF64A is slightly larger or almost equal to the cationic head of choline (13). Therefore, AF64A is "recognized" by the HAChT system, since the aziridinium moiety in AF64A is rather stable at physiological pH (19, 27; A. Fisher and I. Hanin, unpublished).

AF64A is most probably targeted toward the HAChT and is not "used up" on its way toward the cholinergic neurons on other neuronal systems. In addition, AF64A could conceivably be transported via the HAChT system into cholinergic neurons (34). Only part of the HAChT system might be alkylated on nucleophilic sites on the choline carrier, since alkylation (i.e. a covalent bond formation) is probably a much slower reaction than the transport process itself. [That the transport of choline via the HAChT is an extremely fast process is evident from a variety of studies (101).] This would allow for an accumulation of the neurotoxin into the cholinergic neurons (mainly terminals) (22, 23, 37).

Once inside the cholinergic neurons, the compound could disrupt fundamental metabolic processes required for viability. This possible mechanism of cholinotoxicity and cytotoxicity of AF64A is evident from studies in which cholinergic and noncholinergic neuroblastoma cell lines, and various partially purified enzymes, were reacted with AF64A in vitro, revealing selective cytotoxicity of this drug against cholinergic substrates only (29, 40). The results indicated that AF64A enters the cell via HAChT and inhibits enzymes involved in choline metabolism but spares enzymes that do not use choline as a substrate or inhibitor.

Eventually, this effect could conceivably cause a decrease in the cellular concentration of phosphatidylcholine that may, in turn, cause disruption of plasma membranes. Such a mechanism may explain, in part, the selective cytotoxic effect of AF64A toward cholinergic neurons. In this regard, we can speculate that AF64A is even more specific for cholinergic neurons than the well-known specific neurotoxin, 6-hydroxydopamine (6OHDA), is for catecholaminergic neurons. The latter neurotoxin can decompose extraneuronally and intraneuronally to a variety of free radicals and H_2O_2 (1–3), which are certainly not as specific for catecholaminergic neurons as AF64A is for cholinergic neurons.

Another related intraneuronal possibility, not contradictory but in fact complementary to the above-mentioned mechanism, is the transformation of AF64A to its acetylated analog, acetylethylcholine aziridinium ion, via ChAT. This compound potentially formed, in situ, could exert toxicity, when accumulated in the presynaptic cytoplasm, by alkylating enzymes involved in vesicular ACh transport, as well as by alkylating other cytoplasmic enzymes (22).

In conclusion, while we have some excellent leads from a variety of studies, the exact mechanism of neurotoxicity and of cytotoxicity induced by AF64A is only partially understood at this time. Further studies are clearly necessary to answer a number of questions.

It is important in this context to point out that AF64A belongs to the class of neurotoxic alkylating agents: AF64A, DSP-4, and xylamine (4). These three alkylating neurotoxins for the presynaptic cholinergic and noradrenergic neurons, respectively, are excellent proof for the notion that alkylating agents of this type are not merely indiscriminately cytotoxic. A careful design of the molecule induces marked specificity, especially if the molecule resembles a substrate molecule such as norepinephrine (for DSP-4 and xylamine) (4), or a precursor such as choline (for AF64A).

COMMENTS REGARDING THE SELECTIVE NEUROTOXICITY OF AF64A

AF64A is a very potent neurotoxin, and on a molar basis is at least as toxic as kainic acid. Therefore, it is clear that certain precautions should be taken when one wants to obtain selective cholinotoxic effects versus nonspecific effects.

Nonspecific effects at the injection site can occur and have been reported in a few studies (28, 30–32, 42). Differences seen among these studies include variations in the size of the necrosis [large (28, 30, 32) or smaller (31, 42)];

different interpretation of the data (31 versus 30); use of different batches of AF64A[2] (17, 18, 27, 28, 43); and different experimental conditions.

No pathological changes in the hippocampus, septum, fimbria-fornix, amygdala, or caudate nucleus were found in our studies using conventional histology following AF64A administration (i.c.v.) at doses that induced selective persistent cholinergic hypofunction and memory disorders in rats (46). In addition we did not detect gross nonspecific histological changes with 1–2 nmol of AF64A, administered i.c. into the dorsal hippocampus, a dose that induced a selective, persistent, presynaptic, cholinotoxic effect in this brain area. However, as the dose was increased a proportionally higher incidence of edema, focal hemorrhage, and in extreme cases, liquefactive necrosis was found (35, 37).

It is therefore still not entirely clear to us whether or not AF64A actually causes a destruction of cholinergic neurons, or whether this agent modifies their functional status. The accumulated histochemical studies are not conclusive at this stage, and much work has yet to be done in this particular area of investigation.

A few general comments should be made in this context regarding the specificity of neurotoxicity of AF64A, as well as of other neurotoxins:

Cavitary lesions along the cannula tract bordered by a narrow zone of gliosis is a *common* feature rather than an exception in the case of use of all the neurotoxins. This is seen with 6OHDA (102–109), kainic acid (110–113), and with 5,6- or 5,7-dihydroxytryptamine [5,6- or 5,7-DHT (114)]. Sometimes these lesions are evident, sometimes they are undetected, depending on the experimental techniques used. Selectivity toward a certain neurotransmitter neuronal system should therefore be defined in such a way that at areas remote from these so-called cavitations only this one neuronal system is impaired while other neurotransmitter systems (in the same area) are spared. Such a condition can be fulfilled by AF64A and to a certain degree with 6OHDA, and with 5,6- or 5,7-DHT, but not with an electrolytic or mechanical lesion. Interestingly, with 6OHDA for instance, nonspecific effects were reported at areas remote from the site of injection (103).

Following any lesion, even if it is selective for a particular neuronal population, secondary changes in tissue morphology will also occur. Death of this neuronal population could lead to extensive gliosis, tissue shrinkage, and if the brain region is adjacent to the ventricles, ventricular enlargement that sometimes might cause deformation of the entire structure in this region. This effect sometimes can be misinterpreted as being a nonspecific lesion, reminiscent of electrolytic lesions, for example.

---

[2]Batches of AF64A used in our studies are identical to the compound sold by Research Biochemicals Inc. (RBI), USA, and are free of potential cytotoxic impurities such as $EtN(CH_2CH_2Cl)_2$ that could be a source of nonspecific-induced damage in the brain. We do not know whether other batches of AF64A, prepared by others, are free of such impurities.

Nonspecific destruction of tissue may also occur due to artifacts of tissue preparation. If we assume that AF64A would specifically alter the membrane morphology in cholinergic neurons (by impairing processes in which choline is either a substrate or inhibitor), and decrease its phosphatidylcholine content, for example (29, 40), then it is possible that the membrane fluidity and fragility might change. This could reveal macroscopically liquefactive tissues in the affected brain area. Once the chemical consistency of these membranes is changed, infusion of chemicals usually used for fixation (formaldehyde and/or glutaraldehyde) could osmotically disrupt these membranes, eventually leading to marked cavitations. Thus, in fact, an experimental method used in histological evaluations could even cause an artifact in interpretation of the data.

For all of the above reasons, in each case that AF64A is employed in a new application, it is recommended that comprehensive histological as well as neurochemical evaluations be conducted to allow reliable interpretation of the data. If by both these methods nonspecific effects are revealed above a certain dose, this dose should be adjusted in order to obtain specific cholinotoxic effects.

SUMMARY

In this review we have described and critiqued several commonly used proposed animal models for SDAT. In particular, we have focussed on the AF64A-treated animal. Major pertinent neurochemical and behavioral data obtained so far with AF64A have been presented, and these effects have been compared with neurochemical and behavioral changes in the SDAT patient. We have commented on the possible mechanism(s) of action of AF64A in vivo, and have also presented some observations and speculations concerning the selectivity of action of AF64A as a specific presynaptic cholinotoxin.

Much work has yet to be done with all the available animal models, including the AF64A-treated animal, before one could definitively state which one is the ideal model for SDAT. Data obtained to date with the AF64A-treated animal are nevertheless most encouraging. Despite some caveats, AF64A is a valuable neurochemical tool with which one can induce a persistent cholinergic deficiency of presynaptic origin.

As with all new tools, however, one must always exercise due care to use it properly, and interpret the results obtained following its administration with caution.

ACKNOWLEDGMENT

Supported in part by NIMH grant #MH34893 to I.H.

Literature Cited

1. Kostrzewa, R. M., Jacobowitz, D. M. 1974. Pharmacological actions of 6-hydroxydopamine. *Pharmacol. Rev.* 26: 199–288
2. Rotman, A. 1977. Minireview. The mechanisms of action of neurocytotoxic compounds. *Life Sci.* 21:891–900
3. Johnsson, G. 1980. Chemical neurotoxins as denervation tools in neurobiology. *Ann. Rev. Neurosci.* 3:169–87
4. Jaim-Etcheverry, G., Zieher, L. M. 1983. 1-chloroethylamines: New chemical tools for the study of noradrenergic neurons. *Trends Pharmacol. Sci.* 4:473–75
5. Wolf, G., Stricker, E. M., Zigmond, M. J. 1978. Brain lesions: induction, analysis and the problem of recovery of function. In *Recovery of Function from Brain Damage*, ed. S. Fingler, pp. 91–112. New York: Plenum
6. Zigmond, M. J., Stricker, E. M. 1977. Behavioral and neurochemical effects of central catecholamine depletion: a possible model for "subclinical" brain damage. In *Animal Models in Psychiatry and Neurology*, ed. I. Hanin, E. Usdin, pp. 415–29. New York: Pergamon
7. McGeer, E. G., McGeer, P. L. 1981. Neurotoxins as tools in neurobiology. *Intern. Rev. Neurobiol.* 22:173–204
8. McGeer, P. L., McGeer, E. G. 1982. Kainic acid: the neurotoxic breakthrough. *CRC Critical Rev. Toxicol.* 10:1–26
9. Coyle, J. T., Schwarcz, R., Bennett, J. P., Campochiaro, P. 1977. Clinical, neuropathologic and pharmacologic aspects of Huntington's disease: correlates with a new animal model. *Prog. Neuro-Psychopharmacol.* 1:13–30
10. Yamamura, H. I., Hruska, R. E., Schwarcz, R., Coyle, J. T. 1977. Effect of striatal kainic acid lesions on muscarinic cholinergic receptor binding: correlation with Huntington's Disease. See Ref. 6, pp. 415–19
11. Coyle, J. T. 1983. Neurotoxic action of kainic acid. *J. Neurochem.* 41:1–11
12. Nadler, J. V. 1979. Minireview. Kainic acid: neurophysiological and neurotoxic actions. *Life Sci.* 24:289–300
13. Fisher, A., Hanin, I. 1980. Minireview: Choline analogs as potential tools in developing selective animal models of central cholinergic hypofunction. *Life Sci.* 27:1615–34
14. Fisher, A., Mantione, C. R., Bech, H.,

Hanin, I. 1981. Atropine potentiates AF64A-induced pharmacological effects in mice *in vivo*. *Fed. Proc.* 40:269
15. Mantione, C. R., Fisher, A., Hanin, I. 1981. Biochemical heterogeneity of high affinity choline transport (HAChT) system demonstrated in mouse brain using ethylcholine mustard aziridinium (AF64A). *Trans. Am. Soc. Neurochem.* 12:219
16. Mantione, C. R., Fisher, A., Hanin, I. 1981. The AF64A-treated mouse: possible model for central cholinergic hypofunction. *Science* 213:579–80
17. Fisher, A., Mantione, C. R., Abraham, D. J., Hanin, I. 1982. Long-term central cholinergic hypofunction induced in mice by ethylcholine aziridinium ion (AF64A) *in vivo*. *J. Pharmacol. Exp. Ther.* 222:140–45
18. Rylett, B. J., Colhoun, E. H. 1980. Kinetic data on the inhibition of high affinity choline transport into rat brain synaptosomes by choline-like compounds and nitrogen mustard analogs. *J. Neurochem.* 34:713–19
19. Rylett, R. J., Colhoun, E. H. 1982. Monoethylcholine mustard aziridinium ion, a cholinergic neurochemical probe: comparison with choline mustard aziridinium ion. *Soc. Neurosci. Abstr.* 8: 772
20. Hanin, I., Mantione, C. R., Fisher, A. 1982. AF64A-induced neurotoxicity: A potential animal model in Alzheimer's disease. In *Alzheimer's Disease: A Report of Progress in Research*, ed. S. Corkin, K. L. Davis, J. H. Growdon, E. Usdin, R. J. Wurtman, 19:267–70. New York: Raven
21. Coyle, J. T., Sandberg, K., Fisher, A., Hanin, I. 1982. AF64A: Selective cholinergic neurotoxin in rat striatum. *Trans. Am. Soc. Neurochem.* 13:271
22. Mantione, C. R., Fisher, A., Hanin, I. 1984. Current topics. III. Possible mechanisms involved in the presynaptic cholinotoxicity due to AF64A *in vivo*. *Life Sci.* 35:33–41
23. Arst, D. S., Berger, T. W., Fisher, A., Hanin, I. 1983. AF64A reduces acetylcholinesterase (AChE) staining, and uncovers AChE-positive cell bodies in rat hippocampus, *in vivo*. *Fed. Proc.* 42:657
24. Mantione, C. R., DeGroat, W. C., Fisher, A., Hanin, I. 1983. Selective inhibition of peripheral cholinergic transmission in the cat produced by

AF64A. *J. Pharmacol. Exp. Ther.* 225:616–22

25. Mantione, C. R., Zigmond, M. J., Fisher, A., Hanin, I. 1983. Selective lesioning of rat hippocampal cholinergic neurons following localized injection of AF64A. *J. Neurochem.* 41:251–55

26. Hanin, I., Coyle, J. T., DeGroat, W. C., Fisher, A., Mantione, C. R. 1983. Chemically induced cholinotoxicity *in vivo:* Studies utilizing ethylcholine aziridinium ion (AF64A). In *Banbury Report: Biological Aspects of Alzheimer's Disease,* ed. R. Katzman, pp. 243–53. New York: Cold Spring Harbor Lab.

27. Caulfield, M. P., May, P. J., Pedder, E. K., Prince, A. K. 1983. Behavioral studies with ethylcholine mustard aziridinium (ECMA). *Proc. Br. Pharmacol. Soc.* 79:287P

28. Asante, J. W., Cross, A. J., Peakin, J. K. W., Johnson, J. A., Slater, H. R. 1983. Evaluation of ethylcholine mustard aziridinium (ECMA) as a specific neurotoxin of brain cholinergic neurons. *Br. J. Pharmacol.* 80:573P

29. Sandberg, K., Schnaar, R. L., Hanin, I., Fisher, A., Coyle, J. T. 1983. Disruption of choline metabolism: a proposed mechanism for the cytotoxic effect of AF64A, a cholinergic neuron-specific neurotoxin. *Soc. Neurosci. Abstr.* 9:961

30. Jarrard, L. E., Kant, G. J., Meyerhoff, J. L., Levy, A. 1984. Behavioral and neurochemical effects of intraventricular AF64A administration in rats. *Pharmacol. Biochem. Behav.* 21:273–80

31. Sandberg, K., Hanin, I., Fisher, I., Coyle, J. T. 1984. Selective cholinergic neurotoxin: AF64A's effects in rat striatum. *Brain Res.* 293:49–55

32. Levy, A., Kant, G. J., Meyerhoff, J. L., Jarrard, L. E. 1984. Noncholinergic neurotoxic effects of AF64A in substantia nigra. *Brain Res.* 305:169–72

33. Sandberg, K., Sanberg, P. R., Hanin, I., Fisher, A., Coyle, J. T. 1984. Cholinergic lesion of the striatum impairs acquisition and retention of passive avoidance response. *Behav. Neurosci.* 98:162–65

34. Curti, D., Marchbanks, R. M. 1984. Kinetics of irreversible inhibition of choline transport in synaptosomes by ethylcholine mustard aziridinium. *J. Membr. Biol.* 82:259–68

35. Sandberg, K., Sanberg, P. R., Coyle, J. T. 1984. Effects of intrastriatal injections of the cholinergic neurotoxin AF64A on spontaneous nocturnal locomotor behavior in the rat. *Brain Res.* 299:339–43

36. Lehr, E., Kuhn, F. J., Hinzen, D. H.

1984. AF64A neurotoxicity: behavioral and electrophysiological alterations in rats. *Soc. Neurosci. Abstr.* 10:775

37. Kasa, P., Farkas, Z., Szerdahelyi, P., Rakonczay, Z., Fisher, A., et al. 1984. Effect of cholinotoxin (AF64A) in the central nervous system: morphological and biochemical studies. In *Regulation of Transmitter Function: Basic and Clinical Aspects,* ed. E. S. Vizi, K. Magyar, pp. 289–93. Budapest: Akademiai Kiado

38. Walsh, T. J., Tilson, H. A., DeHaven, D. L., Mailman, R. B., Fisher, A., et al. 1984. AF64A, a cholinergic neurotoxin, selectively depletes acetylcholine in hippocampus and cortex, and produces long-term passive avoidance and radial-arm maze deficits in the rat. *Brain Res.* 321:91–102

39. Potter, P. E., Harsing, L. G. Jr., Kakucska, I., Gaal, Gy., Vizi, E. S., Fisher, A., Hanin, I. 1985. Effects of AF64A on hippocampal cholinergic and monoaminergic systems *in vivo. Fed. Proc.* 44:897

40. Sandberg, K., Schnaar, R. L., McKinney, M., Hanin, I., Fisher, A. 1985. AF64A: an active site directed irreversible inhibitor of choline acetyltransferase. *J. Neurochem.* 44:439–45

41. Arbogast, R. E., Kozlowski, M. R. 1984. Reduction of cortical choline acetyltransferase activity following injections of ethylcholine mustard aziridinium ion (AF64A) into the nucleus basalis of Meynert. *Soc. Neurosci. Abstr.* 10:1185

42. McGurk, S. R., Butcher, L. L. 1985. Neuropathology following intracerebral infusions of ethylcholine mustard aziridinium (AF64A). *Fed. Proc.* 44:897

43. Casamenti, F., Branco, L., Pedata, F., Pepeu, G. 1986. Biochemical and behavioral effects of AF64A in the rat. In *Dynamics of Cholinergic Function,* ed. I. Hanin. New York: Plenum. In press

44. Brandeis, R., Pittel, Z., Lachman, C., Heldman, E., Luz, S., et al. 1986. AF64A-induced cholinotoxicity: behavioral and biochemical correlates. In *Alzheimer's and Parkinson's Disease: Strategies for Research and Development,* ed. A. Fisher, I. Hanin, C. Lachman. New York: Plenum. In press

45. Leventer, S., McKeag, D., Clancy, M., Wulfert, E., Hanin, I. 1985. Intracerebroventricular AF64A reduces ACh release from rat hippocampal slices. *Neuropharmacology* 24:453–59

46. Terry, R. D., Davies, P. 1983. Some morphologic and biochemical aspects of Alzheimer's Disease. In *Aging of the Brain,* ed. D. Samuel, E. Giacobini, G.

Filogamo, G. Giacobini, A. Vernadakis, 20:47–59. New York: Raven

47. Growdon, J. H., Wurtman, R. J. 1983. The future of cholinergic precursor treatment of Alzheimer's disease. See Ref. 26, pp. 451–59

48. Coyle, J. T., Price, D. L., Delong, M. R. 1983. Alzheimer's disease: a disorder of cortical cholinergic innervation. *Science* 219:1184–90

49. Perry, E. K., Tomlinson, B. E., Blessed, G., Bergman, K., Gibson, P. H., et al. 1978. Correlation of cholinergic abnormalities with senile plaques and mental test scores in senile dementia. *Br. Med. J.* 2:1457–59

50. Kitt, C. A., Price, D. L., Struble, R. G., Cork, L. C., Wainer, B. H., et al. 1984. Evidence for cholinergic neurites in senile plaques. *Science* 226:1443–45

51. Davies, P. 1979. Neurotransmitter-related enzymes in senile dementia of the Alzheimer type. *Brain Res.* 171:318–27

52. Davis, K. L., Yamamura, H. I. 1978. Minireview: Cholinergic underactivity in human memory disorders. *Life Sci.* 23:1729–34

53. Davies, P. 1983. Neurotransmitters and neuropeptides in Alzheimer's disease. See Ref. 26, pp. 255–65

54. Bartus, R. T., Dean, R. L., Beer, B., Lippa, A. S. 1982. The cholinergic hypothesis of geriatric memory dysfunction: a critical review. *Science* 217:408–17

55. Francis, P. T., Palmer, A. M., Sims, N. R., Bowen, D. M., Davison, A. N., et al. 1985. Neurochemical studies of early-onset Alzheimer's disease. *N. Engl. J. Med.* 313:7–11

56. Bartus, R. T., Flicker, C., Dean, R. L. 1983. Logical principles for the development of animal models of age-related memory impairments. In *Assessment in Geriatric Psychopharmacology*, ed. T. Grook, S. Ferris, R. T. Bartus, pp. 263–99. New Canaan, Conn: Powley Assoc.

57. Sims, N. R., Bowen, D. M., Allen, S. J., Smith, C. C. T., Neary, D., et al. 1983. Presynaptic cholinergic dysfunction in patients with dementia. *J. Neurochem.* 40:503–9

58. Rylett, R. J., Ball, M. J., Colhoun, E. H. 1983. Evidence for high affinity choline transport in synaptosomes prepared from hippocampus and neocortex of patients with Alzheimer's disease. *Brain Res.* 289:169–75

59. Richter, J. A., Perry, E. K., Tomlinson, B. E. 1980. Acetylcholine and choline levels in postmortem human brain tissue: preliminary observations in Alzheimer's disease. *Life Sci.* 26:1683–89

60. Davies, P., Verth, A. W. 1978. Regional distribution of muscarinic acetylcholine receptors in normal and Alzheimer's type dementia brains. *Brain. Res.* 13:385–92

61. Reisine, T. D., Yamamura, H. I., Bird, E. E., Sokes, E., Enna, S. J. 1978. Pre- and post-synaptic neurochemical alterations in Alzheimer's disease. *Brain Res.* 159:477–81

62. Nordberg, A., Larsson, C., Adolfsson, R., Alafuzoff, I., Winblad, B. 1983. Muscarinic receptor compensation in hippocampus of Alzheimer's patients. *J. Neural Transm.* 56:13–19

63. Mash, D. C., Flynn, D. D., Potter, L. T. 1985. Loss of M2 muscarine receptors in the cerebral cortex in Alzheimer's disease and experimental cholinergic denervation. *Science* 228:1115–17

64. Vickroy, T. W., Leventer, S. L., Watson, M., Roeske, W. K., Hanin, I., et al. 1985. Selective reduction of central cholinergic parameters following ethylcholine mustard aziridinium (AF64A) administration. *The Pharmacologist* 27: 133

65. Bowen, D. M., Francis, P. T., Palmer, A. M. 1986. Cholinergic and non-cholinergic hypothesis for Alzheimer's disease: the biochemical evidence. See Ref. 44. In press

66. Thal, L. J., Fuld, P. A., Masur, D. M., Sharpless, N. S. 1983. Oral physostigmine and lecithin improve memory in Alzheimer disease. *Ann. Neurol.* 13: 491–96

67. Davis, K. L., Mohs, R. C., Davis, B. M., Horwath, T. S., Greenwald, B. S., et al. 1983. Oral physostigmine in Alzheimer's disease. *Psychopharmacol. Bull.* 19:451–53

68. Harbaugh, R. E., Roberts, D. W., Saunders, R. L., Reeder, T. M. 1984. Preliminary report: intracranial cholinergic drug infusion in patients with Alzheimer's disease. *Neurosurgery* 15:514–18

69. Bartus, R. T., Dean, R. L., Beer, B. 1980. Memory deficits in aged cebus monkeys and facilitation with central cholinomimetics. *Neurobiol. Aging* 1: 145–52

70. Struble, R. G., Cork, L. C., Price, D. L. Jr., Price, D. L., Davis, R. T. 1983. Distribution of neuritic plaques in the cortex of aged rhesus monkeys. *Soc. Neurosci. Abstr.* 9:927

71. Constantinidis, J. 1978. Is Alzheimer's disease a major form of senile dementia? Clinical, anatomical, and genetic data. In

Alzheimer's Disease: Senile Dementia and Related Disorders, ed. R. Katzman, R. D. Terry, K. L. Bick, pp. 15–25. New York: Raven

72. Coyle, J., McKinney, M., Johnston, M. V., Hedreen, J. C. 1983. Synaptic neurochemistry of the basal forebrain cholinergic projection. Psychopharmacol. Bull. 19:441–47

73. Rigter, H. 1983. Pitfalls in behavioural ageing research in animals. In Aging of the Brain, ed. W. H. Gispen, J. Traber, 7:197–207. Amsterdam: Elsevier

74. Gibson, G. E., Peterson, C. 1983. Pharmacologic models of age-related deficits. See Ref. 56, pp. 323–43

75. Ridley, R. M., Barratt, N. G., Baker, H. F. 1984. Cholinergic learning deficit in the marmoset produced by scopolamine and icv hemicholinium. Psychopharmacologia 83:340–45

76. Caulfield, M. P., Fortune, D. H., Roberts, P. M., Stubley, J. K. 1981. Intracerebroventricular hemicholinium-3 (HC-3) impairs learning of a passive avoidance task in mice. Br. J. Pharmacol. 74:865P

77. Perl, D. P., Brody, A. R. 1980. Alzheimer's disease: X-ray spectrometric evidence of aluminum accumulation in neurofibrillary tangle-bearing neurons. Science 208:297–99

78. Klatzo, I., Wisniewski, H. M., Streicher, E. 1965. Experimental production of neurofibrillary degeneration. J. Neuropathol. Exp. Neurol. 24:187–99

79. Crapper, D. R., Dalton, A. J. 1973. Alterations in short-term retention, conditioned avoidance response acquisition and motivation following aluminum induced neurofibrillary-degeneration. Physiol. Behav. 10:925–33

80. Lee, M. H., Rabe, A., Shek, J., Wisniewski, H. M. 1984. Intracranial aluminum produces avoidance learning deficit in immature rabbits. Soc. Neurosci. Abstr. 10:997

81. Wisniewski, H. M., Iqbal, K., McDermott, J. R. 1980. Aluminum-induced neurofibrillary changes: its relationship to senile dementia of Alzheimer's type. Neurotoxicology 1:121–24

82. McDermott, J. R., Smith, A. I., Iqbal, K., Wisniewski, H. M. 1979. Brain aluminum in aging and Alzheimer disease. Neurology 29:908–14

83. Fibiger, H. C. 1982. The organization and some projections of cholinergic neurons of the mammalian forebrain. Brain Res. Rev. 4:327–88

84. Fibiger, H. C., Murray, C. L., Phillips, A. G. 1983. Lesions of the nucleus basa-

lis magnocellularis impair long-term memory in rats. Soc. Neurosci. Abstr. 9:332

85. Stewart, G., Price, M. T., Olney, J. W. 1983. N-Methylaspartate, a useful excitotoxin for lesioning substantia innominata neurons in the rat. Soc. Neurosci. Abstr. 9:355

86. El-Defrawy, S. R., Coloma, F., Jhamandas, K., Boegman, R. J., Beninger, R. J., et al. 1984. Functional and neurochemical cortical cholinergic impairment following neurotoxic lesions of the nucleus basalis magnocellularis (nbM) the rat. Soc. Neurosci. Abstr. 10:1187

87. Friedman, E., Lerer, B., Kuster, J. 1983. Loss of cholinergic neurons in the rat neocortex produces deficits in passive avoidance learning. Pharmacol. Biochem. Behav. 19:309–12

88. Kohler, C., Schwarcz, R., Fuxe, K. 1979. Intrahippocampal injections of ibotenic acid provide histological evidence for a neurotoxic mechanism different from kainic acid. Neurosci. Lett. 15:223–28

89. Guldin, W.O., Markowitsch, H. J. 1982. Epidural kainate, but not ibotenate, produces lesions in local and distant regions of the brain: A comparison of the intracerebral actions of kainic acid and ibotenic acid. J. Neurosci. Methods 5: 83–93

90. Flicker, C., Dean, R. L., Watkins, D. L., Fisher, S. K., Bartus, R. T. 1983. Behavioral and neurochemical effects following neurotoxic lesions of a major cholinergic input to the cerebral-cortex in the rat. Pharmacol. Biochem. Behav. 18:973–81

91. Wenk, G. L., Olton, D. S. 1984. Recovery of neocortical cholineacetyltransferase activity following ibotenic acid injection into the nucleus basalis of Meynert in rats. Brain Res. 293:184–86

92. Hepler, D., Wenk, G., Olton, D., Lehmann, J., Coyle, J. T. 1983. Lesions in nucleus basalis of Meynert and medial septal area of rats produce similar memory impairments in three behavioral tasks. Soc. Neurosci. Abstr. 9:639

93. Aigner, T., Aggleton, J., Mitchell, S., Price, D., DeLong, M., et al. 1983. Effects of scopolamine on recognition memory in monkeys after ibotenic acid injections into the nucleus basalis of Meynert. Soc. Neurosci. Abstr. 9:826

94. Hepler, D., Olton, D., Wenk, G. 1984. Lesions in the nucleus basalis magnocellularis and medial septal area of rats impair spatial working memory in a T-maze task. Soc. Neurosci. Abstr. 10:135

95. Davidson, M., Haroutunian, V., Mohs, R. C., Davis, B. M., Harvath, T. B., et al. 1986. Human and animal studies with cholinergic agents: how clinically exploitable is the cholinergic deficiency in Alzheimer's disease? See Ref. 44. In press

96. McKinney, M., Davies, P., Coyle, J. T. 1982. Somatostatin is not colocalized in cholinergic neurons innervating the cerebral cortex-hippocampal formation. *Brain Res.* 243:169–74

97. Pontecorvo, M. J., Flicker, C., Bartus, R. T. 1986. Cholinergic dysfunction and memory: implications for the development of animal models of aging and dementia. See Ref. 43. In press

98. Salamone, J. D., Beart, P. M., Alpert, J. E., Iversen, S. D. 1984. Impairment in T-maze reinforced alteration performance following nucleus basalis magnocellularis lesions in rats. *Behav. Brain Res.* 13:63–70

99. Berman, R. F., Crosland, R., Jenden, D. J., Altman, H. J. 1984. Failure of oxotremorine to improve memory in rats with lesions of the nucleus basalis of Meynert. *Soc. Neurosci. Abstr.* 10:776

100. Crosland, R. D., Berman, R. F., Altman, H. J., Jenden, D. J. 1984. Reduced cortical choline acetyltransferase activity and impaired passive avoidance behavior in rats as a function of time after lesioning of the nucleus-basalis of Meynert. *Soc. Neurosci. Abstr.* 10:776

101. Jope, R. 1979. High affinity choline transport and acetyl CoA production in brain and their roles in the regulation of acetylcholine synthesis. *Brain Res. Rev.* 1:313–44

102. Poirier, L. J., Langelier, P., Roberge, A., Bouncher, R., Kitsikis, A. 1972. Non-specific histopathological changes induced by the intracerebral injection of 6-hydroxydopamine (6-OH-DA). *J. Neurol. Sci.* 16:401–16

103. Butcher, L. L., Eastgate, S. M., Hodge, G. K. 1984. Evidence that punctate intracerebral administration of 6-hydroxydopamine fails to produce selective neuronal degeneration. *Naunyn-Schmiedeberg's Arch. Pharmacol.* 285:31–40

104. Butcher, L. L., Hodge, G. K., Schaeffer, J. C. 1975. Degenerative processes after intraventricular infusion of 6-hydroxydopamine. In *Chemical Tools in Catecholamine Research,* ed. G. Jonsson, T. Malmfors, C. Sachs, 1:83–90. New York: American Elsevier

105. Marshall, J. F., Gotthelf, T. 1979. Sensory inattention in rats with 6-hydroxydopamine-induced degeneration of ascending dopaminergic-neurons—apomorphine-induced reversal of deficits. *Exp. Neurol.* 65:398–411

106. Hokfelt, T., Ungerstedt, U. 1973. Specificity of 6-hydroxydopamine induced degeneration of central monoamine neurons—electron and fluorescence microscopic study with special reference to intracerebral injection on nigro-striatal dopamine system. *Brain Res.* 60:269–97

107. Ungerstedt, U. 1971. Histochemical studies on the effect of intracerebral injections of 6-hydroxydopamine on monoamine neurons in the rat brain. In *6-Hydroxydopamine and Catecholamine Neurons,* ed. T. Malmfors, H. Thoenen, pp. 101–28. Amsterdam: North-Holland

108. Sachs, C., Jonsson, C. 1975. Mechanisms of action of 6-hydroxydopamine. *Biochem. Pharmacol.* 24:1–8

109. Kelly, P. H., Joyce, E. M., Minneman, K. P., Phillipson, O. T. 1977. Specificity of 6-hydroxydopamine-induced destruction of mesolimbic or nigro-striatal dopamine-containing terminals. *Brain Res.* 122:382–87

110. Meibach, R. C., Brown, L., Brooks, F. H. 1978. Histofluorescence of kainic acid-induced striatal lesions. *Brain Res.* 148:219–23

111. Herndon, R. M., Coyle, J. T., Addics, E. 1980. Ultrastructural analysis of kainic acid lesion of cerebellar cortex. *Neuroscience* 5:1013–26

112. Krammer, E. B., Lischka, M. F., Karobath, M., Schonbeck, G. 1979. Is there a selectivity of neuronal degeneration induced by intrastriatal injection of kainic acid? *Brain Res.* 177:577–82

113. Nagy, J. I., Vincent, S. R., Lehmann, J., Fibiger, H. C., McGeer, E. G. 1978. The use of kainic acid in the localization of enzymes in the substantia nigra. *Brain Res.* 149:431–41

114. Lorens, S. A., Gulberg, H. C., Hole, K., Kohler, C., Srebro, B. 1976. Activity, avoidance learning and regional 5-hydroxytryptamine following intrabrain stem 5,7-dihydroxytryptamine and electrolytic midbrain raphe lesions in the rat. *Brain Res.* 100:97–113

Ann. Rev. Pharmacol. Toxicol. 1986. 26:183–200

PHARMACOLOGICAL ASPECTS OF METABOLIC PROCESSES IN THE PULMONARY MICROCIRCULATION

C. Norman Gillis

Departments of Anesthesiology and Pharmacology, Yale University School of Medicine, New Haven, Connecticut 06510

INTRODUCTION

Lung pharmacology is concerned with both therapeutic and toxic effects of drugs on lung cells and cellular processes. Increasingly in the last several years, those interested in this field have also focused their attention on actions of lung on drugs and toxins reaching it via the air space or blood—the pharmacokinetic (metabolic or nonrespiratory) function of lung (1, 2). These occur in many cells of the lung; however, particularly intimate contact of the delicate alveolar-capillary unit with both the external environment and blood makes this site a frequent focus of injury due to environmental or vascular insults, such as hyperoxia, xenobiotic toxicity, septicemia, and adult respiratory distress in man (1, 2, 2a). This, coupled with the intense metabolic activity known to occur in cells of the alveolar-capillary membrane, has generated much effort to understand mechanisms and the significance of lung metabolic functions.

In carrying out these functions, the lung acts as a highly efficient "biochemical filter" for central venous blood. This reflects primarily two actions. First, the pulmonary circulation is interposed between the right and the left heart, and therefore all circulating blood passes through the lungs about once per minute. Secondly, within the lung, blood interacts with the very large metabolically active endothelial surface, which is now recognized as the site of many pharmacokinetic functions (1–4). Alveolar epithelium is an equally active site for degradation or activation of many xenobiotic substances (2), especially those whose route of access is via the airway.

183

0362-1642/86/0415-0183$02.00

Prominent among pharmacokinetic functions is removal[1], biosynthesis, and release of several vasoactive hormones that have significant effects on cardiovascular regulation, both in normal and disease states. These substances include biogenic amines, prostaglandins, leukotrienes, and peptides. Thus, aortic blood can differ markedly from central venous blood in its content of substances that profoundly alter the physiological status of the cardiovascular and other systems. An informative review of xenobiotic uptake and metabolism was recently published (2). Accordingly, this topic will be given only limited consideration. The main purpose of this chapter is to consider recent developments concerning pharmacokinetic processes that affect endogenous "substrates."

PHARMACOKINETIC LUNG FUNCTIONS

Recent review articles (2, 5, 6, 7) provide detailed information on mechanisms whereby the lung removes endogenous substances from pulmonary blood. Important features of these metabolic functions include the following. (*a*) Endogenous substrates for lung metabolism have profound physiologic effects, either per se or by modulating other effector mechanisms. Many are involved in critical regulatory processes, including homeostasis, capillary permeability change, endothelial interaction with platelets and leukocytes, and the inflammatory process. (*b*) Removal frequently results in loss of biological activity, but usually not in binding of unchanged substrate (in contrast to many xenobiotics). (*c*) There is considerable specificity of removal, even among close chemical congeners. (*d*) Good evidence now links many of the processes to the microvascular endothelium, although there are other sites of removal. Major classes of endogenous substrate for removal include biogenic amines, prostaglandins, peptides, and adenine nucleotides.

Biogenic Amines

Removal of the biogenic amines [norepinephrine (NE), and 5-hydroxytryptamine (5-HT)] in mammalian lungs is achieved by a carrier-mediated, temperature- and drug-sensitive transport process, followed by intracellular degradation by monoamine oxidase (MAO) and catechol-O-methyl transferase (COMT) in the case of NE (7). Removal of biogenic amines has characteristics of both neuronal and extraneuronal NE uptake (7), occurs rapidly, and can effectively reduce pulmonary arterial blood concentration of these amines in a single transpulmonary passage. While they cannot account for this rapid

---

[1] The term *removal* is used throughout this chapter to connote a net reduction in concentration of drug or vasoactive substance in lung effluent (whether in vitro or in vivo) compared to that in central venous blood or pulmonary arterial outflow.

removal, other processes such as uptake into platelets, adrenergic nerve endings (8), and neuroepithelial cells are important for pulmonary retention of biogenic amines over the longer period (9). It was recently shown that NE removed by perfused rat lung, in which endothelial and other sites of MAO and COMT were blocked, enters three kinetically defined pools identified (10) as vascular, extracellular, and a "slowly effluxing pool." The latter is blocked by cocaine and thus may reflect adrenergic nerve endings. Interestingly, entry into a slowly effluxing pool is also characteristic of xenobiotics (2), although the corresponding morphological site is the macrophage (2) rather than adrenergic nerves. Although removal of 5-HT involves a transport phenomenon, the nature of the carrier or its binding site for the amine is unknown. There may also be a subcellular site for 5-HT removal, since high affinity, temperature-sensitive binding of 5-HT to purified mitochondrial preparations has been reported (11). The latter binding sites may be serotonin receptors that subserve some as yet unknown action, presumably in mitochondria (11), although high affinity binding sites per se need not necessarily be coupled with a physiological function. Transport of biogenic amines from blood is the rate-limiting step in overall removal (5–7) and is blocked by a variety of drugs, including inhibitors of both adrenergic neuronal and non-neuronal uptake systems, as well as certain adrenergic blocking agents (7). Some structural specificity for 5-HT and NE (12) transport is evident, although this topic has been relatively little studied. N-acetyl-5-methoxytryptamine (melatonin) is not taken up by lung (13), and alpha-methyl serotonin has a lower affinity for removal than serotonin itself (14).

Serotonin congeners that inhibit uptake of the parent biogenic amine by rat lung slices have been studied (15). The indole ring system and an amine side chain were essential for activity. Structures with increased ionization of the indole hydroxyl group had greater inhibitory activity. However, it is unclear whether, in the lung slice, 5-HT removal occurs into endothelial cells (i.e. the normal vascular route) or whether other cells are equally involved. In contrast to the biogenic amines, inactivation of phenylethylamine (12), mescaline (16), and octopamine (12) reflects solely deamination by isoenzymes of monoamine oxidase. A possible role for lung in regulating circulating concentrations of mescaline and perhaps other psychotomimetic amines seems to merit consideration. Serotonin and NE are found in the lung (17, 18) and thus de novo biosynthesis of these amines seems probable. The rich adrenergic innervation of the lung suggests that neuronal regulation of metabolic functions is possible, either by causing local change in amine concentration, or by influencing hemodynamic factors such as blood flow.

Several studies suggest that altered biogenic amine removal might be linked to cardiovascular regulation. A surprisingly high incidence of primary pulmonary hypertension was reported among patients using the anorectic drug aminorex (19), which also decreases 5-HT removal by rat lung (20). Some of these patients were successfully treated by use of a serotonin antagonist, supporting the likelihood of increased "free" 5-HT (consequent to diminished removal) as the mechanism. Severe systemic hypertension after cardiopulmonary bypass (CPB) in man has been linked to increased circulating NE concentrations (21). We recently reported that lung NE removal was decreased after prolonged (3–4 hr) CPB in dogs (22), a finding similar to our observation with another substrate, prostaglandin E_1 (23). Also, patients with pulmonary hypertension had no net transpulmonary NE gradient (24, 25). These studies suggest it would be profitable to explore further the link between pulmonary vascular disease and experimentally or disease-induced change in lung metabolic functions (24, 25).

Prostaglandins

Prostaglandins of the E and F series also are extensively removed by mammalian lungs (26–28). A carrier-mediated, energy-requiring process has been implicated (29–31), although there is also rapid degradation by 15-hydroxy-prostaglandin-dehydrogenase (PGDH) and other enzymes (29–31). Although prostaglandin removal is drug-sensitive, both in vivo (32) and in vitro (29–31, 33, 34), the rate-limiting step in the process is unclear. Studies with perfused lung (29–31, 33, 34) are consistent with an endothelial site, but large vessel endothelial cells in culture do not transport prostaglandins. This negative finding might reflect either the relatively small number of cells used or the absence of this property in cells from large vessels.

To define, adequately, the rate-limiting step in postaglandin removal one needs inhibitors that act specifically either on transport or enzymatic degradation. Unfortunately, available antagonists affect both processes simultaneously. Studies have been reported of structural requirements among sulfasalazine analogues for inhibition of $PGF_{2\alpha}$ degradation by NAD^+-dependent PGDH in preparations of bovine lung and human placenta (35). Requirements for optimal inhibition were two aromatic rings and acetyl and hydroxyl moieties at positions 1 and 2 in the salicyl C-ring system. Further study of structural requirements for prostaglandin transport and enzymatic degradation by PGDH are essential to define more clearly the mechanism of prostaglandin removal and the consequences of its inhibition.

Specificity is also evident in prostaglandin removal since thromboxane and prostacyclin pass through the pulmonary circulation unchanged—although they are taken up by skeletal muscle (36). There is therefore a parallel between PGI_2 and epinephrine (37), both of which are taken up by skeletal muscle but escape significant degradation in the lung.

Peptides

Both bradykinin and angiotensin I (AI) are substrates for kininase II or angiotensin converting enzyme (ACE). This membrane-bound enzyme hydrolyzes peptidyl dipeptide bonds from the carboxyl terminal of bradykinin and AI, resulting in biological inactivation of the former and conversion of the latter to angiotensin II. Angiotensin II is not normally metabolized by the lung, which is consistent with its role as a "circulating" hormone (38). However in pathophysiological states, including edema, it may be hydrolyzed, perhaps because it is exposed to normally intracellular angiotensinases (28).

Several other biologically relevant peptides also escape degradation by the lung. Thus, vasoactive intestinal polypeptide (VIP), found in autonomic nerves of airway and vascular smooth muscle cells (5, 28), bombasin, which occurs in endocrine cells of fetal lung (28), and oxytocin all escape lung inactivation (1, 28). Substance P is reported to be hydrolyzed by cultured endothelial cells (39) but not by intact lung (28).

An aminopeptidase in human vascular endothelial cells hydrolyzes leu-enkephalins (40). Degradation of both leu[5]- and met[5]-enkephalin by perfused lung was established by studies that employed rat colon bioassay (43) and high performance liquid chromatographic techniques (41) to identify metabolites formed. Over 95% of the initial enkephalin radioactivity was recovered in the perfusion medium. This is reminiscent of earlier studies with bradykinin (42) and indicates that neither parent compound nor the metabolites are stored in the tissue. The inhibition of ACE by captopril, or of aminopeptidase by bestatin, diminished met-enkephalen metabolism (43). Interestingly, inhibition of enkephalinase with thiorphan did not affect metabolism. Thus, at least in rat lung, both leu[5]- and met[5]-enkephalin are metabolized by two enzymes—ACE and an aminopeptidase, perhaps the recently described peptidyl dipeptidase (44), which is distinct from ACE. These observations suggest a role for lung metabolism in modulating physiological and pharmacological functions of these opiate peptides, including control of arterial concentrations of enkephalins released into the circulation in, for example, canine endotoxin shock (44a). In fact, increased rat pulmonary vascular resistance, in response to leu-enkephalin, was enhanced by a combination of captopril and bestatin (44b).

BENZ-PHE-ALA-PRO   Since the introduction of hipp-his-leu (45) to measure ACE activity, these synthetic substrates have attracted much interest because they are technically easier to use than the natural peptides. One such compound is benzoyl-phenylalanyl-alanyl-proline (BPAP), synthesized and first used to measure ACE of endothelial cells in culture (54). BPAP has found application in the measurement of lung ACE both in this laboratory (46–50) and others (51–53). The attractiveness of tritiated BPAP to measure ACE lies in the fact that it is rapidly hydrolyzed (46, 48) by ACE to yield tritiated benz-phe, which is easily separated from the parent compound (54). Also, BPAP lacks significant cardiovascular effects (46, 48, 49) and thus does not alter perfusion characteristics of the lung during its use. Hydrolysis of BPAP in vivo is inhibited, in a dose-dependent manner, by bradykinin or captopril (46, 48). The apparent K_m for hydrolysis in vivo is about 9 μM (49), which is close to that reported with cultured cells (54).

INSULIN REMOVAL   Purified hog lung ACE cleaves dipeptides from the B-chain of insulin (55). Also, insulin is an effective inhibitor of both plasma and lung ACE (55). Recently, it was reported that aortic (56) and pulmonary arterial (56a) endothelial cells in culture transport insulin by an energy-dependent, receptor-mediated process. Transport in the cultured cell was relatively slow (15% in 2 hr, when aortic cells were incubated with 1 ng insulin/ml). Binding of insulin could be the first step in the process leading to transfer of the hormone from blood to target cells. Lung binding may reflect merely the large endothelial surface area present. On the other hand, it is tempting to imagine the lung exerting some regulatory role in the physiological function of insulin.

NATRIURETIC ATRIAL FACTOR   The natriuretic atrial factor (NAF), a potent vasodilator of pre-contracted vessels (57), binds specifically to high affinity sites on membrane preparations of rat mesenteric and renal vessels (58). However, the capacity of these sites is low, an observation consistent with only modest uptake of NAF by large pulmonary vessels and small systemic vessels (57). Yet we observed 67 ± 4% single-pass removal of 3-[^{125}I]-iodotyrosyl [28] NAF by rabbit lung in situ (M. Turrin & C. N. Gillis, unpublished observations). The nature of this avid removal is unknown. However, the lung is ideally suited to contribute to the regulation of systemic physiological actions of NAF released from the right heart.

ADENINE NUCLEOTIDES   Adenine nucleotides are substrates for 5'-nucleotidase and ATPase that degrade ADP to AMP and then to adenosine (6). Adenosine itself is a substrate for carrier-mediated transport into endothelial cells (59–61) and is an important mediator of regional blood flow. Thus, knowledge of its pharmacokinetics in the pulmonary (and extrapulmonary) vascular bed is of considerable interest. Aortic (61) and pulmonary arterial (62) endothelial cells or isolated perfused lungs (63, 64) remove adenosine from culture or perfusion medium, respectively. The biological significance of this property, in vivo, has been questioned, since red blood cell transport of adenosine appears to have a potentially greater role in removal of blood-borne nucleotide than pulmonary vascular endothelium (59, 60). Much less is known about abluminal endothelial transport of adenosine. It has been suggested (65) that endothelium plays an integral role in modifying interstitial concentrations of adenosine, an important link between tissue metabolism and vascular smooth muscle activity.

XENOBIOTICS   In addition to the endogenous substrates mentioned, many xenobiotics are also removed during their transpulmonary passage. Many of these compounds are lipophilic basic amines (e.g. propranolol, lidocaine) and their removal by lung reflects both high lipid solubility and specific binding sites (2, 67).

Because of the avid removal and subsequent release of unchanged xenobiotics, including important drugs in clinical use such as beta-blocking agents, local anesthetics, and antihypertensives, it has been suggested that the lung could act as a "capacitor," preventing sudden increases in systemic levels of these compounds (66, 67). If so, previously bound drug might be displaced by a second agent, with consequent liberation of relatively large (and potentially toxic) concentrations of the first drug [e.g. propranolol (66,67)] into the coronary, cerebral, and other critical vascular beds. Recent reports of competition between bupivacaine and serotonin (68) and of Fentanyl uptake by the lung (69) raise similar possibilities. In general, however, this apparently critical area of clinical pharmacology has not received the systematic study it merits.

ENDOTHELIAL BIOSYNTHESIS OF VASODILATORS AND PULMONARY HEMODYNAMICS

Endothelial cells in culture synthesize many vasoactive substances, both spontaneously and in response to pharmacological challenge. Whether similar synthetic properties are present (or are biologically important) in vivo is uncertain. Nevertheless, it is appropriate to emphasize that release of substances by lung could have significant effects not only on systemic vessels "downstream" from the lungs but also on pulmonary vasculature per se. Two specific examples merit further consideration.

Prostacyclin

It was recently reported that release of prostacyclin (PGI_2) by cultured aortic endothelial cells was greatly enhanced by exposure to shear stress, either pulsatile or nonpulsatile (70). Bovine pulmonary arterial endothelial cells and perfused rat lung (71) release more PGI_2 in response to shear stress or altered flow, respectively. Studies of this type could shed light on the role of the lung in modifying events downstream, including cardiac function, pulmonary and peripheral vascular tone as well as platelet aggregation. Furthermore, the pattern of pulse wave and shear stress might affect metabolic processes in the lung by influencing synthesis of PGI_2—or that of other mediators, including EDRF (see below). For example, PGI_2 is reported to depress 5-HT clearance (72) and thromboxane apparently can diminish PGE_2 inactivation by rat lung (73). Therefore, the possibility exists that such interactions may represent a method of indirect control over lung metabolic functions.

Endothelial-Derived Relaxing Factor (EDRF)

Some vasoactive hormones, including acetylcholine and bradykinin, are thought to dilate vascular smooth muscle by releasing a diffusible vasodilator substance (74). This mechanism clearly occurs in large diameter systemic or pulmonary blood vessels, in which it has been demonstrated that there is a basal release of the compound. It is much less certain whether this also applies to precapillary resistance vessels. Also in question is the chemical identity of EDRF, although it is not a product of cyclo-oxygenase activity (74). It seems reasonable to question whether basal release of EDRF, especially if it occurs in lung microvasculature, contributes to the normally low resistance of the pulmonary circuit. Might hypoxic vasoconstriction occur, therefore, because such release, or de novo synthesis, is reduced? If so, can we then suggest that the pathophysiology of acute respiratory failure [secondary to loss of hypoxic vasoconstriction (2a)] might also involve impaired release of EDRF? Indeed, this suggestion has been offered in discussing the fact that bradykinin constricts, rather than dilates, canine pulmonary vessels from which the endothelium was physically removed (76). Certain drugs that inhibit EDRF synthesis and release may increase pulmonary vascular resistance by a similar mechanism. The opposite drug action, namely local promotion of EDRF synthesis and release, could represent a unique approach to the pharmacotherapy of increased pulmonary vascular resistance. Indeed, when the structure of EDRF is elucidated, it is likely that analogs of the molecule will be attractive candidates for therapy of both systemic and pulmonary hypertension.

FUNCTIONAL ASPECTS OF ACE INHIBITION

Interest in peptide hydrolysis by lung ACE increased with development of a new class of antihypertensive drugs that inhibit the enzyme. These drugs also have effects other than ACE inhibition, including release of arachidonic acid derivatives (77)—presumably via local or systemic elevation of kinin concentration. Nevertheless, there is good correlation between inhibition of lung, vascular, central nervous system, or renal ACE in vitro and the antihypertensive effects of these drugs (78, 79). Recently we found (47) that pulmonary ACE activity in conscious rabbits was depressed for over six days after a single i.v. dose of captopril (2 mg/kg). During this period, systemic arterial pressure correlated closely with inhibition of pulmonary ACE. In contrast, there was an early, pronounced fall in plasma ACE; however, 24 hours later, when plasma ACE activity had returned to control levels, systemic blood pressure was at its nadir. This hypotensive effect could involve decreased arterial AII or increased arterial bradykinin (secondary to inhibition of pulmonary ACE) as well as additional mechanisms.

Lung Removal of ACE Inhibitors

Uptake and binding of ACE inhibitors has been studied with a view to defining the location and function of ACE in the lung as well as the pharmacological actions of these drugs. ^{3}H-Captopril binds with high affinity to a single site in membrane preparations of rat lung and choroid plexus in vitro (80). Binding parallels ACE activity, determined in the same preparation. Furthermore, binding of ^{3}H-captopril and ACE activity were inhibited in a parallel, dose-dependent manner by several other carboxylate ACE inhibitors, suggesting that under the conditions of this assay in vitro, captopril binds selectively, only to ACE (80).

Whether this is also true in vivo was recently studied in this laboratory. We found (81) that 40% of a bolus injection of captopril (10 nmoles/kg) was removed by lungs of anesthetized rabbits. Uptake was saturable, decreasing to 6% when 70 nmole of captopril were given, and was specific since the drug inhibited hydrolysis of BPAP in vivo, but captopril failed to affect the uptake of 5-HT given in the same bolus. This study (81) suggested that lung removal of captopril in vivo was due primarily to binding of the drug to endothelial ACE, as was also found in vitro (80).

Because of the specificity evident in the binding of captopril to ACE, we recently began to study lung removal (i.e. specific binding) of another ACE inhibitor in preparation for the design of techniques for "in-line" measurement of lung metabolic functions (see below). We used a new ACE inhibitor, (N-[1-(S)-carboxy-(4-OH-3-^{125}I-phenyl)-ethyl-L-ala-L-pro) or CPAP, kindly supplied by Drs. Ryan and Chung of the University of Miami. With rabbit lungs perfused in situ, we found (82) that this compound was rapidly taken up (67%) in a single pass. The process was inhibited in dose-dependent fashion by unlabelled CPAP or by captopril. This compound was also shown (82) to be equipotent with captopril in inhibiting hydrolysis of BPAP by rabbit lungs. In a similar study (83), the same compound was used to determine that hypoxia had no direct effect on the activity of ACE in the rabbit lung.

In-line Measurement of Lung Metabolic Functions

The fact that ^{125}I-CPAP is photon emitting allowed us to begin development of a system for measurement of its removal in-line. Such a system offers the hope of virtually instantaneous measurement of a process that could provide data about an enzyme present on the microvascular surface of lung as well as other organs. Furthermore, if successful, this method could allow study of modifications during experimental changes imposed in the lung. In the system developed (84), we used a bolus injection, double indicator dilution technique. The bolus contained ^{125}I-CPAP and also ^{99m}Tc-sulfur colloid, as an intravascular reference. Lung effluent, sampled from the carotid artery of an anesthetized rabbit, is passed through a flow cell, in which these photon-emitting isotopes are detected by a sodium iodide crystal, the output of which was directed to counting equipment that allowed separation of the two isotopes on the basis of their photopeak energies. Output was passed through a buffered interface to a microcomputer. Custom software was used to record radioactivity in the arterial outflow as a continuous function of time, for about 25 seconds after administration of the bolus injection. Data were stored in the computer and used to calculate cardiac output, mean transit times, and volumes of distribution of both isotopes.

Cardiac outputs calculated with this system compared closely with those determined simultaneously by direct Fick method, and the slope relating both values was not significantly different from 1. Also, instantaneous and integral removal curves are available at the same time. Figure 1 shows the fractional concentration curves so obtained after the administration of 0.1 μg (left) and 10.0 μg (right) of CPAP/kg to an anesthetized rabbit. It can be seen that (a) the integral removal was about 45% in this animal after 0.1 μg CPAP and (b) that removal was reduced to zero by use of 10 μg cold CPAP/kg. Thus, in-line determination of CPAP removal reveals similar behavior to experiments in situ. The fact that removal is apparently somewhat lower in the in-line system may be due to the much higher blood flow in the intact, anesthetized animal.

ALTERED ENDOTHELIAL REMOVAL FUNCTION AND LUNG INJURY

This topic has been extensively reviewed during the last three years (2, 85–87) and the interested reader is referred to these papers for more detailed discussion. Endothelial cells of the lung are often early sites of injury caused by a variety of substances, including oxygen, bleomycin, and monocrotaline, and experimental or disease-associated conditions, such as radiation injury (85–87). The mechanism of such injury is uncertain, but it has now been reported that normobaric hyperoxia decreases fluidity in the hydrophobic core of the plasma membrane in cultured pulmonary endothelial cells (87a). Such effects, coupled with the close association of lung removal functions with the microvascular endothelium, led to the proposal that acute lung injury might modify the latter process (85). If so, it was reasoned, measurement of metabolic functions may provide early reflection of injury to the pulmonary endothelium.

There is now considerable support for this hypothesis from experiments in a

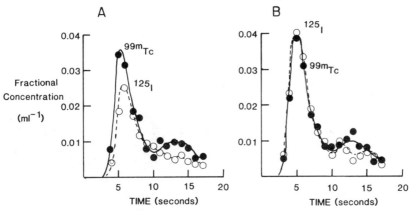

Figure 1 Indicator dilution data obtained, in-line, from an anesthetized rabbit. Panel *A* presents the fractional concentration curves obtained after rapid i.v. injection of a bolus containing ^{99m}Tc-sulfur colloid as intravascular reference and 0.1 μg (total dose) of the ACE inhibitor, CPAP (see text). Integral removal was 45%. Panel *B* shows corresponding data after injection of bolus containing 10 μg of CPAP per kg. Notice that the two curves are coincident, implying that removal was zero in the presence of excess cold CPAP.

number of animal models of lung injury, including each of the models mentioned above (85–87). In virtually all cases, the predominant effect of acute injury is to lower removal of the substrate tested. The most frequently employed substrates for removal were 5-HT, prostaglandins, and synthetic substrates for ACE. Furthermore, in many instances altered removal precedes morphological or clinical evidence of injury (85, 88). Studies designed to evaluate this link in man revealed that 5-HT (89, 90) or PGE_1 (91) removal is relatively well preserved after short periods of cardiopulmonary bypass. In contrast, patients with adult respiratory distress syndrome (ARDS) had significantly reduced single-pass removal of $^3H\text{-}PGE_1$ (91), $^{14}C\text{-}5\text{-}HT$ (91, 91a); those suffering from emphysema also showed diminished ^3H-propranolol removal (92). The transpulmonary gradient for endogenous NE (25) and prostaglandin $F_{2\alpha}$ (93) is decreased in adults with primary pulmonary hypertension. The NE gradient was zero in children with pulmonary hypertension secondary to congenital heart disease; however, surgical correction of the underlying lesion caused prompt recovery of NE removal (24).

INTERPRETATION OF REDUCED REMOVAL IN THE INJURED LUNG

Experimental and disease-associated lung injury (see above) is often associated with altered blood flow rate and nonuniform perfusion of the lung that may alter quantitative measurements of removal (86). Thus it is critically important to distinguish altered removal due to hemodynamic changes from that due to intrinsic endothelial injury. There is presently no fully accepted method for reliably achieving this separation in vivo. However, Rickaby et al (34, 94–96) used the rapid injection multiple indicator dilution method in a promising approach to this difficult problem. Reasoning that data from this type of experiment contain information about both convective (hemodynamic) and endothelial transport (kinetic) processes in the lung, they developed a mathematical formulation (97, 98) for lung removal processes, assuming that Michaelis Menten kinetics governs the interaction between substrate and transport (or surface enzyme) site. In this method, the injected bolus contains an intravascular reference indicator, trace amounts of radiolabeled substrate, and varying amounts of unlabeled substrate. The total amount of substrate is adjusted to provide, in a single traverse of the lung circulation, a profile of intracapillary concentrations such that the kinetics of the unidirectional removal process ranges from first order to nearly zero order.

Several studies indicate that this technique can separate altered endothelial cell functions (i.e. due to injury) from those produced by changes in lung perfusion both in vitro (34, 95, 99) and in vivo (32, 49, 50). First, varying flow rate in isolated perfused dog lung did not change the calculated apparent V_{max} (96), which indirectly reflects the number of transport sites. Also the apparent K_m was unchanged, unless flow rates less than 50% of normal were used. Varying the pH of perfusion medium over the range 7.2–7.8 did not change 5-HT kinetic parameters (100). There was fair agreement in calculated values for the apparent V_{max} and K_m for 5-HT removal, determined simultaneously in the same lung preparation, after steady infusion and bolus injections of the amine (101). Embolization of lungs with large (550 μm) glass beads, which reduced vascular volume and surface area, significantly reduced V_{max} for 5-HT removal but did not alter the K_m (94). Similarly, the apparent V_{max} for PGE$_1$ is reduced after embolization (102), probably again as a result of decreased surface area.

This model (34, 95), originally proposed for transport functions, seems equally applicable to substances removed only by enzymatic processes (48–50, 102a, 103). Thus, similar estimates have been reported for apparent K_m and V_{max} for BPAP hydrolysis whether studied by indicator dilution techniques (48–50, 59, 103) or by steady-state techniques in isolated perfused lungs (48, 102a, 99). The apparent kinetics for BPAP removal were unaffected by large changes in pulmonary perfusion. However, V_{max} was significantly reduced at high transpulmonary pressures (and lung volumes), presumably because alveolar vessels were compressed in this state (104) and thus reduced perfused surface area.

Although the apparent kinetics for lung metabolic functions appears to be largely independant of flow, less is known about the predictive value of the model in analyzing the mechanism of drug inhibition. Imipramine, which antagonizes 5-HT removal, doubled the K_m for the process and reduced V_{max} (94). Under the usual conditions for analysis in vitro, these are changes consistent with a mixed inhibitor mechanism. However, since imipramine is taken up by lung tissue (67), thereby creating uncertainty about its local concentration in relation to the 5-HT transport site (105), the precise nature of its inhibitory effect on the chemical kinetics of the amine transport remains to be elucidated. In particular, although increases in apparent K_m are suggestive of competition for carrier receptor sites, a literal interpretation of the estimated organ value of K_m as a function only of chemical affinity is an oversimplification. Nevertheless, this model has provided a useful basis on which to begin efforts to separate endothelial functional change due to injury from effects associated with strictly hemodynamic factors. Dawson et al reported (106) in a later study that 5-HT removal was lowered if surface area was sufficiently reduced, but was unaffected by oleic acid injury. This is consistent with data in patients showing that, unless lung microvascular surface area was decreased by atelectasis, 5-HT removal was unaffected by cardiopulmonary bypass (90). Thus it seems that relatively small quantitative reduction in 5-HT removal, for example, may actually reflect a functional loss of major portions of perfused endothelial surface [see also reference (86)].

As an alternative experimental approach, removal can be measured during steady infusions of a substrate (48, 101, 107, 108). In this case, the transpulmonary gradient can be determined directly and will measure the rate of removal if return of unchanged material to the vascular space is sufficiently slow. Since steady infusion appears impractical for clinical application, the bolus injection technique seems a more realistic means to measure lung metabolic functions in vivo. Certainly there is a need to expand greatly our understanding of the quantitative interpretation of data derived by the latter technique. Nevertheless, currently available data amply justify continued use of the bolus injection method to study microvascular and endothelial metabolic function in vivo as well as in the clinical setting.

ACKNOWLEDGMENTS

I am grateful to Dr. Bruce R. Pitt for helpful discussions during the preparation of this paper. Original investigations in the author's laboratory were supported, in part, by Grants HL 13315, HL 27207, and HL 07410 from the National Heart, Lung, and Blood Institute.

Literature Cited

1. Bakhle, Y. S., Vane, J. R. 1974. Pharmacokinetic function of the pulmonary circulation. *Physiol. Rev.* 54:1007–54
2. Bend, J. R., Serabjit-Singh, C. J., Philpot, R. M. 1985. The pulmonary uptake, accumulation and metabolism of xenobiotics. *Ann. Rev. Pharmacol.* 25:97–125
2a. Rinaldi, J. E., Rogers, R. M. 1982. Adult respiratory distress syndrome: changing concepts of lung injury and repair. *N. Eng. J. Med.* 306:900–9
3. Gillis, C. N., Roth, J. A. 1976. Pulmonary disposition of circulation vasoactive hormones. *Biochem. Pharmacol.* 25:2547–53
4. Junod, A. F. 1977. Metabolism of vasoactive agents in lung. *Am. Rev. Respir. Dis.* 115:51–57
5. Said, S. I. 1982. Metabolic functions of the pulmonary circulation. *Circ. Res.* 50:325–33
6. Ryan, U. S., Ryan, J. W. 1984. Cell biology of pulmonary endothelium. *Circulation* 70(Suppl. 3):46–62
7. Gillis, C. N., Pitt, B. R. 1982. The fate of circulating amines within the pulmonary circulation. *Ann. Rev. Physiol.* 44:269–81
8. Bosin, T. R., Lahr, P. D. 1981. Mechanisms influencing the disposition of serotonin in mouse lung. *Biochem. Pharmacol.* 30:3187–93
9. Gillis, C. N. 1985. Peripheral metabolism of serotonin. In *Serotonin and the Cardiovascular System*, ed. P. M. Vanhoutte, pp. 27–36. New York: Raven
10. Metting, P. J., Levin, J. A., Samuels, J. T. 1985. Compartmental analysis of the efflux of 1-[^{3}H]norepinephrine from isolated perfused rat lung. *J. Appl. Physiol.* 58:244–50
11. Das, D. K., Steinberg, M. 1985. Specific binding of serotonin in rat lung. *Am. J. Physiol.* 248:E58–E63
12. Gillis, C. N., Roth, J. A. 1977. The fate of biogenic monoamines in perfused lung. *Br. J. Pharmacol.* 59:585–90
13. Kopin, I. J., Pare, C. M. B., Axelrod, J., Weissbach, H. 1961. The fate of melatonin in animals. *J. Biol. Chem.* 236:3072–75
14. Alabaster, V. A. 1977. Inactivation of endogenous amines in the lung. In *Metabolic Functions of the Lung: Lung Biology in Health and Disease*, ed. C. Lenfant, 4:3–31. New York: Dekker
15. Mais, D. E., Bosin, T. R. 1981. Structural specificity of the inhibition of seroto-

nin accumulation in rat lung slices. *Res. Commun. Chem. Pathol. Pharmacol.* 34:241–49
16. Roth, R. A., Roth, J. A., Gillis, C. N. 1977. Disposition of ^{14}C-mescaline by rabbit lung. *J. Pharmacol. Exp. Ther.* 200:394–401
17. Sadavongvivad, C. 1970. Pharmacological significance of biogenic amines in the lungs: 5-hydroxytryptamine. *Br. J. Pharmacol.* 38:353–65
18. Aviado, D. M., Sadavongvivad, C. 1970. Pharmacological significance of biogenic amines in the lungs: noradrenaline and dopamine. *Br. J. Pharmacol.* 38:374–85
19. Steinberg, H., Fisher, A. 1977. Serotonin in the lung. In *Serotonin in Health and Disease*, ed. W. B. Essman, pp. 69–109. New York: Spectrum
20. Seiler, K. U., Wassermann, O., Wensky, H. 1976. On the role of serotonin in the pathogenesis of pulmonary hypertension induced by anorectic drugs: an experimental study in the isolated perfused rat lung. *Clin. Exp. Pharmacol. Physiol.* 3:323–30
21. Wallach, R., Karp, R. B., Reves, J. G., Oparil, S., Smith, L. R., James, T. N. 1980. Pathogenesis of paroxysmal hypertension developing during and after coronary bypass surgery: a study of hemodynamic and humoral factors. *Am. J. Cardiol.* 46:559–65
22. Pitt, B. R., Gillis, C. N., Hammond, G. L. 1984. Depression of pulmonary metabolic function by cardiopulmonary bypass procedures increases levels of circulating norepinephrine. *Ann. Thorac. Surg.* 38:508–13
23. Pitt, B. R., Hammond, G. L., Gillis, C. N. 1982. Depressed pulmonary removal of ^{3}H-prostaglandin E$_1$ after prolonged cardiopulmonary bypass. *J. Appl. Physiol.* 52:887–92
24. Gewitz, M., Pitt, B. R., Laks, H., Hammond, G. L., Talner, N., Gillis, C. N. 1982. Reversible effect of pulmonary hypertension on extraction of endogenous catecholamines by the pulmonary vasculature. *Pediatr. Pharmacol.* 2:57–63
25. Sole, M. J., Drobac, M., Schwartz, L., Hussain, M. N., Vaughan-Neil, E. F. 1979. The extraction of circulating catecholamines by the lungs in normal man and in patients with pulmonary hypertension. *Circulation* 60:160–63
26. Ferreira, S. H., Vane, J. R. 1967. Prostaglandins: their disappearance from and

release into the circulation. *Nature* 216:868–73

27. Hammond, G. L., Cronau, L. H., Whittaker, D., Gillis, C. N. 1977. Fate of prostaglandins E_1 and A_1 in the human pulmonary circulation. *Surgery* 81:716–22

28. Said, S. I. 1982. Pulmonary metabolism of prostaglandins and vasoactive peptides. *Ann. Rev. Physiol.* 44:257–68

29. Anderson, M. W., Eling, T. E. 1976. Prostaglandin removal and metabolism by isolated perfused rat lung. *Prostaglandins* 11:645–77

30. Bito, L. Z., Baroody, R. A., Reitz, M. E. 1977. Dependence of pulmonary prostaglandin metabolism on carrier-mediated transport processes. *Am. J. Physiol.* 232:E382–87

31. Bito, L. Z., Baroody, R. A. 1975. Inhibition of pulmonary prostaglandin metabolism by inhibitors of prostaglandin biotransport (probenecid and bromocresol green). *Prostaglandins* 10:633–39

32. Pitt, B. R., Forder, J. R., Gillis, C. N. 1983. Drug-induced impairment of pulmonary ^3H prostaglandin E_1 removal in vivo. *J. Pharmacol. Exp. Ther.* 227:531–37

33. Hook, R., Gillis, C. N. 1975. Removal and metabolism of prostaglandin E_1 by rabbit lung. *Prostaglandins* 9:193–201

34. Linehan, J. H., Dawson, C. A. 1979. A kinetic model of prostaglandin metabolism in the lung. *J. Appl. Physiol.* 47:404–11

35. Berry, C. N., Hoult, J. R. S., Peers, S. H., Agback, H. 1983. Inhibition of prostaglandin 15-hydroxydehydrogenase by sulphasalazine and a novel series of potent analogues. *Biochem. Pharmacol.* 32:2863–71

36. Dusting, G. J., Moncada, S., Vane, J. R. 1978. Recirculation of prostacyclin in the dog. *Br. J. Pharmacol.* 64:315–20

37. Pitt, B. R., Hammond, G. L., Gillis, C. N. 1982. Comparison of pulmonary and extrapulmonary extraction of biogenic amines. *J. Appl. Physiol.* 52:1545–51

38. Vane, J. R. 1969. The release and fate of vaso-active hormones in the circulation. *Br. J. Pharmacol.* 35:209–42

39. Johnson, A. R., Erdos, E. G. 1977. Metabolism of vasoactive peptides by human endothelial cells in culture. Angiotensin I converting enzyme (kininase II) and angiotensinase. *J. Clin. Invest.* 59:684–95

40. Erdos, E. G., Johnson, A. R., Boyden, N. T. 1978. Hydrolysis of enkephalin by cultured human endothelial cells and by purified peptidyl dipeptidase. *Biochem. Pharmacol.* 27:843–48

41. Gillespie, M. N., Krechniak, J. W., Crooks, P. A., Altiere, R. J., Olson, J. W. 1985. Pulmonary metabolism of exogenous enkephalins in isolated perfused rat lungs. *J. Pharmacol. Exp. Ther.* 232:675–81

42. Ryan, J. W. 1982. Processing of endogenous polypeptides by the lung. *Ann. Rev. Physiol.* 44:241–55

43. Manwaring, D., Mullane, K. 1984. Disappearance of enkephalins in the isolated perfused rat lung. *Life Sci.* 34:

44. Benuck, M., Berg, M. J., Marks, N. 1981. A distinct peptidyl dipeptidase that degrades enkephalin: exceptionally high activity in rabbit kidney. *Life Sci.* 28:2643–50

44a. Evans, S. F., Medbank, S., Hinds, C. J., Tomlin, S. J., Varley, J. G., Rees, L. H. 1984. Plasma levels and biochemical characterization of circulating met-enkephalin in canine endotoxic shock. *Life Sci.* 34:1481–86

44b. Crooks, P. A., Bowdy, B. D., Reinsel, C. N., Iwamoto, E. T., Gillespie, M. N. 1984. Structure activity evidence against opiate receptor involvement in leu-enkephalin-induced pulmonary vasoconstriction. *Biochem. Pharmacol.* 33:4095–98

45. Cushman, D. W., Cheung, H. S. 1971. Spectrophotometric assay and properties of the angiotensin converting enzyme of rabbit lung. *Biochem. Pharmacol.* 20:1637–48

46. Catravas, J. D., Gillis, C. N. 1981. Metabolism of ^3H-benzoyl-phenylalanyl-alanyl-proline by pulmonary angiotensin converting enzyme *in vivo:* Effects of bradykinin, SQ14225, or acute hypoxia. *J. Pharmacol. Exp. Ther.* 217:263–70

47. Chen, X., Pitt, B. R., Moalli, R., Gillis, C. N. 1984. Correlation between lung and plasma angiotensin converting enzyme and the hypotensive effect of captopril in conscious rabbits. *J. Pharmacol. Exp. Ther.* 229:649–53

48. Ashton, J. H., Pitt, B. R., Gillis, C. N. 1985. Apparent kinetics of angiotensin converting enzyme: hydrolysis of $[^3H]$ benzoyl-phenylalanyl-alanyl-proline in the isolated perfused lung. *J. Pharmacol. Exp. Ther.* 232:602–7

49. Howell, R. E., Moalli, R., Gillis, C. N. 1984. Analysis of rabbit pulmonary angiotensin converting enzyme kinetics in vivo. *J. Pharmacol. Exp. Ther.* 228:154–60

50. Moalli, R., Man, P., Hasan, F. M., Faruggia, R., Teplitz, C., Gillis, C. N.

1984. Pulmonary metabolic functions in rabbits given *E. coli* endotoxin. *Fed. Proc.* 43:405

51. Ryan, J. W. 1983. Assay of peptidase and protease enzymes *in vivo*. *Biochem. Pharmacol.* 32:2127–37

52. Rubin, D. B., Mason, R. J., Bodds, L. J. 1982. Angiotensin converting enzyme substrates hydrolysed by fibroblasts and vascular endothelial cells. *Exp. Lung Res.* 3:137–45

53. Jackson, R. M., Pisarello, J. B. 1984. Hypoxia pre-adaptation prevents oxygen-induced depression of lung angiotensin converting enzyme. *Am. Rev. Respir. Dis.* 130:424–28

54. Ryan, U. S., Clements, E., Habliston, D., Ryan, J. W. 1978. Isolation and culture of pulmonary endothelial cells. *Tissue Cell.* 10:535–54

55. Igic, R., Erdos, E. G., Yeh, H. S. J., Sorrells, K., Nakajima, T. 1972. Angiotensin I converting enzyme of the lung. *Circ. Res. 31(3)II51–61*

56. King, G. L., Johnson, S. M. 1985. Receptor mediated transport of insulin accross endothelial cells. *Science* 227:1583–86

56a. Dernovsek, K. D., Bar, R. S. 1985. Processing of cell-bound insulin by capillary and macrovascular endothelial cells in culture. *Am. J. Physiol.* 248:E244–51

57. Maack, T., Camargo, M. J. F., Laragh, J. F., Atlas, S. A. 1985. Atrial natriuretic factor: structure and function. *Kidney Int.* 27:607–16

58. Schiffrin, E. L., Chartier, L., Thibault, G., St-Louis, J., Cantin, M., Genest, J. 1985. Vascular and adrenal receptors for atrial natriuretic factor in the rat. *Circ. Res.* 56:801–7

59. Catravas, J. D., White, R. E. 1984. Kinetics of pulmonary angiotensin converting enzyme and 5'-nucleotidase in vivo. *J. Appl. Physiol.* 57:1173–81

60. Catravas, J. D. 1984. Removal of adenosine from the rabbit pulmonary circulation in vivo and in situ. *Circ. Res.* 54:603–11

61. Pearson, J. D., Carleton, J. S., Hutchings, A., Gordon, J. L. 1978. Uptake and metabolism of adenosine by pig aortic endothelial and smooth muscle cells in culture. *Biochem. J.* 170:265–71

62. Dieterle, Y., Ody, C., Ehrensberger, A., Stalder, H., Junod, A. F. 1978. Metabolism and uptake of adenosine triphosphate and adenosine by porcine aortic and pulmonary endothelial cells and fibroblasts in culture. *Circ. Res.* 42:869–76

63. Hellewell, P. G., Pearson, J. D. 1983.

Metabolism of circulating adenosine by the porcine isolated perfused lung. *Circ. Res.* 53:1–7

64. Bakhle, Y. S., Chelliah, R. 1983. Metabolism and uptake of adenosine in rat isolated lung and its inhibition. *Br. J. Pharmacol.* 79:509–15

65. Bassingthwaighte, J. B., Wang, C. Y., King, R. B. 1985. Modeling adenosine metabolism by endothelial cells. *Fed. Proc.* 44:1263

66. Dollery, C. T., Junod, A. F. 1976. Concentration of +/− propranolol in isolated perfused lungs of rat. *Br. J. Pharmacol.* 57:67–71

67. Junod, A. F. 1975. Mechanisms of drug accumulation in the lung. In *Lung Metabolism*, ed. A. F. Junod, R. de Haller, pp. 219–31. New York: Academic

68. Rothstein, P., Cole, J., Pitt, B. R. 1984. Pulmonary extraction of bupivacaine is dose-dependent. *Anesthesiology* 61:A236

69. Roerig, D., Bunke, S., Dawson, C. A., Kotrly, K., Kampine, J. P. 1985. Inhibition of Fentanyl uptake in the isolated perfused rat lung by propranolol. *Fed. Proc.* 44:1758

70. Frangos, J. A., Eskin, S. G., McIntire, L. V., Ives, C. L. 1985. Flow effects on prostacyclin production by cultured human endothelial cells. *Science* 227:1477–79

71. Grondelle, A., Worthen, G. S., Ellis, D., Mathias, M. M., Murphy, R. C., et al. 1984. Altering hydrodynamic variables influences PGI_2 production by isolated lungs and endothelial cells. *J. Appl. Physiol.* 57:388–95

72. Utsunomiya, T., Krausz, M. M., Shepro, D., Hechtman, H. B. 1981. Prostaglandin control of plasma and plalelet 5-hydroxytryptamine in normal and embolized animals. *Am. J. Physiol.* 241:H766–71

73. Boura, A. L. A., Murphy, R. D. 1978. Thromboxane B_2 inhibits prostaglandin E_2 inactivation by the rat isolated perfused lung. *Clin. Exp. Pharmacol. Physiol.* 5:387–92

74. Furchgott, R. F. 1984. Role of endothelium in the responses of vascular smooth muscle to drugs. *Ann. Rev. Pharmacol.* 24:175–97

75. Deleted in proof

76. Chand, N., Altura, B. M. 1981. Acetylcholine and bradykinin relax intrapulmonary arteries by acting on endothelial cells: role in lung vascular disease. *Science* 213:1376–79

77. McGiff, J. C. 1981. Interactions of prostaglandins with the kallikrein-kinin and

renin-angiotensin systems. *Clin. Sci.* 59:105–16

78. Cohen, M. L., Kurz, K. D. 1982. Angiotensin converting enzyme inhibition in tissues from spontaneously hypertensive rats after treatment with captopril or MK421. *J. Pharmacol. Exp. Ther.* 220:63–69

79. deOliveiraSalgado, M. C., Krieger, E. M. 1983. Acute changes in the renin-angiotensin system modify bradykinin and angiotensin reactivity and metabolism in conscious rats. *Hypertension* 5:V172–76 (Suppl.)

80. Strittmatter, S. M., Kapiloff, M. S., Snyder, S. H. 1983. ^{3}H-Captopril binding to membrane associated angiotensin converting enzyme. *Biochem. Biophys. Res. Commun.* 112:1027–33

81. Howell, R. E., Moalli, R., Gillis, C. N. 1985. Captopril removal by rabbit lung *in vivo. Biochem. Pharmacol.* 34:2371–75

82. Turrin, M., Pitt, B. R., Ryan, J. W., Chung, A., Clark, M. B., Gillis, C. N. 1985. Uptake of RAC (N-[1-(S)-carboxy - (4 - OH - 3- ^{125}I - phenyl - ethyl-L-ala-L-pro), an inhibitor of angiotensin converting enzyme (ACE) by rabbit lungs, *in situ. Fed. Proc.* 44:1890

83. Mason, G. R., Effros, R. M., Huszcuk, A., Chung, A., Ryan, J. W. 1985. Pulmonary vascular uptake of an angiotensin converting enzyme inhibitor is uninfluenced by hypoxia. *Fed. Proc.* 44:1757

84. Pitt, B. R., Woodford, M., Gillis, C. N. 1985. In-line measurement of pulmonary metabolic function in vivo. *Fed. Proc.* 44:1890

85. Gillis, C. N., Catravas, J. D. 1982. Altered removal of vasoactive substances in the injured lung: Detection of lung microvascular injury. *Ann. NY Acad. Sci.* 384:458–74

86. Gillis, C. N., Pitt, B. R. 1986. The pulmonary microcirculation and metabolic functions of the lung. In *Current Topics in Pulmonary Pharmacology and Toxicology*, ed. M. Hollinger. Philadelphia: Praeger. In press

87. Block, E. R. 1984. Early metabolic changes in response to lung injury: extrapolation from animals to humans. *J. Toxicol. Environ. Health* 13:369–86

87a. Block, E. R., Parel, J. M., Angelides, K. J., Sheridan, N. P., Garg, L. C. 1986. Hyperoxia reduces plasma membrane fluidity: a mechanism for endothelial cell dysfunction. *J. Appl. Physiol.* In press

88. Dobuler, K. J., Catravas, J. D., Gillis, C. N. 1982. Early detection of oxygen-induced lung injury in conscious rabbits:

Reduced activity of angiotensin converting enzyme and removal of 5-hydroxytryptamine in vivo. *Am. Rev. Respir. Dis.* 126:534–39

89. Gillis, C. N., Cronau, L. H., Mandel, S., Hammond, G. L. 1979. Indicator dilution measurement of 5-hydroxytryptamine clearance by human-lung. *J. Appl. Physiol.* 46:1178–83

90. Dargent, F., Neidhart, P., Bachmann, M., Suter, P. M., Junod, A. F. 1985. Simultaneous measurement of serotonin and propanolol pulmonary extraction in patients after extracorporeal circulation and surgery. *Am. Rev. Respir. Dis.* 131:242–45

91. Gillis, C. N., Pitt, B. R., Hammond, G. L. 1983. Depressed pulmonary removal of prostaglandin E_1 in patients with respiratory failure. *Circulation* 68:401

91a. Morel, D. R., Dargent, F., Bachman, M., Suter, P. M., Jurod, A. F. 1985. Pulmonary extraction of serotonin and propanolol in patients with adult respiratory distress syndrome. *Am. Rev. Respir. Dis.* 132:479–84

92. Pang, J. A., Butland, R. J. A., Brooks, N., Cattell, M., Geddes, D. M. 1982. Impaired lung uptake of propranolol in human pulmonary emphysema. *Am. Rev. Respir. Dis.* 125:194–98

93. Jose, P., Niederhauser, U., Piper, P. J., Robinson, C., Smith, A. P. 1976. Degradation of prostaglandin $F_{2\alpha}$ in the human pulmonary circulation. *Thorax* 31:713–19

94. Rickaby, D. A., Dawson, C. A., Linehan, J. H. 1984. Influence of embolism and imipramine on kinetics of serotonin uptake by dog lung. *J. Appl. Physiol.* 56:1170–77

95. Rickaby, D. A., Linehan, J. H., Bronikowski, T. A., Dawson, C. A. 1981. Kinetics of serotonin uptake in dog lung. *J. Appl. Physiol.* 51:405–14

96. Rickaby, D. A., Dawson, C. A., Linehan, J. H. 1982. Influence of blood and plasma flow rate on kinetics of serotonin uptake by lungs. *J. Appl. Physiol.* 53: 677–84

97. Bronikowski, T. A., Linehan, J. H., Dawson, C. A. 1980. A mathematical analysis of perfusion heterogeneity on indicator extraction. *Math. Biosci.* 52:27–51

98. Bronikowski, T. A., Dawson, C. A., Linehan, J. H., Rickaby, D. A. 1982. A mathematical model of indicator extraction by the pulmonary endothelium via saturation kinetics. *Math. Biosci.* 61: 237–66

99. Linehan, J. H., Dawson, C. A., Wagner-

Weber, V. M. 1981. Prostaglandin E₁ uptake by isolated cat lungs perfused with physiological salt solutions. *J. Appl. Physiol.* 50:428–34

100. Rickaby, D. A., Dawson, C. A., Linehan, J. H. 1984. Kinetics of serotonin uptake by the dog lung is pH independent in the physiological range. *Proc. Soc. Exp. Biol. Med.* 175:361–65

101. Malcorps, C. M., Dawson, C. A., Linehan, J. H., Bronikowski, T. A., Rickaby, D. A., et al. 1984. Lung serotonin uptake kinetics from indicator dilution and constant infusion methods. *J. Appl. Physiol.* 57:720–30

102. Pitt, B. R., Moalli, R., Gillis, C. N. 1984. Apparent kinetics of pulmonary removal of prostaglandin E₁ (PGE₁) after microembolization in anesthetized rabbits. *Am. Rev. Respir. Dis.* 129:A350

102a. Moalli, R., Howell, T. E., Gillis, C.N. 1985. Kinetics of captopril- and enalapril-induced inhibition of pulmonary angiotensin converting enzyme in vivo. *J. Pharmacol. Exp. Ther.* 234:372–77

103. Pitt, B. R., Lister, G. 1984. Kinetics of pulmonary angiotensin-converting enzyme activity in conscious developing lambs. *J. Appl. Physiol.* 57:1158–66

104. Moalli, R., Ashton, J. H., Pitt, B. R., Gillis, C. N. 1983. Effect of airway pressure (P_{aw}) on pulmonary angiotensin converting enzyme (ACE) activity in isolated perfused rabbit lung. *Fed. Proc.* 42:593

105. Straus, O. H., Goldstein, A. 1943. Zone behavior of enzymes. *J. Gen. Physiol.* 26:559–85

106. Dawson, C. A., Christensen, C. W., Rickaby, D. A., Linehan, J. H., Johnston, M. R. 1985. Lung damage and pulmonary uptake of serotonin in intact dogs. *J. Appl. Physiol.* 58:1761–66

107. Iwasawa, Y., Gillis, C. N. 1974. Pharmacological analysis of norepinephrine and 5-hydroxytryptamine uptake from the pulmonary circulation: Differentiation of uptake uptake sites for each amine. *J. Pharmacol. Exp. Ther.* 188:386–93

108. Block, E. R., Fisher, A. B. 1977. Depression of serotonin clearance by rat lungs during oxygen exposure. *J. Appl. Physiol.* 42:33–38

Ann. Rev. Pharmacol. Toxicol. 1986. 26:201–24

LEUKOCYTES AND ISCHEMIA-INDUCED MYOCARDIAL INJURY

Benedict R. Lucchesi

Department of Pharmacology, The University of Michigan Medical School, Ann Arbor, Michigan 48109

Keven M. Mullane

Department of Pharmacology, New York Medical College, Valhalla, New York 10595

THE MEANS OF LIMITING INFARCT SIZE

In the early 1970s Maroko, Braunwald, and others demonstrated the importance of myocardial oxygen supply and demand as a major determinant of the extent of myocardial injury (1–3). A variety of agents that reduced myocardial oxygen demand, B-adrenoceptor antagonists and calcium channel blockers for example, were shown to be beneficial in animal models of myocardial ischemia. The time for clinical testing of agents that improve myocardial oxygenation was said to have come (4). A decade later, however, the limited clinical results have been far from exciting. This approach to reducing ischemia-induced myocardial injury suffers from three major problems.

Implicit in the concept of salvaging ischemic myocardium by altering myocardial oxygen supply and demand is the assumption that myocardial tissue injury results solely from an inability of the coronary vasculature to deliver necessary oxygen and nutrients to maintain myocyte viability. However, we believe that other pathophysiologic processes contribute to irreversible myocardial damage.

It is also assumed that the restoration of coronary blood flow to the ischemic myocardium would, of itself, prevent the development of irreversible damage. However, reperfusion of jeopardized myocardium may lead to cellular processes that extend the area of cell necrosis beyond that which could be attributed

201

to the period of ischemia, alone, and produce long-term functional derangements of the heart (5–8).

Finally, if myocardial damage is solely the result of an imbalance between oxygen supply and demand, then maneuvers designed to limit infarct size will only be effective if given early after the onset of myocardial ischemia. While such treatment has practical limitations clinically, which has probably contributed to the tempered enthusiasm for infarct size limitation (9), the ability to salvage ischemic myocardium at later periods (10, 11), or even after a period of myocardial oxygen deprivation (i.e. after adequate reperfusion) (12, 13), suggests other processes have to be taken into consideration.

In the past three years, several investigative efforts (14–16, 12, 14–19) have independently proposed a role for leukocytes as contributors to ischemia-induced myocardial injury. The tissue damage resulting from myocardial ischemia activates a cascade of events that can broadly be defined as an inflammatory response that occurs independently of any improvement in myocardial oxygenation. If the premise is true, that the inflammatory response and invading leukocytes contribute to the ultimate extent of myocardial injury, then agents directed against the leukocytes may provide a novel means of limiting infarct size and may expand the time frame in which therapy can be initiated and still be effective, since neutrophil infiltration proceeds for up to 24 hr (20, 21).

CAN LEUKOCYTES EXACERBATE ISCHEMIA-INDUCED MYOCARDIAL DAMAGE?

The presence of leukocytes in infarcted myocardium has been demonstrated histologically at autopsy (20, 21) and by the use of radiolabeled cells to clinically define infarcts in patients (22, 23). Owing, in part, to methodological problems whereby the blood pool of radioactivity had to be cleared before accurate scanning, these studies suggested that polymorphonuclear leukocytes (PMN) do not appear until 24 hr after the start of the ischemia event and that they peak at about 72 hr before declining. This led to the belief that PMN infiltration was merely the result of necrosis and reflected the initiation of a repair process. However, the question still remains, can PMNs cause or exacerbate necrosis? For this to be true, neutrophils should be evident much earlier than 24 hr, before the final extent of the infarct has been delineated. Mullane and co-workers (17) found that the activation, margination, and diapedesis of PMNs already became apparent after 60 min of coronary artery occlusion, and over the ensuing 5 hr a large number of PMNs invaded the ischemic area. Enhanced capillary permeability after coronary occlusion is evident within 15–20 min (24). Edema formation appears and is dependent upon an *interaction between* chemotactic factors, such as complement fragment

C_{5a}, the presence of PMNs, and the local generation of a vasodilator prostaglandin (25). All of these requirements are fulfilled in the ischemic myocardium (17, 26–29) and compel one to consider that PMNs are recruited very quickly and may contribute to some early changes associated with myocardial ischemia. Thus temporally, PMN activation and subsequent influx do appear to be related to ischemia-induced myocardial necrosis. In the study of patients at the time of autopsy, Fishbein et al (21) observed a parallel development of PMN infiltration and tissue necrosis, but they did not associate the two processes in the progression of infarction. Although the evidence indicates, therefore, that PMN influx and the development of necrosis are temporally related, this association does not prove causality.

HOW CAN LEUKOCYTES PROMOTE TISSUE DAMAGE?

In vitro studies show that during the process of phagocytosis, PMNs release a variety of mediators that can be considered toxic to tissues. These mediators include oxygen metabolites (free radicals), arachidonic acid metabolites, platelet-activating factor, and lysosomal enzymes.

Oxygen Metabolites and Free Radicals

The activation of neutrophils by a soluble or phagocytic stimulus initiates a "respiratory burst" with a sudden and large increase in oxygen consumption, activation of the hexose monophosphate shunt, and the generation of oxygen metabolites and toxic free radicals, which can be released into the external tissue environment (30, 31). Greater than 90% of the oxygen consumed by neutrophils during this period can be accounted for by superoxide anion (O_2^-) formation, through the action of a NAD(P)H-oxidase located in the cell membrane (32, 33). When two molecules of O_2^- react with each other, one is oxidized and the other is reduced forming hydrogen peroxide (H_2O_2) and oxygen in a dismutation reaction, which can be catalyzed by superoxide dismutase (also present in the leukocyte) (34). Formation of the hydroxyl radical (.OH) requires a trace metal, which, when reduced by O_2^-, can react with H_2O_2 to form .OH and OH^-. Lactoferrin is an iron-binding protein found in the specific granules of neutrophils, which can increase .OH production in vitro (35), presumably by its ability to provide iron for the O_2^-/H_2O_2 system. Lactoferrin is also released into the extracellular environment during neutrophil activation and could represent an important source of mediators of tissue injury. Finally, the reaction of H_2O_2 with the neutrophil myeloperoxidase (contained within the azurophilic granules) produces an enzyme substrate complex that can oxidize various halides, in particular chloride (Cl^-), to produce highly reactive toxic products such as hypochlorous acid (HOCl) (36, 37). For a more detailed account of the formation and role of leukocyte-derived oxygen metabolites, the reader is referred to the excellent review by Fantone & Ward (38).

Oxygen metabolites can directly alter structural components of tissue, producing degradation of glycosaminoglycans, proteoglycans, and collagen (38), together with injury and lysis of a variety of cell types including endothelial cells (39), erythrocytes (40), fibroblasts (41), platetlets (42), and leukocytes (43). These highly reactive oxygen metabolites attack membrane phospholipids and act on unsaturated fatty acids to produce lipid peroxidation, a frequent manifestation of free radical generation, which results in increased membrane fluidity, increased permeability, and loss of membrane integrity (44, 45). Hess and co-workers (46) have described a depression of calcium uptake in the cardiac sarcoplasmic reticulum that is due to the generation of free radicals at pH 6.4. This effect can be reproduced by exogenously formed free radicals that are generated from a xanthine-xanthine oxidase system that, at pH 6.5, produces the superoxide anion and hydroxyl radical. Activated human leukocytes have been shown to depress canine cardiac sarcoplasmic reticulum calcium transport because of their ability to generate superoxide anion, hydrogen peroxide, and hydroxyl radical (47). Myocardial cells in culture show uptake of antimyosin, reflecting sarcolemmal damage, under conditions that promote free radical generation (48). The production of malonyldialdehyde (MDA), indicative of lipid free radical oxidation, is associated with reoxygenation-induced damage of the heart (49). The exogenous generation of superoxide anions via the xanthine-xanthine oxidase system at pH 7.4 also results in increased mitochondrial MDA formation and reduced mitochondrial respiration leading to an increase in cytosolic free calcium and a decrease in ATP (50). These changes in the sarcoplasmic reticulum and mitochondria correlate with the development of irreversible injury. Lipid peroxides can also react with proteins, leading to a loss of enzymatic activity, scission of polypeptide chains, and destruction of some labile amino acids including cysteine and lysine (51). In contrast, phospholipase activity may actually be enhanced (52), leading to the release of unsaturated fatty acids. Thus, the generation of free radicals, and the ensuing lipid peroxidation, can contribute to many different aspects of tissue damage.

The generation of free radicals may be particularly important during reoxygenation of ischemic myocardium, which often enhances the injury (5–8). However, free radicals can be produced even during the period of ischemia, since the pO_2 in the ischemic core is 5–10 mmHg, which is sufficient to sustain 83% of the free radical generation (53). Myocardial ischemia is associated with a decrease in superoxide dismutase and glutathione peroxidase activity (54–57), the two major intracellular enzymes that normally protect the heart from free radical-mediated damage by preventing the increased formation of toxic oxygen metabolites.

While it is apparent from the foregoing that the formation of free radicals can impair cell and mitochondrial membrane integrity, the effects of these chemical species on cardiac function have not been addressed. Recently Jackson and co-workers (58), using isolated hearts perfused with a buffer subjected to electrolysis to generate free radicals, demonstrated an increase in perfusion pressure and a decrease in myocardial contractility—changes indicative of ischemia.

The most persuasive evidence implicating oxygen-derived free radicals in myocardial injury stems from the use of a variety of free radical scavengers to suppress various indices of myocardial dysfunction or damage. These scavengers have included superoxide dismutase and catalase (46, 59–61), superoxide dismutase alone (48, 49, 58, 62), superoxide dismutase plus mannitol (46, 47, 63), dimethyl sulfoxide (48, 64, 65), allopurinol (66), co-enzyme Q10 (67), and glucose-insulin-potassium cardioplegia (68), together with antioxidants such as alpha-tocopherol, selenium, and ascorbate (49, 69, 70). These drugs prevent cardiac enzyme release (48, 49, 59, 68–71, 89), prevent sarcolemmal damage (48) and restore depressed calcium uptake and ATPase activity in the sarcolemma (46, 47, 68), maintain mitochondrial integrity and function (59, 61, 62), and prevent malondialdehyde formation and release (49, 57). In addition, these drugs improve cardiac function (58–60, 63, 72) and quantitatively reduce infarct size (13, 66). The study by Jolly and co-workers (13) in an occlusion-reperfusion model of myocardial damage in the anesthetized dog is particularly pertinent because these workers demonstrated that the administration of superoxide dismutase and catalase during the early reperfusion phase was associated with maximal protection against reperfusion injury that could be divorced from the damage that was the result of myocardial oxygen deprivation (coronary occlusion). These authors postulated that primary myocardial cellular damage due to ischemia is additive to the cardiac cell damage during the reperfusion phase; the latter form of injury is mediated, at least in part, by toxic metabolites of oxygen.

From the foregoing, it is clear that myocardial ischemia and, in particular, reperfusion of the ischemic tissue are accompanied by the formation of oxygen-derived free radicals, which overwhelm diminished endogenous protective mechanisms to exacerbate cell injury and tissue damage. It is important to recognize that cell death is probably a far more violent event than is often imagined, "an explosion rather than a dissolution" (73), since the generation of free radicals (the conversion of a stable to an unstable chemical species) requires an explosive release of energy. The question arises as to the source of oxygen-derived free radicals in myocardial ischemia and/or reperfusion. While it is known that activated neutrophils can generate and release substantial quantities of oxygen metabolites, it is certain that they are not the sole source of these products, since free radical generation and protection by various scavengers is also observed in isolated hearts, perfused with a blood-free medium (49, 50, 54, 55, 57, 67). McCord (74) has demonstrated that ischemia in vivo results in the conversion of xanthine dehydrogenase to xanthine oxidase and that reperfusion of the tissue is accompanied by a burst of O_2^- and H_2O_2 production via this enzyme. Samples of ischemic myocardium biopsied 30 min after coronary occlusion show a greater than 300% increase in xanthine oxidase activity (66), indicating that this mechanism could be an important source of free radicals in myocardial tissue. The relative importance of myocardial xanthine oxidase and the neutrophil NAD(P)H oxidase system to free radical-mediated damage of the ischemic or reperfused myocardium remains to be determined.

Membrane Phospholipids and Lysolipids

A number of studies have focused on examining changes in the integrity of the sarcolemmal membrane since Jennings and co-workers (75, 76) demonstrated that changes in permeability of the sarcolemmal membrane led to the accumulation of tissue calcium, which correlated with the time course of the onset of irreversible injury. These alterations in permeability may be due to free radical generation (46, 77) or the degradation of membrane phospholipds (78). These two events are not mutually exclusive, and changes in membrane phospholipids may well result from free radical attack, while the enhanced lipid peroxidation increases membrane fluidity and permeability. Chien and co-workers (79) found that irreversible ischemic injury in the heart is accompanied by the degradation of membrane phospholipids because of activation of phospholipases and loss of reacylase activity. This can be seen as an increased accumulation of free arachindonate, which parallels the time course of irreversible injury. Moreover, in vitro treatment of sarcolemmal vesicles or cultured myocardial cells with exogenous phospholipases causes damage similar to that seen in vivo (78), while activated neutrophils also release phospholipase A_2 (which cleaves and releases arachidonate from membrane phospholipids) into the external environment (80, 81) and may contribute to this effect. These mechanisms may provide arachidonic acid for its subsequent metabolism to eicosanoids.

Phospholipase attack on membrane phospholipids will not only cleave a fatty acid, such as arachidonic acid, but will leave a lysophospholipid remaining. Normally, reacylation enzymes prevent the accumulation of lysolipids (82); however, during ischemia reacylase activity is low (83), due in part to the depletion of ATP which is required to form the fatty acyl CoA derivatives of the fatty acids to be reincorporated. Consequently, an increase in lysophospho-glycerides has been detected in ischemic tissue in vivo as well as in effluents from ischemic regions (84–86). Corr and co-workers (87, 88) have obtained evidence implicating these lysolipids in electrophysiological derangements accompanying myocardial ischemia.

Neutrophils contain high concentrations of 1-O-alkyl-2-aryl-sn-glycero-3-phosphocholine within the membrane phospholipids (89). Stimulation of the neutrophils activates phospholipase A_2 to liberate arachidonic acid, leaving 1-O-alkyl-2-lyso-sn-glycero-3-phosphocholine, which can subsequently be acetylated to form platelet-activating factor (PAF-acether) (90, 91). PAF-acether promotes neutrophil activation and degranulation and has been implicated in anaphylaxis and inflammation, where it induces vascular leakage and smooth muscle contraction (90, 91). In addition, this mediator can cause cardiac dysfunction and promote arrhythmias (92, 93), and it can exacerbate ischemia-induced myocardial damage (94). Recently, 24-hr infarcted myocardium has been demonstrated to generate PAF-acether, which may reflect the earlier influx and continued presence of functioning neutrophils (95).

Arachidonic Acid Metabolism

The activation of PMNs is accompanied by the release of arachadonic acid (AA) and the formation of a variety of pro-inflammatory metabolites. Arachindonic acid can activate the neutrophil NADPH oxidase, leading to the generation of superoxide anions (96). PMNs metabolize AA primarily via a 5-lipoxygenase enzyme to form 5-HETE and LTB_4 (97, 98). This latter compound is chemotactic for neutrophils (99, 100), promotes leukocyte adhesion to the vascular endothelium (101), and, at high concentrations, acts as a calcium ionophore to increase intracellular calcium and to promote free radical generation and the release of lysosomal enzymes (102). Moreover, in the presence of neutrophils and a vasodilator prostaglandin such as PGI_2, LTB_4 can produce edema (25). LTC_4 may also be formed, which induces coronary vasoconstriction and impairs contractility (103–106). Neutrophils contain a number of other enzymes capable of metabolizing AA, including 15- (107) and 12-lipoxygenases (17) and a cytochrome P450-dependent monooxygenase (108). The importance of the products of these pathways is not clear. Metabolites of AA can be re-esterified into the cell membrane (109), however, and, if this occurs in the myocytes, it may result in alterations in membrane function and permeability. Superoxide anions can also oxygenate arachidonic acid to a potent chemotactic factor (110).

The heart is unusual in that it has a very low capacity to metabolize AA when compared to other organs (7). Indeed almost all of the cyclo-oxygenase activity that is detected is localized to the coronary blood vessels (111) and the epicardial membrane (112), while the myocytes have either nondetectable or negligible cyclo-oxygenase or lipoxygenase activites. Consequently, the finding (17) that infarcted myocardium had an increased capacity to metabolize exogenous AA suggested either the unmasking of dormant enzymes already contained with the tissue or an influx of cells with a very active metabolic pathway. This latter possibility is the most likely, since the profile of metabolites formed by the infarcted myocardium was similar to that observed in purified preparations of neutrophils, whereas the enhanced metabolism could be prevented by pharmacologic interventions that suppressed the neutrophil infiltration into the heart (17). Thus, migrating cells can alter the metabolic profile of the tissue that they invade and give rise to products not normally found in the host tissue and which may influence the activities and function of that tissue. We feel that this is a potentially important concept, the significance of which has yet to be examined.

Lysosomal Enzymes

Wildenthal (113, 114) proposed a "lysosomal hypothesis" whereby myocardial ischemia enhanced the fragility of cardiac lysosomes leading to the leakage of lysosomal enzymes into the cell cytosol, thereby promoting cellular damage. Certainly increased lysosomal permeability and the release of lysosomal-derived cathepsin D can be related temporally to the process of irreversible injury (115). This hypothesis can be extended to consider the lysosomal enzymes released by activated neutrophils that are capable of proteolytic attack on ischemic myocytes as has been demonstrated for the neutrophil-derived lysosomal enzymes that contribute to the degenerative tissue damage associated with rheumatoid arthritis (116). However, the extent of myocardial cell injury caused by proteolytic enzymes is not clear. It appears unlikely that they contribute to a significant extent, since drugs shown to stabilize lysosomes in vitro and prevent the release of cardiac enzymes do not uniformly reduce ischemia-induced myocardial damage. For example, PGE_2 (117), PGI_2 (117), naproxen (118), and ibuprofen (119) suppress the ischemia-induced release of cardiac lysosomal enzymes to a similar extent, whereas only PGI_2 (120, 121) and ibuprofen (122–124), but not PGE_2 (120) or naproxen (125), reduce infarct size. Measuring the formation of tyrosine (an amino acid that is neither synthesized nor degraded by cardiac muscle) as an index of lysosomal protease activity in the myocardium, Bolli and co-workers (126, 127) found that proteolysis actually decreased during 3 hr of ischemia. The subsequent increase in proteolysis correlated with the leukocyte infiltration that increased over 24 hr and was thought to reflect leukocyte-mediated digestion of the necrotic debris rather than an extension of the myocardial injury. Moreover, inhibition of lysosomal protease activity with leupeptin, antipain, pepstatin, and chymostatin totally suppressed proteolysis but did not influence infarct size (128, 129), thus suggesting that lysosomal enzyme activity and the extent of myocardial damage are not linked.

WHAT CAUSES LEUKOCYTE ACTIVATION?

The complement system of plasma proteins is thought to play an important role in the pathogenesis of ischemia-induced myocardial damage. Activated components of complement are potent chemotactic and stimulatory agents for neutrophils and may initiate leukocyte infiltration into the extravascular myocardial tissue (26, 27, 130). Hill & Ward (130) found that coronary artery ligation led to the stimulation of a tissue protease, present in the myocardium, that cleaves the third component of complement into chemotactically active fragments. Subsequently, the localization of complement components has been studied in the ischemic myocardium of the baboon, using immunohistochemical techniques (26, 27). C_3, C_4, and C_5 were found extensively throughout the infarcted myocardium within the myocytes and arteriolar smooth muscle. Electron microscopy revealed C_3 associated with the contractile elements of myocytes as well as nuclear, mitochondrial, and sarcoplasmic reticular membranes (27). Moreover, human heart subcellular membranes, in particular mitochondrial membranes, bind and activate the same complement components in vitro (131). While myocardial infarction in patients is accompanied by a reduction in circulating complement components after 24–48 hrs (132), the complement components are already present in infarcted myocardium within 4 hr (26). Unfortunately, earlier time points have not been examined to determine if there is a temporal correlation with neutrophil activation and infiltration. The presence of complement components within the myocytes places these chemotactic mediators in an ideal position to attract neutrophils from the circulation. The interaction of C_{3b} with a specific receptor on the surface of the neutrophil triggers phagocytosis and the formation of neutrophil-derived mediators (133, 134). Moreover, complement-induced superoxide anion generation can occur independently of phagocytosis (135), thereby promoting free radical-mediated damage. The concept that the complement system is responsible for the neutrophil accumulation is supported by the observation that C_3, C_4, and C_5 localization is more intense at the periphery of the infarct and tends to decrease towards the center of the damaged area (27), a transmural distribution similar to that observed by Mullane et al (136) for the neutrophils using an assay for the neutrophil-specific myeloperoxidase enzyme.

If the complement system does account for the neutrophil activation and infiltration, the question arises as to what triggers complement activation? It is important to recognize that the immunohistochemical demonstration of C_3 in the myocardial fibers was accompanied by histological evidence of ischemic damage with myofibril disintegration, nuclear fragmentation, mitochondrial dense body formation, and the presence of albumin within the same fibers (27).

Thus damage initiated by the ischemic insult activates the complement system, which in turn promotes neutrophil infiltration. The influx of neutrophils into the myocardium is not observed if the ischemia is not of a sufficient duration to initiate the damage. However, marginating neutrophils in the vascular compartment may contribute to some early consequences of ischemia, such as edema (25), but remain within the vasculature until irreversible damage occurs.

The complement-derived anaphylatoxins C3a and C5a may themselves contribute to the cardiac dysfunction accompanying myocardial ischemia. C3a, apart from eliciting chemotaxis, enhancing vascular permeability, and provoking the release of mediators such as histamine, leukotrienes, prostaglandins, and PAF-acether (137), also produces coronary vasoconstriction, left ventricular contractile failure, tachycardia, and impaired atrioventricular conduction when injected into the isolated heart of the guinea pig (138). This profile of ischemia-like responses is attributed to the release of mediators from the heart, including histamine, leukotrienes, and a cyclo-oxygenase product (138).

Finally, the generation of oxygen-derived free radicals can also lead to the formation of chemotactic factors in plasma (139), if the oxygen metabolites are liberated and come into contact with plasma as a result of cellular damage. The importance of free-radical mediated activation of a chemotactic factor is currently unknown.

DOES LEUKOCYTE INHIBITION MODULATE THE DEVELOPMENT OF MYOCARDIAL NECROSIS?

A corollary of the proposal that neutrophils exacerbate ischemia-induced myocardial injury is that agents that abrogate leukocyte activation or infiltration, or prevent the release of specific neutrophil-derived mediators, should similarly reduce the extent of myocardial damage.

That a "heterolytic" or inflammatory process contributes to myocardial injury in addition to the autolytic process of oxygen deprivation has been recognized for over two decades (2, 3). However, results with anti-inflammatory drugs have been inconsistent (11, 12, 123–125, 140–146), which has made it difficult to appreciate the importance or extent of the damage provoked by the inflammatory response. Frequently, studies utilizing anti-inflammatory agents were not accompanied by any monitoring of the inflammatory response to demonstrate the effectiveness of the drug. Identification of the invading leukocytes as a major culprit of the heterolytic damage stemmed from studies by two independent groups of investigators (12, 14, 15, 17). Mullane & Moncada (12) and Jolly & Lucchesi (147) observed a reduction in infarct size with an experimental nonsteroidal anti-inflammatory drug (NSAID), BW755C. Since myocardial protection is not a general property of other NSAIDs, such as aspirin (140), naproxen (125), meclofenamate (141), zomepirac (142), or indomethacin (12, 143), it could not be attributed to an inhibition of the enzyme system cyclo-oxygenase, a known general mechanism of action of NSAIDs (148). However, these latter drugs do not inhibit leukocyte infiltration into an inflammatory lesion (149, 150), and, while they are thought to provide some symptomatic relief in chronic inflammation, by reducing the pain and swelling for example, it is generally considered that they do little to ameliorate the underlying progression of the disease and tissue destruction (150). BW755C, in contrast, suppresses the neutrophil infiltration into inflammatory lesions (149, 151), probably as a result of its ability to inhibit the lipoxygenase pathway of arachidonic acid metabolism (151, 152). Mullane & Moncada (12) suggested that this effect could underly the myocardial protective effects of BW755C, and subsequently they provided evidence to support this proposal (17). Other drugs that inhibit the lipoxygenase enzyme (and consequently neutrophil infiltration), including nafazatrom (19) and dipyridamole (153), also reduce infarct size (19, 154–156).

Meanwhile, Lucchesi and co-workers were examining the effects of another NSAID, ibuprofen. This drug reduces infarct size, independently of any hemodynamic changes, which suggests that it is acting by a mechanism other than to alter myocardial oxygenation (122–124). Lucchesi's group, recognizing that ibuprofen is capable of influencing both platelet and leukocyte behavior, assessed the ability of ibuprofen to alter the accumulation of these blood elements in the ischemic myocardium. They found that the myocardial protection afforded by ibuprofen is accompanied by a selective suppression of neutrophil infiltration (14). Subsequently, the ability of ibuprofen to inhibit the release of a variety of neutrophil-derived mediators, and consequently neutrophil activation and ischemic damage, was demonstrated (157).

Direct studies whereby leukocytes were depleted with either specific antineutrophil antiserum (15) or hydroxyurea (17) confirmed that myocardial damage induced by coronary artery occlusion and reperfusion is reduced when leukocytes, in particular neutrophils, are prevented from invading the ischemic myocardium. Recognition of leukocyte inhibition as an effective means of salvaging ischemic myocardium helps explain the protection observed with a variety of chemically unrelated drugs.

Complement depletion with cobra venom factor attenuates leukocyte infiltration into the heart and diminishes the area of damage (145, 158), thereby further implicating complement fragments as the important chemotactic factors in this response. Aprotinin (Trasylol®), a serine protease inhibitor, also reduces infarct size (145, 159). Hill & Ward (130) provided evidence that a protease was involved in complement activation in the ischemic myocardium, and aprotinin subsequently was found to prevent the release of a chemotactic factor into the coronary sinus blood during ischemia (145). Thus, aprotinin may suppress complement activation and, in turn, leukocyte infiltration and may result in a reduction in ischemic damage. More recently, aprotinin was found to prevent the increased production of oxygen-derived free radicals by PMNs sensitized by exposure to a low oxygen tension (160), thereby offering another leukocyte-dependent mechanism for the beneficial effects of this drug.

Epidemiologic studies have recognized that Greenland Eskimos have a low incidence of cardiovascular diseases such as myocardial infarction (161, 162). This intrinsic myocardial protection is attributed to the diet rich in eicosapenta-enoic acid (EPA, C20:5), obtained from seal meat and fish (161–164). Feeding dogs a diet enriched with fish oil resulted in a smaller infarct size after being subjected to coronary artery occlusion and reperfusion (165). Although not recognized at the time, this myocardial protection may have resulted from an effect on leukocytes. Terano and co-workers (166) found that rats fed EPA accumulated the fatty acid in their neutrophils. Upon stimulation, the EPA is released together with AA. The EPA, which competes with AA, is readily metabolized by the 5-lipoxygenase enzyme to LTB_5. Similar results recently have been obtained in human volunteers fed EPA (167). LTB_5 exhibits only one fifth to one tenth the biological potency of LTB_4 in stimulating neutrophil chemotaxis and aggregation (167, 168), whereas EPA-fed rats also exhibit a diminished inflammatory response (166). Thus EPA also has an "anti-inflammatory" action involving the leukocytes, which could account for its beneficial actions in acute myocardial ischemia.

In summary, a variety of chemically unrelated drugs can reduce infarct size, independently of changes in myocardial oxygenation. The common effect of all of these drugs is to reduce leukocyte infiltration and the ensuing inflammatory response, which suggests that this action accounts for the myocardial protective effects of this diverse group of agents.

MYOCARDIAL SALVAGE OR DELAY?

It was concluded by Chambers and co-workers (144) using another NSAID, flurbiprofen, that although infarct size was reduced at 6 hr, it was not reduced after 24 hr, so the drug merely delayed the development of damage rather than limiting its ultimate size. Although drugs that delay myocardial injury may be important in their own right and may extend the time frame in which other strategies can be gainfully employed to limit infarct size, it is apparent that many of the drugs demonstrated to influence leukocyte behavior do actually reduce the area of necrosis. Ibuprofen persistently reduces infarct size at 6 hr, 24 hr (124), 48 hr (123), and 72 hr (169). Neutropenia maintained with specific antiserum reduces the extent of damage induced by circumflex coronary artery occlusion for 90 min, whether measured 6 hr (15) or 24 hr after reperfusion (16)—as does BW755C (12, 147). Finally, complement depletion in the rat with cobra venom factor retarded the development of necrosis for 21 days

(170). These studies indicate that drugs that are directed against the in-flammatory response and that suppress leukocyte infiltration can permanently salvage the ischemic myocardium. The failure of flurbiprofen to reduce infarct size at 24 hr may have resulted from an ineffective dose to inhibit leukocyte invasion, since no means was used to determine the effective (anti-inflammatory) concentrations of the drug.

MECHANISMS UNDERLYING THE MYOCARDIAL PROTECTIVE EFFECTS OF DRUGS DIRECTED AGAINST LEUKOCYTES

The initial studies highlighting the ability of drugs directed against the leuko-cytes to limit the area of ischemic damage utilized an occlusion-reperfusion model of myocardial injury (12, 14, 15, 17, 18, 154). Reperfusion is thought to exacerbate some biochemical and functional derangements of ischemia (5–8). Moreover, reperfusion of the ischemic region improves the likelihood of leukocytes reaching the area of injury and may accelerate their influx. Howev-er, the participation of the leukocytes in myocardial damage is not restricted to reperfusion models. Total occlusion of a coronary artery also is accompanied by a rapid leukocyte infiltration (17, 171), in particular at the periphery of the infarct, while infarct size is still reduced by drug-induced leukopenia (172).

A number of possible mechanisms could explain the beneficial effects of the anti-leukocyte agents. The release of pro-inflammatory mediators potentially deleterious to the ischemic myocardium has been addressed. Clearly, drugs that suppress either the activation or infiltration of leukocytes into the ischemic myocardium will prevent the formation and release of all these mediators at the site at which they could do harm. Indeed, it has not been possible to delineate the importance of any one group of leukocyte-derived mediators in the process of myocardial tissue injury, since it appears that cellular infiltration is the first property to be lost when drugs directed against leukocyte-derived mediators are administered in vivo (17, 19).

Another mechanism that could account for the beneficial effects of drugs directed against the leukocytes is the improvement of blood flow to the ischem-ic myocardium. Jacob and co-workers (173, 174) have proposed that the aggregation of leukocytes could block coronary vessels and contribute to myocardial ischemia. Engler and co-workers (175) showed that leukocytes obstructed 60% of the capillaries within the ischemic myocardium, thereby preventing the full restoration of blood flow to the previously ischemic zone upon reperfusion. This "no-reflow" phenomenon could exacerbate myocardial damage by maintaining the ischemia despite attempts to restore the oxygen supply. Thus damage due to oxygen deprivation and that induced by activated leukocytes cannot be separated totally but rather are interrelated. Capillary plugging and leukocyte aggregation indicate an activated state of the cells that can be prevented by various anti-leukocyte drugs such as dexamethasone, which attenuate the "no-reflow" phenomenon (176). Leukocyte depletion prevents the progressive increase in coronary vascular resistance observed during ischemia and thus enhances blood flow to the ischemic zone (177). Consequently, leukocytes can exert deleterious effects on the coronary microcirculation during both myocardial ischemia and reperfusion.

INFLAMMATION, LEUKOCYTES, AND MYOCARDIAL REPAIR

The primary role of the invading neutrophils is not to destroy host tissue but rather to clear the cellular debris as the first step in a healing process in which a fibrous scar tissue of great tensile strength is deposited to replace the nonfunctional necrotic tissue (20, 21, 178). If site clearance is impaired, the necrotic mass becomes surrounded by a fibrous caspsule that prevents healing and can lead to ventricular wall thinning, dysfunction, and risk of ventricular wall aneurysm or rupture (170, 179–181). Measurements of proteolysis, as a reflection of the digestion of necrotic debris by neutrophils, show a dramatic increase within 48 hr of coronary occlusion, which correlates with leukocyte infiltration. Proteolysis may be prevented by the steroidal anti-inflammatory agent, methylprednisolone, implying retardation of the removal of necrotic tissue (182). Leukopenia, induced by whole body irradiation, reduces collagen degradation in the infarct zone after 24 hr of coronary occlusion (127). High doses of methylprednisolone, which suppress the inflammatory response induced by myocardial injury, slow the removal of necrotic myocytes, resulting in "mummification" of the infarct, and impaired myocardial healing (179). Moreover, multiple doses of methylprednisolone administered to patients with acute myocardial infarction have been associated with an increased incidence of ventricular aneurysm and rupture (183, 184)—effects attributed to inadequate repair of the infarct. The NSAIDs ibuprofen (185) and indomethacin (186) also were found to increase the incidence of scar thinning after myocardial infarction in experimental models, suggesting that retardation of the healing process may be a common property of drugs that inhibit the inflammatory process.

If anti-inflammatory or anti-leukocyte agents impair the healing process in the myocardium, they will be of limited use in the management of patients with acute myocardial ischemia and an evolving myocardial infarct. However, scar thinning does not correlate with the ability of the drug to suppress leukocyte infiltration, since only ibuprofen, and not indomethacin, attenuates the cellular response (14, 17, 157). Cobra venom factor and methylprednisolone attenuate neutrophil invasion and diminish myocardial damage to the same extent, yet only the latter is associated with impaired healing (170). Even agents that provoke scar thinning—ibuprofen and methylprednisolone—can be administered for a shorter period to achieve the same degree of myocardial protection without producing wall thinning and the associated ventricular dysfunction (170, 185).

These studies indicate that there is no clear relationship between inhibition of the early neutrophil infiltration and subsequent impairment of the healing process. Rather, it appears that the neutrophil response can be manipulated successfully without automatically resulting in scar thinning. Recently, Roberts and co-workers (187) suggested that inhibition of the mononuclear cell infiltration, not the neutrophil invasion, is associated with left ventricular scar thinning. Consequently, the chronic inflammatory resonse, characterized by mononuclear cells, may be involved primarily in the repair process, while selective inhibition of the acute response, associated with PMNs, may protect the ischemic myocardium without compromising the healing phase. Further studies in this important area are mandated.

CLINICAL SIGNIFICANCE

There is a direct correlation between the extent of myocardial injury and both short- and long-term prognosis in patients with acute myocardial infarction (3, 188). The recognition of an inflammatory response as a contributing factor to ischemia-induced myocardial injury, and, in particular, reperfusion-induced damage, may provide a means of treatment even if the patient's hospital admission is delayed a few hours. Anti-inflammatory steroids have been demonstrated to be effective even when administered 6 hr after coronary occlusion (11), and BW755C is beneficial when given during reperfusion, after the one hour period of ischemia is over (12). Second, the thrombolytic agents such as streptokinase and tissue plasminogen activator represent a therapeutic breakthrough whereby blood flow to ischemic regions of the myocardium can be restored. The increasing application of thrombolytic therapy and/or coronary angioplasty has prompted awareness of reperfusion-induced injury and ventricular dysfunction (189–192). The use of free radical scavengers or antineutrophil agents coupled with procedures for the restoration of coronary artery blood flow, given either immediately before or during the time of reperfusion, may reduce complications associated with the extension of myocardial injury and cell death.

Finally, a contribution of leukocytes to the initiation of ischemic heart disease should also be considered, since there is a positive correlation between the circulating leukocytes count and the incidence of myocardial infarction (193–195), while the converse is also true (196). Moreover, smoking, which increases the leukocyte count, is also associated with an increased incidence of myocardial infarction (193, 194). Furthermore, cigarette smoke can activate the alternative pathway of complement (197). A high proportion of patients with unstable angina who succumbed to sudden coronary death were found to have a clustered infiltration of inflammatory cells in the adventitia of the coronary artery, which may be related to coronary artery vasospasm (198).

ACKNOWLEDGMENTS

Dr. Mullane's studies cited in this review were supported in part by a Grant-In-Aid from the American Heart Association, with funds contributed in part by the American Heart Association, Westchester/Putnam Chapter. K. M. Mullane is the recipient of a Pharmaceutical Manufacturer's Association Faculty Development Award. Dr. Lucchesi's studies cited in this review were supported by a Grant from The National Institute of Health, NHLBI, HL-19782.

Literature Cited

1. Maroko, P. R., Kjekshus, J. K., Sobel, B. E., Watanabe, T., Lovell, J. W., et al. 1971. Factors influencing infarct size following experimental coronary artery occlusions. *Circulation* 43:67–82

2. Maroko, P. R., Braunwald, E. 1973. Modification of myocardial infarct size after coronary occlusion. *Ann. Intern. Med.* 79:720–33

3. Gillepsie, T., Sobel, B. 1977. A rationale for therapy of acute myocardial infarction. Limitation of infarct size. *Adv. Intern. Med.* 22:319–53

4. Braunwald, E., Maroko, P. R. 1974. The reduction of infarct size—an idea whose time (for testing) has come. *Circulation* 50:206

5. Hearse, D. J., Humphrey, S. M., Nayler, W. G., Slade, A., Gorder, D. 1975. Ultrastructural damage associated with reoxygenation of the anoxic myocardium. *J. Mol. Cell. Cardiol.* 7:315–24

6. Hearse, D. J. 1977. Reperfusion of the ischemic myocardium. *J. Mol. Cell. Cardiol.* 9:605–16

7. Meerbaum, S., Corday, E. 1975. Symposium on reperfusion during acute myocardial infarction—Parts 1 and 2. *Am. J. Cardiol.* 36:211–61, 368–406

8. Corday, E., Meerbaum, S. 1983. Symposium on the present status of reperfusion of the acutely ischemic myocardium. Part 1. *J. Am. Coll. Cardiol.* 1:1031–36

9. Oliver, M. 1984. Has the study of infarct size limitation done any good? In *Therapeutic Approaches to Myocardial Infarct Size Limitation*, ed. D. J. Hearse, D. M. Yellon, pp. sciii–vi. New York: Raven

10. Hillis, L. D., Fishbein, M. C., Braunwald, E., Maroko, P. R. 1977. The influence of the time interval between coronary artery occlusion and the administration of hyaluronidase on salvage of ischemic myocaredium in dogs. *Circ. Res.* 41:26–31

11. Libby, P., Maroko, P. R., Bloor, C. M., Sobel, B. E., Braunwald, E. 1973. Reduction of experimental myocardial infarct size by corticosteroid administration. *J. Clin. Invest.* 52:599–607

12. Mullane, K. M., Moncada, S. 1982. The salvage of ischemic myocardium by BW755C in anesthetized dogs. *Prostaglandins* 24:255–66

13. Jolly, S. R., Kane, W. J., Bailie, M. B., Abrams, G. D., Lucchesi, B. R. 1984. Canine myocardial reperfusion injury: its reduction by the combined administration of superoxide dismutase and catalase. *Circ. Res.* 54:277–85

14. Romson, J. L., Hook, B. G., Rigot, V. H., Schork, M. A., Swanson, D. P., Lucchesi, B. R. 1982. The effect of ibuprofen on accumulation of indium-111-labeled platelets and leukocytes in experimental myocardial infarction. *Circulation* 66:1002–11

15. Romson, J. L., Hook, B. G., Kunkel, S. L., Abrams, G. D., Schork, M. A., Lucchesi, B. R. 1983. Reduction of the extent of ischemic myocardial injury by neutrophil depletion in the dog. *Circulation* 67:1016–23

16. Lucchesi, B. R., Romson, J. L., Jolly, S. R. 1984. Do leukocytes influence infarct size? See Ref. 9, pp. 219–48

17. Mullane, K. M., Read, N., Salmon, J. A., Moncada, S. 1984. Role of leuko-

cytes in acute myocardial infarction in anesthetized dogs: relationship to myocardial salvage by anti-inflammatory drugs. *J. Pharmacol. Exp. Ther.* 228: 510–22

18. Mullane, K. M., Moncada, S. 1983. Cytoprotection with prostacylin and dual enzyme inhibitors. In *Mechanism of Drug Action*, ed. T. P. Singer, P. E. Mansour, R. N. Ondarza, pp. 229–42. New York: Academic

19. Bednar, M., Smith, B., Pinto, A., Mullane, K. M. 1985. Nafazatrom-induced salvage of ischemic myocardium in anesthetized dogs is mediated through inhibition of neutrophil function. *Circ. Res.* 57:131–41

20. Mallory, G., White, P., Salcedo-Salger, J. 1939. The speed of healing of myocardial infarction. A study of the pathologic anatomy in seventy-two cases. *Am. Heart J.* 18:647–71

21. Fishbein, M. C., Maclean, D., Maroko, P. R. 1978. Histopathologic evolution of myocardial infarction. *Chest* 73:843–49

22. Weiss, E. S., Ahmed, S. A., Thakur, M. L., Welch, M. J., Coleman, R. E., Sobel, B. E. 1977. Imaging of the inflammatory response in ischemic canine myocardium with ¹¹¹-indium-labeled leukocytes. *Am. J. Cardiol.* 40:195–99

23. Thakur, M. L., Gottschalk, A., Zaret, B. L. 1979. Imaging experimental myocardial infarction with indium-111-labeled autologous leukocytes: effects of infarct age and residual regional myocardial blood flow. *Circulation* 60:297–305

24. Tillmanns, H., Kubler, W. 1984. What happens in the microcirculation? See Ref. 9, pp. 107–24

25. Wedmore, C. V., Williams, T. J., 1981. Control of vascular permeability by polymorphonuclear leukocytes in inflammation. *Nature* 289:646–50

26. Pinckard, R. N., O'Rourke, R. A., Crawford, M. H., Grover, F., McManus, L. M., et al. 1980. Complement localization and mediation of ischemic injury in baboon myocardium. *J. Clin. Invest.* 66:1050–56

27. McManus, L. M., Kolb, W. P., Crawford, M. H., O'Rourke, R. A., Grover, F. L., Pinckard, R. N. 1983. Complement localization in ischemic baboon myocardium. *Lab. Invest.* 48:436–77

28. Coker, S. J., Parratt, J. R., Ledingham, I. McA., Zeitlin, I. J. 1981. Early release of thromboxane and 6-keto-PGF₁ from the ischemic canine myocardium: relation to early post-infarction arrhythmias. *Nature* 291:323–24

29. Sakai, K., Ito, T., Ogowa, K. 1982.

Roles of endogenous protacyclin and thromboxane A₂ in the ischemic canine heart. *J. Cardiovasc. Pharmacol.* 4:129–35

30. Roos, D. 1980. The metabolic response to phagocytosis. In *The Cell Biology of Inflammation*, ed. G. Weissman, pp. 337–87. Elsevier/North Holland: Biomedical.

31. Babior, B. M. 1984. The respiratory burst of phagocytes. *J. Clin. Invest.* 73:599–601

32. Roos, D. J., Hamon-Muller, W. T., Weening, R. J. 1976. Effect of cytochalasin-B on the oxidative metabolism of human peripheral blood granulocytes. *Biochem. Biophys. Res. Commun.* 68: 43–50

33. McPhail, L. C., DeChatelet, L. R., Shirley, P. S. 1976. Further characterization of NADPH oxidase activity of human polymorphonuclear leukocytes. *J. Clin. Invest.* 58:774–80

34. Salin, M. C., McCord, J. M. 1974. Superoxide dismutases in polymorphonuclear leukocytes. *J. Clin. Invest.* 54: 1005–9

35. Ambruso, D. R., Johnston, R. B. 1981. Lactoferrin enhances hydroxyl radical production by human neutrophils, neutrophil particulate fractions and an enzymatic generating system. *J. Clin. Invest.* 67:352–60

36. Klebanoff, S. J. 1968. Myeloperoxidase-halide-hydrogen peroxide antibacterial system. *J. Bacteriol.* 95:2131–38

37. Harrison, J. E., Schultz, J. 1976. Studies on the chlorinating activity of myeloperoxidase. *J. Biol. Chem.* 251:1371–74

38. Fantone, J. C., Ward, P. A. 1982. Role of oxygen-derived free radicals and metabolites in leukocyte-dependent inflammatory reactions. *Am. J. Pathol.* 107:394–418

39. Sachs, T., Moldow, L. F., Craddock, P. R., Bowers, J. K., Jacob, H. S. 1978. Oxygen radical mediated endothelial cell damage by complement stimulated granulocytes: an in vitro model of immune vascular damage. *J. Clin. Invest.* 61: 1161–67

40. Weiss, S. J. 1979. Neutrophil-generated hydroxyl radicals destroy RBC targets. *Clin. Res.* 27:466A (Abstr.)

41. Simon, R. H., Scoggin, C. H., Patterson, D. 1981. Hydrogen peroxide causes the fatal injury to human fibroblasts exposed to oxygen radicals. *J. Biol. Chem.* 256:7181–86

42. Clark, R. A., Klebanoff, S. J. 1979. Myeloperoxidase-mediated-platelet release reaction. *J. Clin. Invest.* 63:177–83

43. Baehner, R. L., Boxer, L. A., Allen, J. M., Davis, J. 1977. Autooxidation as a basis for altered function by polymorphonuclear leukocytes. *Blood* 50:327–35

44. Mead, J. F. 1976. Free radical mechanisms of lipid damage and consequences for cellular membranes. See Ref. 45, pp. 51–68

45. Pryor, W. A. 1976. The role of free radical reactions in biological systems: free radical initiated reactions. In *Free Radicals in Biology,* ed. W. A. Pryor, 1:1–49. New York: Academic

46. Hess, M. L., Okabe, E., Ash, P., Kontos, H. A. 1984. Free radical mediation of the effects of acidosis on calcium transport by cardiac sarcoplasmic reticulum in whole heart hemogenates. *Cardiovasc. Res.* 18:149–57

47. Rowe, G. T., Manson, N. H., Caplan, M., Hess, M. L. 1983. Hydrogen peroxide and hydroxyl radical mediation of activated leukocyte depression of cardiac sarcoplasmic reticulum. Participation of the cyclooxygenase pathway. *Circ. Res.* 53:584–91

48. Scott, J. A., Khaw, B. A., Locke, E., Haber, E., Homey, C. 1985. The role of free radical-mediated processes in oxygen-related damage in cultured murine myocardial cells. *Circ. Res.* 56:72–77

49. Gaudel, Y., Duvelleroy, M. A. 1984. Role of oxygen radicals in cardiac injury due to reoxygenation. *J. Mol. Cell. Cardiol.* 16:459–70

50. Guarnieri, C., Ceroni, C., Muscari, C., Flamigni, F. 1982. Influence of oxygen radicals on heart metabolism. In *Advances in Heart Metabolism,* ed. C. M. Calderara, P. Harris, pp. 423–32. Bologna: CLUEB

51. Rechnagel, R. O. 1967. Carbon retrachloride hepatotoxicity. *Pharmacol. Rev.* 19:145–208

52. Meerson, F. Z., Kagan, V. E., Kozlov, Yu. P., Belkina, L. M., Arkhipenko, Yu. V. 1982. The role of lipid peroxidation in pathogensis of ischemic damage and the antioxidant protection of the heart. *Basic Res. Cardiol.* 77:465–85

53. Rao, P. S., Cohen, M. V., Mueller, H. S. 1983. Production of free radicals and lipid peroxides in early experimental myocardial ischemia. *J. Mol. Cell. Cardiol.* 15:713–16

54. Guarnieri, C., Flamigni, F., Russoni-Calderara, C. 1979. Glutathione peroxidase activity and release of glutathione from oxygen-deficient perfused rat heart. *Biochem. Biophys. Res. Commun.* 89:678–84

55. Guarnieri, C., Flamigni, F., Calderara,

C. M. 1980. Role of oxygen in the cellular damage induced by reoxygenation of hypoxic heart. *J. Mol. Cell. Cardiol.* 12:797–808

56. Rao, P. S., Mueller, H. S. 1983. Lipid peroxidation and acute myocardial ischemia. *Adv. Exp. Med. Biol.* 161:347–64

57. Julicher, R. H. M., Tijburg, L. B. M., Sterrenberg, L., Bast, A., Koomen, J. M., Noordhoek, J. 1984. Decreased defence against free-radicals in rat heart during normal reperfusion after hypoxic, ischemic and calcium-free perfusion. *Life Sci.* 35:1281–88

58. Jackson, C. V., Mickelson, J., Lucchesi, B. R. 1985. Electrolysis and its effects on the myocardial performance of the isolated Langendorff-perfused rabbit heart. *Fed. Proc.* 44:731 (Abstr.)

59. Shlafer, M., Kane, P. F., Kirsh, M. M. 1982. Superoxide dismutase plus catalase enhances the efficacy of hypothermic cardioplegia to protect the globally ischemic, reperfused heart. *J. Thorac. Cardiovasc. Surg.* 83:830–39

60. Shlafer, M., Kane, P. F., Wiggins, V. Y., Kirsh, M. M. 1982. Possible role for cytotoxic oxygen metabolites in the pathogenesis of cardiac ischemic injury. *Circulation* 66(2):I85–92

61. Otani, H., Tanaka, H., Inoue, T., Umemoto, M., Omoto, K., et al. 1984. In vitro study on contribution of oxidative metabolism of isolated rabbit heart mitrochondria to myocardial reperfusion injury. *Circ. Res.* 55:168–75

62. Burton, K. P., McCord, J. M., Ghai, G. 1984. Myocardial alteration due to free-radical generation. *Am. J. Physiol.* 246:H776–83

63. Stewart, J. R., Blackwell, W. H., Crute, S. L., Loughlin, V., Hess, M. L., Greenfield, L. J. 1982. Prevention of myocardial ischemia/reperfusion injury with oxygen free-radical scavengers. *Surg. Forum* 33:317–20

64. Shlafer, M., Kane, P. F., Kirsh, M. M. 1982. Effect of dimethyl sulfoxide on the globally ischemic heart: Possible relevance to hypothermic organ preservation. *Cryobiology* 19:61–69

65. Ganok, C. E., Simms, M., Safavi, S. 1982. Effects of dimethylsulfoxide (DMSO) on the oxygen paradox in perfused rat hearts. *Am. J. Pathol.* 109:270–76

66. Chambers, D. E., Parks, D. A., Patterson, G., Roy, R., McCord, J. M., et al. 1985. Xanthine oxidase as a source of free-radical damage in myocardial ischemia. *J. Mol. Cell. Cardiol.* 17:145–52

67. Nakamwa, Y., Takahashi, M., Hayashi,

J., Mori, H., Ogawa, S., et al. 1982. Protection of ischemic myocardium with coenxyme Q_{10}. *Cardiovasc. Res.* 16: 132–37

68. Hess, M. L., Okabe, E., Poland, J., Warner, M., Stewart, J. R., Greenfield, J. 1983. Glucose, insulin, potassium protection during the course of hypothermic global ischemia and reperfusion: A new proposed mechanism by the scavenging of free-radicals. *J. Cardiovasc. Pharm.* 5:35–43

69. Caldarera, C. M., Davalli, P., Guarnieri, C. 1978. Effect of α-tocopherol and sodium selenite on post-anoxic reoxygenated rat hearts. *J. Mol. Cell. Cardiol.* 10 (Suppl 1):16 (Abstr.)

70. Guarnieri, C., Ferrari, R., Visiolo, O., Caldarera, C. M., Naylor, W. G. 1978. Effect of tocopherol on hypoxic perfused and re-oxygenated rabbit heart muscle. *J. Mol. Cell. Cardiol.* 10:893–906

71. Lefer, A. M., Araki, H., Okamatsu, S. 1981. Beneficial actions of a free-radical scavenger in traumatic shock and myocardial ischemia. *Circ. Shock* 8:273–82

72. Lucas, S. K., Gardner, T. J., Flaherty, J. T., Bulkley, B. H., Elmer, E. B., Gott, V. L. 1980. Beneficial effects of mannitol administration during reperfusion after ischemic arrest. *Circulation* 62 (Suppl. 1):34–41

73. Dormandy, T. L. 1983. An approach to free-radicals. *Lancet* 2:1010–14

74. McCord, J. M. 1985. Oxygen-derived free-radicals in postischemic tissue injury. *N. Engl. J. Med.* 312:159–63

75. Jennings, R. B., Hawkins, H. K., Lowe, J. E., Hill, M. L., Klotman, S., Reimer, K. A. 1978. Relation between high energy phosphate and lethal injury in myocardial ischemia in the dog. *Am. J. Pathol.* 92:187–214

76. Jennings, R. B., Reimer, K. A. 1981. Lethal myocardial ischemic injury. *Am. J. Pathol.* 102:241–55

77. Hess, M. L., Manson, N. H. 1984. Molecular oxygen: friend and foe. The role of the oxygen free-radical system in the calcium paradox, the oxygen paradox and ischemia/reperfusion injury. *J. Mol. Cell. Cardiol.* 16:969–85

78. Chien, K. R., Reeves, J. P., Buja, L. M., Bonte, R., Parkey, R. W., Willerson, J. T. 1981. Phospholipid alterations in canine ischemic myocardium. Temporal and topographical correlations with Tc-99-PPi accumulation and an in vitro sarcolemmal Ca^{++} permeability defect. *Circ. Res.* 48:711–19

79. Chien, K. R., Han, A., Sen, A., Buja, L.

M., Willerson, J. T. 1984. Accumulation of unesterified arachidonic acid in ischemic canine myocardium. Relationship to a phophatidylcholine deacylation-reacylation cycle and the depletion of membrance phopholipids. *Circ. Res.* 54:313–22

80. Lanni, C., Becker, E. L. 1983. Release of phospholipase A_2 activity from rabbit peritoneal neutrophils by F-Met-Leu-Phe. *Am. J. Pathol.* 113:90–94

81. Mullane, K. M., Flower, R. J. 1980. The interaction of anti-inflammatory drugs with arachidonic acid metabolism. *Mater. Med. Pol.* 3:195–206

82. Gross, R. W., Sobel, B. E. 1982. Lysophophatidyl choline metabolism in the rabbit heart. *J. Biol. Chem.* 257: 6702–8

83. Chien, K. R., Han, A., Bush, L. R., Buja, L. M., Willerson, J. T. 1983. Accumulation of unesterfied arachidonate in ischemic canine myocardium: evidence of defective reacylasion of membrane phopholipids. *Clin. Res.* 31:485A (Abstr.)

84. Sobel, B. E., Corr, P. B., Robison, A. K., Goldstein, R. A., Witkowski, F. X., Klein, M. S. 1978. Accumulation of lysophosphoglycerides with arrhythmogenic properties in ischemic myocardium. *J. Clin. Invest.* 62:546–53

85. Snyder, D. W., Crafford, W. A. Jr., Glaskow, J. L., Rankin, D., Sobel, B. E., Corr, P. B. 1981. Lysophosphoglycerides in ischemic myocardial effluents and potentiation of their arrhythmogenic effects. *Am. J. Physiol.* 241:H700–7

86. Shakh, N. A., Downar, E. 1981. Time course of changes in porcine myocardial phospholipid levels during ischemia. A reassessment of the lysolipid hypothesis. *Circ. Res.* 49:316–25

87. Corr, P. B., Cain, M. E., Witkowski, F. X., Price, D. A., Sobel, B. E. 1979. Potential arrhythmogenic electrophysiological derangements in canine Parkinje fibers induced by lysophosphoglyorides. *Circ. Res.* 44:822–32

88. Corr, P. B., Sobel, B. E. 1983. Arrhythmogenic properties of phospholipid metabolites associated with myocardial ischemia. *Fed. Proc.* 42:2454–59

89. Sugiura, T., Oruna, Y., Sekiguchi, M., Waku, K. 1982. Ether phospholipids in guinea pig polymorphonuclear leukocytes and macrophages. Occurrence of high levels of 1-O-alkyl-2-aryl-sn-glycero-3-phosphocholine. *Biochim. Biophys. Acta* 712:515–22

90. Benveniste, J., Jouvin, E., Pirotzky, E.,

Arnoux, B., Mencia-Huerta, J. M., et al. 1981. Platelet-activating factor (PAF-acether): Molecular aspects of its release and pharmacological actions. *Int. Arch. Allergy Appl. Immunol.* 66 (Suppl. 1): 121–26

91. O'Flaherty, J. T., Wykle, R. L., Miller, C. H., Lewis, J. C., Waite, M., et al. 1981. 1-O-alkyl-sn-glyceryl-3-phosphorylcholines: a novel class of neutrophil stimulants. *Am. J. Pathol.* 103:70–79

92. Levi, R., Burke, J. A., Guo, Z-G., Hattori, Y., Hoppens, C. M., et al. 1984. Acetyl glyceryl ether phosphorylcholine (AGEPC). A putative mediator of cardiac anaphylaxis in the guinea pig. *Circ. Res.* 54:117–24

93. Kenzora, J. L., Perez, J. E., Bergmann, S. R., Lange, L. G. 1984. Effects of acetyl glyceryl ether of phosphorylcholine (platelet activating factor) on ventricular preload, afterload and contractility in dogs. *J. Clin. Invest.* 74:1193–1203

94. Lepran, I., Lefer, A. M. 1985. Ischemic aggravating effects of platelet-activating factor in acute myocardial ischemia. *Basic Res. Cardiol.* 80:135–41

95. Annable, C. R., McManus, L. M., Carey, K. D., Pinckard, R. N. 1985. Isolation of platelet-activating factor (PAF) from ischemic baboon myocardium. *Fed. Proc.* 44:1271 (Abstr.)

96. Curnutte, J. T. 1985. Activation of human neutrophil nicotinamide adenine dinucleotide phosphate, reduced (triphosphopyridine nucleotide, reduced) oxidase by arachidonic acid in a cell-free system. *J. Clin. Invest.* 75:1740–43

97. Borgeat, P., Samuelsson, B. 1979. Transformation of arachidonic acid by rabbit polymorphonuclear leukocytes. *J. Biol. Chem.* 254:2643–46

98. Borgeat, P., Samuelsson, B. 1979. Arachidonic acid metabolism in polymorphonuclear leukocytes: effects of ionophore A23187. *Proc. Natl. Acad. Sci. USA* 76:2148–52

99. Palmer, R. M. J., Stepney, R. J., Higgs, G. A., Eakins, K. E. 1980. Cheomkinetic activity of arachidonic acid lipoxygenase products on leukocytes of different species. *Prostaglandins* 20:411–18

100. Linbom, L., Hedqvist, P., Dahler, S-E., Lindgren, J. A., Arfors, K. E. 1982. Leukotriene B$_4$ induces extravasation and migration of polymorphonuclear leukocytes in vivo. *Acta Physiol. Scand.* 116: 105–8

101. Gimbrone, M. A., Brock, A. F., Schafer, A. I. 1984. Leukotriene B$_4$ stimulates

polymorphonuclear leukocyte adhesion to cultered vascular endothelial cells. *J. Clin. Invest.* 74:1552–55

102. Serhan, C. N., Radin, A., Smolen, J. E., Korchak, H., Samuelsson, B., Weissmann, G. 1982. Leukotrieve B$_4$ is a complete secretagogue in human neutrophils: a kinetic analysis. *Biochem. Biophys. Res. Commun.* 107:1006–12

103. Burke, J. A., Levi, R., Guo, Z-G., Corey, E. J. 1982. Leukotrienes C$_4$, D$_4$ and E$_4$: effects on human and guinea-pig cardiac preparations in vitro. *J. Pharmacol. Exp. Ther.* 221:235–41

104. Michelassi, F., Landa, L., Hill, R. D., Lowenstein, E., Watkins, W. D., et al. 1982. Leukotriene D$_4$: a potent coronary artery vasocontractor associated with impaired ventricular contraction. *Science* 217:841–43

105. Ezra, D., Boyd, L. M., Feuerstein, G., and Goldstein, R. E. 1983. Coronary constriction by leukotriene C$_4$, D$_4$ and E$_4$ in the intact pig heart. *Am. J. Cardiol.* 51:1451–54

106. Panzenbeck, M. J., Kaley, G. 1983. Leukotriene D$_4$ reduces coronary blood flow in the anesthetized dog. *Prostaglandins* 25:661–70

107. Narumiya, S., Salmon, J. A., Cottee, F. H., Weatherly, B. C., Flower, R. J. 1981. Arachidonic acid 15-lipoxygenase from rabbit peritoneal polymorphonuclear leukocytes. Partial purification and properties. *J. Biol. Chem.* 256:9583–92

108. Bednar, M. M., Schwartzman, M., Ibraham, N. G., McGiff, J. C., Mullane, K. M. 1984. Conversion of arachidonic acid to two novel products by cytochrome P450-dependent mixed-function oxidase in polymorphonuclear leukocytes. *Biochem. Biophys. Res. Commun.* 123:581–88

109. Stenson, W. F., Parker, C. W. 1979. Metabolism of arachidonic acid in ionophore-stimulated neutrophils. Esterification of a hydroxylated metabolite into phospholipids. *J. Clin. Invest.* 64:1457–65

110. Perez, H. D., Weksler, B. B., Goldstein, I. M. 1980. Generation of a chemostatic lipid from arachidonic acid by exposure to a superoxide-generating system. *Inflammation* 4:313–27

111. Gerritsen, M. E., Printz, M. P. 1981. Sites of prostaglandin synthesis in the bovine heart and isolated bovine coronary microvessels. *Circ. Res.* 49:1152–63

112. Dusting, G. J., Nolan, R. D., Woodman, O. L., Martin, T. J. 1983. Prostacyclin produced by the pericardium and its in-

fluence on coronary vascular tone. *Am. J. Cardiol.* 52:28A–35A

113. Wildenthal, K. 1975. Lysosomes and lysosomal enzymes in the heart. In *Lysosomes in Biology and Pathology*, ed. J. T. Dingle, R. T. Dean, 4:167–90. North Holland: Amsterdam

114. Wildenthal, K. 1978. Lysosomal alterations in ischemic myocardium: Result or cause of myocellular damage? *J. Mol. Cell. Cardiol.* 10:595–603

115. Decker, R. S., Wildenthal, K. 1978. Sequential lysosomal alterations during cardiac ischemia. 2. Ultrastructural and cytochemical changes. *Lab. Invest.* 38: 663–73

116. Weissmann, G. 1982. Activation of neutrophils and the lesions of rheumatoid arthritis. *J. Lab. Clin. Med.* 100:322–32

117. Ogletree, M. L., Lefer, A. M. 1978. Prostaglandin-induced preservation of the ischemic myocardium. *Circ. Res.* 42:218–24

118. Smith, E. F. III, Lefer, A. M. 1981. Stabilization of cardiac lysosomal and cellular membranes in protection of ischemia myocardium due to coronary occlusion: Efficacy of the monsteroidal anti-inflammatory agent, naproxen. *Am. Heart J.* 101:394–402

119. Lefer, A. M., Crossley, K. 1980. Mechanism of the optimal protective effects of ibuprofen in acute myocardial ischemia. *Adv. Shock Res.* 3:133–42

120. Jugdutt, B. I., Hutchins, G. M., Bulkley, B. H., Becker, L. C. 1981. Dissimilar effects of prostacyclin, prostaglandin E_1, and prostaglandin E_2 on myocardial infarct size after coronary occlusion in conscious dogs. *Circ. Res.* 49:685–700

121. Ribeiro, L. G. T., Brandon, T. A., Hopkins, D. G., Reduto, L. A., Taylor, A. A., Miller, R. R. 1981. Prostacyclin in experimental myocardial blood flow, infarct size and mortality. *Am. J. Cardiol.* 47:835–40

122. Romson, J. L., Bush, L. R., Haack, D. W., Lucchesi, B. R. 1980. The beneficial effects of oral ibuprofen on coronary artery thrombosis and myocardial ischemia in the conscious dog. *J. Pharmacol. Exp. Ther.* 215:271–78

123. Jugdutt, B. I., Hutchins, G. M., Bulkley, B. H., Becker, L. C. 1980. Salvage of ischemic myocardium by ibuprofen during infarction in the conscious dog. *Am. J. Cardiol.* 46:74–82

124. Romson, J. L., Bush, L. R., Jolly, S. R., Lucchesi, B. R. 1982. Cardioprotective effects of ibuprofen in experimental regional and global myocardial ischemia. *J. Cardiovasc. Pharm.* 4:187–96

125. Bolli, R., Goldstein, R. E., Davenport, N., Epstein, S. E. 1981. Influence of sulfinpyrazone and naproxen on infarct size in the dog. *Am. J. Cardiol.* 47:841–47

126. Bolli, R., Davenport, N. J., Goldstein, R. E., Epstein, S. E. 1983. Myocardiala proteolysis during acute myocardial ischemia. *Cardiovasc. Res.* 17:274–81

127. Cannon, R. O., Butany, J. W., McManus, B. M., Speir, E., Kravitz, A. B., et al. 1983. Early degradation of collagen after acute myocardial infarction in the rate. *Am. J. Cardiol.* 52:390–95

128. Bolli, R., Cannon, R. O., Speir, E., Goldstein, R. E., Epstein, S. E. 1983. Role of cellular proteinases in acute myocardial infarction. I. Proteolysis in nonischemic and ischemic rat mayocardium and the effects of antipain, leupeptin, pepstatin and cheymostatin adminstered in vivo. *J. Am. Coll. Cardiol.* 2:671–80

129. Bolli, R., Cannon, R. O., Speir, E., Goldstein, R. E., Epstein, S. E. 1983. Role of cellular proteinases in acute myocardial infarction. 2. Influence of in vivo suppression of myocardial proteolysis by antipain, leupeptin and pepstatin on myocardial infarct size in the rat. *J. Am. Coll. Cardiol.* 2:681–88

130. Hill, J. H., Ward, P. A. 1971. The phlogistic role of C3 leukotactic fragments in myocardial infarcts of rats. *J. Exp. Med.* 133:885–900

131. Giclas, P. C., Pinckard, R. N., Olson, M. S. 1979. In vitro activation of complement by isolated human heart subcellular membranes. *J. Immunol.* 122: 146–51

132. Pinckard, R. N., Olson, M. S., Giclas, P. C., Terry, R., Boyer, J. T., O'Rourke, R. A. 1975. Consumption of classical complement components by heart subcellular membranes in vitro and in patients after acute myocardial infarction. *J. Clin. Invest.* 56:740–50

133. Goldstein, I., Hoffstein, S., Gallin, J., Weissmann, G. 1973. Mechanism of lysosomal enzyme release from human leukocytes: microtubule assembly and membrane fusion induced by a component of complement. *Proc. Natl. Acad. Sci. USA* 70:2916–20

134. Estensen, R. D., White, J. G., Holmes, B. 1974. Specific degranulation of human polymorphonuclear leukocytes. *Nature* 248:347–48

135. Goldstein, I. M., Roos, D., Kaplan, H. B., Weissmann, G. 1975. Complement and immunoglobulins stimulate superoxide production by human leukocytes in-

dependently of phagocytosis. *J. Clin. Invest.* 56:1155–63

136. Mullane, K. E., Kraemer, R., Smith, B. 1985. Myeloperoxidase activity as a quantitative assessment of neutrophil infiltration into ischemic myocardium. *J. Pharmacol. Methods* 14:157–67

137. Hugli, T. E. 1983. The chemistry and biology of C3a, C4a and C5a and their effects on cells. In *Biological Response, Mediators and Modulators*, ed. T. J. August, pp. 99–116. New York: Academic

138. Hachfeld Del Balzo, U., Levi, R., Polley, M. J. 1985. Cardiac dysfunction caused by purified human C3a anaphylatoxin. *Proc. Natl. Acad. Sci. USA* 82:886–90

139. Tainer, J. A., Turner, S. R., Lynn, W. S. 1975. New aspects of chemotaxis: Specific target cell attraction by lipid and lipoprotein fractions of *Escherichia coli* chemotactic factor. *Am. J. Pathol.* 81:401–10

140. Bonow, R. O., Lipson, L. C., Sheehan, F. H., Capurro, N. L., Isner, J. M., et al. 1981. Lack of effect of aspirin on myocardial infarct size in the dog. *Am. J. Cardiol.* 47:258–64

141. Ogletree, M. L., Lefer, A. M. 1976. Influence of nonsteroidal anti-inflammatory agents on myocardial ischemia in the cat. *J. Pharmacol. Exp. Ther.* 197:582–93

142. Hook, B. G., Romson, J. L., Jolly, S. R., Bailie, M. B., Lucchesi, B. R. 1982. Effect of zomepirac on experimental coronary artery thrombosis and ischemic myocardial injury in the conscious dog. *J. Cardiovasc. Pharm.* 5:302–8

143. Jugdutt, B. I., Hutchins, G. M., Bulkley, B. H., Pitt, B., Becker, L. C. 1979. Effect of indomethacin on collateral blood flow and infarct size in the conscious dog. *Circulation* 59:734–43

144. Chambers, D. E., Yellow, D. M., Hearse, D. J., Downey, J. M. 1983. Effects of flubiprofen in altering the size of myocardial infarcts in dogs: reduction or delay? *Am. J. Cardiol.* 51:884–90

145. Hartmann, J. R., Robinson, J. A., Gunnar, R. M. 1977. Chemotactic activity in the coronary sinus after experimental myocardial infarction: effects of pharmacologic interventions on ischemic injury. *Am. J. Cardiol.* 40:550–55

146. Vogel, W. M., Zannoni, V. G., Abrams, G. D., Lucchesi, B. R. 1977. Inability of methylprednisolone sodium succidnate to decrease infarct size or preserve enzyme activity measured 24 hours after coronary occlusion in the dog. *Circulation* 55:588–95

147. Jolly, S. R., Lucchesi, B. R. 1983. Effect of BW755C in an occlusion-reperfusion model of ischemic myocardial injury. *Am. Heart J.* 106:8–13

148. Moncada, S., Vane, J. R. 1979. Mode of action aspirin-like drugs. *Adv. Intern. Med.* 24:1–22

149. Higgs, G. A., Eakins, K. E., Mugridge, K. G., Moncada, S., Vane, J. R. 1980. The effects of non-steroid anti-inflammatory drugs on leukocyte migration in carrageenin-induced inflammation. *Eur. J. Pharmacol.* 66:81–86

150. Higgs, G. A., Palmer, R. M. J., Eakins, K. E., Moncada, S. 1981. Arachidonic acid metabolism as a source of inflammatory mediators and its inhibition as a mechanism of action for anti-inflammatory drugs. *Mol. Aspects Med.* 4:275–301

151. Salmon, J. A., Simmons, P. M., Moncada, S. 1983. The effects of BW755c and other anti-inflammatory drugs on eicosanoid concentrations and leukocyte accumulation in experimentally-induced acute inflamation. *J. Pharm. Pharmacol.* 35:808–13

152. Higgs, G. A., Flower, R. J., Vane, J. R. 1979. A new approach to anti-inflammatory drugs. *Biochem. Pharmacol.* 28:1959–61

153. Carter, G. W., Dyer, R., Young, P. 1985. Dipyridamole: a potent and specific 5-lipooxygenase inhibitor. *Fed. Proc.* 44:904 (Abstr.)

154. Shea, M. J., Murtagh, J. J., Jolly, S. R., Abrams, G. D., Pitt, B., Lucchesi, B. R. 1984. Beneficial effects of nafazatrom on ischemic reperfused myocardium. *Eur. J. Pharmacol.* 102:63–70

155. Fiedler, V. B. 1984. Reduction of acute myocardial ischemia in rabbit hearts by nafazatrom. *J. Cardiovasc. Pharm.* 6:318–24

156. Blumenthal, D. S., Hutchins, G. M., Jugdutt, B. I., Becker, L. C. 1981. Salvage of ischemic myocardium by dipyridamole in the conscious dog. *Circulation* 64:915–23

157. Flynn, P. J., Becker, W. K., Vercellotti, G. M., Weisdorf, D. J., Craddock, P. R., et al. 1984. Ibuprofen inhibits granulocyte responses to inflammatory mediators. A proposed mechanism for reduction of experimental myocardial infarct size. *Inflammation* 8:33–44

158. Maroko, P. R., Carpenter, C. B., Chiariello, M., Fishbein, M. C., Radvany, P., et al. 1978. Reduction by cobra venom factor of myocardial necrosis after coronary artery occlusion. *J. Clin. Invest.* 61:661–70

159. Diaz, P. E., Fishbein, M. C., Davis, M. A., Askenazi, J., Maroko, P. R. 1977. Effect of the kallikrein inhibitor aprotinin on myocardial ischemic injury after coronary occlusion in the dog. *Am. J. Cardiol.* 40:541–49

160. Hallett, M. B., Shandall, A., Young, H. L. 1985. Mechanism of protection against "reperfusion injury" by aprotinin. Roles of polymorphonuclear leukocytes and oxygen radicals. *Biochem. Pharmacol.* 34:1757–61

161. Dyerberg, J., Bang, H. O., Moncada, S., Vane, J. R. 1978. Eicosapentaenoic acid and prevention of thrombosis and atherosclerosis? *Lancet* 1:117–19

162. Editorial. 1983. *Eskimo Diet Diseases* 1:1139

163. Dyerberg, J., Bang, H. O. 1979. Haemostatic function and platelet polyunsaturated fatty acids in Eskimos. *Lancet* 2:433–35

164. Dyerberg, J., Bang, H. O., Hjorne, N. 1975. Fatty-acid composition of plasmalipids in Greenland Eskimos. *Am. J. Clin. Nutr.* 28:958–66

165. Culp, B. R., Lands, W. E. M., Lucchesi, B. R., Pitt, B., Romson, J. 1980. The effect of dietary supplementation of fish oil on experimental myocardial infarction. *Prostaglandins* 20:1021–31

166. Terano, T., Salmon, J. A., Moncada, S. 1984. Effect of orally administered eicosapentaenoic acid (EPA) on the formation of leukotriene B_4 and leukotrieve B_5 by rat leukocytes. *Biochem. Pharmacol.* 33:3071–76

167. Lee, T. H., Hoover, R. L., Williams, J. D., Sperling, R. I., Ravalese J. III, et al. 1985. Effect of dietary enrichment with eicosapentaenoic and decosahexaenoic acid on in vitro neutrophil and monocyte leukotriene generation and neutrophil function. *N. Engl. J. Med.* 312:1217–24

168. Terano, T., Salmon, J. A., Moncada, S. 1984. Biosynthesis and biological activity of leukotriene B_5. *Prostaglandins* 27:217–32

169. Kirlin, P. C., Romson, J. L., Pitt, B., Abrams, G. D., Schork, M. A., Lucchesi, B. R. 1982. Ibuprofen-mediated infarct size reduction: effects on regional myocardial function in canine myocardial infarction. *Am. J. Cardiol.* 50:849–56

170. MacLean, D., Fishbein, M. C., Braunwald, E., Maroko, P. R. 1978. Long-term preservation of ischemic myocardium after experimental coronary artery occlusion. *J. Clin. Invest.* 61:541–51

171. McCluskey, E. R., Murphree, S., Saffitz, J. E., Morrison, A. R., Needleman,

P. 1985. Temporal changes in 12-HETE formation in two models of canine myocardial infarction. *Prostaglandins* 29:387–403

172. Ksiezycka, E., Hastie, R., Maroko, P. R. 1983. Reduction in myocardial damage after experimental coronary artery occlusion by two techniques which deplete neutrophils. *Circulation* 68:185 (Abstr.)

173. Jacob, H. S. 1983. Neutrophil activation as a mechanism of tissue injury. *Semin. Arthritis Rheum.* 13 (Suppl. 1):144–47

174. Jacob, H. S., Craddock, P. R., Hammerschmidt, D. E., Moldow, C. F. 1980. Complement-induced granulocyte aggregation. An unsuspected mechanism of disease. *N. Engl. J. Med.* 302:789–94

175. Engler, R., Schmid-Schonbein, G. W., Pavelec, R. S. 1983. Leukcoyte capillary plugging in myocardial ischemia and reperfusion in the dog. *Am. J. Pathol.* 111:98–111

176. Nellis, S. H., Roberts, B. H., Kinney, E. L., Field, J., Ummat, A., Zelis, R. 1980. Beneficial effect of dexamethasone on the "no reflow" phenomenon in canine myocardium. *Cardiovasc. Res.* 14:137–41

177. Engler, R., Dahlgren, M., Schmid-Schoenbein, G., Dobbs, A. 1984. Leukocyte depletion prevents progressive flow impairment to ischemic myocardium. *Circulation* 70 (Suppl. II):228 (Abstr.)

178. Karsner, H. T., Dwyer, J. E. 1916. Studies in infarction. 6. Experimental infarction of the myocardium, myocardial regeneration and cicatrization. *J. Med. Res.* 29:21–40

179. Kloner, J. A., Fishbein, M. C., Lew, H., Maroko, P. R., Braunwald, E. 1978. Mummification of the infarcted myocardium by high dose corticosteroids. *Circulation* 57:56–63

180. Hutchins, G. M., Bulkley, B. H. 1978. Infarct expansion versus extension: two different complications of acute myocardial infarction. *Am. J. Cardiol.* 41:1127–32

181. Schuster, E. H., Bulkley, B. H. 1979. Expansion of transmural myocardial infarction: a pathophysiologic factor in cardiac rupture. *Circulation* 60:1532–38

182. Bolli, R. 1982. Protection of ischemic myocardium in experimental animals and in man: a review. *Cardiovasc. Res. Cent. Bull.* 21:1–33

183. Bulkley, B. H., Roberts, W. C. 1974. Steroid therapy during acute myocardial infarction. A cause of delayed healing of

ventricular aneurysm. *Am. J. Med.* 56: 244–50

184. Roberts, R., Demello, V., Sobel, B. E. 1976. Deleterious effects of methyprednisolone in patients with myocardial infarction. *Circulation* 53 (Suppl. 1):I204–7

185. Brown, E. J. Jr., Kloner, R. A., Schoen, F. J., Hammerman, H., Hale, S., Braunwald, E. 1983. Scar thinning due to ibuprofen administration after experimental myocardial infarction. *Am. J. Cardiol.* 51:877–83

186. Hammerman, H., Kloner, R. A., Schoen, F. J., Brown, E. J. Jr., Hale, S., Braunwald, E. 1983. Indomethacin-induced scar thinning after experimental myocardial infarction. *Circulation* 67: 1290–95

187. Roberts, Ch. S., MacLean, D., Maroko, P., Kloner, R. A. 1985. Relation of early mononuclear and polymorphonuclear cell infiltration to late scar thickness after experimentally induced myocardial infarction in the rat. *Basic Res. Cardiol.* 80:202–9

188. Sobel, B., Bresnahan, G., Shell, W., Yoder, R. 1972. Estimation of infarct size in man and its relation to prognosis. *Circulation* 46:640–48

189. Braunwald, E. 1985. The aggressive treatment of acute myocardial infarction. *Circulation* 71:1087–92

190. Khaja, F., Walton, J. A. Jr., Brymer, J. F., Lo, E., Osterberger, L., et al. 1983. Intracoronary fibrinolytic therapy in acute myocardial infarction. *N. Engl. J. Med.* 308:1305–11

191. Kennedy, J. W., Ritchie, J. L., Davis, K. B., Fritz, J. K. 1983. Western Washington randomized trial of intracoronary streptokinase in acute myocardial infarction. *N. Engl. J. Med.* 309:1477–82

192. Sheehan, F. H., Mathey, D. G., Schofer, J., Dodge, H. T., Bolson, E. L. 1985. Factors that determine recovery of left ventricular function after thrombolysis in patients with acute myocardial infarction. *Circulation* 71:1121–28

193. Friedman, G. D., Klatsky, A. L., Siegelaub, A. B. 1974. The leukocyte count as a predictor of myocardial infarction. *New Engl. J. Med.* 290:1275–78

194. Zalokar, J. B., Richard, J. L., Claude, J. R. 1981. Leukocyte count, smoking, and myocardial infarction. *New Engl. J. Med.* 304:465–68

195. Kostis, J. B., Turkevich, D., Sharp, J. 1984. Association between leukocyte count and the presence and extent of coronary atherosclerosis as determined by coronary arteriography. *Am. J. Cardiol.* 53:997–99

196. Shoenfeld, Y., Pinkhas, J., Beilinson Medical Center. 1981. Leukopenia and low incidence of myocardial infarction. *New Engl. J. Med.* 304:1606

197. Kew, R. R., Ghebrehiwet, B., Janoff, A. 1985. Cigarette smoke can activate the alterative pathway of complement in vitro by modifying the third component of complement. *J. Clin. Invest.* 75:1000–7

198. Kohchi, K., Takebayashi, S., Hiroki, T., Nobuyoshi, M. 1985. Significance of adventitial inflammation of the coronary artery in patients with unstable angina: results at autopsy. *Circulation* 71:709–16

Ann. Rev. Pharmacol. Toxicol. 1986. 26:225–58

PHARMACOLOGY OF CALCIUM CHANNELS AND SMOOTH MUSCLE

Leon Hurwitz

Department of Pharmacology, School of Medicine, University of New Mexico, Albuquerque, New Mexico 87131

INTRODUCTION

A number of diverse cellular functions (contraction, secretion, etc.) are known to be regulated by fluctuations in the free calcium ion concentration in the cytosol (1). One important source of these divalent ions is the calcium reservoir in the extracellular fluid (1). Calcium ions can be mobilized from this external pool by the operation of calcium channels that are anchored in the plasma membrane (1). The obvious involvement of these membrane-bound ion channels in the regulation of essential cellular functions has generated considerable interest in and exploration of their functional characteristics. This article deals with three aspects of the operation of calcium channels. The first section contains a qualitative description of the functional properties of different types of calcium channels. This is followed by an overview of the manner in which pharmacological agents may modify the functional behavior of calcium channels. Lastly, a discussion of the various types of calcium channels that appear to exist in smooth muscle cells is presented.

FUNCTIONAL CHARACTERISTICS OF CALCIUM CHANNELS

Ion Permeation

A calcium channel residing in the membrane of a eukaryotic cell is viewed as being a macromolecular structure consisting essentially of one or more glycoproteins (2, 3, 4). Its configuration is presumed to be roughly cylindrical with an aqueous pore at its center (2, 3). The permeation of extracellular calcium ions through the pore into the cytosol is accomplished via several discrete steps.

225

The initial step consists of a reversible interaction between the divalent ion and a calcium binding site (calcium coordination site) that is thought to be located at or near the surface of the channel (5–8). Alternatively, the initial reaction may be viewed as the passage of the divalent ion over some energy barrier requiring some level of free energy of activation, followed by the descent of the ion into an energy well that is reflected by a net loss of free energy (8, 9). The occupation by the cation of a relatively deep energy well would be analogous to the cation exhibiting a relatively high affinity for the channel coordination site and vice versa.

Because the movement of a cation through the aqueous pore of a calcium channel must be preceded by a reversible interaction with a channel binding site, several dynamic aspects of ion permeation simulate those observed in enzymatic reactions that obey Michaelis-Menten kinetics (5, 6, 7). Thus, the interaction between some particular cation and the channel binding site may be characterized by an apparent dissociation constant that remains invariable as long as other conditions (i.e. membrane potential, temperature, etc.) are not modified. Furthermore, the relationship between the rate of cation permeation through a population of calcium channels and the extracellular cation concentration defines a simple, hyperbolic saturation curve. These functional properties of the calcium channel were first described by Hagiwara and Takahashi (7) who utilized the maximum slope of the action potential as a measure of the maximum current flowing through the calcium channels of barnacle muscle. Beirao and Lakshminarayanaiah (10) obtained similar results with voltage clamp measurements in barnacle muscle.

Based on the manner in which inorganic cations and calcium channels interact, one element of the driving force that energizes the inward movement of permeant cations is the level of saturation of the binding sites in or on the calcium channels. The second element is the interaction between the electric field within the membrane and the charged ion moving across the membrane. Because intracellular concentrations of calcium ions are generally very low, outwardly directed driving forces are correspondingly low. Within the aqueous pore of the calcium channel the driving force acting to propel the permeant cation inward will be countered by steric configurations and reactive groups or, in other terms, by energy barriers that act to impede the flow of ions through the channel. It appears that one of these barriers may be sufficiently high and uniquely structured to permit some types of cations to pass through, but halt any further forward movement of others. Such a barrier has the capacity to confer a selective action on the channel, and thereby restrict the types of ion species that will be permitted to traverse the cell membrane via this pathway. In view of its functional role in the channel, this barrier has been labeled the selectivity filter (3, 9, 11). In addition to establishing the ion specificity of the channel, the selectivity filter, as well as other energy barriers, serve to regulate the speed at which a permeant cation will move through the aqueous pore of the channel (9, 11). Some cations such as Ca, Ba and Sr penetrate the calcium channel relatively rapidly (5, 6). Others such as Zn, Mn and Cd move through the channel at a much slower speed (5, 6). This rate process will determine the maximum possible electrical current that a particular ion species can generate by moving through a population of calcium channels under a given set of conditions.

When the relationship between current flow and the extracellular ion concentration produces a simple, hyperbolic saturation curve, there is implicit in these dynamics the concept that only one ion may interact with and move through the channel in any given instant. This concept has been challenged by Hess and Tsien (12) who studied calcium channels in single ventricular cells obtained from the hearts of guinea pigs. These workers found that the inhibition of barium currents by calcium ion and the inhibition of sodium currents by calcium ion resulted, in each case, in a very different estimated dissociation constant for the calcium ion-channel binding site complex. Their results, therefore, are inconsistent with the notion that calcium competes with these other cations for a single channel binding site. In addition, they measured the total current produced by mixtures of calcium and barium ions placed in the extracellular medium. The two divalent ions were mixed in various proportions, although their total concentration was held constant at 10 mM. Under these conditions, the total current passing through a population of single ion channels (i.e. channels in which only one ion is present within the pore at any given time) would be expected to be higher than the current produced by the presence of 10 mM of the slower moving cation alone. Hess and Tsien found, instead, that the measured current reached a minimum level when the cation mixture was 70% barium ion and 30% calcium ion.

In order to account for the experimental data they obtained, these investigators envisioned the operation of a single file calcium channel that possesses a sequence of three energy barriers within its aqueous pore. Moreover, the three energy barriers are separated by two distinct energy wells (or two binding sites). Such a channel may contain a single cation that occupies either one of its two energy wells or it may contain two cations simultaneously that occupy both energy wells. When both energy wells are occupied, there is a significant repulsive force between the two cations that facilitates the evacuation of a cation from one or the other of the two energy wells into the surrounding medium (i.e. evacuation into the extracellular medium from one energy well and into the cytosol from the other). The experimental data obtained also dictate that this channel must interact with calcium ions somewhat differently than it does with barium ions. Two differences were built into the hypothetical model of the calcium channel. First, the two energy wells that may be occupied by calcium ions were considered to be deeper than those occupied by barium ions (i.e. calcium ions have a relatively greater affinity for the two binding sites than do barium ions). Second, the rate of movement of calcium ions through the channel was considered to be lower than that of barium ions (i.e. calcium ions must traverse a higher energy barrier [selectivity filter] during their passage through the channel).

Given these structural and functional properties of the calcium channel, one can readily explain the unusually low level of total current flow in the presence of 7 mM barium ions and 3 mM calcium ions. In qualitative terms, the interaction between these extracellular cations and the calcium channels will produce a variety of cation-calcium channel complexes. One of these complexes, which will be present in some fraction of the total population, will consist of a channel in which the energy well closer to the extracellular medium will be empty whereas the energy well closer to the cytosol will be occupied by a calcium ion. Extracellular barium ions that approach the unoccupied energy well of such a channel will establish a repulsive force between itself and the calcium ion occupying the second energy well or binding site. Since calcium ions have a higher affinity for these binding sites than do barium ions, it is likely that the barium ion, rather than the calcium ion, will be repelled and thus will be unable to react with and occupy the empty site. In effect, the presence of calcium ions will cause the barium ions to exhibit a lesser affinity for *unoccupied* channel sites than they would have had calcium ions been absent. As a consequence, the level of current generated by the 7 mM barium ions, in this situation, will be lower than one would expect from 7 mM barium ions that were merely competing with 3 mM calcium ions for open channel sites in single ion channels. This model of the calcium channel also explains why sodium ion, which exhibits a low affinity for the calcium channel binding sites, appears to be an impermeant ion in the presence of calcium ions, but readily permeates the channels in the absence of calcium ions. (12, 13).

Ventricular cells from guinea pig heart are not the only cells that appear to possess multi-ion calcium channels (i.e. a channel that may, at any instant, contain more than one ion in its pore). Evidence for multi-ion calcium channels has also been found in skeletal muscle fibers (13) and rat brain synaptosomes (14). Channels such as those that reside in ventricular cells from the guinea pig heart (multi-ion channels) do not adhere to a simple hyperbolic relationship between the current flow and the extracellular calcium ion concentration. Yet this type of relationship, which is usually characteristic of saturable single ion channels, was observed by several investigators who studied calcium channels in barnacle muscle (7, 10). Hille has pointed out that multi-ion channels may appear to obey such a relationship if the range of extracellular ion concentrations examined is not sufficiently broad (9). On the other hand, there may, indeed, be fundamental differences in ion permeation mechanisms among various calcium channels that reside in different types of cells or in different animal species.

Types of Calcium Channels

Regardless of the mechanism by which ion permeation occurs in calcium channels, those cations that have the capacity to traverse the selectivity filter and pass through the channel pore can only do so when the channel is in an open conformation. Calcium channels assume this open conformation when conditions are suitable and an appropriate stimulus is applied (see below). In the absence of these essential elements the gating mechanisms of calcium channels maintain the great majority of the channels in a closed conformation. Although it is difficult to generalize, calcium channels found in a number of different types of cells appear to have a gating mechanism that is similar to that of the sodium channel in that it operates to transform the channel into any one of three different conformations or states (15–19). One of these is the open conformation and is referred to as the activated state. The other two are closed conformations and are referred to as: (a) the deactivated state and (b) the inactivated state.

Based on the type of excitatory stimulus required to convert a channel to the activated state, calcium channels have been divided into two broad groups (20–22). One group is voltage sensitive and will convert to the activated state when the membrane potential has been reduced to an appropriate level. The other group appears to be closely associated with specific receptors in the plasma membrane. Its conversion to the activated state can be brought about by interactions between these receptors and neurotransmitters or hormones that can activate the receptor molecules. Many excitable cells possess both types of calcium channels in their plasma membranes.

Voltage-Dependent Calcium Channels

ACTIVATION   By employing an experimental technique and procedure that will rapidly change the membrane potential and hold it to any desired level (voltage clamp technique), it has been possible to examine the relationship that exists between the level of the membrane potential and the magnitude of the current flowing through voltage sensitive calcium channels. Experiments (23–26) have shown that the membrane potential must first be reduced to some threshold point (i.e. brought to some more positive level) before any calcium current becomes detectable. The voltage change required is usually greater than that needed to turn on the membrane depolarizing sodium current (25). As the membrane potential is made increasingly more positive beyond the threshold point, an increasingly larger inward calcium current will be induced (23–25). This progressive increase in calcium current is a consequence of a progressive increase in ionic conductance (i.e. decrease in electrical resistance) that reflects the activation of increasing numbers of calcium channels (25, 27). At the same time, part of the inwardly directed driving force, namely the interaction between calcium ions and the electric field within the membrane, will become weaker as membrane potential becomes more positive (25, 27). This factor will serve to reduce the flow of inward current. As long as the changes made in the membrane potential are moderate, increases in ionic conductance appear to have a greater influence on current flow than do decreases in driving force. This is evidenced by the progressive increase in calcium current. At some point, however, the change in membrane potential will become large enough to activate a relatively high percentage of the calcium channel population. Further elevations in the positivity of the membrane potential should then have an opposite effect; that is, the continued reduction in driving force should exert a greater influence on current flow than should continued small increases in ionic conductance. In keeping with these concepts, experimental investigations have demonstrated that as membrane potential is made increasingly more positive the inward calcium current will rise progressively until it reaches a peak magnitude (23–25). From that point on, it will fall progressively (23, 25).

The manner in which depolarization (increase in positivity) of the cell membrane increases the conductance of voltage-sensitive calcium channels relates to the stochastic behavior of calcium channels (28, 29). At any given membrane potential all calcium channels in the membrane will fluctuate between the deactivated state and the activated state. In general, a channel will be either in a closed conformation or in a fully activated conformation, although patch clamp studies have demonstrated that channels may, in some cases, exhibit more than one activated state in which there are differing magnitudes of current flow (28). It follows that any single calcium channel observed over some span of time will be in an open conformation for part of that time and in a closed conformation for part of that time. In any single instant there will be some probability that the channel will be in the activated state or in the deactivated state. When dealing with a population of calcium channels in which all individual units behave in the same fashion, the probability that any single channel will be in the activated state translates into an average or mean fraction of the total population that will be in the activated state (28). An adjustment in membrane potential to a more positive level will, therefore, increase the mean fraction of a calcium channel population that exists in the activated state (and the mean ionic conductance) expressly by increasing the probability that individual channels will assume the activated conformation.

The transformation of a channel from the deactivated state to the activated state appears to require the repositioning of charged gating particles or components within the channel (5). The process is both voltage dependent and time dependent (25). Hagiwara and Ohmori (31) determined the rate at which channel activation rose to a new steady state level following a change in membrane potential to a more positive level. The measurements were made on calcium channels in clonal cells (GH_3) isolated from a rat anterior pituitary adenoma. Their results disclosed a process in which the fraction of activated channels in the total population increased progressively along a complex curve with respect to time. An analysis of the curve showed it to be consistent with a mechanism of activation that included the following series of reversible reactions:

$$C_1 \underset{\beta_1}{\overset{\alpha_1}{\rightleftharpoons}} C_2 \underset{\beta_2}{\overset{\alpha_2}{\rightleftharpoons}} O$$

where C_1 represents the density of channels (i.e. the number of channels per unit area of membrane) that are in an initial deactivated state; C_2 represents the density of channels in a second conformation, in which the channels are still in a deactivated state; O represents the density of channels in an activated state; and the quantities (α_1), (α_2), (β_1) and (β_2) represent first order rate constants. Moreover (α_1) equals (α_2) and (β_1) equals (β_2). Under these conditions, the mean fraction of the channels that will be in each of the three conformations, under steady state conditions, will depend upon the ratio of the first order rate constants, (α/β). If, for example, (α/β) equalled 2, the mean distribution observed under steady state conditions would be: approximately 14.3% of the population in state C_1; approximately 28.6%, in state C_2, and approximately 57.1%, in state O. Moreover as discussed above, these data indicate that in a uniform population of channels, each individual channel would have a 57.1% chance of being in the activated state in any single instant of time. The increased probability that a calcium channel will be found in the activated state following a reduction in membrane potential is, therefore, the consequence of an increase in the ratio (α/β) that is induced by the voltage change.

Although the probability factor and its underlying determinant, the ratio (α/β), govern the proportion of time that a single channel will be in the activated state, these factors do not reveal the number of times that a channel will fluctuate between states in any designated time frame. The latter process is regulated by the absolute magnitudes of the rate constants (α) and (β) (29). The operation of a large (β), for example, will mean that the transformation of a channel from state O to state C_2 will occur at a rapid rate. Thus, a channel, after assuming the open state conformation, will remain in that state for an average length of time equal to the inverse of (β). Similarly, the state C_1 will have an average time span equal to the inverse of (α) and the state C_2 will have an average time span equal to the inverse of ($\alpha + \beta$). In more general terms, forward and backward transformations that occur rapidly lead to an increased frequency of fluctuations. When considering a whole population of channels, comparatively large first order rate constants will speed the approach to a new steady state level, once the appropriate stimulus has been applied (29).

Reuter (30) has noted that voltage-dependent calcium channels typically open in bursts and that burst lengths increase with membrane depolarization. However, the mean duration of channel openings is only moderately voltage dependent. This observation fits well with the notion of a three state model in which the calcium channel fluctuates for a time between a closed state (C_2) and an open state (O) (bursts of activity) and then between one closed state (C_2) and another closed state (C_1) (interval between bursts). It is also consistent with the concept that a reduction in membrane potential induces large increases in the magnitudes of the alpha rate constants, but only moderate changes in the magnitudes of the beta rate constants. The resulting increase in the ratio (α/β) increases the probability that the channel will convert to the activated state and thereby increases the mean ionic conductance and the mean inward calcium current that flows through a population of calcium channels. By contrast, the amplitude of the inward calcium current conducted through a single open channel will be reduced somewhat by membrane depolarization because the inward driving force has been diminished.

Calcium channels in tissues other than GH_3 cells appear to be activated via a similar two step process (i.e. transformation of C_1 to C_2 and C_2 to O). Nonetheless, evidence for a two step gating mechanism has not been a consistent finding. Studies carried out on a variety of cell types have characterized the gating mechanism of calcium channels as a process consisting of a single reversible transformation from a closed to an open state up to as many as six reversible transformations (5, 15). Hagiwara and Ohmori (31) contend that these findings may, indeed, indicate that there are several different types of calcium channels in biological tissues or, alternatively, that the experimental procedures used to characterize the activation process did not produce equally reliable data in all cell types.

In a study performed by Fenwick et al (32) on chromaffin cells, the concept of a two step transformation was retained, but the rate constants were found to have different magnitudes. At a membrane potential of -5mV, and an extracellular concentration of 95mM Ba^{++}, the rate constant (α_1) was found to be equal to 61 s^{-1}, (α_2) equalled 345 s^{-1}, β_1 equalled 606 s^{-1} and (β_2) equalled 1230 s^{-1}. This model defines a gating process in which individual channels exhibit bursts of activity, characterized by relatively high frequency fluctuations between a closed and an open state (i.e. fluctuations between C_2 and O). This activity is interspersed with long periods of quiescence (i.e. fluctuations between C_2 and C_1). The comparatively low magnitude of (α_1) is largely responsible for the long periods of quiescence.

Hess et al (33), working with calcium channels in cardiac muscle cells, uncovered three different modes of gating behavior. At a test membrane potential in the moderately negative range, individual channels were observed to exhibit brief openings which occurred in rapid bursts. The gating mechanism underlying these activation-deactivation events involved the two step transformation process, $C_1 \rightleftharpoons C_2 \rightleftharpoons O$. A probability factor of .3 or less was also noted. This type of channel behavior was labeled mode 1. On occasion, although very infrequently, the channels underwent a spontaneous, short-lived, reversible modification. During this brief period the two step activation process was still operative, but the magnitudes of the first order rate constants were significantly altered. As a result the channels remained in the open state for relatively long periods of time and were closed for only short periods of time. The probability factor rose to a magnitude greater than .7. This type of channel behavior was labeled mode 2. At other times individual channels underwent some sort of modification that caused them to remain closed for an extended period of time. This quiescent pattern was labeled mode 0. Calcium channels in several other cell types have also been found to exhibit a mixture of modes 0, 1, and 2 (33, 34).

Variations in gating behavior detected in calcium channels of GH_3 cells (derived from a rat pituitary adenoma) were interpreted as having an entirely different basis (35). In this case, the differences in gating behavior were attributed to the operation of two distinctly different populations of calcium channels in the same cell. This conclusion was reached, in part, by quickly changing the membrane potential from a level of +10mV to a level of −80mV and measuring the time required for the calcium channels to close. Speed of closure was determined by monitoring the time dependent decay of the calcium "tail" current. It was found that the "tail" current decayed in two phases. One of these, the fast phase, had a time constant (inverse of rate constant) of 110 μsec; the other, the slow phase, had a time constant of 2.7 msec. These data may be interpreted to indicate that some fraction of the calcium channels in the cell membrane closes at a rapid rate while another fraction closes at a relatively slow rate. Further work showed that the fast deactivating fraction differs from the slow deactivating fraction in several respects. Relative to the slow deactivating channels, the fast deactivating channels are activated slightly more rapidly, are activated at more positive voltages, have a greater barium to calcium selectivity ratio, and are considerably more resistant to inactivation by a prolonged depolarizing pulse. These findings were taken as evidence for the existence and operation of two distinctly different populations of calcium channels in the same cell. Multiple types of calcium channels have also been uncovered in chick dorsal root ganglion cells (36), neuroblastoma cells (37, 38), Neanthes egg cells (39), as well as other kinds of cells.

INACTIVATION   It is clear from the evidence available that there are a number of different types of voltage-dependent calcium channels, each reacting to a reduction in membrane potential in its own unique fashion. In all cases, however, a reduction in membrane potential serves to elevate the conductance of a population of calcium channels. The elevation in conductance is a direct consequence of the opening of channel gates. If the reduction in membrane potential is maintained for some period of time, it may not necessarily lead to a sustained high level of channel conductance. The calcium channels may undergo a gradual modification that causes them to exhibit increasingly lower levels of conductance with time. The gradual diminution in ionic conductance seen in the face of a persistent excitatory stimulus is brought about by a mechanism that transforms the channel into a conformation termed the inactivated state. A calcium channel in an inactivated state, like one in a deactivated state, is in a closed conformation and will not permit a flow of ions through its aqueous pore. The specific stimulus that initiates the conversion of a calcium channel from the deactivated or activated state to the inactivated state differs in different types of calcium channels. Current evidence indicates that there are four major types of voltage-dependent calcium channels based on the distinctive factors or conditions that induce or do not induce each of them to assume the inactivated conformation.

In a few cell types the stimulus that initiates the inactivation of calcium channels is the same one that initiates the inactivation of sodium channels. In both cases a time-dependent inactivation occurs when the cell membrane has been adequately depolarized. It has been shown that an increasingly greater reduction in membrane potential, within a restricted voltage range, will generate an increasingly larger rate constant involved in the speed of transformation of calcium channels into the inactivated state (40, 41). At membrane potentials more negative than those in the restricted voltage range (within limits) the rate constant appears to have a very small magnitude; at membrane potentials less negative than those in the restricted voltage range the rate constant has an invariable high magnitude (40, 41). In addition, the mean fraction of the calcium channels that assume the inactivated state during steady state conditions will become increasingly greater as the reduction in membrane potential is increased within a specified voltage range (40, 42). At potentials more negative than this specified voltage range a negligible number of calcium channels assume the inactivated state; at potentials less negative than the specified voltage range essentially all the calcium channels are transformed into the inactivated state (40, 42). In general, the voltage-dependent inactivation of calcium channels exhibits slower kinetics and occurs within a more positive membrane potential range than does the voltage-dependent inactivation of sodium channels (43).

In many tissues, voltage-sensitive calcium channels, although rapidly activated by reductions in membrane potential, are not subsequently inactivated by a maintained low level of membrane potential. The inactivating stimulus in these channels is free intracellular calcium (43–46). Eckert and Chad (43), in an effort to account for the kinetic behavior of the calcium-dependent inactivation process, have developed a working model of the reactions involved. In their scheme, free intracellular calcium ions react reversibly with calcium channel binding sites. The stoichiometry is $1:1$ (no cooperativity). Each calcium ion-calcium channel interaction leads, hypothetically, to an enzymatic de-phosphorylation of a channel component and thereby produces an inactivated channel (43, 47). Intracellular calcium ions are assumed to have an affinity for channel binding sites whether the calcium channel is in the activated or the deactivated state. Thus, the following interactions are thought to occur:

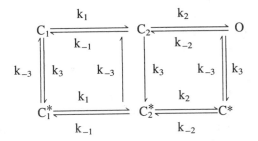

where C_1, C_2 and O have their usual meanings (see above), the asterisks denote inactivated states and the various k's represent first order rate constants. The horizontal transitions in the above scheme are voltage-dependent; the vertical transitions are calcium dependent.

Since the inactivation of calcium channels is purported to be a consequence of a reversible interaction between calcium channel binding sites and in-tracellular calcium ions, the degree to which a calcium channel population will become inactivated should be dependent upon the concentration of free calcium ions in the cytosol. The mean fraction of the channel population that assumes the inactivated state, in this case, will be a hyperbolic function of the free calcium ion concentration in the cytosol. Although the intracellular calcium ion concentration of excitable cells in the resting state is usually very low, one can induce a large increase in the intracellular level of calcium ions by lowering the membrane potential sufficiently to initiate a substantial influx of calcium into the cell. If the resultant influx of calcium ions produces a progressive rise in the intracellular calcium ion concentration that, ideally, is linear with respect to time, then the mean fraction of the calcium channel population that becomes inactivated will increase as a hyperbolic function of time. This means that the rate of inactivation of calcium channels, shortly after the cell membrane has been depolarized, will be relatively rapid. However, as time passes and the free calcium ions in the cytosol reach a high level, further inactivation of the calcium channels will proceed relatively slowly.

The hyperbolic increase in the fraction of inactivated calcium channels that occurs with the progression of time may be viewed as the basic dynamics of the calcium-dependent inactivation process. It can, however, be modified by a number of factors. One such factor is the temporal variation in the inward calcium current. For a comparatively short span of time immediately following an excitatory reduction in membrane potential a time-dependent elevation will occur in the average number of calcium channels that assume the activated state. During this period, the inward calcium current will quickly rise from a negligible level to a relatively high level. Once this change has been achieved the current flow, in the absence of any other modifying influence, will display a constant amplitude, signifying the attainment of new steady-state conditions for the activation of the calcium channels. The attainment of these steady-state conditions cannot be detected experimentally because the calcium-dependent inactivation reaction, superimposed on the activation process, causes a continuous diminution of the inward calcium current. As a result, the calcium current, following membrane depolarization, will exhibit a sharp rise in amplitude, reach a peak (below the steady state level for activation) and then exhibit a relatively slow fall in amplitude. This swing in the calcium current is unlikely to produce an increase in the intracellular calcium ion concentration that is linear with respect to time. In addition, there are several intracellular processes and reactions that undoubtedly alter the free calcium ion concentration in the cytosol. These include: (a) diffusion of calcium ions away from their sites of interaction with calcium channels, (b) interactions between calcium ions and intracellular binding sites, and (c) sequestration and/or extrusion of calcium ions by energy-dependent calcium pumps (43). Despite the influence of these modifying factors, the rate of the calcium-dependent inactivation process has been observed to be biphasic, i.e. characterized by two different time constants (43, 48, 49). Initially, one sees a fast phase of inactivation that appears to reflect, at least in part, the steep limb of a hyperbolic curve and, subsequently, a slow phase of inactivation that seems to reflect, in part, the shallow limb of a hyperbolic curve. If, as a result of the progressive inactivation of calcium channels, the inward calcium current dwindles to a point that the rate of entry of calcium ions equals the rate of removal of calcium ions from the site of action, the calcium-dependent inactivation process will display a steady state mode (44).

Studies have shown that the entry of strontium ions or barium ions into the cytosol of various cell types is less effective in producing calcium channel inactivation than is the entry of calcium ions. Barium ion produces much less inactivation than does calcium ion and strontium ion is intermediate (43, 46, 50–53).

Calcium channels in which inactivation is both voltage-dependent and calcium-dependent have also been uncovered. The channels of snail neurons (23) and possibly cardiac muscle (15) fit into this category. Eckert and Tillotson (52) have speculated that in cells that contain this type of calcium channel, the intracellular calcium ion, by binding to the inner surface of the cell membrane, may change the surface potential. The change in surface potential would then bring about a hyperpolarizing displacement of a voltage-sensitive gating process. Such a mechanism would be both voltage dependent and calcium dependent.

Lastly, there is a group of voltage-dependent calcium channels in which neither the voltage-dependent nor the calcium-dependent inactivation process operates or operates effectively. The channels in this group are, at most, only slightly inactivated or very slowly inactivated. Channels that exhibit these characteristics have been found in squid synaptic terminals (55, 56), adrenal chromaffin cells (57), photoreceptor inner segments (58), nerve cell bodies of Helix (59, 60), frog skeletal muscle fibers (61), type II channels in the egg cell of the worm, *Neanthes arenacedentata* (39) and other cell types.

Receptor-Operated Calcium Channels

Those calcium channels closely linked to membrane receptors and activated by agonist-receptor interactions have been labeled receptor-operated channels. Although they play an important role in the functional behavior of smooth muscle and many secretory cells, the receptor-operated calcium channels have received much less scrutiny than have calcium channels activated by membrane depolarization. Because of the lack of experimental data characterizing receptor-operated calcium channels, their specific properties remain largely unknown.

PHARMACOLOGY OF CALCIUM CHANNELS

Indirect Acting Agents

A wide variety of chemical substances can affect calcium channels indirectly by modifying the conditions that regulate calcium channel function. These include drugs that induce or prevent changes in membrane potential, drugs that alter the extracellular and/or intracellular concentrations of calcium ion, drugs that modify biochemical reactions involved in the operation of calcium channels (i.e. phosphorylation and dephosphorylation reactions, etc.) and drugs that activate or prevent the activation of membrane receptors closely linked to calcium channels. Often a single agent will elicit a series of cellular responses affecting more than one type of calcium channel. For example, acetylcholine, by complexing with and activating cholinergic receptors in a smooth muscle cell, will activate the receptor-operated channels that are directly associated with these membrane receptors. The resulting increase in inward calcium current as well as increases in other ionic currents induced by the activation of cholinergic receptors serve to reduce the membrane potential (20). The latter effect may, in turn, be of sufficient magnitude to initiate the activation of voltage-dependent calcium channels that reside in the same smooth muscle cell (20). It is of interest to note that the indirect modification of voltage-dependent calcium channel behavior by various neurotransmitters and hormones constitutes, in many instances, the normal physiological mechanism for regulating calcium channel function.

Inorganic Ions

A number of inorganic cations can interact with calcium channels in a direct and reversible manner. As a consequence, they exert a strong influence on the operation of activated channels. The type of influence that a particular inorganic cation will exert depends upon two factors. One is the affinity of the cation for the channel binding site involved in the first step in ion permeation (see above). The other is the speed at which the cation travels through the aqueous pore (i.e. the height of the energy barrier [selectivity filter] that the cation encounters) to reach the cytosol. Divalent cations, such as strontium and barium, which exhibit reasonably high affinities for the channel binding site and can traverse the channel pore more rapidly than calcium ion, act as excellent calcium substitutes (25). Depending on the extracellular concentrations employed, they can generate currents either equal to or greater than the one produced by calcium ion. Divalent cations, such as cobalt, nickel, cadmium, and manganese, exhibit reasonably high affinities for the channel binding site, but traverse the channel pore at low or even negligible speeds (25). These cations behave as potent competitive inhibitors of ion permeation through calcium channels. Monovalent cations, such as sodium (62–64), potassium (62–65), and caesium (65) also exhibit an affinity for the calcium channel binding site and can penetrate its aqueous pore. They have the capacity, therefore, to carry substantial currents through calcium channels. The trivalent ion, lanthanum, interacts rather strongly with calcium binding sites and has been found to be an excellent inhibitor of ionic currents conducted by calcium channels (5, 7, 25).

Organic Calcium Channel Blockers and Stimulators

In 1964, Fleckenstein reported that the chemical agents, verapamil and prenylamine, had the same inhibitory effect on cardiac muscle as did the withdrawal of extracellular calcium ions (66). Since that time a large number of organic compounds, of widely different chemical structures, have been found to have a similar inhibitory effect (67, 68). This effect stems, ultimately, from the direct actions of these compounds on calcium channels. The members of this group of compounds were originally called calcium antagonists because their inhibitory effects could be reversed by increasing the calcium ion concentration in the extracellular medium. More recently, they have also been referred to as calcium entry blocking agents or calcium channel blockers.

SUBGROUPS   The calcium entry blocking agents have been divided into three subgroups (67). Group I consists of nifedipine and related 1,4 dihydropyridines. Group II contains the calcium blockers verapamil, D600, diltiazem, and diclofurime which, for the most part, have unrelated chemical structures. Group III is made up of diphenylalkylamine compounds such as cinnarizine, fendiline, flunarizine, and prenylamine. The compounds in groups I and II exhibit potent and selective actions on calcium channels in cardiac muscle, whereas group III compounds appear to be less selective, causing a diminution in activity of both calcium and sodium channels in cardiac muscle (69). It has been shown, moreover, that verapamil, D600, and diltiazem, namely group II compounds, have approximately equiactive effects on calcium channels in cardiac muscle and vascular smooth muscle (69), while nifedipine and related dihydropyridines, as well as flunarizine and cinnarizine, exert preferential effects on vascular smooth muscle (68, 69).

SITES OF ACTION   The manner in which the organic calcium entry blocking agents inhibit voltage-dependent calcium channels in cardiac cells and other types of cells (nerve, smooth muscle, secretory, etc.) does not appear to be unique. Local anesthetic agents inhibit sodium channels in a similar fashion (70, 71). As a first step, the calcium channel blocking agent presumably enters or crosses the cell membrane in order to gain access to the appropriate site of action in or on the channel (70). This concept is supported by several lines of evidence. First, the calcium blockers were found to be sufficiently lipophilic to penetrate the cell membrane and enter the cytosol (72). Second, a highly polar N-methyl quaternized derivative of D600 was observed to have no effect on the action potential of guinea-pig ventricular myocytes when applied externally, but lowered and shortened the calcium-dependent plateau of the action potential when applied intracellularly (73). On the other hand, D600 produced the latter effect when applied either internally or externally. It was inferred, therefore, that externally applied D600 had to cross the cell membrane before acting (73).

Although the inhibitory effects of the organic calcium channel blockers can be reversed by increasing the extracellular calcium ion concentration, a simple competition between the blocking agent and extracellular calcium for the channel coordination site involved in ion permeation is not a likely possibility. This conclusion is based on experiments that show that cadmium ion blocks barium currents more strongly than it does calcium currents, as would be expected from the relative affinities of these two current-carrying ions for the coordination binding site (see above), whereas the organic calcium blockers have the opposite effect (74).

Numerous radioligand binding studies have been performed for the purpose of characterizing the channel binding sites that interact with the organic calcium blockers. Often the calcium blockers have been observed to complex with two specific groups of membrane sites; a low affinity-high capacity group and a high affinity-low capacity group (75, 76). In many cases, particularly in those studies performed on smooth muscle, the correlation between the concentrations of blocking agent required to produce functional blockade of calcium channels and the concentrations at which substantial binding takes place was found to be very good (68). Other studies have disclosed a poor correlation. In cardiac muscle, skeletal muscle and brain tissue (68, 4) binding of the inhibitory agent to a high affinity site occurs at concentrations well below those required to affect ion permeation through calcium channels. This finding has been rationalized, to some extent, by the proposal that calcium channels in membrane fragments frequently used for binding studies are in an inactivated state, the conformational state that displays the highest affinity for calcium blockers (67, 70). This proposal seems to be borne out by work performed by Kunze and Hawkes (75). These investigators measured the binding of ^{3}H nitrendipine to membrane preparations of PC12 (pheochromocytoma) cells. They found that the apparent dissociation constant (K_D) and the total number of binding sites (B_{max}) were similar to values obtained in whole cells. When a calcium current was produced in the whole cell by a voltage step to $+10$ mV from a holding potential of -100mV, the inhibitory dose 50 (IC_{50}) of nitrendipine was 10^{-6} M. When the holding potential was lowered from -100 mV to -20 mV, a membrane potential at which the steady state inactivation of calcium channels rises to 50%, the inhibitory dose 50 (IC_{50}) of nitrendipine decreased to 130 nM. They also calculated the dissociation constant for the binding of nitrendipine to inactivated channels and found it to be 8 nM, a value very similar to the K_D for the nitrendipine-high affinity site complex. Moreover, the total number of calcium channels calculated from electrophysiological studies agreed with the value calculated from data delineating the binding of nitrendipine to high affinity sites. On the other hand, a study carried out on intact frog sartorius muscle led to the conclusion that this muscle contains many more dihydropyridine binding sites than it does calcium channels (78).

The binding of dihydropyridine derivatives to membrane sites may be altered by introducing other organic calcium blocking agents. A number of calcium blockers including verapamil and diltiazem appear to interact with a common membrane site different from but allosterically linked to the dihydropyridine binding site (79). By interacting with the common site verapamil can decrease, whereas diltiazem can increase, the binding of a dihydropyridine blocking agent to its membrane sites (79).

Despite the functional antagonism that exists between extracellular calcium ions and calcium blockers, the binding of ^{3}H dihydropyridine derivatives to membrane sites is not reduced by low to moderate concentrations of calcium ion. Only very high levels of inorganic divalent ions have been observed to reduce drug binding (80, 81). In addition to these observations, Krafte et al (82) have demonstrated that an elevation in the concentration of Ca^{++}, Sr^{++}, Ba^{++}, or Mg^{++} will cause a depolarizing shift in the calcium channel in-activation-voltage curve both in single cells and in multicellular Purkinje fibers; that is, the fraction of the channel population found in the inactivated state at a given membrane potential is reduced. The divalent ion-induced shift in the inactivation curve also occurs in the presence of nisoldipine. Since the magnitude of the shift is the same order whether or not nisoldipine is present, these investigators concluded that the antagonistic actions of the divalent ions are due, in part, to a nonspecific modification of a negative membrane surface charge.

MODES OF ACTION

Use-dependent blockade   A prominent feature of the blockade produced by calcium channel blocking agents is use dependence (70, 71, 74, 83–85). In a cell stimulated repeatedly (i.e. one whose membrane is depolarized repeatedly for short periods), a drug exhibiting use dependence will induce an increasingly greater degree of inhibition with each successive stimulation until a steady-state level of inhibition is reached. Use dependence will theoretically be observed when an inhibitory agent exhibits little or no affinity for an ion channel in the deactivated state, but interacts to a significant degree with an activated or an inactivated ion channel or both (70, 71, 86). The activation and inactivation of ion channels initiated by membrane depolarization will, therefore, lead to an inhibitory agent-ion channel interaction and a consequent blockade of ion permeation. If the duration of the depolarization is very brief, a state of equilibrium for the interaction may not be achieved. Moreover, a return to resting conditions will be followed by a dissociation of bound inhibitory agent that may or may not reach completion before the next membrane depolarization is elicited. In the latter instance some bound inhibitory agent will be retained and more will become bound during the second depolarization. This will result in a greater degree of blockade than had occurred during the first depolarization. The process will continue until the quantity of inhibitory agent that becomes bound to activated and/or inactivated channels during a period of activity (i.e. when the membrane is depolarized) is equal to the quantity dissociating from deactivated channels during a period of rest (i.e. when the membrane is polarized to resting level). At that point the blockade of ion permeation will remain at a constant level.

Given these circumstances, a prerequisite for demonstrating use-dependent blockade should be the selection of a frequency of stimulation high enough to prevent the complete dissociation of the inhibitory agent-ion channel complex during a period of rest. The selection of a suitable frequency will obviously depend upon the rate at which the blocking agent in question reacts with and dissociates from the ion channels under the conditions that prevail. There are reports in the literature that do, indeed, show that an increase in the frequency of stimulation enhances the progression of use-dependent blockade of calcium channels induced by several different kinds of organic calcium blockers (83, 84, 85) and, further, that the use of very low frequencies essentially abolishes this type of blockade (83, 85).

Use-dependent blockade is also influenced by the magnitude of the membrane potential during periods of rest. As the negativity of the membrane potential is reduced, within a limited voltage range, the extent to which inactivated and activated cardiac calcium channels are transformed to the deactivated state will be reduced (5, 23–25, 30, 31, 40, 42). In addition, the presence of a calcium blocking agent that exhibits a preferential affinity for activated and/or inactivated channels will produce a further shift in the steady-state distribution of ion channels between the deactivated state and other conformational states; that is, the fraction of ion channels found in the deactivated state at a given membrane potential will be reduced (67, 86). Consequently, the dissociation of an inhibitory agent from ion channels should be more rapid in a strongly polarized membrane (one with a large negative membrane potential) during periods of rest than in a membrane brought to a less negative potential during periods of rest (71). In keeping with these concepts, hyperpolarization of the membrane has been shown to reduce or abolish use-dependent blockade of calcium channels induced by calcium entry blocking agents (83, 85, 87).

An effort has been made to determine which conformational states of the calcium channel form firm complexes with the channel blockers. In a study carried out by Lee and Tsien (74), a barium current was elicited in ventricular myocytes by a prolonged depolarizing pulse (600 msec). In the absence of any inhibitory agent this current underwent a slight inactivation. The presence of nitrendipine or D600 hastened the decay of the barium current. This effect was attributed to a blockade of activated channels. Diltiazem did not hasten the decay of the barium current and was judged to have little effect on activated calcium channels. Kanaya et al (84) showed that diltiazem and verapamil produced a stronger block of calcium current when the duration of a depolarizing conditioning impulse was increased from 100 msec to 2–3 sec. Moreover, the diltiazem-induced block could not be enhanced by increasing the voltage of a 30 msec conditioning pulse (too little time for much inactivation to occur) from -30 mV to $+80$ mV. Based on these data, the investigators concluded that the affinity of diltiazem for inactivated channels is greater than its affinity for activated channels. These studies as well as others indicate that some calcium blockers such as diltiazem interact primarily with inactivated calcium channels, whereas blocking agents such as verapamil, D600, and nitrendipine also interact with activated calcium channels.

Actions of dihydropyridine compounds   In some respects, the pharmacological actions of the dihydropyridine compounds differ sharply from those of other blocking agents. Members of the dihydropyridine group such as nitrendipine (74), nisoldipine (88), nifedipine (89), and nimodipine (89) have been observed to produce a blockade of calcium current that fails to exhibit more than minimal use dependency. In addition, Kass (88) has reported that the blockade of calcium current in cardiac tissue induced by nisoldipine, unlike that produced by D600, could not be removed by holding the membrane at a relatively negative potential for up to 2 minutes. There is, however, an indication that the dihydropyridine blockers dissociate from calcium channel sites relatively quickly (74). On this basis, the suggestion has been made that stimulation frequencies employed in past studies may have been too low to demonstrate use-dependent block with the dihydropyridines (70). Additional work will be needed to ascertain the validity of this contention.

The dihydropyridine derivatives, Bay K 8644 and CGP 28392, have been shown to have the unique capacity to enhance rather than block current flow through calcium channels (90, 91). In Purkinje fibers, Bay K 8644 induced a shift in the peak inward current-voltage curve (see above) toward a more negative voltage range and increased peak inward currents (92). Kokubun and Reuter (91) found that this type of drug increases single channel current somewhat, but the primary basis for its excitatory effect is a prolongation of the mean open time of the calcium channel. The characteristic burst behavior seen in control experiments was transformed, in the presence of the drug, to a much longer channel opening with only a few, brief interruptions. As a result, the fraction of the total calcium channel population that assumed the open channel conformation at some specified membrane potential was substantially increased (i.e. the probability factor was increased). The presence of Bay K 8644 or CGP 28392 also shortened the time constant for the brief closures that occur during bursts and lengthened slightly the time constant for the long interval between bursts. It is of interest that the dihydropyridine blocking agents, nimodipine, nitrendipine, and nifedipine, like Bay K 8644 and CGP 28392, increase the time constant for the long intervals of closure between bursts. With the former agents, however, the increase in the duration and number of long intervals of closure appear to be more pronounced than any modification induced in the open state of the channel. The net outcome, therefore, is a reduction in overall calcium current (91). If a cardiac cell preparation is depolarized or stimulated at a high rate the excitatory agent Bay K 8644 will exert an inhibitory effect on the calcium channels (92). High concentrations of the drug will also inhibit the channels (92). Consequently, it has been referred to as a partial agonist (92).

Hess et al (33) consider these effects of the dihydropyridines to be a reflection of their modulating action on the naturally occurring behavior of calcium channel gates. As indicated previously (see above) these investigators discovered that the gating mechanism of a calcium channel may undergo spontaneous transitions among three distinctly different modes. Mode 1, characterized by brief openings that occur in rapid bursts, is the most probable gating form that calcium channels assume. However, in the presence of an inhibitory dihydropyridine such as nimodipine, the channel gates display an increased likelihood of converting to mode 0 which leads to prolonged periods of channel closure. By contrast, Bay K 8644, an excitatory dihydropyridine, enhances the likelihood that a channel will exhibit mode 2 behavior, namely long lasting channel openings and very brief channel closings. They also noted that any particular drug such as nitrendipine or Bay K 8644, at an appropriate concentration, may increase the occurrence of both mode 0 and mode 2 behavior. Whether the resultant effect is inhibitory or excitatory will depend upon which mode change is the more dominant. These observations led to the contention that dihydropyridine compounds cannot possibly modify calcium currents by physically plugging the channel pore. Such a mechanism would not explain the agonist-like (excitatory) component of nitrendipine's net inhibitory action. The idea that agonist and antagonist actions of nitrendipine may occur at different binding sites seems improbable because Bay K 8644 competes for all nitrendipine binding sites (93). The experimental results point, instead, to a mechanism of action involving the modulation of calcium channel gating. It would appear, moreover, that the antagonistic actions of the dihydropyridine agents simulate the action of the voltage-dependent inactivation process (conversion to mode 0) and serve to reinforce and to be reinforced by the action of this potential-dependent inactivation process.

The effects of dihydropyridine agents have also been studied in GH4Cl pituitary cells that possess two different populations of calcium channels. One set of calcium channels undergoes little or no inactivation, while the other set inactivates rapidly. It was found that nimodipine preferentially blocked and Bay K 8644 preferentially enhanced the current in the noninactivating calcium channels (94).

Neurohormones

The membranes of cardiac cells contain neurohormone receptors known to play an important regulatory role in the operation of voltage-dependent calcium channels. Excitation of beta adrenergic receptors in these membranes increase (95), whereas excitation of muscarinic cholinergic receptors decrease (96, 97) the amplitude of calcium currents initiated by membrane depolarization. Drugs such as norepinephrine, epinephrine, and isoproterenol which excite beta adrenergic receptors are, therefore, powerful calcium channel stimulants. The sequence of events that leads to an increase in the calcium current by these drugs begins with a reversible interaction between the drug and the membrane receptor. This interaction induces the activation of adenylate cyclase. As a consequence, the level of cyclic AMP in the cytoplasm increases. The elevation in the level of cyclic AMP activates a cyclic AMP-dependent protein kinase resulting in the phosphorylation of membrane proteins presumed to be part of or linked, in some manner, to potential calcium channels (31, 98, 99). In ventricular heart cells of the frog, phosphorylation of these critical proteins increased the average number of voltage-sensitive calcium channels that could be transformed to the open state. The net result was a larger inward calcium current. Single channel current remained unaltered and the probability that a channel would assume the activated conformation at some given membrane potential increased to a moderate degree (about a 50% increase). The major change was an increase in the average number of functional calcium channels in the cell (about a threefold increase at a membrane potential of $+10$ mV) (100).

The reduction in calcium current brought about by the interaction of cholinergic agonists, such as acetylcholine, and cholinergic receptors in cardiac cells may possibly involve cyclic GMP (101–103). However, the series of reactions that lead to this inhibitory effect is not yet clearly understood.

CALCIUM CHANNELS IN SMOOTH MUSCLE

Evidence for Two Calcium Channel Types

The calcium ions that initiate a mechanical response in smooth muscle cells may be mobilized from calcium reservoirs within the cell and/or from the calcium pool (both free and loosely bound calcium) in the external environment (22). There are two major routes by which calcium ions from the latter pool may traverse the cell membrane and thereby gain access to the contractile apparatus. One pathway is the receptor-operated calcium channel system; the other is the voltage-dependent calcium channel system (20–22). To some extent, extracellular calcium ions may also reach the cytosol via a small membrane leak (22) and perhaps via a sodium-calcium exchange mechanism (104).

Several lines of evidence support the view that receptor-operated calcium channels in smooth muscle cells constitute a separate group of membrane elements that can be distinguished from voltage dependent-channels. In 1958 Evans et al (105) reported that isolated smooth muscle preparations that were completely depolarized in a bathing medium containing a high concentration of K_2SO_4 could still undergo contractions in response to an agonist. Durbin and Jenkinson (106) observed that the size of the contractions induced were directly related to the concentration of calcium ions in the bathing medium. In addition, Robertson (107) noted that in the depolarized longitudinal muscle from rabbit ileum ^{45}Ca uptake could be markedly increased by acetylcholine. Subsequently, several groups of investigators (108–110) showed that certain normally polarized vascular tissue (i.e. rabbit ear artery, rabbit main pulmonary artery, porcine coronary artery and others) could be stimulated to contract by concentrations of an agonist that did not produce any significant change in membrane potential. However, the extent to which the agonist-induced contractions, under these conditions, resulted from the influx of calcium ions through activated voltage-independent calcium channels or the release of calcium ions from internal stores is not clear. Using a pharmacological approach Meisheri et al (21) demonstrated that, in the rabbit aorta, calcium influx stimulated by a depolarizing high potassium medium could be preferentially inhibited by D600, whereas calcium influx stimulated by norepinephrine could be preferentially inhibited by amrinone. They also observed that the calcium fluxes stimulated by the high potassium medium and by norephinephrine were additive. In sum, these experimental results favor the proposal that receptor-operated calcium channels constitute one population and that voltage-dependent calcium channels constitute another population of membrane elements. Whether or not membrane potential exerts any essential or modulating influence on the activation of receptor-operated calcium channels is still unresolved.

Receptor-Operated Calcium Channels

Golenhofen and colleagues have reported the existence of two different types of agonist- (i.e. acetylcholine, epinephrine) controlled calcium activation systems (111). One, which they labeled the P system, is activated in association with regenerative potential changes in the membrane; the other, labeled the T system, seems to be less dependent upon electrical activity in the membrane. Agonist-activation of the P system elicits phasic contractions in smooth muscle cells; agonist-activation of the T system elicits tonic contractions in smooth muscle cells. The two systems can also be distinguished by their differing responses to various inhibitory agents. The P system is preferentially suppressed by verapamil, D600, and nifedipine, whereas the T system is more strongly inhibited by sodium nitroprusside. Golenhofen notes that the molecular basis of the P-T differentiation is not yet clear. There is evidence to indicate that both systems can operate with calcium ions from a variety of sources. It seems reasonable to assume, however, that the phasic contractions they observed are induced, at least in part, by action potentials that reflect the operation of voltage-dependent calcium channels. These channels are presumably activated by the increase in ionic conductance (supposedly Na and Ca conductance) and consequent membrane depolarization brought about by the agonist.

Little is known about the functional characteristics of receptor-operated calcium channels or about the manner in which they are linked to membrane receptors in the smooth muscle cell. The proposal has been made that a receptor-induced breakdown of inositol phospholipids is responsible for the opening of calcium channel gates (112). The specific membrane substrates that are broken down following an agonist-receptor interaction are phosphatidylinositol and polyphosphoinositides (113). Much experimental data have been generated, some of which support (113–116) and some of which question the validity of (117–119) this proposal. Recently, the metabolic degradation of a fraction of the total inositol phospholipid pool, namely the polyphosphoinositides, has been considered as a possible intermediary event that links receptor activation to a physiological response (113). The polyphosphoinositides of interest are phosphatidylinositol 4-phosphate and phosphatidylinositol 4,5 biphosphate, particularly the latter (113). The smooth muscle of the iris is an example of a cell in which activation of muscarinic, cholinergic, and alpha$_1$ adrenergic receptors induce an extremely rapid breakdown of phosphatidylinositol 4,5 bisphosphate but not phosphatadylinositol or phosphatidylinositol 4 phosphate (120–122). It should be noted, however, that interest in the relationship between the rapid breakdown of phosphatidylinositol 4,5-bisphosphate and calcium mobilization is focused primarily on the release of calcium ions from internal cellular stores (113, 123–125). It stems from observations that inositol 1,4,5-trisphosphate, a hydrolytic product of phosphatidylinositol 4,5-bisphosphate (113), can induce the release of calcium from nonmitochondrial stores in permeabilized leaky pancreatic acinar cells (123) and saponin-treated hepatic cells (124, 126, 127) and from microsomal fractions of rat insulinoma (128). The role of inositol phospholipid turnover, if any, in the external calcium influx often required to sustain a physiological response, is still not understood (113).

Agonist-receptor interactions that lead to an elevation in cyclic nucleotides also have a questionable influence on the influx of calcium ions in smooth muscle cells. Ousterhout and Sperelakis (103) have examined the effects of dibutyryl cAMP, dibutyryl cGMP, and 8-bromo-cGMP on calcium channel function in vascular smooth muscle. Cultured smooth muscle cells were prepared from rat aortas by enzyme dispersion and reaggregation. Calcium-dependent action potentials were elicited in these aortic reaggregates by electrical stimulation in the presence of tetraethylammonium (TEA). They found that .1 mM dibutyryl cAMP depressed and .5–1.0 mM dibutyryl cAMP abolished the TEA-induced action potentials. By contrast, 1 mM dibutyryl cGMP and .1–1.0 mM 8-bromo-cGMP had no appreciable effect on these action potentials. In an intact preparation of rabbit pulmonary artery, however, .1–2.0 mM dibutyryl cAMP was observed to have little or no effect on TEA-induced action potentials. Based on these results, Ousterhout and

Sperelakis suggest that cAMP, but not cGMP, may regulate the function of voltage-dependent calcium channels in rat aortic smooth muscle cells. Obviously, more work is needed to clarify the role that cyclic nucleotides may play in the operation of both receptor-operated and voltage-dependent calcium channels in smooth muscle cells.

Voltage-Dependent Calcium Channels

A number of studies have been performed that collectively indicate that several different types of voltage-dependent calcium channels reside in smooth muscle cells. Working with uterine smooth muscle of the guinea pig, Hamon and Vassort have characterized an inward current that appears to flow through calcium channels that are both activated and inactivated by reductions in membrane potential (129). This inward current has been shown to be sensitive to the inhibitory actions of Mn, Co, La (130–132), and D600 (131, 132) and to be unaffected by drastic reductions in the extracellular sodium ion concentration (131, 133, 134) or by the presence of the sodium channel blocker, tetrodotoxin (131, 135, 136). A relatively small diminution in membrane potential was sufficient to induce this calcium channel current to attain a detectable amplitude, indicating a low threshold of activation. Peak current amplitude occurred at 50 mV depolarization (i.e. a reduction in membrane potential from a resting level of −55 mV to a level of −5 mV). Inactivation of the channels conducting this inward current was investigated by noting the effect that a prior conditioning impulse of one second duration had on the amplitude of the inward current induced by a 38 mV depolarization. These investigators found that conditioning impulses of increasingly greater positive potential levels caused the subsequent current initiated by the 38 mV depolarization to exhibit increasingly smaller amplitudes. Their results demonstrated that the inward conductance underwent steady-state inactivation the level of which was dependent on the membrane potential. The relationship between membrane potential and inactivation of these calcium channels was observed to have a form similar to that used by Hodgkin and Huxley (137) to describe inactivation of sodium channels. Calcium channels in smooth muscle that are rapidly activated and inactivated by reductions in membrane potential are assumed to be involved in the development of action potentials (and consequent increases in muscle tension) in those smooth muscles that exhibit this kind of electrical activity. There is ample evidence to indicate that action potentials in smooth muscle cells can be inhibited by organic (138, 139) and inorganic (140–142) calcium blockers, can be modified by variations in the extracellular calcium ion concentration (140–144), and are not greatly affected by drastic reductions in the extracellular sodium ion concentration (140, 143–146) or by the sodium channel blocker, tetrodotoxin (147, 148).

It has been known for many years that many smooth muscle preparations can also be stimulated to contract by exposing them to a membrane-depolarizing high potassium bathing medium. Some smooth muscles characteristically undergo a monophasic mechanical response; others undergo a biphasic or even more complex mechanical response in the presence of a high potassium medium (20). The longitudinal muscle of the guinea pig ileum, for example, exhibits a biphasic response (149–151). The initial component of the response, termed the phasic response, consists of a very rapid but transitory increase in muscle tension. This tension change is usually followed by some degree of relaxation. Subsequently, the longitudinal muscle will undergo a second, less rapid, but more sustained increase in muscle tension. The second tension change, termed the tonic response, after reaching a peak level, will gradually diminish in amplitude over a prolonged period of time (90–120 min).

Whether a smooth muscle preparation exhibits a monophasic or more complex contraction, experience has shown that these potassium-induced tension changes are usually quite sensitive to the inhibitory actions of both inorganic (149, 151, 152–154) and organic (150, 155–161) calcium blockers. The mechanical response can be prevented by adding a calcium entry blocking agent to the high potassium bathing solution (151, 160) or aborted by adding such an agent after the contraction has been induced (151, 162). It can also be abolished by removing calcium ions from the high potassium bathing solution and reinstated by adding calcium ions back to the solution (150). These findings support the notion that an essential step in the development of a potassium-induced contraction is the influx of calcium ions from the extracellular environment. Additional support for this notion stems from experiments demonstrating that the potassium-induced biphasic mechanical response of the longitudinal muscle from the guinea pig ileum is associated with a cobalt-sensitive biphasic influx of calcium ions. The initial phase of the calcium influx is rapid and very transient; the latter phase is considerably slower and more sustained (152). Data showing that calcium fluxes accompany potassium-induced tension changes have also been obtained in other types of smooth muscle (160, 163).

Based on experiments performed on the longitudinal muscle of the guinea pig ileum, Hurwitz et al (150, 151) have advanced the proposal that a high potassium bathing medium activates at least two different types of voltage-dependent (or potassium-activated) calcium channels in the smooth muscle cell. The data that led to this proposal was obtained, to a large extent, by monitoring changes in muscle tension. A significant disclosure was the finding that a relaxed longitudinal muscle that had been incubated in a calcium-deficient, high potassium bathing medium (140 mM KCl) for 10 minutes or more could be induced to undergo a characteristic biphasic mechanical response by introducing 1.8 mM $CaCl_2$ into the bathing medium. This finding demonstrated that both components of the mechanical response can be elicited in smooth muscle cells that have been depolarized for an extended period of time. The inference drawn is that the calcium channels associated with this complex mechanical response cannot be rapidly inactivated by large reductions in membrane potential. A series of experiments was also performed to test the relative effects of various interventions on the biphasic mechanical response. The results obtained showed that both components could be inhibited by organic and inorganic calcium blocking agents, but could not be modified by the anticholinergic agent, atropine. However, the initial phasic component exhibited a preferential sensitivity to the inhibitory effect of small concentrations (6–20 μM) of lanthanum ion and to an inhibitory action exerted by moderate concentrations (1.8 mM) of calcium ions. Indeed, the relatively brief duration of the phasic component was attributed to the somewhat latent inactivating effect of calcium ions present in the bathing medium. By contrast, the tonic component displayed a preferential sensitivity to the inhibitory effect induced by incubating the muscle for a very long period (70–80 min) in a calcium-deficient, high potassium bathing medium before adding 1.8 mM $CaCl_2$ to elicit the biphasic response. The influx of calcium ions associated with the tonic component of the mechanical response was also inhibited more strongly by this procedure than was the influx of calcium ions associated with the phasic component (152). Other data pointing to differences between these two components have also been reported. Cameron and Lewis (164) found that low doses (15 μg/ml) of a toxin obtained from the stonefish produced an appreciable inhibition of the phasic response but had a lesser effect on the tonic response. Rangachari et al (165) have noted that a selective inhibition of the phasic response could be achieved by replacing chloride ion in the bathing medium with sulphate ion. Taken as a whole, the available evidence favors the contention that the biphasic mechanical response induced by a high potassium medium in the longitudinal muscle of the guinea pig ileum reflects the operation of two different voltage-dependent calcium channel systems. Those channels associated with the initial phasic component of the response permit a rapid, but transient inward movement of calcium ions and are quickly inactivated by the presence of calcium ions. Those channels associated with the subsequent tonic component of the response permit a much slower but more sustained inward movement of calcium ions and are slowly inactivated by prolonged exposure to the high potassium bathing medium. Hogestatt and Andersson (166), working with cerebral arteries from the rat, have suggested that the operation of two different voltage-dependent calcium channel systems may also be responsible for the potassium-induced biphasic contractions seen in their vascular smooth muscle preparation.

Although the physiological role of the calcium channels that become functional in a high potassium bathing medium is uncertain, Ratz and Flaim (167) raise the possibility that calcium channels of the type encountered in a high potassium medium may play an important role in smooth muscle cells that normally contract in response to graded depolarizations of the plasma membrane. A channel that exhibits an increasingly greater probability of assuming the activated state as membrane potential is reduced, and does not readily undergo inactivation in a depolarized cell, would be well suited to deliver calcium ions to the cytoplasm during graded, well sustained depolarizations of the cell membrane.

Summary of Multiple Calcium Channel Types in Smooth Muscle

It would appear, therefore, that the types of voltage-dependent calcium channels that may be present in smooth muscle cells include those that are rapidly inactivated by reductions in membrane potential, those that are inactivated by the presence of calcium ions and/or those that are not readily inactivated by a diminution in membrane potential or the presence of calcium ions. A number of observations favor the assumption that any single smooth muscle cell may harbor several different types of voltage-dependent calcium channels. Visceral smooth muscles (uterine, intestinal, etc.), for example, will, under normal physiological conditions, undergo an increase in muscle tension following a stimulus-induced initiation or increase in the frequency of trains of action potentials (20, 168). These same cells can also be stimulated to develop complex, well sustained increases in muscle tension by immersing them in a membrane-depolarizing, high potassium bathing medium (20). In addition to harboring multiple types of voltage-dependent calcium channels, smooth muscle cells contain receptor-operated calcium channels, the functions of which are regulated, at least in part, by agonist-receptor interactions. In early experiments performed on various smooth muscle preparations, voltage-dependent calcium channels, as a group, seemed to differ from receptor-operated calcium channels in being much more sensitive to the inhibitory actions of calcium channel blockers (21, 169, 170). More recent work has uncovered a number of exceptions to this general observation. Examples of receptor-operated channels that are equally sensitive or even more sensitive to the actions of calcium blockers than are voltage-dependent channels have been noted in the literature (171–173).

Literature Cited

1. Rubin, R. P. 1982. *Calcium and Cellular Secretion*, New York: Plenum Press
2. Hille, B. 1984. Na and K channels of axons. In *Ionic Channels of Excitable Membranes*, pp. 58–75. Sunderland, Massachusetts: Sinauer Associates
3. Lakshminarayanaiah, N. 1981. Calcium channels in the barnacle muscle membrane. In *New Perspectives on Calcium Antagonists*, ed. G. B. Weiss, pp. 19–33. Baltimore: Williams & Wilkins
4. Towart, R., Schramm, M. 1984. Recent advances in the pharmacology of the calcium channel. *Trends Pharmacol. Sci.* 5:111–13
5. Hagiwara, S., Byerly, L. 1981. Calcium channel. *Ann. Rev. Neurosci.* 4:69–125
6. Hagiwara, S., Byerly, L. 1981. Mem-

brane biophysics of calcium currents. *Fed. Proc.* 40:2220–25

7. Hagiwara, S., Takahashi, K. 1967. Surface density of calcium ions and calcium spikes in the barnacle muscle fiber membrane. *J. Gen. Physiol.* 50:583–601

8. Hille, B. 1984. Elementary properties of ions in solution. See Ref. 2, pp. 151–80

9. Hille, B. 1984. Selective permeability: Saturation and binding. See Ref. 2, pp. 249–71

10. Beirao, P. S., Lakshminarayanaiah, N. 1979. Calcium carrying system in the giant muscle fiber of the barnacle species, *Balanus nubilus*. *J. Physiol.* 293:319–27

11. Hille, B. 1984. Selective permeability: Independence. See Ref. 2, pp. 226–48

12. Hess, P., Tsien, R. W. 1984. Mechanism of ion permeation through calcium channels. *Nature* 309:453–56

13. Almers, W., McCleskey, E. W. 1984. Non-selective conductance in calcium channels of frog muscle: Calcium selectivity in a single-file pore. *J. Physiol.* 353:585–608

14. Nelson, M. T. 1985. Divalent cation interactions with single calcium channels from rat brain. *Biophys. J.* 47:67a

15. Tsien, R. W. 1983. Calcium channels in excitable cell membranes. *Ann. Rev. Physiol.* 45:341–58

16. Kass, R. S., Scheuer, T. 1982. Calcium ions and cardiac electrophysiology. In *Calcium Blockers*, ed. S. F. Flaim and R. Zelis, pp. 3–19. Baltimore: Urban and Schwarzenberg

17. Beeler, G. W. Jr., Reuter, H. 1970. Membrane calcium current in ventricular myocardial fibers. *J. Physiol.* 207:191–209

18. New, W., Trautwein, W. 1972. Inward membrane currents in mammalian myocardium. *Pfluegers Arch.* 334:1–23

19. Trautwein, W., McDonald, T. F., Tripathi, O. 1975. Calcium conductance and tension in mammalian ventricular muscle. *Pfluegers Arch.* 354:55–74

20. Bolton, T. B. 1979. Mechanisms of action of transmitter and other substances on smooth muscle. *Physiol. Rev.* 59:606–718

21. Meisheri, K. D., Hwang, O., Van Breeman, C. 1981. Evidence for two separate Ca^{2+} pathways in smooth muscle plasmalemma. *J. Membr. Biol.* 59:19–25

22. Van Breemen, C., Aaronson, P. I., Cauvin, C. A., Loutzenhiser, R. D., Mangel, A. W., Saida, K. 1982. The calcium cycle in arterial smooth muscle. See Ref. 16, pp. 53–63

23. Brown, A. M., Morimoto, K., Tsuda,

Y., Wilson, D. L. 1981. Calcium current-dependent and voltage-dependent inactivation of calcium channels in Helix aspersa. *J. Physiol.* 320:193–218

24. Inomata, H., Kao, C. Y. 1976. Ionic currents in the guinea-pig taenia coli. *J. Physiol.* 255:347–378

25. Hille, B. 1984. Calcium channels. See Ref. 2, pp. 76–98

26. Lakshminarayanaiah, N., Beirao, P. S. 1979. Calcium system of a grant barnacle muscle fiber. *Proc. West Pharmacol. Soc.* 22:301–07

27. Hille, B., 1984. Introduction. See Ref. 2, pp. 1–19

28. Hille, B., 1984. Counting channels. See Ref. 2, pp. 205–25

29. Hille, B., 1984. Endplate channels and other electrically inexcitable channels. See Ref. 2, pp. 117–47

30. Reuter, H. 1983. Calcium channel modulation by neurotransmitters, enzymes and drugs. *Nature* 301:569–574

31. Hagiwara, S., Ohmori, H. 1982. Studies of Ca channels in rat clonal pituitary cells with patch electrode voltage clamp. *J. Physiol.* 331:231–52

32. Fenwick, E. M., Marty, A., Neher, E. 1982. Sodium and calcium channels in bovine chromaffin cells. *J. Physiol.* 331:599–635

33. Hess, P., Lansman, J. B., Tsien, R. W. 1984. Different modes of Ca channel gating behavior favored by dihydropyridine Ca agonists and antagonists. *Nature* 311:538–44

34. Fox, A. P., Hess, P., Lansman, J. B., Nowycky, M. C., Tsien, R. W. 1984. Slow variations in the gating properties of single calcium channels in guinea pig heart cells, chick neurones and neuroblastoma cells. *J. Physiol.* 353:75P

35. Armstrong, C. M., Matteson, D. R. 1985. Two distinct populations of calcium channels in a clonal line of pituitary cells. *Science* 227:65–67

36. Nowycky, M. C., Fox, A. P., Tsien, R. W. 1985. Three types of calcium channels in chick dorsal root ganglion cells. *Biophys. J.* 47:67a

37. Tsunoo, A., Yoshii, M., Narahashi, T. 1985. Differential block of two types of calcium channels in neuroblastoma cells. *Biophys. J.* 47:433a

38. Yoshii, M., Tsunoo, A., Narahashi, T. 1985. Different properties in two types of calcium channels in neuroblastoma cells. *Biophys. J.* 47:433a

39. Fox, A. P., Krasne, S. 1982. Relaxation due to depletion in an egg cell calcium current. *Biophys. J.* 37:20a

40. Fukushima, Y., Hagiwara, S. 1983. Vol-

tage-gated Ca^{2+} channel in mouse myeloma cells. *Proc. Natl. Acad. Sci. USA* 80:2240–42

41. Fox, A. P. 1981. Voltage-dependent inactivation of a calcium channel. *Proc. Natl. Acad. Sci. USA* 78:953–56

42. Reuter, H. 1979. Properties of two inward membrane currents in the heart. *Ann. Rev. Physiol.* 41:413–24

43. Eckert, R., Chad, J. E. 1984. Inactivation of Ca channels. *Prog. Biophys. Mol. Biol.* 44:215–67

44. Chad, J., Eckert, R., Ewald, D. 1984. Kinetics of calcium dependent inactivation of calcium current in voltage clamped neurones of *Aplysia californica*. *J. Physiol.* 347:279–300

45. Kostyuk, P. G., Krishtal, O. A. 1977. Effects of calcium and calcium-chelating agents on the inward and outward current in the membrane of mollusc neurones. *J. Physiol.* 270:569–580

46. Tillotson, D. 1979. Inactivation of Ca conductance dependent on entry of Ca ions in Molluscan neurons. *Proc. Nat. Acad. Sci. USA* 76:1497–1500

47. Chad, J., Eckert, R. 1985. Calcineurin, a calcium-dependent phosphatase, enhances Ca-mediated inactivation of Ca current in perfused snail neurons. *Biophys. J.* 47:266a

48. Kostyuk, P. G. 1980. Calcium ionic channels in electrically excitable membrane. *Neuroscience* 5:945–59

49. Nagura, I. S. 1977. Long lasting inward current in snail neurons in barium solutions in voltage clamp conditions. *J. Membr. Biol.* 35:239–56

50. Brehm, P., Eckert, R. 1978. Calcium entry leads to inactivation of calcium channel in Paramecium. *Science* 202: 1203–1206

51. Mentrard, D., Vassort, G., Fischmeister, R. 1984. Calcium mediated inactivation of the calcium conductance in caesium loaded frog heart cells. *J. Gen Physiol.* 83:105–31

52. Eckert, R., Tillotson, D. 1981. Calcium mediated inactivation of the calcium conductance in caesium loaded giant neurones of *Aplysia californica*. *J. Physiol.* 314:265–80

53. Ashcroft, F. M., Stanfield, P. R. 1982. Calcium inactivation in skeletal muscle fibers of the stick insect *Carausius morosus*. *J. Physiol.* 330:349–72

54. Deleted in proof.

55. Llinas, R., Steinberg, I. Z., Walton, K. 1981. Presynaptic calcium currents in squid giant synapse. *Biophys. J.* 33:289–322

56. Augustine, G., Eckert, R., Zucker, R.

57. Hamill, O. P., Marty, A., Neher, E., Sakmann, B., Sigworth, F. J. 1981. Improved patch-clamp techniques for high-resolution current recording from cells and cell-free membrane patches. *Pfluegers Arch.* 391:85–100

58. Corey, D. P., Dubinsky, J., Schwartz, E. A. 1982. The calcium current of rod-photoreceptor inner segments recorded with a whole cell patch clamp. *Soc. Neurosci. Abstr.* 8:944

59. Eckert, R., Lux, H. D. 1975. A non-inactivating inward current recorded during small depolarizing voltage steps in snail pacemaker neurons. *Brain Res.* 83:486–89

60. Eckert, R., Lux, H. D. 1976. A voltage-sensitive persistent calcium conductance in neuronal somata of Helix. *J. Physiol.* 254:129–51

61. Almers, W., Fink, R., Palade, P. T. 1981. Calcium depletion in frog muscle tubules: the decline of calcium current under maintained depolarization. *J. Physiol.* 312:177–207

62. Reuter, H., Scholz, H. 1977. A study of the ion selectivity and the kinetic properties of the calcium dependent slow inward current in mammalian cardiac muscle. *J. Physiol.* 264:17–47

63. Reuter, H., Scholz, H. 1977. The regulation of Ca conductance of cardiac muscle by adrenaline. *J. Physiol.* 264:49–62

64. Lee, K. S., Lee, E. W., Tsien, R. W. 1981. Slow inward current carried by Ca^{2+} or Ba^{2+} in single isolated heart cells. *Biophys. J.* 33:143a

65. Lee, K. S., Tsien, R. W. 1982. Reversal of current through calcium channels in dialyzed single heart cells. *Nature* 297:498–501

66. Fleckenstein, A. 1964. Die Bendeutung der energiereichen Phosphate bei der Kontraktilitat und tonus des Myokards. *Verh. Dtsch. Ges. Inn. Med.* 70:81–99

67. Spedding, M. 1985. Calcium antagonist subgroups. *Trends Pharmacol. Sci.* 6: 109–14

68. Janis, R. A., Triggle, D. J. 1983. New developments in Ca^{2+} channel antagonists. *J. Med. Chem.* 26:775–85

69. Fleckenstein, A. 1981. Fundamental actions of calcium antagonists on myocardial and cardiac pacemaker cell membranes. See Ref. 3, pp. 59–81

70. Hondeghem, L. M., Katzung, B. G. 1984. Antiarrhythmic agents: The modulated receptor mechanism of action of sodium and calcium channel-blocking

drugs. *Ann. Rev. Pharmacol. Toxicol.* 24:387–423
71. McDonald, T. F., Pelzer, D., Trautwein, W. 1980. On the mechanism of slow calcium channel block in heart. *Pfluegers Arch.* 385:175–79
72. Pang, D. C., Sperelakis, N. 1983. Nifedipine, diltiazem, bepridil and verapamil uptakes into cardiac and smooth muscles. *Eur. J. Pharmacol.* 87:199–207
73. Hescheler, J., Pelzer, D., Trube, G., Trautwein, W. 1982. Does the organic calcium channel blocker D600 act from inside or outside on the cardiac cell membrane? *Pfluegers Arch.* 393:287–91
74. Lee, K. S., Tsien, R. W. 1983. Mechanism of calcium channel blockade by verapamil, D600, diltiazem and nitrendipine in single dialysed heart cells. *Nature* 302:790–94
75. Kunze, D. L., Hawkes, M. J., Hamilton, S. L., Brown, A. M. 1985. Binding and pharmacological studies of nitrendipine on PC 12 cells. *Biophys. J.* 47:264a
76. Shrikhande, A. V., Sarmiento, J. G., Janis, R. A., Rutledge, E. Triggle D. J. 1985. Characteristics of binding of Bay K 8644 to high and low affinity sites on cardiac membranes. *Biophys. J.* 47:265a
77. Deleted in proof
78. Schwartz, L. M., McClesky, E. W., Almers, W. 1985. Specific binding of dihydropyrindines to intact frog sartorius muscle: Binding is voltage dependent, but most binding sites are not functional Ca channels. *Biophys. J.* 47:512a
79. Murphy, K. M. M., Gould, R. J., Largent, B. L., Snyder, S. H. 1983. A unitary mechanism of calcium antagonist drug action. *Proc. Nat. Acad. Sci. USA* 80:860–64
80. Ehlert, F. J., Roeske, W. R., Itoga, E., Yamamura, H. I. 1982. The binding of [^{3}H] nitrendipine to receptors for calcium channel antagonists in the heart, cerebral cortex and ileum of rats. *Life Sci.* 30: 2191–2202
81. Gould, R. J., Murphy, K. M. M., Snyder, S. H. 1982. [^{3}H] nitrendipine-labeled calcium channels discriminate inorganic calcium agonists and antagonists. *Proc. Nat. Acad. Sci. USA* 79:3656–60
82. Krafte, D., Coplin, B., Bennett, P., Kass R. S. 1985. Surface charge modification influences blocking activity of dihydropyridine Ca channel antagonists. *Biophys. J.* 467:512a
83. Ehara, T., Kaufmann, R. 1978. The voltage and time-dependent effects of (−l)-verapamil on the slow inward current in isolated cat ventricular myocardium. *J. Pharmacol. Exp. Ther.* 207:49–55

84. Kanaya, S., Arlock, P., Katzung, B. G., Hondeghem, L. M. 1983. Diltiazem and Verapamil preferentially block inactivated calcium channels. *J. Mol. Cell. Cardiol.* 15:145–48
85. Pelzer, D., Trautwein, W., McDonald, T. F. 1982. Calcium channel block and recovery from block in mammalian ventricular muscle treated with organic channel inhibitors. *Pfluegers Arch.* 394:97–105
86. Hille, B., 1984. Mechanisms of block. See Ref. 2, pp. 272–302
87. Trautwein, W., Pelzer, D., McDonald, T. F., Osterrieder, W. 1981. AQA 39, a new bradycardic agent which blocks myocardial calcium (Ca^{2+}) channels in a frequency- and voltage-dependent manner. *Naunyn-Schmiedeberg's Arch. Pharmacol.* 317:228–32
88. Kass, R. S. 1982. Nisoldipine: A new, more selective, calcium current block in cardiac Purkinje fibers. *J. Pharmacol. Exp. Ther.* 223:446–56
89. Hachisu, M., Pappano, A. J. 1983. A comparative study of the blockade of calcium-dependent action potentials by verapamil, nifedipine and nimodipine in ventricular muscle. *J. Pharmacol. Exp. Ther.* 225:112–20
90. Schramm, M., Thomas, G., Towart, R., Frankowiak, G. 1983. Novel dihydropyridines with positive inotropic action through activation of Ca^{2+} channels. *Nature* 303:535–37
91. Kokubun, S., Reuter, H. 1984. Dihydropyridine derivatives prolong the open state of Ca channels in cultured cardiac cells. *Proc. Nat. Acad. Sci. USA* 81: 4824–27
92. Sanguinetti, M. C., Kass, R. S. 1985. Voltage selects activity of the Ca channel modulator Bay K8644. *Biophys. J.* 47: 513a
93. Janis, R. A., Sarmiento, J. G., Maurer, S. C., Bolger, G. T., Triggle, D. J. 1984. Characteristics of the binding of [^{3}H] nitrendipine to rabbit ventricular membranes: Modification by other Ca^{++} channel antagonists and by Ca^{++} channel agonist Bay K 8644. *J. Pharmacol. Exp. Ther.* 231:8–15
94. Cohen, C. J., McCarthy, R. T. 1985. Differential effects of dihydropyridines on two populations of Ca channels in anterior pituitary cells. *Biophys. J.* 47: 513a
95. Kass, R. S., Wiegers, S. E. 1982. Ionic basis of concentration-related effects of noradrenaline on the action potential of cardiac Purkinje fibres. *J. Physiol.* 322: 541–58

96. Giles, W., Noble, S. J. 1976. Changes in membrane currents in bullfrog atrium produced by acetylcholine. *J. Physiol.* 261:103–23
97. TenEick, R., Nawrath, H., McDonald, T. F., Trautwein, W. 1976. On the mechanism of the negative inotropic effect of acetylcholine. *Pfluegers Arch.* 361:207–213
98. Rinaldi, M. L., Capony, J. P., Demaille, J. G. 1982. The cyclic AMP-dependent modulation of cardiac sarcolemmal slow calcium channels. *J. Molec. Cell. Cardiol.* 14:279–289
99. Osterrieder, W., Brum, G., Hescheler, J., Trautwein, W., Flockerzi, V., Hofmann, F. 1982. Injection of subunits of cyclic AMP-dependent protein kinase into cardiac myocytes modulates Ca^{++} current. *Nature* 298:576–78
100. Bean, B. P., Nowycky, M. C., Tsien, R. W. 1984. Beta adrenergic modulation of calcium channels in frog ventricular heart cells. *Nature* 307:371–75
101. Trautwein, W., Taniguchi, J., Noma, A. 1982. The effect of intracellular cyclic nucleotides and calcium on the action potential and acetylcholine response of isolated cardiac cells. *Pfluegers Arch.* 392:307–14
102. Kohlhardt, M., Haap, K. 1978. 8-Bromo-guanosine-3',5'-monophosphate mimics the effects of acetylcholine on slow response action potential and contractile force in mammalian atrial myocardium. *J. Mol. Cell. Cardiol.* 10:573–86
103. Ousterhout, J. M., Sperelakis, N. 1985. Role of cyclic nucleotides in regulation of slow channel function in vascular smooth muscle. *Biophys. J.* 47:266a
104. Aickin, C. C., Brading, A. F., Burdyga, Th. V. 1984. Evidence for sodium-calcium exchange in the guinea-pig ureter. *J. Physiol.* 347:411–430
105. Evans, D. H. L., Schild, H. O., Thesleff, S. 1958. Effects of drugs on depolarized plain muscle. *J. Physiol.* 143:474–85
106. Durbin, R. P., Jenkinson, D. H. 1961. The calcium dependence of tension development in depolarized smooth muscle. *J. Physiol.* 157:90–96
107. Robertson, P. A. 1960. Calcium and contractility in depolarized smooth muscle. *Nature* 186:316–17
108. Su, C., Bevan, J. A., Ursillo, R. C. 1964. Electrical quiescence of pulmonary artery smooth muscle during sympathomimetic stimulation. *Circ. Res.* 15:20–27
109. Droogmans, G., Raeymakers, L., Casteels, R. 1977. Electro- and pharma-comechanical coupling in the smooth muscle cells of the rabbit ear artery. *J. Gen. Physiol.* 70:129–48
110. Ito, Y., Kitamura, K., Kuriyama, H. 1979. Effects of acetylcholine and catecholamines on the smooth muscle cell of the porcine coronary artery. *J. Physiol.* 294:595–611
111. Golenhofen, K. 1981. Differentiation of calcium activation processes in smooth muscle using selective antagonists. In *Smooth Muscle*, ed. E. Bulbring, A. F. Brading, A. W. Jones and T. Tomita, pp. 157–70. Austin: Univ. Texas Press
112. Michell, R. H. 1975. Inositol phospholipids and cell surface receptor function. *Biochem. Biophys. Acta* 415:81–147
113. Hirasawa, K., Nishizuka, Y. 1985. Phosphatidylinositol turnover in receptor mechanism and signal transduction. *Ann. Rev. Pharmacol. Toxicol.* 25:147–70
114. Jafferji, S. S., Michell, R. H. 1976b. Effects of calcium-antagonistic drugs on the stimulation by carbamoylcholine and histamine of phosphatidylinositol turnover in longitudinal smooth muscle of guinea-pig ileum. *Biochem. J.* 160:163–69
115. Fain, J. N., Berridge, M. J. 1979. Relationship between hormonal activation of phosphatidylinositol hydrolysis, fluid secretion and calcium flux in the blowfly salivary gland. *Biochem. J.* 178:45–58
116. Berridge, M. J., Fain, J. N. 1979. Inhibition of phosphatidylinositol synthesis and the inactivation of calcium entry after prolonged exposure of the blowfly salivary gland to 5-hydroxytryptamine. *Biochem. J.* 178:59–69
117. Hawthorne, J. N. 1982. Is phosphatidylinositol now out of the calcium gate? *Nature* 295:281–82
118. Farese, R. V., Larson, R. E., Sabir, M. A. 1980. Effects of Ca^{2+} ionophore A23187 and Ca^{2+} deficiency on pancreatic phospholipids and amylase release in vitro. *Biochim. Biophys. Acta* 633:479–84
119. Cockroft, S., Bennett, J. P., Gomperts, B. D. 1980. Stimulus-secretion coupling in rabbit neutrophils is not mediated by phosphatidylinositol breakdown. *Nature* 288:275–77
120. Abdel-Latif, A. A., Akhtar, R. A., Hawthorne, J. N. 1977. Acetylcholine increases the breakdown of triphosphoinositide of rabbit iris muscle prelabelled with [^{32}P] phosphate. *Biochem. J.* 162:61–73
121. Akhtar, R. A., Abdel-Latif, A. A. 1978. Calcium ion requirement for acetylcho-

line-stimulated breakdown of triphosphoinositide in rabbit iris smooth muscle. *J. Pharmacol. Exp. Ther.* 204:655–68

122. Akhtar, R. A., Abdel-Latif, A. A. 1980. Requirement for calcium ions in acetylcholine-stimulated phosphodiesteratic cleavage of phosphatidyl-myo-inositol 4,5 biphasphate in rabbit iris smooth muscle. *Biochem. J.* 192:783–91

123. Streb, H., Irvine, R. F., Berridge, M. J., Schultz, I. 1983. Release of Ca^{2+} from a nonmitochondrial intracellular store in pancreatic acinar cells by inositol-1,4,5-trisphosphate. *Nature* 306:67–69

124. Burgess, G. M., Godfrey, P. P., McKinney, J. S., Berridge, M. J., Irvine, R. F., Putney, J. W. Jr. 1984. The second messenger linking receptor activation to internal Ca release in liver. *Nature* 309:63–66

125. Berridge, M. J. 1984. Inositol triphosphate and diacylglycerol as second messengers. *Biochem. J.* 220:345–60

126. Joseph, S. K., Thomas, A. P., Williams, R. J., Irvine, R. F., Williamson, J. R. 1984. Myo-inositol 1,4,5-triphosphate. *J. Biol. Chem.* 259:3077–81

127. Thomas, A. P., Alexander, J., Williamson, J. R. 1984. Relationship between inositol polyphosphate production and the increase of cytosolic free Ca^{2+} induced by vasopressin in isolated hepatocytes. *J. Biol. Chem.* 259:5574–84

128. Prentki, M., Biden, T. J., Janjic, D., Irvine, R. F., Berridge, M. J., Wollheim, C. B. 1984. Rapid mobilization of Ca^{2+} from rat insulinoma microsomes by inositol-4,5-triphosphate. *Nature* 309:562–64

129. Vassort, G. 1981. Ionic currents in longitudinal muscle of the uterus. See Ref. 111, pp. 353–66

130. Anderson, N. C., Ramonl, F., Snyder, A. 1971. Studies on calcium and sodium in uterine smooth muscle excitation under current clamp and voltage-clamp conditions. *J. Gen. Physiol.* 58:322–39

131. Mironneau, J. 1973. Excitation-contraction coupling in voltage clamped uterine smooth muscle. *J. Physiol.* (Lond.) 233:127–41

132. Vassort, G. 1975. Voltage-clamp analysis of transmembrane ionic currents in guinea-pig myometrium: evidence for an initial potassium activation triggered by calcium enflux. *J. Physiol.* (Lond.) 252:713–34

133. Mironneau, J. 1974. Voltage clamp analysis of the ionic currents in uterine smooth muscle using the double sucrose gap method. *Pfluegers Arch. Gesamte Physiol. Menschen Tiere* 352:197–210

134. Vassort, G. 1974. Initial ionic currents in guinea-pig myometrium. *J. Physiol.* 237:50–51P

135. Anderson, N. C. 1969. Voltage-clamp studies on uterine smooth muscle. *J. Gen. Physiol.* 54:145–65

136. Kao, C. Y. 1971. Some new leads into the physiology of mammalian smooth muscles. In *Research in Physiology*, ed. F. F. Kao, K. Koizumi, M. Vassalle, pp. 365–72. Bologna: Aulo Gaggi

137. Hodgkin, A. L., Huxley, A. F. 1952. A quantitative description of membrane current and its application to conduction and excitation in nerve. *J. Physiol.* 117:500–44

138. Golenhofen, K., Lammel, E. 1972. Selective suppression of some components of spontaneous activity in various types of smooth muscle by iproveratril (verapamil). *Pfluegers Arch. Gesamte Physiol. Menschen Tiere* 331:233–43

139. Riemer, J., Dorfler, F., Mayer, C.-J., Ulbrecht, G. 1974. Calcium-antagonistic effects on the spontaneous activity of guinea-pig taenia coli. *Pfluegers Arch. Gesamte Physiol. Menschen Tiere* 351:241–58

140. Brading, A. F., Bulbring, E., Tomita, T. 1969. The effect of sodium and calcium on the action potential of the smooth muscle of the guinea pig taenia coli. *J. Physiol.* 200:637–54

141. Osa, T. 1973. The effects of sodium, calcium and manganese on the electrical and mechanical activities of the myometrial smooth muscle of pregnant mice. *Jap. J. Physiol.* 23:113–33

142. Osa, T. 1974. Modification of the mechanical response of the smooth muscles of pregnant mouse myometrium and guinea-pig ileum by cadmium and manganese ions. *Jap. J. Physiol.* 24:101–17

143. Holman, M. E. 1958. Membrane potentials recorded with high-resistance microelectrodes and the effects of changes in ionic environment on the electrical and mechanical activity of the smooth muscle of the taenia coli of guinea-pig. *J. Physiol.* 141:464–488

144. Bulbring, E., Kurijama, H. 1963. Effect of changes in the external sodium and calcium concentrations on spontaneous electrical activity in smooth muscle of guinea-pig taenia coli. *J. Physiol.* 166:29–58

145. Kuriyama, H., Tomita, T. 1970. The ac-

tion potential in the smooth muscle of the guinea-pig taenia coli and ureter studied by the double sucrose-gap method. *J. Gen. Physiol.* 55:147–162

146. Holman, M. E. 1957. The effect of changes in sodium chloride concentration of the smooth muscle of guinea-pig's taenia coli. *J. Physiol.* 136:569–84

147. Nonomura, Y., Hotta, Y., Ohoshi, H. 1966. Tetrodotoxin and manganese ions: effects on electrical activity and tension in taenia coli of guinea-pig. *Science* 152:97–99

148. Tomita, T. 1981. Electrical activity (spikes and slow waves) in gastrointestinal smooth muscles. See Ref. 111, pp. 127–56

149. Triggle, C. R., Triggle, D. R. 1976. An analysis of the actions of cations of the lanthanide series on the mechanical response of guinea pig ileal longitudinal smooth muscle. *J. Physiol.* 254:39–54

150. Hurwitz, L., McGuffee, L. J., Little, S. A., Blumberg, H. 1980. Evidence for two distinct types of potassium-activated calcium channels in an intestinal smooth muscle. *J. Pharmacol. Exp. Ther.* 214:574–80

151. Hurwitz, L., McGuffee, L. J., Smith, P. M., Little, S. A. 1982. Specific inhibition of calcium channels by calcium ions in smooth muscle. *J. Pharmacol. Exp. Ther.* 220:382–88

152. Little, S. A., Teaf, E., Hurwitz, L. 1985. Cobalt-sensitive biphasic uptake of calcium ions in potassium-depolarized smooth muscle. *J. Pharmacol. Exp. Ther.* 232:746–53

153. Swamy, V. C., Triggle, C. R., Triggle, D. J. 1976. The effects of lanthanum and thulium on the mechanical responses of rat vas deferens. *J. Physiol.* 254:55–62

154. Shino, H. 1976. Mechanisms of the contracting action of K, acetylcholine and Ba and of the antispasmodic action of Cd and Mn on the pyloric antrum strip of rats stomach, particularly in relation to Ca. *Folia Pharmacol. Jpn.* 72:95–104

155. Haeusler, G. 1972. Differential effect of verapamil on excitation-contraction coupling in smooth muscle and on excitation-secretion coupling in adrenergic nerve terminals. *J. Pharmacol. Exp. Ther.* 180:672–82

156. Riemer, J., Dorfler, F., Mayer, C.-J., Ulbrecht, G. 1974. Calcium-antagonistic effects on the spontaneous activity of guinea-pig taenia coli. *Pfluegers Arch.* 351:241–58

157. Magaribuchi, T., Nakajima, H., Kiyomoto, A. 1977. Effects of diltiazem and lanthanum ion on the potassium contracture of isolated guinea-pig smooth muscle. *Jpn. J. Pharmacol.* 27:333–39

158. Nagao, T., Ikeo, T., Sato, M. 1977. Influence of calcium ions on responses to diltiazem in coronary arteries. Short communications. *Jpn. J. Pharmacol.* 27:330–32

159. Fleckenstein, A., Nakayama, K., Fleckenstein-Grun, G., Byon, Y. K. 1976. Interactions of H ions, Ca-antagonistic drugs and cardiac glycosides with excitation-contraction coupling of vascular smooth muscle pp 117–123. In *Ionic Actions on Vascular Smooth Muscle*, ed. by E. Betz, Berlin: Springer

160. Godfraind, T. 1983. Actions of nifedipine on calcium fluxes and contraction in isolated rat arteries. *J. Pharmacol. Exp. Ther.* 224:443–450

161. Kuriyama, H., Mishima, K., Suzuki, H. 1975. Some differences in contractile response of isolated longitudinal and circular muscle from the guinea-pig stomach. *J. Physiol.* 251:317–31

162. Goodman, F. R. 1981. Calcium-channel blockers and respiratory smooth muscle, See Ref. 3, pp. 217–33

163. Mayer, C. J., Van Breemen, C., Casteels, R. 1972. The action of Lanthanum and D600 on the calcium exchange in the smooth muscle cells of the guinea-pig taenia coli. *Pfluegers Arch.* 377:333–50

164. Cameron, A. M., Lewis, R. J. 1982. The antispasmogenic action on guinea-pig ileum of a fraction obtained from the toxic skin secretion of the stonefish, *Synanceia trachynis. Toxicon* 20:991–1000

165. Rangachari, P. K., Triggle, C. R., Daniel, E. E. 1982. Chloride removal selectively inhibits phasic contractions of guinea pig ileal longitudinal smooth muscle. *Can. J. Physiol. Pharmacol.* 60:1741–44

166. Hogestatt, E. D., Andersson, K.-E. 1984. Mechanisms behind the biphasic contractile response to potassium depolarization in isolated rat cerebral arteries. *J. Pharmacol. Exp. Ther.* 228:187–95

167. Ratz, P. H., Flaim, S. F. 1982. Species and blood vessel specificity in the use of calcium for contraction. See Ref. 16, pp. 77–98

168. Burnstock, G., Holman, M. E., Prosser, C. L. 1963. Electrophysiology of smooth muscle. *Physiol. Rev.* 43:482–527

169. Schumann, H. J., Gorlitz, B. D., Wagner, J. 1975. *Naunyn. Schiemedeberg's Arch. Pharmacol.* 289:409–18

170. Van Breeman, C., Huang, Meisheri, K. D. 1981. The mechanism of inhibitory action of diltiazem on vascular smooth muscle contractility. *J. Pharmacol. Exp. Ther.* 218:459–63

171. Kondo, K., Suzuki, H., Okuno, T., Suda, M., Saruta, T. 1980. Effects of nifedipine, diltiazem and verapamil on the vasconstrictor responses to norepinephrine and potassium ions in the rat mesenteric artery. *Arch. Int. Pharmacodyn. Ther.* 245:211–17

172. Bevan, J. A. 1983. Diltiazem selectivity inhibits cerebrovascular intrinsic but not extrinsic myogenic tone. *Circ. Res.* 52(Suppl.):104–109

173. Walus, K. M., Fondacaro, J. D., Jacobson, E. D. 1981. Effects of calcium and its antagonists on the canine mesenteric circulation. *Circ. Res.* 48:692–700

Ann. Rev. Pharmacol. Toxicol. 1986. 26:259–91

THE METABOLISM OF XENOBIOTICS BY CERTAIN EXTRAHEPATIC ORGANS AND ITS RELATION TO TOXICITY*

Theodore E. Gram[1], Laud K. Okine[2], and Rosalinda A. Gram[2]

Toxicology Branch, DTP[1] and Laboratory of Experimental Therapeutics and Metabolism, DTP[2] National Cancer Institute, National Institutes of Health, Bethesda, Maryland 20205

INTRODUCTION

Considerable interest has developed in recent years in the bioactivation of xenobiotics in extrahepatic organs and in the accompanying toxic effects in these organs. However, the presence of covalently bound xenobiotic in, for example, kidney, coupled with selective pathologic changes in kidney, is not prima facie evidence for the generation of a toxic chemical species in that target organ. There is now abundant and further accumulating evidence that many reactive intermediates may be formed in liver and that they are sufficiently stable to diffuse back into the venous blood and be distributed to other organs where they may be covalently bound and produce tissue injury. Thus, one must exercise caution in equating high concentrations of covalently bound xenobiotics in specific organs and pathologic changes in those organs with in situ activation of the xenobiotic.

Williams (1) considered the metabolism of foreign chemical compounds, or xenobiotics, to occur via four chemical mechanisms: namely oxidation, reduction, and hydrolysis (Phase I reactions); and synthesis (conjugation) (Phase II reactions). Many excellent reviews (2–5) are available that discuss the specific types of reactions included with these categories, and they are not repeated here. It suffices to state that most of the reactions that fall within the scope of this review are oxidative reactions of a special type; in general they are catalyzed by enzyme systems known as monooxygenases or mixed function

---

oxidases. These enzymes present in the microsomal fraction of most mammalian organs and tissues, nonmammalian species, bacteria, molds, and plants usually require NADPH and an electron transport chain consisting of a flavoprotein—commonly referred to as NADPH cytochrome c (P-450) reductase—and a family of hemoprotein isozymes known collectively as cytochromes P-450. In most instances, interaction of this enzyme system with xenobiotics results in biological inactivation of the xenobiotic ("detoxication") and increased rate of clearance from the body. However, in other instances—those of specific interest to us here—xenobiotic substrates that are themselves biologically inert or of a low order of biological activity are converted by the monooxygenase system to highly reactive metabolic intermediates that form adducts with vital cellular macromolecules (DNA, RNA, proteins, lipids). These interactions may lead to a variety of detrimental biological consequences, including cellular necrosis, mutagenesis, and malignant transformations.

Because of its large mass and its richness in monooxygenases, much of the early work, relating bioactivation of xenobiotics to various toxic effects, was performed with, and concentrated upon, liver (6). More recently, however, an abundant literature has accumulated on the bioactivation of xenobiotics in extrahepatic organs with resulting toxicity either in situ or in distant sites that are the primary loci of toxicity.

Finally, we wish to emphasize that the primary purpose of this paper is not to review extrahepatic drug metabolism per se; many excellent reviews (7–9) and monographs (e.g. 10) perform that function quite adequately. The thrust of this paper instead determines if organ-specific toxicity has a metabolic basis, why it is selective (formation of a specific toxic metabolite, unusual sensitivity of that organ to a common metabolite, prolonged retention, etc), and, where possible, what biochemical mechanism(s) account for the selective toxicity.

The literature review for this manuscript was completed in February 1985.

RESPIRATORY TRACT

Level of the Respiratory Tree

NASAL EPITHELIUM   Although the field of inhalation toxicology has proliferated immensely in the past ten years, systematic study of the metabolism of xenobiotics by the most proximal segments of the respiratory tree did not appear until 1982. Dahl and his co-workers (11) detected easily measurable levels of microsomal cytochrome P-450 and its related monooxygenases in nasal epithelium and ethmo- and maxilloturbinate membranes from dogs. The nasal carcinogen hexamethylphosphoramide was metabolized by nasal enzymes to another nasal carcinogen, formaldehyde. Later work from the same laboratory described the presence of cytochrome P-450, p-nitroansole O-demethylase, and aniline hydroxylase in nasal membranes of six common laboratory species (12). Rabbit, guinea pig, and hamster were richest in these enzymes. Cytochrome P-450 levels in rat nasal epithelium were 1.6 times that of lung (per mg protein) (13). Brittebo and co-workers (14, 15) reported the metabolism of carcinogenic nitrosamines and of aminopyrine by nasal mucosa of mice and rats; they suggested a correlation between intranasal metabolism of a variety of substituted nitrosamines and their carcinogenicity in situ. Monooxygenases in nasal turbinates of dogs and rats catalyzed the activation of benzo[α]pyrene, 2-aminoanthracene (16), and 1-nitropyrene to bacterial mutagens in selected strains of *Salmonella typhimurium* (17).

In view of the established nasal carcinogenicity of formaldehyde, Dahl & Hadley (18) examined 32 potential substrates that might be metabolized to formaldehyde by rat nasal mucosa. Substrates demethylated at similar rates by nasal and liver microsomes were methamphetamine, propylhexedrine, cocaine, nicotine, dimethylaniline, and hexamethylphosphoramide. Rat nasal epithelium was found to oxidize benzo[α]pyrene to dihydrodiols, quinones, and phenols 10 times more rapidly than lung microsomes (19). Autoradiographic studies with [ethyl-^{14}C] phenacetin in rats (20) revealed that 5 minutes after an i.v. injection, radioactivity was highly concentrated in nasal mucosa—specifically subepithelial glands—associated with olfactory epithelium and also trachea. Incubation of tissue slices with phenacetin revealed that the O-deethylase capacity of nasal mucosa of rats was 10 times that of liver and over twenty times that of lung. Nasal mucosa of rabbits was approximately 7 times as rich in O-deethylase activity as liver. These activities were markedly inhibited by the monooxygenase inhibitors metyrapone and SKF 525-A. Injection of mice with [^{14}C]-chlorobenzene followed by autoradiography demonstrated covalent binding of the material that was selectively concentrated in the nasal and tracheo-bronchial epithelium. In the nose, radioactivity was bound to the subepithelial glands (Bowman's glands) underneath areas of olfactory epithelium (21).

TRACHEA   Like the nasal mucosa, the most common form of toxic insult to the tracheobronchial tree resulting from interaction with xenobiotics is malignant transformation. Recent reviews are available (22, 23), and because of the extensive size of the literature and the relative homogeneity of its toxic manifestations (carcinogenesis), we review the field briefly here.

Kaufman et al (24) incubated hamster tracheas with [^{3}H]-benzo[α]pyrene (BP), then isolated the tracheal epithelial cells, purified their DNA, and found it to contain covalently bound [^{3}H]-BP. Binding was enhanced if the tracheas were taken from hamsters previously exposed to BP plus Fe_2O_3. The authors concluded that tracheal epithelium is able to metabolize BP and that metabolism is required for the inducible binding of BP to tracheal epithelial DNA. Later carcinogenesis studies clearly demonstrated that in golden hamsters, the tracheal epithelium is the target tissue for the development of tumors by polycyclic hydrocarbons such as BP (25). Tracheal organ cultures and isolated tracheal microsomes catalyzed the binding of [³H]-BP to DNA in vitro. HPLC analysis revealed a variety of metabolic products such as phenols, quinones, tetrols, and diols (including the 7,8-dihydrodiol), subsequently shown to be the penultimate carcinogenic species.

When cloned hamster tracheal epithelial cells were incubated with [³H]-BP, adducts with DNA were formed (26). The cells formed the ultimate carcinogen, 7,8-dihydro-7,8-dihydroxy BP-9,10-epoxide, which reacted with deoxyadenosine, deoxycytosine, and deoxyguanosine; the DNA-carcinogen adducts were partially repaired during the course of the incubation. In addition to these biochemical events (27, 28), it was reported that incubation of rat tracheal organ culture in media containing 7,12-dimethybenz-[α]anthracene (DMBA), benz[α]anthracene, BP, or 3-methylcholanthrene (3-MC) produced morphologic alterations consisting of hyperplasia, metaplasia, and other general cytotoxic features. Following intratracheal administration of BP-Fe$_2$O$_3$ to rats and hamsters, there was a striking species difference in the distribution of lesions (29). In hamsters, squamous metaplasia of the trachea and large bronchi were observed, while in rats squamous nodules of bronchioalveolar origin developed. These differences correlated with penetration and persistence of BP in hamster tracheal epithelium but not in rat. Interestingly, when BP was incubated with tracheal organ cultures (23), binding to DNA in hamster trachea was 17 times greater than in rat trachea; this appears to correlate nicely with the relative species specificity for BP carcinogensis.

A vast literature exists on the organotropy of nitrosamines, specifically diethylnitrosamine (DEN) for the respiratory tract of the hamster (30). Although the bronchiolar nonciliated epithelial (Clara) cell is clearly the cellular site of covalent binding of [³H]-DEN and both metaplastic and neoplastic transformations, it should be noted that the mucous cells of the trachea and the ciliated and Clara cells of the bronchi are also cellular targets (31, 32).

BRONCHI   The capacity of human bronchus to metabolize and covalently bind carcinogenic aromatic hydrocarbons was reported by Harris et al (33). Specimens of bronchi (1 cm^2) were cultured for one week and then incubated with [³H]-BP. Total binding of BP depended on its concentration, incubation time, and temperature. [³H]-BP and its metabolites were bound to cellular macromolecules and to DNA isolated from bronchial mucosa. The cell types involved were predominantly ciliated and mucous cells. Earlier work by this group had shown that cultured human bronchial epithelium could also metabolize 7,12-dibenz[α,h]anthracene to molecular species that bound tightly to macromolecules including DNA. The same group demonstrated that cultured human bronchial epithelium catalyzed the demethylation of dimethylnitrosamine and 1,2-dimethylhydrazine to products that bound to both cellular DNA and protein (34). Bronchial DNA was methylated in both the O-6 and N-7 positions of guanine. Autrup et al (35) reported that cultured human bronchial epithelium in vitro converted [^{3}H]-BP to 7,8-dihydroxy-7,8-dihydro BP (the "dihydrodiol"), the penultimate carcinogenic species of BP. Aryl hydrocarbon hydroxylase (AHH) is a microsomal enzyme that catalyzes the oxidation of BP to metabolic products (phenols, quinones, epoxides; for review see Ref. 4) that ultimately bind covalently to DNA and initiate carcinogensis. Kahng et al (36) found that exposure of bronchial epithelium during culture to benz[α]anthracene induced AHH activity and the binding of [^{3}H]-BP to the epithelial DNA by as much as 29-fold.

BRONCHIOLES, ALVEOLI, AND VASCULAR ENDOTHELIUM   A number of excellent reviews have appeared on the role of metabolic activation of xenobiotics in lung injury (37, 39). Most of these involve attack of a reactive electrophilic intermediate on bronchiolar nonciliated (Clara) epithelial cells, alveolar type I or type II cells, or vascular endothelium. There are at least three general mechanisms by which xenobiotics elicit lung injury; others and/or combinations undoubtedly exist of which we are currently unaware. The first involves activation of the xenobiotic to a chemically reactive species that may covalently bind to vital macromolecules, frequently in a specific cell type, and cause malignant transformation or necrosis. This reactive intermediate may be formed in situ and act directly in the lung or be formed elsewhere (e.g. liver) and be transported to lung, where it exerts its toxic action. The second mechanism involves xenobiotics with appropriate redox characteristics that accept an electron from, for example, NADPH, with the formation of a free radical, such as R-ṄO$_2^-$. These radicals can transfer the electron to dioxygen (O$_2$), resulting in formation of another free radical called superoxide anion radical, O$_2^-$; through a series of redox steps, O$_2^-$ may give rise to ^{1}O$_2$ (singlet oxygen), H$_2$O$_2$, or ·OH$^-$, all four of which are toxic in varying degrees. Finally a few xenobiotics (bleomycin, O$_2$) attack the tight junctions between capillary endothelial cells causing leakage of serous, serofibrinous, or even hemorrhagic exudate into the alveolar space.

Pulmonary Toxicity of Oxygen

If adult rats are placed in 100% O$_2$ at 1 atmosphere pressure, virtually 100% of the animals are dead within 60–72 hours. The cause of death is pulmonary insufficiency resulting from massive fibrinous pulmonary edema (40). Microscopically one finds that the initial lesion is loosening and then necrosis of capillary endothelial cells followed by loss of type I alveolar epithelial cells. Interestingly, if rats are initially exposed to 85% O_2 (1 atm) for five or more days, they acquire tolerance and are able to survive for prolonged periods in 100% O_2. The chemical and biochemical mechanisms of acute O_2 toxicity and the origins of tolerance are reviewed extensively elsewhere (41, 42). Dioxygen (O_2) is thought to be toxic to tissues including lung because of its ability to generate free radicals (43). Dioxygen readily undergoes one electron reduction in biological systems with the formation of $O_2^{\cdot-}$, superoxide radical anion (41). This reaction may occur nonenzymatically or may be catalyzed by numerous enzymes such as NADPH cytochrome P-450 reductase, xanthine oxidase, and several mitochondrial enzymes. Once formed, superoxide may produce a number of further reduction products known collectively as reactive oxygen or oxyradicals. Superoxide may produce damage to mammalian cells and tissues either directly (i.e. by inactivating enzymes) or indirectly by stimulating lipid peroxidation. The sequential four-electron reduction of dioxygen may be depicted as

$$O_2 \xrightarrow{e^-} O_2^{\cdot-} \xrightarrow{e^-} H_2O_2 \xrightarrow{e^-} \cdot OH \xrightarrow{e^-} H_2O$$

Superoxide, hydrogen peroxide, singlet oxygen, and especially the highly reactive hydroxy radical ($\cdot OH$) are individually and collectively toxic to tissues and cells. Normally, tissues have defense mechanisms that protect them against the toxic effects of oxyradicals (44). Among these are superoxide dismutase (SOD), catalase, and glutathione peroxidase, together with tissue stores of α-tocopherol, reduced glutathione (GSH), and ascorbate. However, when these defenses are overwhelmed as in oxygen toxicity or paraquat poisoning (see below), toxic levels of various oxyradicals accumulate in tissues.

That oxyradicals are directly capable of evoking tissue damage was cleverly demonstrated by Johnson et al (45). Xanthine and xanthine oxidase (which together generate $O_2^{\cdot-}$) when instilled into the trachea of rats produced acute lung injury that was not produced by either of the two components singly or by saline. The lung injury was markedly reduced by intratracheal SOD (which degrades $O_2^{\cdot-}$) but not by catalase. Similar administration of glucose and glucose oxidase (which generate H_2O_2) produced lung injury of lesser magnitude; this was prevented by catalase that degrades H_2O_2. Finally, intratracheal administration of glucose and glucose oxidase plus lactoperoxidase, which presumably generate $^1O_2$ or HOCl, resulted in massive pulmonary edema and a fibrinous exudate in the alveolar space. Fourteen days later, the lungs were markedly hypercellular and exhibited extensive interstitial fibrosis. The progression to pulmonary fibrosis suggests that oxygen metabolites may be an important vector in the pathogenesis of interstitial pulmonary fibrosis.

Toxicity of Paraquat and Other Agents that Generate Reactive Oxygen Radicals

Paraquat, also known as methyl viologen, has been used as a redox reagent in chemistry for some years; it can accept an electron and be converted to a free radical; in the process it is transformed from colorless to blue. Its tremendous economic utility as a broad spectrum herbicide led to its widespread use and to the discovery that it is a lung toxin in animals and man.

Parenteral administration of paraquat to most mammalian species results in its selective accumulation in lung relative to other organs; 30 hours after dosing, there was six to seven times more paraquat in lung than in plasma of rats (46). Similarly, incubation of lung slices with paraquat reveals the remarkable capacity of this organ to concentrate the xenobiotic (46); slice/medium ratios ranging from $5:1$ to $15:1$ can be obtained. Accumulation does not occur by covalent binding. Paraquat uptake by lung is an active, energy-dependent uptake process that occurs against a concentration gradient and can be blocked in the usual ways; anaerobiosis, cold, iodoacetate, etc, and also by a variety of other amines that are themselves actively accumulated by lung slices, such as 5-hydroxytryptamine, norepinephrine, spermine, propanolol, imipramine, chlorpromazine, diphenhydramine, and chlorphentermine (37).

Liver or lung microsomes incubated aerobically with NADPH slowly oxidize NADPH; addition of paraquat results in massive increases in the rates of NADPH oxidation and oxygen uptake (47). Associated with this oxidative burst, one discovers a marked increase in O_2^- formation. These reactions are not blocked by carbon monoxide (CO) and are therefore not cytochrome P-450 dependent (48).

It is currently held that the mechanism by which paraquat damages tissues (lung, kidney, liver) is as follows:

$$PQ^{+2} \xrightarrow[\text{NADPH cytochrome } c \text{ reductase}]{\text{NADPH}} PQ^{+} \xrightarrow{\quad\quad\quad\quad} PQ^{+2}$$

$$O_2 \searrow O_2^-$$
$$\downarrow$$
$$H_2O_2$$
$$\downarrow$$
$$\cdot OH$$

In the presence of microsomes and NADPH, paraquat undergoes one-electron reduction to its free radical. This reaction is catalyzed by NADPH cytochrome c reductase (49). Under aerobic conditions, the paraquat free radical immediately transfers its electron to dioxygen with the formation of O_2^- and the regeneration of the paraquat cation. The net result of these reactions is that a reduction-oxidation cycle is set up in which paraquat functions catalytically, NADPH is consumed (NADPH/NADP falls) (47), and most importantly, enormous quantities of O_2^- are generated. Since oxyradicals (see the section on O_2 toxicity) are (a) themselves toxic and (b) able to stimulate lipid peroxidation that is destructive to biomembranes and also yields products (hydroxynonenals) that are cytotoxic (50), it is not possible at this time to identify the more toxic of these coincidental events.

As noted above, mammalian organisms have a variety of endogenous mechanisms to protect themselves from oxidant stress, the generation of large amounts of oxyradicals, and it is not until these defenses are overwhelmed that oxidant toxicity occurs. For example, superoxide dismutase (SOD) degrades O_2^-, catalase degrades H_2O_2, and glutathione peroxidase converts fatty acid hydroperoxides to alcohols (41, 42). In addition, tissue stores of α-tocopherol, reduced glutathione (GSH), and ascorbate scavenge oxyradicals. The toxicity of paraquat, defined either in terms of LD_{50} or LT_{50}, can be manipulated with the knowledge of these oxidant protective mechanisms. For example, hyperoxia (e.g. 100% O_2) markedly increases paraquat toxicity while hypoxia (10% O_2) reduces it (51). Depletion of tissue GSH stores by pretreatment with diethylmaleate or vitamin E deficiency dramatically increases paraquat toxicity. Similarly, selenium deficiency produced by dietary means also increases paraquat toxicity. Selenium is a component of glutathione peroxidase. There are two final points regarding paraquat worthy of note. All mammalian species studied to date except the rabbit, respond to paraquat with pulmonary lesions (52, 53). It is not clear whether the rabbit lung is absolutely refractory to the effects of paraquat or whether a higher dose is required in it than in other species. Finally, there is no convincing evidence to date that, other than the cyclic reduction and oxidation undergone by paraquat, there is any net biotransformation of the compound in vivo or in vitro.

The pathologic changes induced by paraquat in mammalian lung have been described in great detail (54). Animals receiving lethal doses of paraquat die in three phases; the most acute deaths (4–18 hours) result from massive pulmonary edema and hemorrhage into the alveolar space. A second group of animals die in 3–6 days from renal failure resulting from widespread necrosis of proximal renal tubular epithelium. Finally, depending on the dose and the species (14–20 days or longer in humans), death results from chronic respiratory failure coincident with massive pulmonary fibrosis. The latter stage, referred to as the proliferative phase (54), begins with the influx into lung of large numbers of fibroblasts with abundant rough endoplasmic reticulum. Fibroblastic activity results in the synthesis and deposition of large amounts of collagen into the extracellular space. The increased septal cellularity and increases in interstitial and intra-alveolar collagen eventually obliterate the alveolar and bronchiolar spaces, and the lung becomes a solid glandular-like organ incapable of either inflation or gas exchange. When the thorax is opened, the "paraquat lung" fails to collapse, exhibits a solid, rubbery consistency, and sinks in water.

Nitrofurantoin is an agent used clinically to treat urinary tract infections. Its use, particularly when administered chronically, is accompanied by pulmonary reactions, once thought to be "hypersensitivity reactions" (55), ranging from cough and dyspnea to infiltrates, effusion, and pulmonary fibrosis, which can be confirmed by pulmonary biopsy. Administration of large doses of nitrofurantoin to rats produced severe respiratory compromise that caused death in 12–36 hours. Tachypnea and cyanosis were conspicuous symptoms; at autopsy the lungs were grossly distended, edematous, and hemorrhagic. Histologically, there was widespread interstitial and alveolar edema, vascular congestion, and hemorrhagic consolidation (56). Perhaps more importantly, the lethality of nitrofurantoin could be manipulated broadly by factors known to be involved in lipid peroxidation. For example, the lethality and pulmonary damage produced by nitrofurantoin were significantly enhanced in rats maintained in 100% oxygen after drug administration (56). Similarly, the lethality was greatly enhanced in rats maintained on a vitamin E deficient diet that was rich in polyunsaturated fat (corn oil). The LD_{50} of nitrofurantoin in this group was 35 mg/kg compared to 400 mg/kg in controls. If vitamin E–deficient rats were repleted with vitamin E, the lethality of nitrofurantoin returned to that of controls.

These findings should be integrated with those of Mason & Holtzman (57) that under aerobic conditions and in the presence of NADPH, microsomes catalyze a one-electron reduction of the nitro group of nitrofurantoin to yield a nitro free radical $(R\text{-}NO_2^-)$ that spontaneously reacts with oxygen to regenerate the parent nitro compound and simultaneously reduces oxygen to $O_2^{-\cdot}$. Although covalent binding of nitrofurantoin can be demonstrated under anaerobic conditions in vitro, under aerobic conditions little covalent binding occurs but large amounts of superoxide are formed in the presence of lung microsomes, NADPH, and nitrofurantoin. Thus it seems likely that the pneumotoxicity of nitrofurantoin is mediated through superoxide and its secondary metabolites, H_2O_2 and $\cdot OH^-$. The mechanism of toxicity therefore seems to bear a strong resemblance to that of paraquat and high concentrations of oxygen itself.

Pulmonary Toxicity of Covalently Bound Xenobiotics

Recent lengthy reviews (38, 58) have explored this area in exquisite detail, and space limitations do not permit reiteration here. Table 1 lists some of the xenobiotics that have been shown to undergo oxidation to reactive intermediates either in lung or elsewhere, to bind covalently in lung, and to produce toxicities. Some xenobiotics that produce lung injury by as yet unknown mechanisms are noted as well.

Table 1   Some xenobiotics that undergo metabolic activation and bind covalently in lung and/or produce pulmonary injury.

Agent	Covalent binding in lung demonstrated	Reference
Polycyclic aromatic hydrocarbons (benzo[α]pyrene, 3-methylcholanthrene)	+	62
Naphthalenes (naphthalene, 2-methylnapthalene)	+	64, 65
4-Ipomeanol	+	66
3-Methylfuran	+	67
Bromobenzene	+	68
3-methylindole	+	69
Butylated hydroxytoluene (BHT)	+	70
Carbon tetrachloride	+	71
1,1-Dichloroethylene (DCE)	+	72
0,0,S-Trimethylphosphorothioate (contaminant of malathion)	+	73
p-Xylene	+	74
α-Naphthylthiourea (ANTU)	+	58
Pyrollizidine alkaloids (monocrotaline)	+	58
Methylcyclopentadiethyl Mn tricarbonyl		
Bleomycins		
Nitrosoureas		
Mitomycin C		
Melphalan		
Cyclophosphamide	+	75, 76

Space limitations preclude discussion of all the agents in Table 1; because so much information is available on 4-ipomeanol and because many of the agents are thought to act through similar mechanisms, 4-ipomeanol is discussed here as a prototype of metabolically activated pulmonary toxins.

4-Ipomeanol [1-(3-furyl)-4 hydroxy-pentanone] is a natural product secreted by moldy sweet potatoes. Cattle consuming such sweet potatoes developed severe, occasionally fatal pulmonary insufficiency; necropsy revealed severe pulmonary edema and hemorrhage. Most of the published data on the biochemical toxicology of 4-ipomeanol are from the laboratory of Boyd and his co-workers (58).

Administration of 4-ipomeanol to rats, rabbits, guinea pigs, and hamsters results in an organ- and cell-specific lesion, viz, selective necrosis of the nonciliated bronchiolar (Clara) cells of the lung. Larger doses cause less specific effects in which ciliated bronchiolar cells are also involved and which eventually affect the alveolar epithelium and vascular endothelial cells. Larger doses evoke massive intra-alveolar edema and hemorrhage, together with pleural effusion. Higher doses produce hepatic and renal lesions. In contrast to rabbits, rats, and other species that display pulmonary lesions in response to 4-ipomeanol, adult male mice exhibit renal cortical necrosis as a primary lesion; female mice and immature mice of either sex are remarkably resistant to this renal insult. Taking advantage of an interesting phylogenetic peculiarity, Buckpitt et al (59) demonstrated that birds (Japanese quail, chickens), whose respiratory tracts lack Clara cells, fail to develop lung damage after 4-ipomeanol. Instead these species develop severe hepatic injury with no evidence of pulmonary involvement such as necrosis, edema, or hemorrhage. In accord with these findings microsomes prepared from lung and liver of rats, guinea pigs, hamsters, and rabbits catalyzed the metabolic activation and covalent binding of 4-ipomeanol in vitro as did microsomes from kidneys of adult male mice. In each case, metabolic activation in vitro correlated with target organ toxicity in vivo. Similarly chicken liver microsomes activated and covalently bound 4-ipomeanol in vitro, while chicken lung microsomes were devoid of activity.

Following parenteral administration of [14C] or [3H]-labeled 4-ipomeanol to rats or rabbits, covalently bound radioactivity is selectively concentrated in lung; smaller amounts are found in liver, kidney, and gut. For example, in rats 24 hr after i.p. administration of 4-ipomeanol (covalently bound material expressed per gram wet weight of organ), liver had 40% that of lung, kidney 25%, and ileum less than 10%. Cell fractionation studies showed that covalently bound material was not concentrated in any particular fraction; in the microsomal fractions, binding was to protein, not phospholipid or RNA. Autoradiography of lungs removed from animals treated 2–4 hours earlier with [3H]-ipomeanol revealed that the covalently bound material was exclusively distributed in Clara cells; adjacent ciliated cells of alveolar epithelial cells were minimally labeled. The covalent binding by Clara cells preceded morphologic evidence of injury by about 12 hours; 16 hours after injection of 4-ipomeanol, Clara cells were undergoing pyknosis and massive cytoplasmic vacualization; necrotic cells were sloughing away from the basal lamina into the bronchiolar lumen.

In vitro studies revealed that when [14C] 4-ipomeanol was incubated with NADPH and subcellular fractions of rat lung and liver, the microsomal fractions were clearly most active in catalyzing covalent binding (60). That metabolic activation of 4-ipomeanol was required before covalent binding could occur was demonstrated by the observations that heat denaturation of microsomes or incubation at 2° essentially abolished binding. Maximum binding occurred in the presence of microsomes, O_2, and NADPH; covalent binding was inhibited by CO, SKF 525-A, and piperonyl butoxide (which implies a role for cytochrome P-450), and also by the presence of cytochrome c or an antibody to NADPH cytochrome c reductase (which clearly indicates participation of the latter enzyme). Covalent binding in vitro was also reduced by the presence of reduced glutathione (GSH), which suggests an active electrophile as a metabolic intermediate. Similarly, depletion of tissue stores of GSH in vivo by pretreatment with diethylmaleate markedly increased covalent binding of 4-ipomeanol. Interestingly, it was found that an antibody to cytochrome b_5 blocked the covalent binding of 4-ipomeanol to rat lung microsomes but not to rat liver microsomes. Relatively poor correlation occurred between total levels of cytochrome P-450 and covalent binding; for example, liver and kidney had higher cytochrome P-450 content then lung but lower covalent binding. On the other hand, lung damage and lethal toxicity correlated well with the amount of covalent binding. An interesting tolerance could be produced to 4-ipomeanol; administration of multiple small doses of the agent increased the acute LD_{50} by about threefold or more. This was not due to inactivation of the monooxygenase system, which activates 4-ipomeanol to the reactive electrophilic species as was shown to explain a similar tolerance to CCl_4 (61).

Knowledge as to the chemical nature of the covalent binding species of xenobiotics has been scanty. Only in the past five years has the dihydrodiol epoxide of benzo[α]pyrene been identified as the active species (62) of the hydrocarbon that actually binds to DNA. Studies on the mechanism of furan binding in lung have utilized the analog 3-methylfuran, which has many of the same biological effects as 4-ipomeanol itself, for example pulmonary toxicity and covalent binding. Recent work in Boyd's laboratory (63) showed that in the presence of NADPH and microsomes from rat lung or liver, 3-methylfuran undergoes ring opening at the oxygen with the formation of 2-methyl-2-butene-1,4-dial. The latter compound binds covalently to microsomes and presumably mediates the toxicity of 3-methylfuran. This finding confirms earlier work on structural studies in the 4-ipomeanol series showing that the presence of the furan ring was essential for metabolic activation and covalent binding to microsomes.

Until recent years it was widely believed that electrophilic metabolic intermediates were so reactive that they reacted with biomolecules at or very near their sites of formation. However, recent work has made it clear that active metabolites of bromobenzene, naphthalene, 1,1-dichloroethylene, and undoubtedly other compounds are sufficiently stable so that they may diffuse out of cells and be carried to organs throughout the body where they bind covalently and may exert toxic effects.

KIDNEY

A number of organic compounds are known to be metabolically activated and cause nephrotoxicity. They are discussed in detail elsewhere (77, 78).

Chloroform

Chloroform ($CHCl_3$) is both hepatotoxic and nephrotoxic in most animal species. $CHCl_3$-induced hepatic damage is manifested predominantly as centrilobular necrosis while the renal lesion is necrosis of the proximal tubules. Renal damage is reflected functionally by proteinuria, glucosuria, and increased blood urea nitrogen. In vitro, renal $CHCl_3$ toxicity is accompanied by reduced ability of renal cortical slices to accumulate organic ions such as p-aminohippurate and tetraethylammonium (77).

Administration of [^{14}C]-$CHCl_3$ to mice produced proximal renal tubular necrosis that was accompanied by extensive covalent binding of radiolabel in both kidney and liver. Autoradiograms revealed that in kidney the covalent binding was predominantly localized over the necrotic tubules. Covalent binding of $CHCl_3$ in liver of male and female mice was similar, whereas binding in kidney of male mice was nearly 10 times greater than in females (79).

Abundant experimental work has confirmed that, in mice, $CHCl_3$ nephrotoxicity occurs only in males while the hepatotoxicity is similar in both sexes. The sex difference in nephrotoxicity is apparently mediated by testosterone; immature or castrated male mice are not susceptible to $CHCl_3$ nephrotoxicity whereas female mice or castrated males injected with testosterone are susceptible (80). The high renal sensitivity of male mice to the toxic effects of $CHCl_3$ has been found to correlate with levels of renal cytochrome P-450 and P-450-linked monooxygenases that are 3–5 times higher in males than in females (80). An additional important clue to the possible involvement of metabolism in $CHCl_3$ nephrotoxicity was the observation that $CDCl_3$ was much less toxic than $CHCl_3$ when incubated with kidney slices from male mice. Organic ion uptake by slices was reduced 15–25% by $CDCl_3$ and 70–90% by $CHCl_3$ (81). Incubation of microsomes from the renal cortex of male mice in the presence of [^{14}C]-$CHCl_3$, NADPH, and O_2 resulted in the formation of [^{14}C]-CO_2 and covalently bound material. Microsomes from female mice were inactive.

That the reaction in male kidneys required NADPH and O_2 and was inhibited by CO, SKF 525-A, and metyrapone suggested a cytochrome P-450–dependent mechanism (82). Later work revealed that renal homogenates or microsomes from male mice oxidize $CHCl_3$ in a P-450–dependent reaction to trichloromethanol (HO-C-Cl_3) that is unstable and spontaneously dehydrochlorinates to yield phosgene ($Cl_2C{=}O$) (83). This step is rate-limiting, and since the C-D bond is stronger than the C-H bond, $CDCl_3$ is less toxic than $CHCl_3$. Phosgene, a highly toxic electrophile, may react with tissue components or with water to give CO_2 and HCl. It can also react with two moles of GSH to form diglutathionyl dithiocarbonate, which in the presence of renal γ-glutamyltranspeptidase and other factors can be converted to the cyclized product 2-oxothiazolidine-4-carboxylic acid (OTZ). Renal glutathione levels are depleted in the process, and pretreatment with diethylmaleate markedly potentiates $CHCl_3$ nephrotoxicity in male mice but not in female mice (84, 85).

Thus, available data suggest that the nephrotoxic species resulting from $CHCl_3$ administration to animals may be phosgene, which is likely formed within the kidney.

Hexachloro-1,3-butadiene

1,1,2,3,4,4-hexachloro-1,3-butadiene (HCBD) is a relatively selective nephrotoxin which when administered to rats causes marked diuresis (i.e. reduced urinary concentrating ability), glucosuria, proteinuria, and increased urinary excretion of alkaline phosphatase and N-acetyl β-glucosaminidase (77). Microscopically one observes selective necrosis of the straight segment (S_3 cells) of the proximal tubules located in the outer zone of the medulla that are characterized by loss of the brush border. Although HCBD is a potent nephrotoxin in rats, it has little morphologic or functional effect in liver. In rats, there is a dramatic sex difference in response to HCBD. For example, a marked depletion of hepatic GSH was observed in male rats after HCBD, whereas no depletion was found in kidney (86). In contrast, female rats, which are much more susceptible to the nephrotoxic effects of this compound, display minimal depletion of hepatic GSH but significant depletion in kidney. Finally, pretreatment of male rats with diethylmaleate, which reduces both hepatic and renal GSH, markedly enhanced the nephrotoxicity of HCBD.

Studies in vitro (87) revealed that incubation of HCBD with glutathione and microsomes or cytosol from either male or female rats resulted in a marked reduction in the GSH concentration. Addition of NADPH to this mixture did not enhance the rate of GSH consumption, which suggests that prior activation of HCBD by a cytochrome P-450 mechanism was not required. Chromatographic and mass spectral analysis of the incubation media allowed characterization of a metabolite, S-(1,1,2,3,4-pentachloro-1,3-butadienyl) glutathione, which indicates formation of an adduct between HCBD and GSH with the elimination of one chlorine. This conjugate was formed at a much faster rate by hepatic microsomes than cytosol (in the presence of exogenous GSH); hence microsomal glutathione S-transferase, as opposed to one of the several cytosolic forms, may predominate in the formation of this adduct, at least in vitro. Adduct formation was uninfluenced by N_2, CO, or the absence of NADPH; the only cofactor requirement was GSH. Glutathione adducts were also formed by renal cytosol from male and female rats but at much slower rates than hepatic fractions.

The toxicology of HCBD and its GSH conjugates was investigated in vivo by Nash et al (88). A nephrotoxic dose of HCBD (200 mg/kg) was administered to male rats, and its excretion into bile was monitored; the major biliary metabolites were a HCBD-glutathione conjugate and smaller amounts of the cysteinylglycine conjugate. The biliary metabolites of HCBD were found to be reabsorbed from the gut and excreted by the kidneys. The glutathione conjugate, its synthetic mercapturic acid derivative, and lyophilized bile containing HCBD metabolites were all nephrotoxic when administered orally to rats. Rats prepared with biliary cannulae that were exteriorized, thus diverting bile from the intestine, were completely protected from renal damage when dosed with HCBD. Thus, it appears that the GSH conjugate of HCBD or one of its degradation products (such as the cysteinylglycine or cysteine conjugate or the mercapturic acid excreted in bile and reabsorbed from the gut) is responsible for the renal toxicity of HCBD. Reabsorption of the conjugate from the gut is more likely after degradation to the lower molecular weight, more lipophilic cysteinylglycine or cysteine conjugates.

Recent work has revealed the presence of an enzyme in renal tubular cells known as cysteine conjugate (C-S) or β-lyase that cleaves the cysteine but not GSH or N-acetylcysteine (mercapturic acid) conjugate to form a reactive fragment containing sulfur (89). The nature of the sulfur is not presently known but it could be a mercaptan (R-C-SH), a sulfenic acid (R-C-SOH), or methylation of the mercaptan followed by oxidation at sulfur could result in products such as R-C-S-CH$_3$, R-C-SO-CH$_3$ (methylsulfinyl), or R-C-SO$_2$-CH$_3$ (methylsulfonyl) (90). Conjugates of other xenobiotics and GSH are toxic: incubation of 1,2-dibromothane (a carcinogen) with DNA in the presence of GSH and glutathione S-transferases results in formation of the adduct S-[2-(N^7-guanyl)ethyl]glutathione (91). Furthermore, sulfur-containing metabolites that could arise from S-(2-chloroethyl) glutathione or the nephrotoxic S-(2-chloroethyl) cysteine have been isolated from the urine of rats treated with the nephrotoxin 1,2-dichloroethane (91). Thus, although the precise metabolic product of HCBD responsible for its nephrotoxicity is not known, its S-substituted cysteine conjugates or their further metabolism by β-lyase to yield reactive sulfur-containing moieties are likely to be involved in the renal toxicity. Green et al (92) reported that the cysteine conjugate of HCBD is cleaved by β-lyase to the mercaptan that is oxidized to the sulfenic acid (R-C-S-OH), which is both nephrotoxic and highly mutagenic.

It is worthy of note that Miyajima et al (93) have compared the utility of histological and functional criteria in evaluating the nephrotoxicity of HgCl$_2$, K$_2$Cr$_2$O$_7$ and cephaloridine utilizing relative kidney weight, uptake of the organic ions p-aminohippurate and tetraethylammonium by slices, BUN, and histology. The authors concluded that renal cortical accumulation of organic ions appeared to be the most sensitive of the functional parameters but that quantitative histological evaluation was equally sensitive as an indicator of nephrotoxicity.

Cephaloridine

Cephaloridine, in contrast to various other cephalosporins and structurally related penicillins, undergoes little or no net secretion by the mammalian kidney (94). Nonetheless, cephaloridine is highly cytotoxic to the proximal renal tubules—the outer stripe of the cortex—which is the segment of the nephron responsible for secreting organic anions such as p-aminohippurate. The cytotoxicity of cephaloridine correlates with high renal cortical drug levels and is reduced or completely prevented by probenecid and other inhibitors of organic ion transport that also reduce the cortical concentration of cephaloridine. The massive accumulation of the drug in the proximal tubular cells appears to result from a paradoxical combination of two factors: active secretion of the drug from the peritubular blood into the cells of the proximal tubule, and a highly limited capacity of the tubular cells to transport the drug into the tubular urine. The very high cortical content of cephaloridine appears to represent and result from a relatively trapped cellular pool in the proximal tubules that is larger than that of p-aminohippurate.

There appears to be a good correlation between renal cortical accumulation of cephaloridine and nephrotoxicity. Thus, administration of the drug to rabbits, guinea pigs, and rats results in highest cortical concentration in rabbit and lowest in rat kidneys. This correlates with the susceptibility of each species to cephaloridine nephrotoxicity. In addition, young animals that did not concentrate cephaloridine to the same extent as older animals, were not as susceptible to cephaloridine nephrotoxicity. Further, as pointed out above, probenecid reduces cortical concentration of cephaloridine and also protects against its nephrotoxicity.

Kuo & Hook (95) studied cephaloridine nephrotoxicity in three species using morphologic and functional criteria. They found that the toxicity was rabbit > rat > mouse and also that cephaloridine produced a dose-related depletion of GSH in renal cortex but not in medulla. The relative susceptibility of the three species to renal GSH depletion paralleled species differences in cephaloridine nephrotoxicity. Pretreatment of animals with diethylmaleate potentiated cephaloridine nephrotoxicity; this strongly suggests a correlation between GSH depletion and cephaloridine toxicity. Kuo et al (96) demonstrated differential effects of phenobarbital pretreatment on cephaloridine toxicity in kidneys of rats unresponsive to the inductive effects of phenobarbital and rabbits that exhibit phenobarbital induction. Phenobarbital induced monooxygenase activities in rabbit kidneys and also potentiated cephaloridine toxicity. Similar treatment of rats had no effect on renal enzymes nor did it affect cephaloridine toxicity. These data suggested that cephaloridine may have been bioactivated in kidney, thus enhancing its toxicity. However, further analysis showed that phenobarbital differentially increased cephaloridine concentration in renal cortex of rabbits (approximately twofold) but had no effect in rats. Thus, the potentiating effect of phenobarbital on cephaloridine nephrotoxicity in rabbits was more likely due to the increased renal cortical accumulation of cephaloridine, the parent drug, rather than an effect on bioactivation. This experiment also emphasizes the obvious fact that microsomal enzyme inducers frequently have multiple effects.

Bromobenzene

Reid (97) demonstrated that [^{14}C]-labeled bromobenzene administered to mice or rats produced necrosis of the proximal renal tubules that was associated with substantial covalent binding of radiolabel in the necrotic cells. Prior treatment of animals with piperonyl butoxide blocked both the covalent binding and the necrogenic effects of bromobenzene. It was concluded that an activated metabolite of bromobenzene (not the parent compound) was responsible for the covalent binding and the renal tubular necrosis and that the metabolite was formed in the liver and transported to the kidney. Bromobenzene is now known to be initially activated by a cytochrome P-450 mechanism to its 2,3- and 3,4-oxides, which may then undergo enzymatic and nonenzymatic conversion to a number of products, among them o- and p-bromophenol, which in turn can be converted to 4-bromocatechol, 4-bromoquinone or hydroquinone, or 2-bromoquinone or hydroquinone (98). o-Bromophenol caused a 50% reduction in renal GSH in rats within ninety minutes, whereas hepatic GSH levels were reduced by only 20% after five hr. Thus, renal GSH was far more susceptible to the initial depleting effects of o-bromophenol than hepatic GSH. In rats, o-bromophenol caused severe renal necrosis associated with elevations in BUN levels (2–3-fold). Liver microsomes converted o-bromophenol to covalently bound material while kidney microsomes did not (99). However, in vivo, o-bromophenol covalently bound to kidney protein in amounts four times greater than to liver protein. Phenobarbital treatment increased covalent binding in vivo to kidney and also increased BUN levels but did not increase covalent binding to liver, which indicates that the nephrotoxic metabolite of o-bromophenol may be generated in liver and transported to kidney.

2-Bromohydroquinone was identified as a metabolite of both bromobenzene and o-bromophenol in the rat (98). Administration of 2-bromohydroquinone to rats caused a dose- and time-dependent decrease in hepatic and renal GSH levels, an increase in BUN, and histopathological changes in kidney (proximal tubular necrosis) without causing alterations in liver. The histologic changes in kidney were indistinguishable from those produced by either bromobenzene or o-bromophenol, but the dose of 2-bromoquinone required to produce similar nephrotoxicity was < 10% that of bromobenzene.

Following administration of bromobenzene to mice (100), p- and o-bromophenol were the major urinary metabolites, although m-bromophenol and 4-bromocatechol were also excreted, all as conjugates. 4-Bromocatechol and 3-bromophenolic isomers were all nephrotoxicants, measured in vivo as increased BUN or in vitro as impaired accumulation of organic anions by renal cortical slices; but they were not hepatotoxicants at equal doses. 4-Bromocatechol was the most nephrotoxic of the four compounds both in vitro and in vivo, resulting in a dose-dependent decrease in renal function while hepatic function was altered only slightly at the higher doses. The renal cortical necrosis produced by 4-bromocatechol administration to mice could not be distinguished histologically from that evoked by bromobenzene.

Therefore, depending on the species, it would appear as if 2-bromohydroquinone or 4-bromocatechol or some metabolite—oxidative or conjugative—is the proximate nephrotoxin derived from bromobenzene. This question remains open (see note added in proof at end of text).

Acetaminophen

About the same time that the hepatotoxicity of large doses of acetaminophen was being studied vigorously, McMurtry et al (101) reported that a mechanism similar to that being described in liver was apparently involved in a nephrotoxicity of acetaminophen. Thus, a single large dose of acetaminophen (~1 g/kg) administered to Fischer 344 rats elicited a dose-dependent acute renal necrosis confined primarily to the distal portions of the proximal tubule (pars rectus). Glomeruli and early proximal convolutions were largely unaffected. These doses of acetaminophen caused both hepatic and renal necrosis, markedly depleted target organ GSH, and resulted in large amounts of radiolabeled metabolite being bound to renal and hepatic protein. It was concluded that this tissue injury resulted from the activation of acetaminophen in situ to a chemically reactive species capable of covalently binding to tissue macromolecules. That the metabolic activation occurred in situ was demonstrated by Breen et al (102), who showed, that after administration of ^{3}H-acetaminophen to rats, covalent binding occurred in both kidney and lung, and that the binding in these tissues was unaffected by total hepatectomy.

Newton and co-workers (103) demonstrated a marked strain difference in rats in susceptibility to acetaminophen-produced renal damage. Acetaminophen produced renal necrosis—restricted to the straight segment of the proximal tubule—in Fischer 344 rats but not in Sprague-Dawley rats. Acetaminophen-induced renal functional changes such as elevation in BUN and impairment in the accumulation of p-aminohippurate by renal cortical slices also correlated with strain-dependent histopathologic changes. However, covalent binding of ring-labeled acetaminophen to renal and hepatic microsomal protein in vitro was the same in the two rat strains as was deacetylation of acetaminophen to p-aminophenol. Thus the strain differences in acetaminophen could not be attributed to differences in P-450-linked activation of parent drug or in the deacetylation to the nephrotoxic metabolite, p-aminophenol. Administration of p-aminophenol to Fischer and to Sprague-Dawley rats resulted in renal lesions in both strains indistinguishable from the acetaminophen-induced renal lesion in Fischer rats. However, covalent binding of p-aminophenol to renal microsomes in vitro was much greater in the sensitive Fischer rats than in the resistant Sprague-Dawley strain. In addition, covalent binding of p-aminophenol or a metabolite thereof was 5–10 times greater in kidney than in liver. It was concluded that strain differences in acetaminophen nephrotoxicity in rats might result from strain differences in the intrarenal metabolic activation of the metabolite p-aminophenol to an arylating species (104).

TESTIS

1,2-Dibromo-3-chloropropane

The literature reveals a pronounced dichotomy in our knowledge of the biological properties of 1,2-dibromo-3-chloropropane (DBCP). A rather great deal is known about the clinical effects of the compound both in humans and experimental animals but little information is available at the molecular level.

Other than renal tubular necrosis observed at high doses (105), the predominant effect of DBCP is gonadal hypofunction, seen only in males. DBCP is an effective nematocide when applied to soil or a variety of edible plants such as peaches, citrus fruits, tomatoes, bananas, and pineapples. Male workers employed in the manufacture of this compound were observed to have a severe impairment of spermatogenesis, azoospermia, and elevated plasma FSH and LH levels (106). Oligospermia was found in workers with lower exposure levels. Testicular biopsy showed selective atrophy of the germinal epithelium (spermatocytes and spermatids); Sertoli cells, from which spermatocytes are generated, were histologically normal as were Leydig (androgen-secreting) cells. No necrotic or inflammatory changes were observed in the seminiferous tubules, merely an absence of spermatogenic activity (107). In humans, the severe oligospermia resulting from DBCP exposure was slowly reversible, requiring 18–21 months following discontinuation of exposure; recovery occurred histologically and in sperm counts (108). Rao et al (109) exposed rabbits to concentrations of 0.1, 1, and 10 ppm DBCP by inhalation for 8–14 weeks. Sperm counts and breeding success followed a dose-response curve. Testicular atrophy was noted in the two highest dose groups (the intermediate dose produced 50% loss of testicular weight at 14 weeks).

Serum testosterone levels were comparable to controls or slightly elevated in exposed animals. Reversibility of these testicular alterations was proportional to dose. Animals exposed to the highest concentration of DBCP had oligospermia and abnormal testicular histology 38 weeks after cessation of exposure. It is worth noting that male mice have been reported to be resistant to the testicular effects of DBCP (110).

DBCP might be expected to undergo conjugation with GSH in the presence of glutathione S-transferase, and this reaction has indeed been demonstrated in vitro (111). Jones and co-workers (112) administered DBCP to rats and reported formation of 1-chloro-2,3-propanediol (α-chlorohydrin) and 1-bromo-2,3-propanediol (α-bromohydrin), formed through the intermediacy of the 2,3-epoxide. They also isolated S-(2,3-dihydroxypropyl)cysteine and 1,3-(bis-cysteinyl)propan-2-ol from urine. Sixteen days after i.p. administration of DBCP to male rats (50 mg/kg), testicular weight was reduced by nearly 50%; body weight and kidney weight were unaffected. The isolation of α-chlorohydrin was of great importance since earlier work (113) had shown this compound to be a potent chemosterilant in male rats. Low doses of α-chlorohydrin (10 mg/kg for 14 days) had been shown, based on serial matings, to have pronounced antifertility activity in male rats, activity apparent within 3–6 days after first administration; cessation of exposure was followed by return to normal fertility. This effect was also shown to occur in guinea pigs, hamsters, rhesus monkeys, rams, and boars and was not accompanied by alterations in sperm count, motility, or morphology. The mechanism of this antifertility effect was unexplained. Higher doses of α-chlorohydrin were accompanied by testicular atrophy and a blockage of the efferent ducts of the epididymis resulting in spermatoceles and sperm-granulomata.

Kluwe et al (113a) compared in male rats the gonadal toxicity of DBCP and its metabolites 3-chloro-1,2-propane epoxide (epichlorohydrin), 3-chloro-1,2-propanediol (α-chlorohydrin), and oxalic acid. Although a threefold difference in potency was noted (DBCP was most active, α-chlorohydrin least active), DBCP and its two halogenated metabolites produced similar impairment of testicular function while oxalic acid was inactive. DBCP, epichlorohydrin, and α-chlorohydrin produced progressive testicular atrophy and hyposperma-togenesis; the latter two compounds also produced sperm granulomas, sperma-toceles and an increased number of morphologically abnormal spermatozoa (113a). Following a single dose of DBCP, atrophic seminiferous tubules devoid of spermatazoa persisted for as long as 25 days and testicular atrophy (~50%) persisted as long as 75 days.

Metabolic studies with α-chlorohydrin (3-chloro-1,2-propanediol) in male rats revealed a number of products, among them: loss of chlorine resulting in the formation of 1,2-epoxy-3-propanol (glycidol) followed by conjugation with GSH at the epoxy function resulting in the 1-cysteine and N-acetylcysteine derivatives [S-(2,3-dihydroxypropyl)cysteine] and the mercapturic acid [N-acetyl-S-(2,3-dihydroxypropyl)cysteine] (113).

It should be noted that compounds chemically related to DBCP have been reported to provoke testicular atrophy, aspermatogenesis, epididymal lesions, and other reproductive abnormalities in male animals. Among these are chloro-methane (methyl chloride) (114), 1,2-dibromomethane (115), tris[tris(2,3-

dibromopropyl)phosphate] (116), chlordecone, carbon disulfide, vinyl chloride, and 2-chlorobuta-1,3-diene (chloroprene) (117).

Benzo[α]pyrene

The metabolism of benzo[α]pyrene by the isolated perfused rat testis and by testicular homogenates has been described (118, 119) but no effort was made to relate this metabolism to toxicity.

OVARY

Benzo[α]pyrene

Mattison & Thorgeirsson (120) reported that aryl hydrocarbon hydroxylase (AHH) activity was localized in the microsomal fraction of murine ovary, was NADPH and oxygen dependent, and was inhibited by CO and by an antibody to NADPH cytochrome c reductase. Pretreatment of animals with 3-MC increased ovarian AHH activity in three rat strains (about threefold), and nearly doubled activity in C57B1/ 6N (B6) mice but had no affect in DBA/2N (D2) mice. Interestingly, the toxicity of 3-MC to oocytes in mice and rats was dramatically different. A histologic technique was devised that permitted quantitative analysis of all the oocytes in a whole ovary. It was found that 7 days after a single i.p. dose of 3-MC (80 mg/kg), 87% of the primordial oocytes were destroyed in the ovaries of B6 mice, 69% were destroyed in D2 mice, but there was no change in oocytes in the ovaries of Sprague-Dawley rats. The data were interpreted to suggest that the oocyte toxicity of 3-MC in mice was related to ovarian AHH activity whereas no association was apparent between ovarian AHH activity and oocyte toxicity in the rat. Moreover, in mice, there is a striking relationship between oocyte destruction and ovarian granulosa cell tumor formation (121). Later work confirmed that ovarian AHH activity in D2 mice was relatively unresponsive to pretreatment with 3-MC but was induced 2–3-fold in B6 mice; basal ovarian AHH activity was similar in both strains (122). However, primordial oocytes of both D2 and B6 mice were destroyed by the carcinogenic hydrocarbons 3-MC, BP, and 7,12-dimethylbenz[α]-anthracene (DMBA) but not by the noncarcinogens pyrene, and α- and β-naphthoflavone (Table 2). The rate of oocyte destruction was faster in responsive B6 mice than in nonresponsive D2 mice. Sprague-Dawley rats were consistently less responsive to the destruction of primordial oocytes by BP, 3-MC, and DMBA than either D2 or B6 mice (123).

Pretreatment of female DBA/2N mice with BP reduced their fertility in a dose-dependent manner; mice receiving a single i.p. dose of BP of 200 or 500 mg/kg were completely infertile when mated 14 days later (Table 3) (124). This was in accord with earlier suggestions that tobacco smoke, which contains BP, might decrease fertility and produce a premature menopause (125) in humans.

Table 2 Effect of various polycyclic hydrocarbons on residual primordial oocytes six days after administration to mice[a]

Treatment[b]	Number of primordial oocytes/ovary	
	DBA/2N mice (D2)	C7B1/6N mice(B6)
Control	5240	3700
β-Naphthoflavone	4945	3555
Pyrene	4240	3216
BP	4493	1233[c]
3-MC	2763[c]	33[c]
7,12-Dimethybenz[α]anthracene	897[c]	20[c]

[a]Taken in part from Mattison & Thorgeirsson, with permission (122).
[b]Compounds administered in a single dose, 80 mg/kg, i.p., 6 days prior to sacrifice.
[c]Significantly different from control ($p < .05$).

BP administered to mice also destroyed primordial oocytes in a dose-related manner but did not reduce the ovarian response to pregnant mare's serum gonadotropin, which suggests that BP acted upon primordial oocytes and not upon growing or preovulatory oocytes or follicles (124). Because α-naphthoflavone, a competitive inhibitor of BP metabolism, blocks the destruction of primordial oocytes, it was suggested that this destruction depends in part on the formation of reactive ovotoxic metabolites with destruction occurring more rapidly in mice with higher rates of ovarian metabolism.

Female C57B1/6N(B6) and DBA/2N mice were dosed with 80 mg/kg i.p. of several polycyclic hydrocarbons. BP, 3-MC, and DMBA destroyed primordial oocytes and the rate of destruction was proportional to the (induced) ovarian AHH activity. After treatment with BP or 3-MC only primordial oocyte destruction occurred with no evidence of toxicity in contiguous granulosa or ovarian stromal cells. DMBA was more generally toxic and destroyed large follicles and oocytes in addition to primordial oocytes and primary follicles. Seven weeks after 3-MC, the ovary had the afollicular histologic appearance of ovarian failure. All three of these hydrocarbons (BP, 3-MC, DMBA) are capable of producing premature ovarian failure in rodents (126).

BP in doses ranging from 10 ng to 10 μg was injected (1 μl corn oil) directly into the ovaries of B6 and D2 mice (126a). Bilateral intraovarian injection of BP was ovotoxic in a time- and dose-related manner. Corn oil alone was without effect. Primordial oocyte destruction was maximal eight days after injection in both mouse strains. Unilateral injection destroyed oocytes only in the treated ovary and i.p. administration of α-naphthoflavone inhibited the oocyte destruction by the highest dose (10 μg) of BP in both strains. Fourteen days after bilateral intraovarian injection, approximately 80% of the primordial oocytes had been destroyed in B6 mice and about 50% in D2 mice. Bilateral in-

Table 3   Effect of benzo[α]pyrene (BP) treatment on some reproductive parameters in female DBA/2N mice[a]

BP dose (mg/kg)	Reproductive performance		Primordial oocytes/ovary	Oocyte destruction (% control)
	Total offspring (12 weeks)	Pups/mouse week		
0	137	0.91	4791	0
5	—	—	3940	18
10	91	0.61	3908	19
50	—	—	2086	56
100	28	0.20	580	88
200	0	0	—	—
500	0	0	0	100

[a]Taken in part from Mattison et al with permission (124).

traovarian injection of BP at 10 μg/ovary had no effect on hepatic AHH or cytochrome P-450 content in either D2 or B6 mice (126a).

Cyclophosphamide

Cyclophosphamide is known to produce sterility in female animals exposed either pre- or postnatally (127). Seven days after a single dose of cyclophosphamide (100 mg/kg), 63% of the primordial follicles of C57B1/6N mice were destroyed. In young rats, destruction of primordial oocytes by cyclophosphamide decreased with age as ovarian GSH levels were increasing (128). Studies on oocyte and follicle destruction by cyclophosphamide in Sprague-Dawley rats and in C57B1/6N and DBA/2N mice revealed that primordial oocytes were most sensitive to destruction. Destruction depended on time, dose, strain, and species; B6 mice were most sensitive to this effect. These results are of particular interest in view of the fact that oocyte destruction and premature ovarian failure is a significant side effect in women treated with alkylating agents (129, 130).

BONE MARROW

Benzene

Exposure to chemicals in the plastics, chemical, and rubber industries and in other areas of the workplace remains a significant public health problem in developed areas of the world. Subacute and chronic benzene toxicity is usually manifested as bone marrow hypoplasia in the form of leukopenia, anemia, thrombocytopenia, and pancytopenia, which may progress to aplastic anemia or leukemia (131). Humans appear to be more susceptible to the leukemogenic action of benzene than most animal species; workers exposed chronically to benzene appear to die in approximately equal numbers from aplastic anemia and leukemia (acute myelogenous or aleukemic) (132), while animals usually succumb to bone marrow aplasia.

Benzene exposure—unless otherwise stated, subacute or chronic exposure is to be assumed—elicits generalized bone marrow depression resulting in reduced numbers of circulating erythrocytes, granulocytes, thrombocytes, lymphocytes, and monocytes. There is a general agreement (131) that benzene is preferentially toxic toward progenitor cells of intermediate differentiation while sparing mature nondividing cell types. In the red cell series for example, early erythroblasts are more sensitive to benzene than stem cells, reticulocytes, or mature erythrocytes.

Irons and co-workers (133) reported that in male Fischer 344 rats exposed to benzene, peripheral lymphocytes and differentiating bone marrow precursor cells were the most sensitive cell populations. Benzene exposure resulted in an increase in the relative number of bone marrow precursor cells in G_2 or M phase of the cell cycle and a reduction in the uptake of ^{3}H-thymidine into bone marrow DNA. As noted above, analysis of bone marrow smears indicated an early cytotoxic effect of benzene on cells of intermediate differentiation (promyelocytes, myelocytes, basophilic and polychromatophilic erythroblasts) irrespective of cell line, with a relative sparing of blast forms and mature nondividing cell types.

Current evidence strongly suggests that a benzene metabolite mediates the myelotoxicity of benzene (132). Metabolites of benzene that have been isolated from biological sources such as urine or microsomal incubations include phenol, catechol, hydroquinone, benzoquinone, 1,3,5-trihydroxybenzene, trans,trans-muconic acid, 1,2-dihydro-1,2-dihydroxybenzene (1,2-dihydrodiol)(all isolated either free or as the sulfate or glucuronide conjugates), and phenylmercapturic acid. The evidence favoring a metabolite as the myelotoxic species, rather than benzene itself, has been reviewed elsewhere (132). Andrews et al (134) reported AHH activity in the bone marrow (femurs, tibia) of rabbits that was localized in the microsomal fraction, was NADPH dependent, was inhibited by CO, and was inducible by pretreatment with 3-MC. Fractionation of the bone marrow revealed that most of the total activity was localized in white cells, i.e. immature granular leukocytes.

Later work (135) showed that benzene could be hydroxylated to phenol and an unidentified metabolite by an analogous in vitro system from rabbit bone marrow that contained cytochrome P-450 and NADPH cytochrome c reductase. Irons et al (136) reported that benzene could be metabolized and covalently bound in bone marrow in situ. Fischer 344 rats received ^{14}C-benzene instilled directly into the bone marrow space of the distal head of the femur, and the hind limb was subjected to perfusion with whole rat blood for up to sixty minutes. Blood and bone marrow were analyzed for benzene and metabolites and the authors found phenol, catechol, hydroquinone, and unknown metabolites covalently bound to bone marrow. Gollmer et al (137) compared the benzene monooxygenase system of bone marrow with that of liver from rabbits and demonstrated that pretreatment with benzene did not affect O-dealkylation in bone marrow but stimulated benzene metabolism and covalent binding of ^{14}C-benzene metabolites. It was also concluded that bone marrow and liver develop separate patterns of cytochrome P-450 isozymes.

Data presented to this point established that both liver and bone marrow possess monooxygenase systems that metabolize and activate benzene to reactive intermediates able to bind covalently to tissue macromolecules. The question remaining was the relative importance of liver and bone marrow in the production of myelotoxic benzene metabolites. This question was largely resolved in a series of publications from Snyders laboratory. Administration of benzene to control (sham-operated) rats caused a 50% inhibition in the incorporation of ^{59}Fe into erythrocytes, an index of erythrogenesis, and urinary excretion of benzene metabolites (138). Partial hepatectomy (75%) decreased the metabolism of benzene by 70% and completely protected animals against benzene-induced hemopoietic toxicity when compared to sham-operated animals that received benzene.

This finding that partial hepatectomy decreases whole body benzene metabolism and protects against benzene hemopoietic toxicity indicates that the liver may play a primary role in the development of benzene-induced bone marrow toxicity. Further support for this view came from the finding that benzene metabolism (covalent binding) and toxicity correlated well in mice of different strains (139). [14]C benzene administration to DBA/2N mice produced greater inhibition of ^{59}Fe incorporation into erythrocytes and higher amounts of covalently bound material (^{14}C) in bone marrow and liver than in the less sensitive C57/B6 strain. The concept relating metabolism of benzene to bone marrow hypoplasia was further supported by Andrews et al (140), who reported that the administration of ^{3}H-benzene to mice resulted in decreased incorporation of ^{59}Fe into erythrocytes and the accumulation of benzene and its metabolites in bone marrow and other tissues. Coadministration of toluene, shown to be a competitive inhibitor of benzene metabolism in vitro, protected mice against benzene-induced depression of red cell ^{59}Fe uptake, reduced the urinary excretion of benzene metabolites, and reduced by 50% or more the accumulation of ^{3}H-benzene metabolites in bone marrow, blood, liver, spleen, and fat without affecting levels of ^{3}H-benzene itself in these tissues. This and other work gives rise to some general principles regarding the link between benzene metabolism and myelotoxicity:

1. The good correlation between reduction in urinary benzene metabolites and reduced bone marrow suppression suggests that benzene metabolism is closely related to its toxicity.

2. Toluene markedly inhibited benzene myelotoxicity and reduced bone marrow levels of benzene metabolites, but it had no effect on those of benzene itself. Thus, benzene metabolites and not benzene per se must mediate bone marrow suppression.

3. Bone marrow accumulated four times more benzene metabolites than liver in the first eight hours after benzene administration. Metabolites in bone marrow persisted far longer than those in fat, spleen, liver, and blood [approximate tissue levels of total benzene metabolites in tissues eight hours after ^{3}H-benzene administration (nmoles/g): bone marrow, 550; liver 25; blood 20; spleen 15; fat 5].

The chemical mechanism of benzene activation (141) utilized a reconstituted system from rabbit liver microsomes. NADPH, cytochrome P-450$_{LM2}$ (form induced by phenobarbital), NADPH cytochrome P-450 reductase, and phospholipids were incubated with ^{14}C-benzene and its conversion to phenol and water-soluble metabolites studied. These reactions were inhibited by catalase, horseradish peroxidase, superoxide dismutase, and several hydroxyl radical scavengers, indicating the participation of H_2O_2, O_2^{-}, and $\cdot OH$ in the process. Microsomal benzene metabolism was inhibited by six different $\cdot OH$ scavengers. Biphenyl was formed in the reconstituted system indicating the cytochrome P-450–dependent production of a hydroxycyclohexadienyl radical as a consequence of interactions between $\cdot OH$ and benzene. The formation of benzene metabolites covalently bound to protein was efficiently inhibited by free radical scavengers but not by epoxide hydrolase.

Returning to the morphological aspects of benzene-induced myeloid cytotoxicity, Wierda et al (142) reported that treatment of mice with benzene produced a dose-dependent inhibition of splenic T- and B-lymphocyte responsiveness to mitogens and a reduction in the capacity of antigen-reactive precursors of B-lymphocytes to generate antibody-producing cells. In addition to studies of the effects of benzene on bone marrow precursors of various circulating blood cells, Gaido & Wierda (143) studied its effects on bone marrow stromal cells since the latter form a supporting matrix for the developing cells and may influence and regulate hemopoetic cell development. Benzene metabolites were examined for their toxicity on mouse bone marrow stromal cell colony formation, and their TD$_{50}$s (given as μM concentration) were as follows: hydroquinone was most toxic (2.5 μM), followed by p-benzoquinone (17 μM), 1,3,5-benzenetriol (59 μM), catechol (124 μM), and phenol (189 μM). Finally, the benzene metabolites, hydroquinone and p-benzoquinone, inhibited mRNA synthesis (measured as RNA polymerase II) by rabbit bone marrow in a concentration dependent manner; they were equipotent and showed IC$_{50}$ values in the range of 6 μM. Catechol and 1,3,5-benzenetriol were less potent with IC$_{50}$ values near 0.1 mM; phenol did not inhibit mRNA synthesis even at concentrations of 1 mM (144).

In a preliminary outline for this review, we included skin, urinary bladder, gastrointestinal tract, adrenal, uterus, placenta, breast, pancreas, and thymus, various white blood cells, and other reticuloendothelial tissues. Space did not permit their inclusion but it is hoped that a subsequent review will do so.

CONCLUSIONS

Because of the attempted scope of this review, it is spotty, incomplete, and in some places less than thorough. We hope to have made the point that in most instances our knowledge of the precise biochemical mechanisms involved in toxic responses at the cellular or tissue level are scantily understood at best. A prominent feature of this ignorance is the current lack of reliable criteria by which we can determine, in cells in situ, cell death in biochemical terms. It is hoped that these many opportunities to gain insight into interesting and important biological problems will attract and appeal to enthusiastic young investigators.

ACKNOWLEDGMENTS

The senior author wishes to express his sincerest appreciation and gratitude to his friends and colleagues who contributed to this project. They assisted in many ways but most profoundly by their advice and by sharing their extensive files and unpublished review articles. I thank them for the strengths of this manuscript and accept the responsibility for its weaknesses. Among them are Alan R. Buckpitt, Howard D. Colby, Alan R. Dahl, Peter Goldman, Jerry B. Hook, Mont R. Juchau, Gopal Krishna, Daniel S. Longnecker, Donald R. Mattison, Roberta J. Pohl, Jan Rydström, Jacqueline H. Smith, Robert Snyder, and Lee W. Wattenberg. We thank Mrs. Beatrice Buddle for her forebearance and her excellent secretarial assistance.

Literature Cited

1. Williams, R. T. 1959. *Detoxication Mechanisms*. New York: Wiley. 796 pp. 2nd ed.
2. Gram, T. E. 1982. Metabolism of drugs. In *Modern Pharmacology*, ed. C. R. Craig, R. E. Stitzel 1:37–54. Boston: Little Brown
3. Lu, A. Y. H., Levin, W. 1974. The resolution and reconstitution of the liver microsomal hydroxylation system. *Biochim. Biophys. Acta* 344:205–40
4. Gelboin, H. V. 1980. Benzo(a)pyrene metabolism, activation, and carcinogenesis: Role and regulation of mixed function oxidases and related enzymes. *Physiol. Rev.* 60:1107–66
5. Lu, A. Y. H., West, S. B. 1980. Multiplicity of mammalian microsomal cytochrome P-450. *Pharmacol. Rev.* 31:277–95
6. Gillette, J. R., Mitchell, J. R., Brodie, B. B. 1974. Biochemical mechanisms of drug toxicity. *Ann. Rev. Pharmacol.* 14:271–88
7. Burke, M. D., Orrenius, S. 1979. Isolation and comparison of endoplasmic reticulum membranes and their mixed function oxidase activities from mammalian extrahepatic tissues. *Pharmacol. Ther.* 7:549–99
8. Bend, J. R., Serabjit-Singh, C. J. 1984. Xenobiotic metabolism by extrahepatic tissues: relationship to target organ and cell toxicity. In *Drug Metabolism and Drug Toxicity*, ed. J. R. Mitchell, M. G. Horning, pp. 99–136. New York: Raven

9. Anders, M. W. 1980. Metabolism of drugs by the kidney. *Kidney Int.* 18:636–47

10. Gram, T. E. 1980. *Extrahepatic Metabolism of Drugs and Other Foreign Compounds.* New York: SP Medical and Scientific Books. 601 pp.

11. Dahl, A. R., Hadley, W. M., Hahn, F. F., Benson, J. M., McClellan, R. O. 1982. Cytochrome P-450–dependent monooxygenases in olfactory epithelium of dogs: Possible role in tumorigenicity. *Science* 216:57–58

12. Hadley, W. M., Dahl, A. R. 1983. Cytochrome P-450–dependent monooxygenase activity in nasal membranes of six species. *Drug Metab. Dispos.* 11:275–76

13. Hadley, W. M., Dahl, A. R. 1982. Cytochrome P-450–dependent monooxygenase activity in rat nasal epithelial membranes. *Toxicol. Lett.* 10:417–22

14. Brittebo, E. B., Löfberg, B., Tjälve, H. 1981. Sites of metabolism of N-nitrosodiethylamine in mice. *Chem. Biol. Interact.* 34:209–21

15. Brittebo, E. B. 1982. N-demethylation of aminopyrine by the nasal mucosa in mice and rats. *Acta Pharmacol. Toxicol.* 51:227–32

16. Bond, J. A., Li, A. P. 1983. Rat nasal tissue activation of benzo(α) pyrene and 2-aminoanthracene to mutagens in *Salmonella typhimurium. Environ. Mutagen.* 5:311–18

17. Bond, J. A. 1983. Bioactivation and biotransformation of 1-nitropyrene in liver, lung and nasal tissues of rats. *Mutat. Res.* 124:315–24

18. Dahl, A. R., Hadley, W. M. 1983. Formaldehyde production promoted by rat nasal cytochrome P-450–dependent monooxygenases with nasal decongestants, essences, solvents, air pollutants, nicotine and cocaine as substrates. *Toxicol. Appl. Pharmacol.* 67:200–5

19. Bond, J. A. 1983. Some biotransformation enzymes responsible for polycyclic aromatic hydrocarbon metabolism in rat nasal turbinates: Effects on enzyme activities of *in vitro* modifiers and intraperitoneal and inhalation exposure of rats to inducing agents. *Cancer Res.* 43:4805–11

20. Brittebo, E. B., Ahlman, M. 1984. Metabolism of a nasal carcinogen, phenacetin, in the mucosa of the upper respiratory tract. *Chem. Biol. Interact.* 50:233–45

21. Brittebo, E. B., Brandt, I. 1984. Metabolism of chlorobenzene in the mucosa of the murine respiratory tract. *Lung* 162:79–88

22. Autrup, H., Grafstrom, R. C., Harris, C. C. 1983. Metabolism of chemical carcinogens by tracheobronchial tissues. In *Organ and Species Specificity in Chemical Carcinogenesis,* ed. R. Langenbach, S. Nesnow, J. M. Rice, pp. 473–95. New York: Plenum

23. Mass, M. J., Kaufman, D. G. 1984. Biochemical studies of the tracheobronchial epithelium. *Environ. Health Perspect.* 56:61–74

24. Kaufman, D. G., Gerta, V. M., Harris, C. C., Smith, J. M., Sporn, M. B., Saffioti, U. 1973. Binding of ^{3}H-labeled benzo(α)pyrene to DNA in hamster tracheal epithelial cells. *Cancer Res.* 33:2837–41

25. Mass, M. J., Kaufman, D. G. 1978. [^{3}H]benzo(α)pyrene metabolism in tracheal epithelial microsomes and tracheal organ cultures. *Cancer Res.* 38:3861–66

26. Eastman, A., Mossman, B. T., Bresnick, E. 1981. Formation and removal of benzo(α)pyrene adducts of DNA in hamster tracheal epithelial cells. *Cancer Res.* 41:2605–10

27. Dirksen, E. R., Crocker, T. T. 1968. Ultrastructural alterations produced by polycyclic aromatic hydrocarbons on rat tracheal epithelium in organ culture. *Cancer Res.* 28:906–23

28. Palekar, L., Kuschner, M., Laskin, S. 1968. Effects of 3-methylcholanthrene on rat trachea in organ culture. *Cancer Res.* 28:2098–2104

29. Schreiber, J., Martin, D. H., Pazmino, N. 1975. Species differences in the effect of benzo(α)pyrene-ferric oxide on the respiratory tract of rats and hamsters. *Cancer Res.* 35:1654–61

30. Reznik-Schüller, H., Reznik, G. 1979. Experimental pulmonary carcinogenesis. *Int. Rev. Exp. Pathol.* 20:211–81

31. Reznik-Schüller, H., Hagne, B. F. 1981. Autoradiographic study of the distribution of bound radioactivity in the respiratory tract of Syrian hamsters given N-[^{3}H]nitrosodiethylamine. *Cancer Res.* 41:2147–50

32. Ohshima, M., Ward, J. M., Singh, G., Katyal, S. L. 1985. Immunocytochemical and morphological evidence for the origin of N-nitrosomethylurea–induced and naturally occurring primary lung tumors in F344/NCr rats. *Cancer Res.* 45:2785–92

33. Harris, C. C., Frank, A. L., van Haften, C., Kaufman, D. G., Connor, R., et al. 1976. Binding of [^{3}H]benzo(α)pyrene to

DNA in cultured human bronchus. *Cancer Res.* 36:1011–18

34. Harris, C. C., Autrup, H., Stoner, G. D., McDowell, E. M., Trump, B. F., Schafer, P. 1977. Metabolism of dimethylnitrosamine and 1,2-dimethylhydrazine in cultured human bronchi. *Cancer Res.* 37:2309–11

35. Autrup, H., Harris, C. C., Stoner, G. D., Selkirk, J. K., Schafer, P. W., Trump, B. F. 1978. Metabolism of [^{3}H]benzo-(α)pyrene by cultured human bronchus and cultured human pulmonary alveolar macrophages. *Lab. Invest.* 38:217–24

36. Kahng, M. W., Smith, M. W., Trump, B. F. 1981. Aryl hydrocarbon hydroxylase in human bronchial epithelium and blood monocyte. *J. Natl. Cancer Inst.* 66:227–32

37. Bend, J. R., Serabjit-Singh, C. J., Philpot, R. M. 1985. The pulmonary uptake, accumulation, and metabolism of xenobiotics. *Ann. Rev. Pharmacol. Toxicol.* 25:97–125

38. Gram, T. E. 1985. The pulmonary mixed-function oxidase system. In *Toxicology of Inhaled Materials,* ed. H. P. Witschi, J. D. Brain, pp. 421–70. Berlin: Springer-Verlag

39. Boyd, M. R. 1976. Role of metabolic activation in the pathogenesis of chemically induced pulmonary disease: mechanism of action of the lung-toxic furan, 4-ipomeanol. *Environ. Health Perspect.* 16:127–38

40. Crapo, J. D., Peters-Golden, M., Marsh-Salin, J., Shelburne, J. S. 1978. Pathologic changes in the lungs of oxygen-adapted rats. A morphometric analysis. *Lab. Invest.* 39:640–53

41. DiGuiseppi, J., Fridovich, I. 1984. The toxicology of molecular oxygen. *CRC Crit. Rev. Toxicol.* 12:315–41

42. Halliwell, B., Gutteridge, J. M. C. 1984. Oxygen toxicity, oxygen radicals, transition metals and disease. *Biochem. J.* 219:1–14

43. Deneke, S. M., Fanburg, B. L. 1982. Oxygen toxicity of the lung: an update. *Br. J. Anaesth.* 54:737–49

44. Frank, L., Massaro, D. 1979. The lung and oxygen toxicity. *Arch. Intern. Med.* 139:347–50

45. Johnson, K. J., Fantone, J. C., Kaplan, J., Ward, P. A. 1981. *In vivo* damage of rat lungs by oxygen metabolites. *J. Clin. Invest.* 67:983–93

46. Smith, L. L., Rose, M. S., Wyatt, I. 1979. The pathology and biochemistry of paraquat. *Ciba Found. Symp.* 65:321–41

47. Witschi, H. P., Kawen, S., Hirai, K-I.,

Coté, M. G. 1977. *In vivo* oxidation of reduced nicotinamide-adenine dinucleotide phosphate by paraquat and diquat in rat lung. *Chem. Biol. Interact.* 19:143–60

48. Ilett, K. F., Stripp, B., Menard, R. H., Reid, W. D., Gillette, J. R. 1974. Studies on the mechanism of the lung toxicity of paraquat: comparison of tissue distribution and some biochemical parameters in rats and rabbits. *Toxicol. Appl. Pharmacol.* 28:216–26

49. Bus, J. S., Gibson, J. E. 1984. Paraquat: Model for oxidant-initiated toxicity. *Environ. Health Perspect.* 55:37–46

50. Benedetti, A., Comporti, M., Esterbauer, H. 1980. Identification of 4-hydroxynonenal as a cytotoxic product originating from the peroxidation of liver microsomal lipids. *Biochim. Biophys. Acta* 620:281–96

51. Smith, L. L., Rose, M. S. 1977. Biochemical changes in lungs exposed to paraquat. In *Biochemical Mechanisms of Paraquat Toxicity,* ed. A. P. Autor, pp. 187–99. New York: Academic

52. Butler, C., Kleinerman, J. 1971. Paraquat in the rabbit. *Br. J. Ind. Med.* 28:67–71

53. Clark, D. G., McElligott, T. F., Hurst, E. W. 1966. The toxicity of paraquat. *Br. J. Ind. Med.* 23:126–32

54. Smith, P., Heath, D. 1976. Paraquat *CRC Crit. Rev. Toxicol.* 4:411–45

55. Sovijarvi, A. R. A., Lemola, M., Stenius, B., Idanpaan-Heikkila, J. 1977. Nitrofurantoin induced acute, subacute, and chronic pulmonary reactions. *Scand. J. Respir. Dis.* 58:41–50

56. Boyd, M. R., Catignani, G. L., Sasame, H. A., Mitchell, J. R., Stiko, A. W. 1979. Acute pulmonary injury in rats by nitrofurantoin and modification by vitamin E, dietary fat, and oxygen. *Am. Rev. Respir. Dis.* 120:93–99

57. Mason, R. P., Holtzman, J. L. 1975. The role of catalytic superoxide formation in the oxygen inhibition of nitroreductase. *Biochem. Biophys. Res. Commun.* 67:1267–74

58. Boyd, M. R. 1980. Biochemical mechanisms in chemical-induced lung injury: roles of metabolic activation. *CRC Crit. Rev. Toxicol.* 7:103–76

59. Buckpitt, A. R., Statham, C. N., Boyd, M. R. 1982. *In vivo* studies on the target tissue metabolism, covalent binding, glutathione depletion and toxicity of 4-ipomeanol in birds, species deficient in pulmonary enzymes for metabolic activation. *Toxicol. Appl. Pharmacol.* 65:38–52

288   GRAM, OKINE, AND GRAM

60. Boyd, M. R., Burka, L. T., Wilson, B. J., Sasame, H. A. 1978. *In vitro* studies on the metabolic activation of the pulmonary toxin 4-ipomeanol by rat lung and liver microsomes. *J. Pharmacol. Exp. Ther.* 207:677–86
61. Glende, E. A. 1972. Carbon tetrachloride-induced protection against carbon tetrachloride toxicity. The role of the liver microsomal drug metabolizing system. *Biochem. Pharmacol.* 21:1697–1702
62. Conney, A. H. 1982. Induction of microsomal enzymes by foreign chemicals and carcinogensis by polycyclic aromatic hydrocarbons. *Cancer Res.* 42:4875–4917
63. Ravindranath, V., Burka, L. T., Boyd, M. R. 1984. Reactive metabolites from the bioactivation of toxic methylfurans. *Science* 224:884–86
64. Griffin, K. A., Johnson, C. B., Breger, R. K., Franklin, R. B. 1982. Effects of inducers and inhibitors of cytochrome P-450–linked monooxygenases on the toxicity, *in vitro* metabolism and *in vivo* irreversible binding of 2-methylnaphthalene in mice. *J. Pharmacol. Exp. Ther.* 221:517–24
65. Buckpitt, A. R., Warren, D. L. 1982. Evidence for hepatic formation, export and covalent binding of reactive naphthalene metabolites in extrahepatic tissues *in vivo*. *J. Pharmacol. Exp. Ther.* 225:8–16
66. Boyd, M. R. 1977. Evidence for the Clara cell as a site of cytochrome P-450–dependent mixed-function oxidase activity in lung. *Nature* 269:713–15
67. Boyd, M. R., Statham, C. N. 1978. Pulmonary bronchiolar alkylation and necrosis by 3-methylfuran, a naturally occurring potential environmental contaminant. *Nature* 272:270–71
68. Reid, W. D., Ilett, K. F., Glick, J. M., Krishna, G. 1973. Metabolism and binding of aromatic hydrocarbons in the lung. Relationship to experimental bronchiolar necrosis. *Ann. Rev. Respir. Dis.* 107:539–51
69. Bray, T. M., Carlson, J. R., Nocerini, M. R. 1984. *In vitro* covalent binding of 3-[^{14}C]methylindole metabolites in goat tissues. *Proc. Soc. Exp. Biol. Med.* 176:48–53
70. Williamson, D., Esterez, P., Witschi, H. 1978. Studies on the pathogenesis of butylated hydroxytoluene-induced lung damage in mice. *Toxicol. Appl. Pharmacol.* 43:577–87
71. Boyd, M. R., Statham, C. N., Longo, N. S. 1979. The pulmonary Clara cell as a target for toxic chemicals requiring

metabolic activation: studies with carbon tetrachloride. *J. Pharmacol. Exp. Ther.* 212:109–14
72. McKenna, M. J., Zempel, J. A., Madrid, E. O., Gehring, P. J. 1978. The pharmacokinetics of [^{14}C]vinylidene chloride in rats following inhalation exposure. *Toxicol. Appl. Pharmacol.* 45:599–610
73. Imamura, T., Hasegawa, L. 1984. Role of metabolic activation, covalent-binding, and glutathione depletion in pulmonary toxicity produced by an impurity of malathion. *Toxicol. Appl. Pharmacol.* 72:476–83
74. Smith, B. R., Plummer, J., Wolf, C. R., Philpot, R. M., Bend, J. R. 1982. p-Xylene metabolism by rabbit lung and liver and its relationship to the selective destruction of pulmonary cytochrome P-450. *J. Pharmacol. Exp. Ther.* 223:736–42
75. Struck, R. F., Kirk, M. C., Witt, M. H., Laster, W. R. 1975. Isolation and mass spectral identification of blood metabolites of cyclophosphamide: evidence for phosphoramide mustard as the biologically active metabolite. *Biomed. Mass. Spectrom.* 2:46–53
76. Patel, J. M., Block, E. R., Hood, C. I. 1984. Biochemical indices of cyclophosphamide-induced lung toxicity. *Toxicol. Appl. Pharmacol.* 76:128–38
77. Rush, G. F., Smith, J. H., Newton, J. F., Hook, J. B. 1984. Chemically induced nephrotoxicity: role of metabolic activation. *CRC Crit. Rev. Toxicol.* 13:99–160
78. Piperno, E. 1981. Detection of drug induced nephrotoxicity with urinalysis and enzyurmia assessment. In *Toxicology of the Kidney*, ed. J. B. Hook, pp. 31–55. New York: Raven
79. Ilett, K. F., Reid, W. D., Sipes, I. G., Krishna, G. 1973. Chloroform toxicity in mice: correlation of renal and hepatic necrosis with covalent binding of metabolites to tissue macromolecules. *Exp. Mol. Pathol.* 19:215–29
80. Smith, J. H., Maita, K., Sleight, S. D., Hook, J. B. 1984. Effect of sex hormone status on chloroform nephrotoxicity and renal mixed function oxidases in mice. *Toxicology* 30:305–16
81. Smith, J. H., Hook, J. B. 1983. Mechanism of chloroform nephrotoxicity. II. *In vitro* evidence of renal metabolism of chloroform in mice. *Toxicol. Appl. Pharmacol.* 70:480–85
82. Smith, J. H., Hook, J. B. 1984. Mechanism of chloroform nephrotoxicity III. Renal and hepatic microsomal metabolism of chloroform in mice. *Toxicol. Appl. Pharmacol.* 73:511–24

83. Branchflower, R. V., Nunn, D. S., Highet, R. J., Smith, J. H., Hook, J. B., Pohl, L. R. 1984. Nephrotoxicity of chloroform: metabolism to phosgene by the mouse kidney. *Toxicol. Appl. Pharmacol.* 72:159–68

84. Kluwe, W. M., Hook, J. B. 1981. Potentiation of acute chloroform nephrotoxicity by the glutathione depletor diethylmaleate and protection by the microsomal enzyme inhibitor piperonyl butoxide. *Toxicol. Appl. Pharmacol.* 59:457–66

85. Smith, J. H., Maita, K., Sleight, S. D., Hook, J. B. 1983. Mechanism of chloroform nephrotoxicity. I. Time course of chloroform toxicity in male and female mice. *Toxicol. Appl. Pharmacol.* 70:467–79

86. Lock, E. A., Ishmael, J. 1981. Hepatic and renal nonprotein sulfhydryl concentration following toxic doses of hexachloro-1,3-butadiene in the rat: The effect of aroclor 1254, phenobaritone, or SKF-525A treatment. *Toxicol. Appl. Pharmacol.* 57:79–87

87. Wolf, C. R., Berry, P. N., Nash, J. A., Green, T., Lock, E. A. 1984. Role of microsomal and cytosolic glutathione S-transferase in the conjugation of hexachloro-1,3-butadiene and its possible relevance to toxicity. *J. Pharmacol. Exp. Ther.* 228:202–8

88. Nash, J. A., King, L. G., Lock, E. A., Green, T. 1984. The metabolism and disposition of hexachloro-1,3-butadiene in the rat and its relevance to nephrotoxicity. *Toxicol. Appl. Pharmacol.* 73:124–37

89. Stevens, J., Jakoby, W. B. 1982. Cysteine conjugate β-lyase. *Mol. Pharmacol.* 23:761–65

90. Bakke, J., Gustafsson, J. A. 1984. Mercapturic acid pathway metabolites of xenobiotics: generation of potentially toxic metabolites during enterohepatic circulation. *Trends Pharmacol. Sci.* 5:517–21

91. Elfarra, A. A., Anders, M. W. 1984. Renal processing of glutathione conjugates: role in nephrotoxicity. *Biochem. Pharmacol.* 33:3729–32

92. Green, T., Nash, J. A., Odum, J., Howard, E. F. 1983. The renal metabolism of a glutathione conjugate of the carcinogen hexachloro-1,-butadiene: evidence for the formation of a mutagenic metabolite in the rat kidney. In *Extrahepatic Drug Metabolism and Chemical Carcinogenesis*, ed. J. Rydström, J. Montelius, M. Bengtsson, pp. 625–26. Amsterdam: Elsevier

93. Miyajima, H., Hewitt, W. R., Coté, M. G., Plaa, G. L. 1983. Relationships between histological and functional indices of acute chemically induced nephrotoxicity. *Fundam. Appl. Toxicol.* 3:543–51

94. Tune, B. M., Fravert, D. 1980. Mechanisms of cephalosporin nephrotoxicity: a comparison of cephaloridine and cephaloglycin. *Kidney Int.* 18:591–600

95. Kuo, C-H., Hook, J. B. 1982. Depletion of renal glutathione content and nephrotoxicity of cephaloridine in rabbits, rats and mice. *Toxicol. Appl. Pharmacol.* 63:292–302

96. Kuo, C-H., Braselton, W. E., Hook, J. B. 1982. Effect of phenobarbital on cephaloridine toxicity and accumulation in rabbit and rat kidneys. *Toxicol. Appl. Pharmacol.* 64:244–54

97. Reid, W. D. 1973. Mechanism of renal necrosis induced by bromobenzene or chlorobenzene. *Exp. Mol. Pathol.* 19:197–214

98. Lau, S. S., Monks, T. J., Gillette, J. R. 1984. Identification of 2-bromohydroquinone as a metabolite of bromobenzene and ortho-bromophenol: implications for bromobenzene-induced nephrotoxicity. *J. Pharmacol. Exp. Ther.* 230:360–66

99. Lau, S. S., Monks, T. J., Greene, K. E., Gillette, J. R. 1984. The role of ortho-bromophenol in the nephrotoxicity of bromobenzene in rats. *Toxicol. Appl. Pharmacol.* 72:539–49

100. Rush, G. F., Newton, J. F., Maita, K., Kuo, C-H., Hook, J. B. 1984. Nephrotoxicity of phenolic bromobenzene metabolites in the mouse. *Toxicology* 30:259–72

101. McMurtry, R. J., Snodgrass, W. R., Mitchell, J. R. 1978. Renal necrosis glutathione depletion and covalent binding after acetaminophen. *Toxicol. Appl. Pharmacol.* 46:87–100

102. Breen, K., Wandscheer, J. C., Peignoux, M., Pessayre, D. 1982. In situ formation of the acetaminophen metabolite covalently bound in kidney and lung. Supportive evidence provided by total hepatectomy. *Biochem. Pharmacol.* 31:115–16

103. Newton, J. F., Yoshimoto, M., Bernstein, J., Rush, G. F., Hook, J. B. 1983. Acetaminophen nephrotoxicity in the rat. I. Strain differences in nephrotoxicity and metabolism. *Toxicol. Appl. Pharmacol.* 69:291–306

104. Newton, J. F., Pasino, D. A., Hook, J. B. 1985. Acetaminophen nephrotoxicity in the rat: Quantitation of renal metabolic

activation *in vivo. Toxicol. Appl. Phar-macol.* 78:39–46
105. Kluwe, W. M. 1981. Acute toxicity of 1,2-dibromo-3-chloropropane in F344 male rat. I. Dose response relationships and differences in routes of exposure. *Toxicol. Appl. Pharmacol.* 59:71–83
106. Potashnik, G., Yanai-Inbar, I., Sacks, M. I., Israeli, R. 1979. Effect of di-bromochloropropane on human testicular function. *Israel J. Med. Sci.* 15:438–42
107. Biava, C. G., Smuckler, G. A., Whor-ton, D. 1978. The testicular morphology of individuals exposed to dibromochloro-propane. *Exp. Mol. Pathol.* 29:448–58
108. Lantz, G. D., Cunningham, G. R., Huckins, C., Lipshultz, L. I. 1981. Recovery from severe oligospermia after exposure to dibromochloropropane. *Fer-til. Steril.* 35:46–53
109. Rao, J. S., Burek, J. D., Murray, F. J., John, J. A., Schwetz, B. A., et al. 1982. Toxicologic and reproductive effects of inhaled 1,2-dibromo-3-chloropropane in male rabbits. *Fundam. Appl. Toxicol.* 2:241–51
110. Oakberg, E. F., Cummings, C. C. 1984. Lack of effect of dibromochloropropane on the mouse testis. *Environ. Mutagen.* 6:621–25
111. MacFarland, R. T., Gandolf, A. J., Sipes, I. G. 1984. Extrahepatic GSH-dependent metabolism of 1,2-dibromo-ethane (DBE) and 1,2-dibromo-3-chloro-propane (DBCP) in the rat and mouse. *Drug. Chem. Toxicol.* 7:213–27
112. Jones, A. R., Fakhouri, G., Gadiel, P. 1979. The metabolism of the soil fumi-gant 1,2-dibromo-3-chloropropane in the rat. *Experientia* 35:1432–34
113. Jones, A. R. 1978. The antifertility ac-tions of α-chlorohydrin in the male rat. *Life Sci.* 23:1625–46
113a. Kluwe, W. M., Gupta, B. N., Lamb, J. C. 1983. The comparative effects of 1,2-dibromo-3-chloropropane (DBCP) and its metabolites, 3-chloro-1,2,propaneox-ide(epichlorohydrin), 3-chloro-1,2-pro-panediol(α-chlorohydrin) and oxalic acid, on the urogenital system of male rats. *Toxicol. Appl. Pharmacol.* 70:67–86
114. Chapin, R. E., White, R. D., Morgan, K. T., Bus, J. S. 1984. Studies of lesions induced in the testis and epididymis of F-344 rats by inhaled methyl chloride. *Toxicol. Appl. Pharmacol.* 76:328–43
115. Wong, L. C. K., Winston, J. M., Hong, C. B., Plotnick, H. 1982. Carcinogenic-ity and toxicity of 1,2-bromoethane in the

rat. *Toxicol. Appl. Pharmacol.* 63:155–65
116. Osterberg, R. E., Bierbower, G. W., Hehir, R. M. 1977. Renal and testicular damage following dermal application of the flame retardant tris(2,3-dibromopro-pyl) phosphate. *J. Toxicol. Environ. Health* 3:979–87
117. Sever, L. E., Hessol, N. A. 1985. Toxic effects of occupational and environmen-tal chemicals on the testes. In *Endocrine Toxicology,* ed. J. A. Thomas, K. S. Korach, J. A. McLachlan, pp. 211–248. New York: Raven
118. Lee, I. P., Nagayama, J. 1980. Metabo-lism of benzo(α)pyrene by the isolated perfused rat testis. *Cancer Res.* 40:3297–3303
119. Nagayama, J., Lee, I. P. 1982. Compari-son of benzo(α)pyrene metabolism by testicular homogenate and the isolated perfused testis of rat following 2,3,7,8-tetrachloro-dibenzo-p-dioxin treatment. *Arch. Toxicol.* 51:121–30
120. Mattison, D. R., Thorgeirsson, S. S. 1978. Gonadal aryl hydrocarbon hy-droxylase in rats and mice. *Cancer Res.* 38:1368–73
121. Mattison, D. R., West, D. M., Menard, R. H. 1979. Differences in benzo(α)py-rene metabolic profile in rat and mouse ovary. *Biochem. Pharmacol.* 28:2101–104
122. Mattison, D. R., Thorgeirsson, S. S. 1979. Ovarian aryl hydrocarbon hy-droxylase activity and primordial oocyte toxicity of polycyclic aromatic hydrocar-bons in mice. *Cancer Res.* 39:3471–75
123. Mattison, D. R. 1979. Difference in sensitivity of rat and mouse primordial oocytes to destruction by polycyclic aromatic hydrocarbons. *Chem. Biol. In-teract.* 28:133–37
124. Mattison, D. R., White, N. B., Nightin-gale, M. R. 1980. The effect of ben-zo(α)pyrene on fertility, primordial oocyte number and ovarian response to pregnant mare's serum gonadotropin. *Pediatr. Pharmacol.* 1:143–51
125. Jick, H., Porter, J., Morrison, A. S. 1977. Relation between smoking and age of natural menopause. *Lancet* 1:1354–55
126. Mattison, D. R. 1980. Morphology of oocyte and follicle destruction by poly-cyclic aromatic hydrocarbons in mice. *Toxicol. Appl. Pharmacol.* 53:249–59
126a. Shiromizu, K., Mattison, D. R. 1984. The effect of intraovarian injection of benzo[α]pyrene on primordial oocyte number and ovarian aryl hydrocarbon

(benzo[α]pyrene)hydroxylase activity. *Toxicol. Appl. Pharmacol.* 76:18–25

127. Mattison, D. R., Chang, L., Thorgeirsson, S. S., Shiromizu, K. 1981. The effects of cyclophosphamide azothioporine and 6-mercaptopurine on oocyte and follicle number in C57BL/6N mice. *Res. Commun. Chem. Pathol. Pharmacol.* 31:155–61

128. Mattison, D. R., Shiromizu, K., Pendergrass, J. A., Thorgeirsson, S. S. 1983. Ontogeny of ovarian glutathione and sensitivity to primordial oocyte destruction by cyclophosphamide. *Pediatr. Pharmacol.* 3:49–55

129. Shiromizu, K., Thorgeirsson, S. S., Mattison, D. R. 1984. Effect of cyclophosphamide on oocyte and follicle number in Sprague-Dawley rats, C57B1/6N and DBA/2N mice. *Pediatr. Pharmacol.* 4:213–21

130. Horning, S. J., Hoppe, R. T., Kaplan, H. S., Rosenberg, S. A. 1981. Female reproductive potential after treatment for Hodgkins disease. *N. Engl. J. Med.* 304:1377–81

131. Snyder, R., Lee, G. W., Kocsis, J. J., Witmer, C. M. 1977. Bone marrow depressant and leukemogenic actions of benzene. *Life Sci.* 21:1709–22

132. Snyder, R., Longacre, S. L., Witmer, C. M., Kocsis, J. J. 1981. Biochemical toxicology of benzene. *Rev. Biochem. Toxicol.* 3:123–53

133. Irons, R. D., Heck, H. D. A., Moore, B. J., Muirhead, K. A. 1979. Effects of short-term benzene administration on bone marrow cell cyle kinetics in the rat. *Toxicol. Appl. Pharmacol.* 51:399–409

134. Andrews, L. S., Sonawane, B. R., Yaffe, S. J. 1976. Characterization and induction of aryl hydrocarbon [benzo(α)pyrene] hydroxylase in rabbit bone marrow. *Res. Commun. Chem. Pathol. Pharmacol.* 15:319–30

135. Andrews, L. S., Sasame, H. A., Gillette, J. R. 1979. ³H-benzene metabolism in rabbit bone marrow. *Life Sci.* 25:567–72

136. Irons, R. D., Dent, J. G., Baker, T. S.,

Rickert, D. E. 1980. Benzene is metabolized and covalently bound in bone marrow *in situ*. *Chem. Biol. Interact.* 30:241–45

137. Gollmer, L., Graf, H., Ullrich, V. 1984. Characterization of the benzene monooxygenase system in rabbit bone marrow. *Biochem. Pharmacol.* 33:3597–3602

138. Sammett, D., Lee, E. W., Kocsis, J. J., Snyder, R. 1979. Partial hepatectomy reduces both metabolism and toxicity of benzene. *J. Toxicol. Environ. Health* 5:785–92

139. Longacre, S. L., Kocsis, J. J., Snyder, R. 1980. Benzene metabolism and toxicity in CD-1 C57/B6 and DBA/2N mice. In *Microsomes Drug Oxidations and Chemical Carcinogenesis*, ed. M. J. Coon, A. H. Conney, R. W. Estabrook, H. V. Gelboin, J. R. Gillette, P. J. O'Brien, 2:897–902. New York: Academic

140. Andrews, L. S., Lee, E. W., Witmer, C. M., Kocsis, J. J., Snyder, R. 1977. Effects of toluene on the metabolism, disposition and hemopoietic toxicity of [³H]benzene. *Biochem. Pharmacol.* 26:293–300

141. Johansson, I., Ingelman-Sundberg, M. 1983. Hydroxyl radical-mediated cytochrome P-450–dependent metabolic activation of benzene in microsomes and reconstituted enzyme systems from rabbit liver. *J. Biol. Chem.* 258:7311–16

142. Wierda, D., Irons, R. D., Greenlee, W. F. 1981. Immunotoxicity in C57BL/6 mice exposed to benzene and aroclor 1254. *Toxicol. Appl. Pharmacol.* 60:410–17

143. Gaido, K., Wierda, D. 1984. *In vitro* effects of benzene metabolites on mouse bone marrow stromal cells. *Toxicol. Appl. Pharmacol.* 76:45–55

144. Post, G. B., Snyder, R., Kalf, G. F. 1984. Inhibition of mRNA synthesis in rabbit bone marrow nuclei *in vitro* by quinone metabolites of benzene. *Chem. Biol. Interact.* 50:203–11

NOTE ADDED IN PROOF   A recent report showed that glutathione conjugates of 2-bromophenol or 2-bromoquinone are the most nephrotoxic compounds yet discovered in the series (> 300 times more toxic than bromobenzene) (Monks, T. J., Lau, S. S., Highet, R. J., Gillette, J. R. 1985. Glutathione conjugates of 2-bromohydroquinone are nephrotoxic. *Drug Metab. Dispos.* 13:553–59).

Ann. Rev. Pharmacol. Toxicol. 1986. 26:293–309

CONTROL BY DRUGS OF RENAL POTASSIUM HANDLING[1]

Heino Velázquez and Fred S. Wright

Departments of Medicine and Physiology, Yale University School of Medicine, New Haven, Connecticut, and Veterans Administration Medical Center, West Haven, Connecticut

INTRODUCTION

The kidney plays a major role in maintaining potassium homeostasis. Investigations during the past thirty years have provided a great deal of information about renal mechanisms involved in the regulation of potassium excretion. Much of this information is summarized in several recent reviews (1–3). Potassium undergoes both glomerular filtration and reabsorptive and secretory transport. Potassium is filtered freely in the large volumes of plasma that are filtered by the glomeruli and that course through the proximal portions of the nephron. Water, organic substances, and electrolytes are extensively reabsorbed from this ultrafiltrate of plasma so that 10% or less of the filtered volume emerges from the loop of Henle. Nearly all of the filtered potassium has been reabsorbed before the luminal fluid reaches the distal tubule. Potassium is added to the luminal fluid by cells of the distal tubule. As a consequence, the concentration of potassium in luminal fluid increases to levels that can exceed the plasma concentration by several fold. The potassium secreted from blood to luminal fluid by the distal cells accounts for most of the potassium that appears in the urine. The gradient for potassium generated in the distal tubule is maintained by the collecting duct system as fluid continues to flow downstream and more water is absorbed. Further secretion of potassium by collecting duct cells contributes to the final regulation of excretion of potassium by the kidney. The distal tubule, strategically located in the distal nephron downstream from the thick ascending limb of Henle's loop and upstream from the collecting duct system, makes a key contribution to the sensitive regulation of the rate at which potassium leaves the body via the kidneys. Under some circumstances, howev-

[1]The US Government has the right to retain a nonexclusive, royalty-free license in and to any copyright covering this paper.

er, this distal location of the potassium secretory mechanism between a segment responsible for diluting luminal fluid and a segment responsible for concentrating luminal fluid can lead to disturbances in the potassium balance of the organism.

In this chapter we review interactions between diuretic drugs and the mechanisms controlling renal potassium excretion. First we summarize briefly some of the ways in which net potassium transport by the kidney can be modified. Determinants of distal potassium transport can exert their influence by acting on distal cells from either the blood side or the lumen side of the epithelium. We then focus on six diuretic drugs and discuss their effects on renal potassium handling and what is known about their mechanism of action. Finally, we consider briefly how changes in plasma levels of aldosterone and vasopressin that occur during changes in volume status can affect distal potassium secretion. These physiologic influences modify the impact of certain diuretic drugs.

DETERMINANTS OF DISTAL POTASSIUM TRANSPORT

The distal tubule is the primary site for potassium secretion from blood to lumen. For the present discussion we define the distal tubule as the portion of the nephron located between the macula densa region and the junction of that tubule with another distal tubule to form the collecting duct. This structure is heterogeneous and contains at least four cell types. Sodium and chloride absorption occurs throughout the distal tubule. Potassium secretion, however, occurs predominantly in the downstream portion, the late distal tubule.

Potassium is transported from plasma and interstitial fluid into distal cells across the basolateral membrane by an ATP driven Na-K exchange pump. Potassium is able to diffuse out of distal cells via conductive pathways in both the basolateral membrane and the luminal membrane. More potassium diffuses across the luminal membrane partly because the electrochemical driving force for potassium is greater: the luminal membrane voltage is less than the basolateral membrane voltage because sodium conductance permits an inward flow of sodium ions that depolarizes the luminal membrane. Thus, net transcellular movement of potassium normally occurs from blood to lumen. This mechanism of active uptake across the basolateral membrane and passive diffusion across the luminal membrane can account for a large part of the potassium secreted, although other mechanisms also influence net potassium transport by distal cells. These include a mechanism for active potassium uptake from lumen to cell (4) and a coupled mechanism for potassium and chloride movement from cell to lumen (5, 6). The rate of net potassium secretion by the distal tubule is regulated by several factors that modify these transport mechanisms.

Factors Acting From the Systemic Circulation

1. A rise in the acidity of plasma causes a decrease in the rate of renal potassium excretion and a decrease in potassium secretion by the distal tubule (7–11). It has been suggested that this decrease in secretion occurs as a result of a shift of hydrogen ions into the cell and potassium ions out of the cell (8, 12). Some evidence also indicates that a decline in the pH of luminal fluid lowers the potassium conductance of the apical cell membrane, which results in decreased potassium secretion (13, 14). If systemic acidosis is prolonged, rates of potassium excretion increase (15, 16). This change appears to be a secondary effect related to increased urine flow rate (11, 16) (see below).

A decrease in acidity of plasma increases the rate of renal potassium excretion and potassium secretion by the distal tubule (8–11, 15). This effect has been attributed to a shift of hydrogen ions out of the cell and of potassium into the cell (8). Metabolic alkalosis is usually associated with an increase in nonchloride anions in plasma, a change that may contribute to an increase in distal potassium secretion (11).

2. States in which plasma aldosterone levels are elevated are sometimes associated with increased rates of potassium excretion and distal potassium secretion (17–20). Aldosterone appears to act first by increasing the permeability of the luminal membrane to sodium, thus depolarizing the luminal membrane and increasing the electrochemical driving force for potassium movement from cell to lumen (21). Later, aldosterone stimulates potassium secretion further by increasing Na-K, ATPase activity in the basolateral membrane and potassium conductance in the luminal membrane (21–23). If a normal or high sodium intake is maintained, potassium wasting will occur (24–26).

3. Antidiuretic hormone (ADH) has been found to increase potassium secretion by the distal tubule under controlled experimental conditions (27). A reciprocal relationship between ADH levels and distal flow rate may serve to keep potassium excretion constant during normal fluctuations of ADH levels (27, 93; see section on influence of volume status on drug action).

4. The rate of distal potassium secretion correlates directly with changes in the plasma potassium concentration (28–30). Systemic events that raise plasma potassium concentration stimulate distal potassium secretion. Potassium secretion continues, but at lower rates when plasma potassium concentration is decreased.

Factors Acting From the Tubule Lumen

1. The rate of flow of luminal fluid is an extremely important determinant of renal potassium excretion and distal potassium secretion (31–34). Increases in fluid flow rate stimulate distal potassium secretion. This effect does not require

a change in sodium transport, sodium concentration, or an increase in the transepithelial voltage (lumen is negative with respect to the interstitium) (31).

2. Net distal potassium secretion depends on the luminal potassium concentration. Decreases in lumen potassium concentration stimulate potassium secretion (31). Increases in lumen potassium concentration reduce net potassium secretion (31).

3. When chloride concentration in lumen fluid is reduced to low levels, distal potassium secretion is stimulated (5, 35). This effect does not appear to depend on the transepithelial voltage or on the particular nonchloride anions that are present when chloride concentration is low (5, 6, 36). It is thought that this increase in potassium secretion is mediated by a mechanism in the luminal membrane of cells of the distal tubule that couples the movement of both potassium and chloride from cell to lumen.

4. An increase or a decrease in the transepithelial voltage (lumen negative) reflects an increased or a decreased electrical driving force for potassium secretion. It sometimes, but not always, correlates with a change in the rate of distal potassium secretion (6, 37–40). It always correlates with a change in the potassium concentration in luminal fluid.

ACTIONS OF DIURETIC DRUGS

Amiloride

Amiloride (*N*-amidino-3,5-diamino-6-
chloropyrazine carboxamide)

Amiloride decreases renal potassium excretion. Because it can counteract influences that tend to produce potassium wasting by the kidney, amiloride has been termed "potassium sparing" (41). Triamterene (2,4,7-triamino-6-phenylpteridine) (42–44) acts in a manner similar to that of amiloride.

Clearance and micropuncture experiments in rats demonstrated a decrease in the renal excretion of potassium when amiloride was administered systemically (37, 44). Sodium excretion increased in some studies (37) but not in others (45, 46). Experiments employing in vivo microperfusion to study the distal tubule of rats showed that amiloride in concentrations of less than 0.1 mM decreases potassium secretion (45, 47), sodium absorption (45, 47), and the transepithelial voltage (39, 40, 48), and increases the rate of calcium absorption (45). The effects on potassium and sodium transport are also present in cortical collecting ducts that are isolated from the kidney and perfused in vitro (49, 50). Amiloride is without effect in the thick ascending limb of Henle's loop (49, 59).

In the distal tubule and the cortical collecting duct, amiloride decreases distal potassium secretion and renal excretion indirectly; it does not act on a potassium transport mechanism directly. Amiloride blocks pathways for sodium ion diffusion in the luminal membrane of cells of the cortical collecting duct. The mechanism of action in distal tubule cells appears to be similar (14, 51). In the absence of amiloride this sodium-conductive pathway partially depolarizes the luminal membrane relative to the basolateral membrane and establishes a favorable electrochemical gradient for potassium movement from cell to lumen. Amiloride decreases distal potassium secretion by hyperpolarizing the luminal membrane and thus decreasing the electrochemical gradient for potassium movement into the lumen. We are not aware of any other setting encountered clinically in which a primary change in the apical membrane voltage (and transepithelial voltage) is the likely explanation for a subsequent change in the rate of potassium secretion by the distal tubule.

Furosemide

Furosemide (4-chloro-*N*-furfuryl-5-sulfamoylanthranilic acid)

Furosemide increases renal potassium excretion. It is used to promote renal sodium and water excretion, and the loss of increased amounts of potassium is not generally a desired effect. Other examples of this class of so-called "high ceiling" diuretics or loop diuretics are bumetanide (3-*N*-butylamino-4-phenoxy-5-sulfamoylbenzoic acid) (52–54), ethacrynic acid ([2,3-dichloro-4-(2-methylenebutyryl)phenoxy]acetic acid) (55, 56), and muzolimine or BAY g 2821 [3-amino-l-(3,4-dichloro-α-methylbenzyl)-2-pyrazolin-5-one] (57–59, 97).

Potassium, sodium, chloride, and water excretion rates increase when furosemide is administered to rats (33, 37). Results of recent microperfusion experiments in rats show that furosemide does not increase the rate of potassium secretion by the distal tubule (60). Bumetanide appears to stimulate net distal potassium secretion by a small amount (61). Results from in vivo micropuncture experiments show that both the potassium concentration and the volume flow rate out of the loop of Henle are increased after furosemide is administered intravenously (37). It is apparent that the rate of potassium absorption by the loop of Henle is greatly decreased. This could contribute directly to the increased rate of renal potassium excretion that is observed (62). As noted earlier, an increase in the concentration of potassium in the lumen of the downstream distal tubule, however, would be expected to decrease the rate of net potassium secretion by this segment. In contrast, the increase in volume flow through the distal tubule would be expected to stimulate net potassium secretion. Thus, the action of furosemide on net potassium transport is complex: a primary inhibition of potassium absorption in the loop of Henle and a secondary stimulation of potassium secretion by the distal tubule are the main factors responsible for the increased urinary potassium loss. This diuretic does not appear to affect potassium transport by the collecting duct (63).

The predominant specific renal effect of furosemide is to inhibit a mechanism mediating the movement of 1 Na, 1 K, and 2 Cl from lumen to cell in the thick ascending limb of Henle's loop (64, 65). The lumen positive voltage decreases towards zero and thus lowers the electrical driving force for passive potassium absorption. Inhibition of potassium absorption via this three-ion cotransporter causes luminal potassium concentration to rise and contributes directly to the increased renal potassium loss (62). Inhibition of sodium and chloride absorption via the cotransporter causes luminal sodium and chloride concentrations to increase and prevents the normal dilution of luminal fluid by this segment. Although furosemide does not affect potassium transport in the distal tubule, it does decrease sodium and chloride transport by this segment (60). The mechanism for sodium and chloride absorption in the distal tubule appears to be different from the mechanism that is found in the thick ascending limb of Henle's loop (47).

Furosemide can also stimulate renal potassium loss by increasing the renal blood flow and filtration rate and thus increasing the flow rate in the distal tubule. This contribution, however, appears to be of minor significance (66–68).

When furosemide is in systemic circulation it binds extensively to plasma proteins. It is effective only from the lumen compartment and reaches its site of action not by filtration at the glomerulus but by secretion by cells of the proximal tubule (63, 69). Probenecid [p-(dipropylsulfamyl)benzoic acid] and indomethacin [1-(p-chlorobenzoyl)-5-methoxy-2-methylindole-3-acetic acid] affect the renal response to furosemide. Probenecid interferes with the organic acid transport mechanism in proximal tubules that also mediates the transport of a wide variety of organic anions, including furosemide and other diuretics, from plasma into luminal fluid (70, 71). The administration of furosemide, together with probenecid, decreases the rate at which furosemide reaches its site of action and prolongs the time course of the effect. However, the magnitude of the diuresis for a given dose of furosemide is not decreased (72). Indomethacin has been reported to decrease the diuretic response to furosemide by a mechanism not related to inhibition of the cyclooxygenase pathway for prostaglandin synthesis or to inhibition of secretory transport of furosemide (73, 98). It may influence the action of furosemide on cells of the thick ascending limb (68, 73).

Acetazolamide

Acetazolamide (5-acetamido-1,3,4-thiadiazole-2-sulfonamide)

$$CH_3CONH \diagdown \overset{S}{\underset{N\text{———}N}{\diagup \diagdown}} \diagup SO_2NH_2$$

Acetazolamide increases renal potassium excretion. It is a diuretic drug that inhibits carbonic anhydrase activity and promotes sodium bicarbonate and fluid excretion. Other examples of this class of diuretics are benzolamide (benzolsulfonamido-5-thia-1-diazol-3,4-sulfonamide) (74, 75) and ethoxolamide (6-ethoxy-2-benzothiazolesulfonamide) (75).

When acetazolamide is administered to rats or dogs, renal potassium loss is stimulated (60, 74, 76, 77). A direct effect of acetazolamide on potassium secretion by the distal tubule has not been demonstrated. This class of diuretic decreases bicarbonate, sodium, and volume absorption in the proximal tubule (74, 77). Thus, more bicarbonate and less chloride is delivered into the loop of Henle. Increased flow rates in the distal tubule result in increased rates of distal potassium secretion and increased renal loss of potassium.

These diuretics act by inhibiting the enzyme carbonic anhydrase of proximal tubule cells (75, 78). The absorption of bicarbonate is thus impaired, and the fluid that is delivered into the loop of Henle and the distal tubule after administering the diuretic has a reduced chloride concentration and increased concentrations of nonchloride anions. It was suggested that distal potassium secretion is stimulated because the increased load of bicarbonate led to an increase in the lumen negative voltage under these conditions (3, 25). In view of more recent evidence, it is unlikely that a rise in luminal bicarbonate increases the lumen negative voltage (5, 36). It is possible but not certain that systemic administration of carbonic anhydrase inhibitors causes lumen chloride concentration in distal tubules to decline sufficiently to stimulate potassium secretion (74). Current evidence supports the conclusion that an increase in lumen flow rate is primarily responsible for the enhanced renal potassium loss after acetazolamide administration.

Hydrochlorothiazide

Hydrochlorothiazide (6-chloro-3,4-dihydro-
2H-1,2,4-benzothiadiazine-7-sulfonamide-1,1-
dioxide)

Hydrochlorothiazide increases renal potassium excretion. This diuretic also increases water and sodium chloride losses but decreases the rate of calcium excretion. Another example is chlorthalidone [2-chloro-5-(1-hydroxy-3-oxo-1-isoindolinlyl)benzenesulfonamide] (99).

The increased rate of potassium loss after hydrochlorothiazide administration does not appear to result from a direct effect on the distal tubule. When thiazide-containing solutions are perfused directly into distal tubules of rats, rates of potassium secretion do not increase (47). However, rates of net sodium, chloride, and water absorption are decreased dramatically after thiazides (46, 47, 79). This effect appears to occur predominantly in the early distal tubule or in distal convoluted tubule cells. In experiments in rats, results from in vivo perfusion of the first part of the distal tubule showed that hydrochlorothiazide decreased net water absorption and net sodium absorption and increased net calcium absorption (46). The diuretic was without effect in the later portion of the distal tubule.

The mechanism by which hydrochlorothiazide increases potassium loss is indirect. It decreases salt and water absorption upstream from the potassium secretory site. Increases in flow rate through the late distal tubule and the collecting duct stimulate rates of potassium secretion. The potassium loss with chlorthalidone appears to be larger than that with hydrochlorothiazide (99). Thiazides can also have a small effect on proximal salt and water absorption because they can inhibit the enzyme carbonic anhydrase (75, 79) (see acetazolamide above).

Spironolactone

Spironolactone decreases potassium excretion when aldosterone is present and is stimulating potassium secretion.

Spironolactone is a competitive antagonist of aldosterone and blocks the stimulating effect of aldosterone on potassium secretion and sodium absorption (58, 80–82). In isolated perfused cortical collecting tubules, spironolactone reduces the ability of aldosterone to stimulate the lumen negative transepithelial

Spironolactone (17-hydroxy-7-
mercapto-3-oxo-17αpregn-4-ene-
21-carboxylic acidγ-lactone,
7-acetate)

voltage (42). Although spironolactone has not always been found to have an effect on the distal tubule of rats (82) or rabbits (42), it is likely that the late portions of the distal tubule are sensitive to this agent. The late portion of the distal tubule, the initial collecting tubule, responds to aldosterone by increasing sodium absorption and potassium secretion, by increasing the lumen negative transepithelial voltage, and by increasing the basolateral membrane area of the principal cells (23, 28, 83). We are not aware of any study that has directly determined the effect of spironolactone on potassium transport by the distal tubule.

Aldosterone binding to specific receptors (19, 81) in the cytoplasm of target cells in the distal nephron leads initially (within hours) to an increase in sodium permeability of the apical membrane followed by an increase (within days) in the potassium conductance of the luminal membrane and in the ATPase activity of the basolateral membrane (21–23). The increase in sodium permeability would be expected to depolarize the apical membrane. This reduction in the cell-negative voltage across the luminal membrane increases the electrochemical driving force for potassium movement from cell to lumen and leads to an increase in net potassium secretion. Continued exposure to aldosterone increases luminal potassium conductance and basolateral ATPase activity, which results in a further increase in net potassium secretion. It appears that a continued high rate of sodium entry into the cell from the luminal compartment is necessary to establish and maintain the higher ATPase levels of cortical collecting tubules (21). Depending on the physiological circumstances, then, the secondary effect on potassium secretion may not always be present. For example, amiloride treatment prevents sodium entry into late distal cells and blocks aldosterone's effect on the ATPase and potassium conductance. Spironolactone prevents aldosterone binding and thus blocks both the initial and delayed aldosterone-stimulated increases in distal potassium secretion.

Indacrinone (Mk 196)

Indacrinone (MK 196) [(6,7-dichloro-2-
methyl-1-oxo-2-phenyl-5-indanyl)oxy]
acetic acid

Indacrinone increases renal potassium excretion. Systemic administration of indacrinone causes diuresis and promotes renal sodium and potassium loss (84, 85). Results from in vivo micropuncture and microperfusion experiments in the rat (84, 86) show that this agent decreases sodium and potassium absorption by the loop of Henle. Sodium absorption, but not potassium secretion, was inhibited in the perfused distal tubule (86). Sodium absorption by the collecting duct also appears to be decreased (84). When indacrinone was applied to segments of the rat medullary thick ascending limb of Henle's loop, which were isolated and perfused in vitro, both the transepithelial voltage (lumen positive) (59, 87) and net chloride absorption were decreased (87).

This diuretic appears to have a complex renal mechanism of action. Its ability to decrease potassium, sodium, and chloride absorption in the loop of Henle and to inhibit the lumen positive voltage suggests that it is inhibiting the furosemide sensitive Na-K-2Cl cotransport mechanism that is known to be present in this segment. The related drug ethacrynic acid (88) also inhibits this cotransport mechanism. In the distal tubule, it is possible that indacrinone affects a mechanism for sodium chloride cotransport (60). Although rates of chloride transport and the transepithelial voltage were not measured, sodium absorption in the distal tubule was reduced without an effect on net potassium secretion (86). We have found that in the distal tubule both furosemide and hydrochlorothiazide also inhibit sodium and chloride absorption without affecting potassium secretion (47, 60). The possibility that sodium chloride cotransport in the distal tubule is inhibited by indacrinone needs to be investigated further.

Finally, indacrinone appears to reduce sodium absorption by the collecting duct (84). Its mechanism of action in this segment is not clear and requires further investigation. A recent report of experiments in toad and frog skin (89) suggests that this agent can block conductive channels for chloride movement. However, at the same time that it blocked chloride conductance in this tissue, it also increased the sodium conductance of the apical membrane. Thus, it stimulated the transepithelial voltage and the short circuit current while decreasing the transepithelial electrical conductance.

Indacrinone enhances renal potassium loss via two mechanisms. First, by inhibiting potassium absorption in the thick ascending limb of Henle's loop it contributes directly to a kaliuresis. Second, because of the decreased solute and water absorption in both the diluting segment and in the distal tubule, potassium secretion is stimulated because of an enhanced fluid flow rate through the distal tubule.

INFLUENCE OF VOLUME STATUS ON DRUG ACTION

We have discussed the mechanisms of action of several drugs and how they affect renal potassium excretion. Most of this information has come from experiments in which a control or a normal state of the organism prevailed. In practice, however, these drugs are used to treat a variety of clinical disorders including hypertension, congestive heart failure, cirrhosis of the liver, idiopathic edema, and the nephrotic syndrome. Diuretic drugs do not generally induce excessive potassium loss when given acutely, and the maintenance of an adequate dietary potassium intake can prevent an imbalance between potassium excretion and intake. In contrast, when diuretics are given chronically, it is sometimes necessary to give potassium supplements to prevent hypokalemia and severe potassium depletion. The etiology of the conditions mentioned above and the treatment regimens applied are beyond the scope of this review and are not discussed.

The effects of diuretic drugs on the renal handling of potassium, however, can be altered dramatically depending on the physiologic state of the organism. Several components of the systems involved in the regulation of body fluid balance are related and interdependent: volume status, aldosterone levels, antidiuretic hormone levels, and rates of potassium secretion by the distal tubule.

Despite the generally accepted view that aldosterone stimulates renal potassium excretion, a number of studies have shown that aldosterone administration is without effect on renal potassium excretion (90–92). Recent results, however, suggest that other variables influencing distal potassium transport are also changed when aldosterone levels are elevated and thus provide a possible explanation for the apparently negative results associated with aldosterone administration. It is well established that flow rate of lumen fluid is an important determinant of distal potassium secretion (31). When aldosterone was infused into rats it was noted that urine flow rates were reduced (28). A decrease in distal flow rate occurring at the same time that aldosterone is promoting distal potassium secretion could result in no net effect on potassium transport (26,

85). Thus, it may be that under normal circumstances fluctuations of aldosterone levels have little effect on renal potassium excretion because of reciprocal changes in tubule flow rate. Disease states in which this counter regulatory system is disturbed could establish conditions in which aldosterone does stimulate distal potassium secretion. If flow rate increases or remains high at a time when the cells of the distal tubule are stimulated by the hormone, the rate of potassium secretion will be enhanced above the control levels. Thus, the use of diuretic drugs under these conditions would greatly stimulate the renal loss of potassium (93). The additional administration of a potassium-sparing diuretic would reduce the overall potassium loss. Spironolactone would prevent the expression of aldosterone's effect on the cells of the distal tubule and would thus decrease the rate of potassium secretion by the distal tubule and the cortical collecting duct.

The volume status of the organism correlates not only with levels of plasma aldosterone but also with levels of vasopressin circulating in plasma. Under conditions of volume contraction, plasma ADH levels are high, water reabsorption by the kidney is maximal, and fluid flow rates are low. To maintain potassium homeostasis during fluctuations of volume status the rates of renal potassium excretion must remain constant. Recent evidence suggests that plasma levels of ADH may influence potassium transport cells of the distal tubule directly and thus contribute to potassium homeostasis (27, 94). In experiments employing Brattleboro rats, which are deficient in ADH, Field and co-workers (27) noted that interruption of the diuresis by administration of ADH did not decrease distal potassium secretion. These results were obtained using free-flow micropuncture techniques in which ion concentrations and fluid flow rates in the distal tubule were permitted to vary. Tubule flow rates and lumen potassium concentrations were not the same in both states. When in vivo microperfusion techniques were employed to maintain constant lumen flow rates, the rate of distal potassium secretion was increased by ADH administration. Thus, it appears that this hormone can have a direct effect on cells of the distal tubule. Under in vivo circumstances the effect is masked because the stimulation of distal potassium secretion by ADH and the reduction of luminal flow rate in the volume-contracted state oppose each other. If ADH levels are high at a time when the organism is not volume contracted, higher rates of potassium secretion are expected because the effect of ADH on potassium-secreting cells is not mitigated by low luminal flow rates. In this setting of inappropriately high ADH (95, 96), the administration of diuretic drugs to correct the water balance would lead to an increased renal potassium loss.

The volume status of the organism, plasma aldosterone levels, and plasma ADH levels all help to determine the magnitude of the renal potassium loss that occurs when diuretics are administered.

SUMMARY

This review has focused on the influence of several diuretic drugs on potassium handling by the kidney. One class of drugs (loop diuretics) acts by directly inhibiting a potassium absorptive mechanism in the luminal membrane of cells of the thick ascending limb of Henle's loop. Two other groups of diuretics affect potassium transport indirectly by inhibiting salt and water absorption upstream from the potassium secretory site in the late distal tubule: carbonic anhydrase inhibitors act in the proximal tubule; thiazides act in the early distal tubule. The subsequent increase in lumen flow rate then stimulates net potassium secretion by the distal tubule. A fourth class of drugs (spironolactone) acts by antagonizing the response of the distal tubule to aldosterone. These drugs decrease the ability of aldosterone to stimulate distal potassium secretion. Finally, a fifth group of drugs (potassium-sparing diuretics) decreases potassium secretion by increasing the luminal membrane voltage and thus decreasing the electrochemical gradient for potassium exit from the cell.

Literature Cited

1. Wright, F. S., Giebisch, G. 1985. Regulation of potassium excretion. In *The Kidney: Physiology and Pathophysiology*, ed. D. W. Seldin, G. Giebisch, pp. 1223–50. New York: Raven
2. Wright, F. S. 1977. Sites and mechanisms of potassium transport along the renal tubule. *Kidney Int.* 11:415–32
3. Giebisch, G., Malnic, G., Berliner, R. W. 1981. Renal transport and control of potassium excretion. In *The Kidney*, ed. B. M. Brenner, F. C. Rector, pp. 408–39. Philadelphia: W. B. Saunders. 2nd ed.
4. Giebisch, G. 1975. Some reflections on the mechanism of renal tubular potassium transport. *Yale J. Biol. Med.* 48:315–36
5. Velázquez, H., Wright, F. S., Good, D. W. 1982. Luminal influences on potassium secretion: chloride replacement with sulfate. *Am. J. Physiol.* 242:F46–55
6. Ellison, D., Velázquez, H. E., Wright, F. S. 1985. Stimulation of distal potassium secretion by low lumen chloride in presence of barium. *Am. J. Physiol.* 248:F638–49
7. Gennari, F. J., Cohen, J. J. 1975. Role of the kidney in potassium homeostasis: lessons from acid-base disturbances. *Kidney Int.* 8:1–5
8. Malnic, G., de Mello-Aires, M., Giebisch, G. 1971. Potassium transport across renal distal tubules during acid-base disturbances. *Am. J. Physiol.* 221:1192–1207

9. Toussaint, C., Vereerstraeten, P. 1962. Effects of blood pH changes on potassium excretion in the dog. *Am. J. Physiol.* 202:768–72
10. Schwartz, W. B., Cohen, J. J. 1978. The nature of the renal response to chronic disorders of acid-base equilibrium. *Am. J. Med.* 64:417–28
11. Stanton, B. A., Giebisch, G. 1982. Effects of pH on potassium transport by renal distal tubule. *Am. J. Physiol.* 242:F544–51
12. Roberts, K. E., Magida, M. G., Pitts, R. F. 1953. Relationship between potassium and bicarbonate in blood and urine. *Am. J. Physiol.* 172:47–54
13. Boudry, J. F., Stoner, L. C., Burg, M. B. 1976. The effect of lumen pH on potassium transport in renal cortical collecting tubules. *Am. J. Physiol.* 230:239–44
14. O'Neil, R. G., Sansom, S. C. 1984. Characterization of apical cell membrane Na^+ and K^+ conductances of cortical collecting duct using microelectrode techniques. *Am. J. Physiol.* 247:F14–24
15. Scott, D., McIntosh, G. H. 1975. Changes in blood composition and in urinary mineral acid excretion in the pig in response to acute acid-base disturbances. *Q. J. Exp. Physiol.* 60:131–40
16. DeSousa, R. C., Harrington, T. J., Ricanate, E. S., Shelkrot, J. W., Schwartz, W. B. 1974. Renal regulation

of acid-base equilibrium during chronic administration of mineral acid. *J. Clin. Invest.* 53:465–76

17. Young, D. B., Jackson, T. E. 1982. Effects of aldosterone on potassium distribution. *Am. J. Physiol.* 243:R526–30

18. Rabinowitz, L. 1979–80. Aldosterone and renal potassium excretion. *Renal Physiol. Basel* 2:229–43

19. Marver, D., Kokko, J. P. 1983. Renal target sites and the mechanism of action of aldosterone. *Miner. Electrolyte Metab* 9:1–18

20. Kassirer, J. P., London, A. M., Goldman, D. M., Schwartz, W. B. 1970. On the pathogenesis of metabolic alkalosis in hyperaldosteronism. *Am. J. Med.* 49:306

21. O'Neil, R. G., Hayhurst, R. A. 1985. Sodium-dependent modulation of the renal Na-K-ATPase: Influence of mineralocorticoids on the cortical collecting duct. *J. Membr. Biol.* 85:169–79

22. Sansom, S. C., O'Neil, R. G. 1985. Mineralocorticoid regulation of apical cell membrane Na^+ and K^+ transport of the cortical collecting duct. *Am. J. Physiol.* 248:F858–68

23. Stanton, B., Giebisch, G., Klein-Robbenhaar, G., Wade, J., DeFronzo, R. A. 1985. Effects of adrenalectomy and chronic adrenal corticosteroid replacement of potassium transport in rat kidney. *J. Clin. Invest.* 75:1317–26

24. George, J. M., Wright, L., Bell, N. H. 1970. The syndrome of primary aldosteronism. *Am. J. Med.* 48:343

25. Cohen, J. J., Gennari, F. J., Harrington, J. T. 1981. Disorders of potassium balance. See Ref. 3, pp. 908–39

26. Seldin, D. W. 1982. Diuretic-induced potassium loss. In *Recent Advances in Diuretic Therapy*, pp. 9–20. Amsterdam: Excerpta Med.

27. Field, M. J., Stanton, B. A., Giebisch, G. H. 1984. Influence of ADH on renal potassium handling: a micropuncture and microperfusion study. *Kidney Int.* 25: 502–11

28. Field, M. J., Stanton, B. A., Giebisch, G. H. 1984. Differential acute effects of aldosterone, dexamethasone, and hyperkalemia on distal tubular potassium secretion in the rat kidney. *J. Clin. Invest.* 74:1792–1802

29. Young, D. B. 1982. Relationship between plasma potassium concentration and renal potassium excretion. *Am. J. Physiol.* 242:F599–F603

30. Stanton, B. A., Giebisch, G. H. 1982. Potassium transport by the renal distal tubule: effects of potassium loading. *Am. J. Physiol.* 243:F487–93

31. Good, D. W., Wright, F. S. 1979. Luminal influences of potassium secretion: Sodium concentration and fluid flow rate. *Am. J. Physiol.* 236:F192–F205

32. Kunau, R. T., Webb, M. L., Borman, S. C. 1974. Characteristics of the relationship between the flow rate of tubular fluid and potassium transport in the distal tubule of the rat. *J. Clin. Invest.* 54:1488–95

33. Dirks, J. H., Seely, J. F. 1970. Effect of saline infusions and furosemide on the dog distal nephron. *Am. J. Physiol.* 219:114–21

34. Khuri, R. N., Wiederholt, M., Strieder, N., Giebisch, G. 1975. Effects of flow rate and potassium intake on distal tubular potassium transfer. *Am. J. Physiol.* 228:1249–61

35. Good, D. H., Velázquez, H., Wright, F. S. 1984. Luminal influences on potassium secretion: low sodium concentration. *Am. J. Physiol.* 246:F609–19

36. Velázquez, H., Wright, F. S., Good, D. W. 1980. Effects of luminal anion composition and acidity on potassium secretion by renal distal tubule. *Fed. Proc.* 39:1079

37. Duarte, C. G., Chomety, F., Giebisch, G. 1971. Effect of amiloride, ouabain and furosemide on distal tubular function in the rat. *Am. J. Physiol.* 221:632–39

38. Good, D. W., Wright, F. S. 1980. Luminal influences on potassium secretion: transepithelial voltage. *Am. J. Physiol.* 239:F289–98

39. Garcia-Filho, E., Malnic, G., Giebisch, G. 1980. Effects of changes in electrical potential difference on tubular potassium transport. *Am. J. Physiol.* 238:F235–46

40. Barratt, L. J. 1976. The effect of amiloride on the transepithelial potential difference of the distal tubule of the rat kidney. *Pfluegers Arch.* 361:251–54

41. Baer, J. E., Jones, C. B., Spitzer, S. A., Russo, H. F. 1967. The potassium sparing and natriuretic activity of N-amidino - 3,4 - diamino - 6 -chloropyrazinecarboxamide hydrochloride dihydrate (amiloride hydrochloride). *J. Pharmacol. Exp. Ther.* 157:472–85

42. Gross, J. B., Kokko, J. P. 1977. Effects of aldosterone and potassium-sparing diuretics on electrical potential differences across the distal nephron. *J. Clin. Invest.* 59:82–89

43. Crabbé, J. 1968. A hypothesis concerning the mode of action of amiloride and triamterene. *Arch. Int. Pharmacodyn. Ther.* 173:474

44. Guignard, J. P., Peters, G. 1970. Effects

of triamterene and amiloride on urinary acidification and potassium excretion in the rat. *Eur. J. Pharmacol.* 10:255–67

45. Constanzo, L. S. 1984. Comparison of calcium and sodium transport in early and late rat distal tubules: effect of amiloride. *Am. J. Physiol.* 246:F937–45

46. Costanzo, L. S. 1985. Localization of diuretic action in microperfused rat distal tubules: Ca and Na transport. *Am. J. Physiol.* 248:F527–35

47. Velázquez, H., Wright, F. S. 1983. Distal tubule pathways for sodium, chloride and potassium transport assessed by diuretics. *Kidney Int.* 23:269

48. Wright, F. S., Velázquez, H. 1983. Enhancement of amiloride action by calcium in rat renal distal tubule. *28th Congr. Int. Union Physiol. Sci., Australia* (Abstr.)

49. Stoner, L. C., Burg, M. B., Orloff, J. 1974. Ion transport in cortical collecting tubule; effect of amiloride. *Am. J. Physiol.* 227:453–59

50. Stokes, J. B. 1982. Ion transport by the cortical and outer medullary collecting tubule. *Kidney Int.* 22:473–84

51. Koeppen, B. M., Biagi, B. A., Giebisch, G. H. 1983. Intracellular microelectrode characterization of the rabbit cortical collecting duct. *Am. J. Physiol.* 244:F35–47

52. Gutsche, H. U., Müller-Ott, K., Brunkhorst, R., Niedermayer, W. 1983. Dose related effects of furosemide, bumetanide and piretanide on the thick ascending limb function in the rat. *Can. J. Physiol. Pharmacol.* 61:159–65

53. Imai, M. 1977. Effect of bumetanide and furosemide on the thick ascending limb of Henle's loop of rabbits and rats perfused in vitro. *Eur. J. Pharmacol.* 41:409–16

54. Ostergaard, E. H., Magnussen, M. P., Nielsen, C. K., Eilertsen, E., Frey, H.-H. 1972. Pharmacological properties of 3-N-butylamino-4-phenoxy-5-sulfamyl-benzoic acid (bumetanide), a new potent diuretic. *Drug. Res.* 22:66–72

55. Goldberg, M., McCurdy, K. K., Flotz, E. L., Bluemle, L. W. 1964. Effect of ethacrynic acid (a new saliuretic agent) on renal diluting and concentrating mechanisms: Evidence for site of action in loop of Henle. *J. Clin. Invest.* 43:201

56. Earley, L. E., Friedler, R. M. 1964. Renal tubular effects of ethacrynic acid. *J. Clin. Invest.* 43:1495

57. Moeller, E., Horstmann, H., Meng, K., Loew, D. 1977. 3-amino-1-(3,4-dichloro-α-methyl-benzyl)-2-pyrazolin-5-one (Bay g 2821), a potent diuretic from

a new substance class. *Experientia* 33:382–83

58. Campen, T. J., Vaughn, D. A., Fanestil, D. D. 1983. Mineralo- and glucocorticoid effects on renal excretion of electrolytes. *Pfluegers Arch.* 399:93–101

59. Schlatter, E., Greger, R., Weidtke, C. 1983. Effect of "high ceiling" diuretics on active salt transport in the cortical thick ascending limb of Henle's loop of rabbit kidney. Correlation of chemical structure and inhibitory potency. *Pfluegers Arch.* 396:210–217

60. Velázquez, H., Good, D. W., Wright, F. S. 1984. Mutual dependence of sodium and chloride absorption by renal distal tubule. *Am. J. Physiol.* 247:F904–11

61. Velázquez, H., Wright, F. S. 1984. Sodium, chloride, and potassium transport by the distal nephron: effect of bumetanide and chlorothiazide. *Kidney Int.* 25:319

62. Burg, M., Green, N. 1973. Effect of ethacrynic acid on the thick ascending limb of Henle's loop. *Kidney Int.* 4:301–8

63. Burg, M. B., Stoner, L., Cardinal, J., Green, N. 1973. Furosemide effect on isolated perfused tubules. *Am. J. Physiol.* 225:119–24

64. Greger, R., Schlatter, E. 1981. Presence of luminal K, a prerequisite for active NaCl transport in the cortical thick ascending limb of Henle's loop of rabbit kidney. *Pfluegers Arch.* 392:92–94

65. Eveloff, J., Kinne, R. K.-H. 1981. Sodium-chloride cotransport in plasma membranes isolated from thick ascending limb of Henle's loop. *Fed. Proc.* 40:356

66. Gerber, J. G., Nies, A. S. 1981. Interaction between furosemide-induced renal vasodilation and the prostaglandin system. *Prostaglandins Med.* 6:135–45

67. Birtch, A. G., Zakheim, R. M., Jones, L. G., Barger, A. C. 1967. Redistribution of renal blood flow produced by furosemide and ethacrynic acid. *Circ. Res.* 21:869–78

68. Brater, D. C. 1983. Pharmacodynamic considerations in the use of diuretics. *Ann. Rev. Pharmacol. Toxicol.* 23:45–62

69. Deetjen, P. 1966. Micropuncture studies on site and mode of diuretic action of furosemide. *Ann. NY Acad. Sci.* 139:408–15

70. Hook, J. B., Williamson, H. E. 1965. Influence of probenecid and alterations in acid-base balance of the saluretic activity of furosemide. *J. Pharmacol. Exp. Ther.* 149:404

71. Honari, J., Blair, A. D., Cutler, R. E. 1977. Effects of probenecid on furose-

mide kinetics and natriuresis in man. *Clin. Pharmacol. Ther.* 22:395

72. Homeida, M., Roberts, C., Branch, R. A. 1977. Influence of probenecid and spironolactone on furosemide kinetics and dynamics in man. *Clin. Pharmacol. Ther.* 22:402–9

73. Chennavasin, P., Seiwell, R., Brater, D. C. 1980. Pharmacokinetic-dynamic analysis of the indomethacin-furosemide interaction in man. *J. Pharmacol. Exp. Ther.* 215:77–81

74. Kunau, R. T. 1972. The influence of the carbonic anhydrase inhibitor, benzolamide (CL-11,366), on the reabsorption of chloride, sodium and bicarbonate in the proximal tubule of the rat. *J. Clin. Invest.* 51:294–306

75. Maren, T. H. 1976. Relations between structure and biological activity of sulfonamides. *Ann. Rev. Pharmacol. Toxicol.* 16:309–27

76. Malnic, G., Klose, R. M., Giebisch, G. 1966. Micropuncture study of distal tubular potassium and sodium transport in rat nephron. *Am. J. Physiol.* 211:529–47

77. Malnic, G., Giebisch, G. 1972. Mechanism of renal hydrogen ion secretion. *Kidney Int.* 1:280

78. Rector, F. C. Jr., Carter, N. W., Seldin, D. W. 1965. The mechanism of bicarbonate reabsorption in the proximal and distal tubules of the kidney. *J. Clin. Invest.* 44:278–90

79. Kunau, R. T., Weller, D. R., Webb, H. L. 1975. Clarification of the site of action of chlorothiazide in the rat nephron. *J. Clin. Invest.* 56:401–7

80. Liddle, G. W. 1966. Aldosterone antagonists and triamterene. *Ann. NY Acad. Sci.* 134:466

81. Edelman, I., Fimognari, G. 1968. On the biochemical mechanisms of action of aldosterone. In *Recent Progress in Hormone Research*, p. 1. New York: Academic

82. Bengele, H. H., McNamara, E. R., Alexander, E. A. 1977. Natriuresis after adrenal enucleation: effect of spironolactone and dexamethasone. *Am. J. Physiol.* 233:F8–12

83. Allen, G. G., Barratt, L. J. 1981. Effect of aldosterone on the transepithelial potential difference of the rat distal tubule. *Kidney Int.* 19:678–86

84. Kauker, M. L. 1977. Clearance and micropuncture studies of the effects of a new indanyloxyacetic acid diuretic on segmental nephron function in rats. *J. Pharmacol. Exp. Ther,* 200:81–87

85. Field, M. J., Giebisch, G. H. 1985. Hormonal control of renal potassium excretion. *Kidney Int.* 27:379–87

86. Field, M. J., Fowler, N., Giebisch, G. H. 1984. Effects of enantiomers of indacrinone (MK-196) on cation transport by the loop of Henle and distal tubule studied by microperfusion in vivo. *J. Pharmacol. Exp. Ther.* 230:62–68

87. Stoner, L. C., Trimble, M. E. 1982. Effects of MK-196 and furosemide on rat medullary thick ascending limbs of Henle in vitro. *J. Pharmacol. Exp. Ther.* 221:715–20

88. Solms, S. J. De, Woltersdorf, O. W. Jr., Cragoe, E. J. Jr., Watson, L. S., Fanelli, G. M. Jr. 1978. (Acylaryloxy)acetic acid diuretics. 2. (2-Alkyl-2-aryl-1-oxo-5-indanyloxy)acetic acids. *J. Med. Chem.* 21:437–43

89. Nagel, W., Beauwens, R., Crabbé, J. 1985. Opposite effects of indacrinone (MK-196) on sodium and chloride conductance of amphibian skin. *Pfluegers Arch.* 403:337–43

90. Cortney, M. A. 1969. Renal tubular transfer of water and electrolytes in adrenalectomized rats. *Am. J. Physiol.* 216:589–98

91. Davis, J. O. 1961. Mechanisms regulating the secretion and metabolism of aldosterone in experimental secondary hyperaldosteronism. *Recent Prog. Horm. Res.* 17:293–352

92. Hierholzer, K., Wiederholt, M., Holzgreve, H., Giebisch, G., Klose, R. M., Windhager, E. E. 1965. Micropuncture study of renal transtubular concentration gradients of sodium and potassium in adrenalectomized rats. *Pfluegers Arch. Gesamte Physiol.* 285:193–210

93. Kelly, R. A., Wilcox, C. S., Souney, P., Mitch, W. E. 1984. Effects of aldosterone and ADH on potassium excretion with furosemide. *Kidney Int.* 25:169

94. Kelly, R. A., Wilcox, C. S., Mitch, W. E., Meyer, T. W., Souney, P. F., et al. 1983. Response of the kidney to furosemide. 2. Effect of captopril on sodium balance. *Kidney Int.* 24:233–39

95. Hantman, B., Rossier, B., Zohlman, R., Schrier, R. 1973. Rapid correction of hyponatremia in the syndrome of inappropriate secretion of antidiuretic hormone: An alternative treatment to hypertonic saline. *Ann. Intern. Med.* 78:870

96. Reineck, H. J., Stein, J. H. 1981. Mechanisms of action and clinical uses of diuretics. See Ref. 3, pp. 1097–1131

97. Loew, D., Ritter, W., Dycka, J. 1977. Comparison of the pharmacodynamic effects of furosemide and BAY g 2821 and correlation of the pharmacodynamics and pharmacokinetics of BAY g 2821 (Muzolimine). *Eur. J. Clin. Pharmacol.* 12:341–44

98. Smith, D. E., Brater, D. C., Lin, E. T., Benet, L. Z. 1979. Attenuation of furosemide's diuretic effect by indomethacin: Pharmacokinetic evaluation. *J. Pharmacokinet. Biopharm.* 7:265–74

99. Ram, C. V. S., Garret, B. N., Kaplan, N. M. 1981. Moderate sodium restriction and various diuretics in the treatment of hypertension. *Arch. Intern. Med.* 141:1015–19

Ann. Rev. Pharmacol. Toxicol. 1986. 26:311–32

PHARMACOLOGY OF THYROTROPIN-RELEASING HORMONE

A. Horita[1,2], M. A. Carino[1], and H. Lai[1]

Departments of Pharmacology[1] and Psychiatry & Behavioral Sciences[2], University of Washington School of Medicine, Seattle, Washington 98195

INTRODUCTION

Thyrotropin-releasing hormone (TRH) was identified as L-pyroglutamyl-L-histidyl-L-proline amide in 1973, and its eventual synthesis enabled researchers to investigate its physiological and pharmacological properties. During the past ten years it has become clear that TRH and its receptors are ubiquitously distributed in the central nervous system (CNS) as well as in several peripheral organs. Studies in which TRH was administered to experimental animals have revealed some intriguing and potentially important clinical actions, most of which are unrelated to its thyrotropin-releasing property. In fact, this property in some instances is looked upon as a side effect, and attempts have been made to synthesize analogues that retain the central, but not the thyrotropin-releasing, properties of TRH (1, 2).

Because of space considerations, the scope of this review has been limited to selected aspects of the pharmacology of TRH. The review of the literature has also been selective and is devoted mostly to papers published after 1982. For a more comprehensive background on the extrapituitary properties of TRH the reader is referred to several earlier publications (3–7).

TRH RECEPTORS

The first studies of extrapituitary TRH binding sites were made as early as 1975 (8), but the lack of a ligand with high specific activity prevented accurate description of their properties. The later availability of [3]H-3MeHis-TRH, a

TRH analogue with higher binding affinity, enabled characterization not only of the properties, but also of the distribution of the receptors. It is now generally agreed that TRH receptors in brain are ubiquitously distributed, but are found in highest densities in limbic structures, especially the amygdala and hypothalamus, and in lower densities in brain stem and cerebellum (9–11). TRH receptors also occur in the spinal cord, with the highest densities in the dorsal and ventral gray matter and lower densities in the dorsal root and ganglia (12, 13). The receptors in the brain and pituitary are very similar (14, 15), but may differ in some ways in their interaction with certain drugs (16).

The receptor is membrane bound, digestible by trypsin and phospholipase, and inactivated by various thiol reagents and metal salts (17, 18). Various drugs have been tested for ability to compete with the radioactive ligand, but thus far only two classes of drugs have been identified that compete at micromolar concentrations. Their pharmacology might be related to TRH-receptor interactions: the dihydrogenated ergot alkaloids and the benzodiazepines. The several components of dihydroergotoxin (DHET) have been found to range in IC_{50} between 10 and 50 μM. Fourteen days of DHET treatment induced an up-regulation of TRH receptors in the cerebral cortex of aged rats, but not in other brain areas (19). The benzodiazepines, particularly chlordiazepoxide, were reported to compete at micromolar concentrations with [3]H-3MeHis-TRH binding to brain and pituitary membranes (20, 21). No relationship was observed between antianxiety potency/benzodiazepine receptor binding and ability to displace the TRH ligand. In fact, flunitrazepam and diazepam, both potent agonists of the benzodiazepine receptor, were considerably weaker than chlordiazepoxide in displacement ability. More recent work demonstrated the presence of regional differences in inhibition of TRH binding by the benzodiazepines (16). The IC_{50}s of chlordiazepoxide and diazepam for [3]H-3MeHis-TRH displacement in membranes from hippocampus, spinal cord, and hypothalamus were 2–25 times greater than in those from the amygdala, retina, and pituitary. Although the significance of these differences is as yet unclear, they suggest the possible existence of multiple classes of TRH receptors.

Some beginnings have been made in solubilizing the TRH receptor from brain. Ogawa et al (22) solubilized the ^{3}H-TRH-bound receptor with Triton X-100. The supernatant was passed through a Sepharose 6B column, and from the elution profiles the molecular weight of the TRH-receptor complex was approximated at 300,000 and the Stoke's radius at 5.8 nm. Johnson et al (23) found that, among a variety of detergents, digitonin alone can solubilize the unbound receptor. They found comparable molecular weights and Stoke's radii as described for the bound receptor, but also demonstrated that the solubilized receptor retains most of its original binding characteristics and therefore must also retain its native conformation. The solubilized receptor demonstrated excellent stability, showing no loss in binding activity even after two months of storage at −20°C.

For a finer localization of receptor sites, several investigators have utilized autoradiographic techniques on rat brain (24–28) and rabbit spinal cord (29). In general these have confirmed results of binding experiments but have made evident differences in density distribution over discrete brain areas, e.g. higher densities in parts of the amygdala, hippocampus, diagonal band of Broca, stria terminalis, and superior colliculus; and lower densities in cortex, brain stem, and spinal cord. High receptor densities were reported in laminae II and substantia gelatinosa in human spinal cord (30).

The various factors that influence brain and spinal cord TRH receptors are now receiving considerable attention. As with many receptor systems, chronic exposure of animals to TRH or its analogues causes down-regulation. Ogawa et al (31) administered 6 mg/kg/day of TRH for 14 days and demonstrated a 20–25% loss of TRH receptor binding sites in hippocampus, hypothalamus, and cerebral cortex, but not in other brain regions investigated. Recovery from down-regulation was seen within one week of discontinuation of TRH treatment. Simasko & Horita (32) also observed down-regulation of TRH receptors in all brain regions investigated after the intracerebroventricular (i.c.v.) infusion of the stable TRH analogue MK-771 continuously via a miniosmotic pump for seven days (5 μg/μl/hr) or periodical administration of it. They found development of tolerance of certain behaviors, such as shaking or large motor movements, which were related temporally to the down-regulation of brain TRH receptors. Other responses, such as tremors, exhibited much less tolerance development. These studies indicate that chronic exposure of the CNS to TRH results in rapid and reversible down-regulation of its receptors, accompanied by development of functional tolerance, the degree of tolerance differing among the responses.

Various toxins and lesioning procedures have also been employed in the functional localization of TRH receptors. Microinjection of kainic acid into the medial septum produced a 35% decrease in density of septal TRH receptors, whereas injections of kainic acid or 6-OHDA into the lateral ventricles or electrolytic lesioning of the fimbria or medial forebrain bundle were ineffectual (33). Manaker et al (34), employing quantitative autoradiographic techniques, found that pretreatment with 6-OHDA would effect variable decreases (25–75%) in TRH receptors in some parts of the brain. From these data and a finding of increased regional TRH levels, the investigators suggested that some TRH receptors are located in presynaptic terminals and that the TRH receptors down-regulate in response to elevated levels of TRH.

In addition to effects on its own receptors, TRH may influence the regulation of other receptors as well. Pirola et al (35, 36) found in both brain and isolated intestine increased densities of muscarinic receptors after a single exposure to TRH. Concomitantly, enhanced responsiveness of both systems to acetylcholine was observed, although TRH itself exerted no direct effect of its own. In contrast to these results, chronic administration of TRH was without effect on central muscarinic receptors (31).

PHARMACOLOGY OF TRH

Behavioral Effects

CONDITIONED BEHAVIOR   The effects of TRH on conditioned behavior in animals have been studied under a variety of performance conditions. In most of the studies TRH was given peripherally (i.p., i.m., or i.v.).

In a reward situation, with FR or FI schedule of reinforcement for food or saccharin solution, TRH and MK-771 decreased the response rate in squirrel monkeys, rabbits, and pigeons (37). Both drugs were equipotent in the squirrel monkeys, whereas MK-771 was twenty times more potent than TRH in rabbits and pigeons. However, under conditions in which responding was maintained by shock termination or presentation, both TRH and MK-771 increased the response rate in the squirrel monkeys. At the same doses of the drugs, responding to food presentation was not affected (38). Thus, the effect of TRH on schedule-controlled behavior is dependent on the consequence (reward or punishment) of the behavior. This conclusion was further confirmed by an experiment in which intramuscular TRH or MK-771 caused a dose-dependent decrease in punished responses maintained by food presentation and a dose-dependent increase in punished responses maintained by shock termination (39). An increase in "punished responding" behavior by a drug is usually indicative of anxiolytic activity; thus, the result would suggest that under certain conditions, TRH has an anxiolytic effect. Related to this effect is a finding (40) of potentiation by TRH (0.03 mg/kg, i.m.) of the rate-increasing effect of pentobarbital, chlordiazepoxide, and ethanol on "punished responding" behavior seen at low doses of these drugs, but it did not affect the rate-decreasing effect observed at higher doses of these drugs.

TRH given intraperitoneally enhanced the acquisition of shuttle-box avoidance behavior (41), apparently by increasing motor activity, and thus intertrial responses. In the same study, the resistance to extinction of the avoidance response was unaffected. A recent study also demonstrated potentiation by TRH (20 mg/kg i.p.) of the conditioned flavor aversion induced by pentobarbital in the rat (42). In a two-choice visual discrimination test, TRH (1 and 50 μg, i.c.v) was found to exert no significant effect on performance (43), but by the signal-detection technique it was found to produce response preservation in the task in a way similar to that produced by peripherally administered amphetamine.

LOCOMOTOR ACTIVITY   Early studies of TRH and locomotor activity have likewise revealed a potentiating effect in animals (44, 45). More recent investigations have dealt, however, with the neural substrates and pharmacology of the locomotor activity-inducing effect of TRH. Both the nucleus accumbens and the hypothalamus are main sites of action, and dopamine appears to play a mediating role. Support for this view has come from several studies. In a recent study (46) in mice, TRH-induced motor activity was inhibited and enhanced by small doses of apomorphine and haloperidol, respectively. These data suggest that TRH-induced motor activity depends on release of dopamine from presynaptic terminals. Other investigators (47, 48) found the response in the rat blocked by pretreatment with the dopamine antagonists haloperidol and α-flupenthixol, as well as by the narcotic antagonist naloxone, and the α_2-adrenergic antagonist yohimbine (47). Narumi & Nagawa (49) observed that haloperidol blocked the locomotor response produced by TRH or DN-1417 injections into the nucleus accumbens, the brain site most sensitive in initiating the response. Sharp et al (50) also reported success in inducing the response by microinjection of TRH into the septum or nucleus accumbens, but not with similar injection into the striatum. Masserano & King (51) observed the response, however, after injection into the hypothalamus, but not after administration into the septum and caudate. The discrepancy in results may proceed from the differences in methods of measuring activity used.

Breese et al (52, 53) recently showed that TRH injections into the medial septum antagonized the locomotor depressant effect of ethanol but did not affect locomotor activity in normal animals even at a dose of 5 µg. These studies are of interest because the septum is a highly sensitive site for the analeptic effect of TRH, and intraseptal TRH injection reverses the effect of pentobarbital on hippocampal acetylcholine turnover but has no significant effect on turnover in conscious animals. Andrew & Sahgal (48) reported on a circadian variation of TRH effects on locomotor activity; the peptide increased locomotor activity when it was injected in the afternoon (13:00–17:00 h) but not when injected in the morning (09:00–12:00 h). This property could be due to the known circadian variation in dopamine activity in the brain. Furthermore, TRH-induced locomotor activity was enhanced in frontal decorticated rats, which indicates an inhibiting role of the frontal cortex (54). This may involve the glutamate innervation from the cortex to the dopamine system of the nucleus accumbens. Thus, it is clear that dopaminergic mechanisms in the nucleus accumbens play a major role in mediating the locomotor effects of TRH.

Biochemical and cellular studies of dopamine functions also support the conclusion that TRH has a selective effect on the mesolimbic dopamine system. For example, Yamada et al (55) reported a TRH enhancement of dopamine turnover rate and synthesis in the nucleus accumbens but not in the olfactory tubercle and striatum. However, it was strange that the powerful TRH analogue MK-771 was without effect on dopamine turnover in the nucleus accumbens. Sharp et al (56), using the in vivo voltammetry technique, also found that TRH and its analogue CG 3509 selectively increased dopamine activity in the mesolimbic system. Further evidence that TRH increases dopamine activity in the nucleus accumbens is given by Kalivas (reported in 7), who found that i.c.v. or intra-accumbens injection of TRH increased the ratio of DOPAC/DA in the nucleus accumbens.

The exact cellular site of action of TRH in the nucleus accumbens is not known. Pinnock et al (57) reported that TRH, when applied iontophoretically, did not affect the activities of neurons in the caudate and nucleus accumbens. In contrast, Hashimoto et al (58) found that TRH and DN-1417 produced both inhibition and excitation on nucleus accumbens neurons, both of which were blocked by haloperidol. However, TRH released ^{3}H-DA from accumbens tissue only at high concentrations (10^{-2} M) (49). These data suggest that TRH does not act directly on dopamine nerve terminals or postsynaptic dopamine receptors to facilitate dopamine mechanisms in the nucleus accumbens.

Other evidence also indicates that TRH could modify dopaminergic function in the striatum. Oki et al (59) found that specific ^{3}H-spiroperidol binding to striatal membrane was reduced if TRH was given 15–150 min before sacrifice. However, TRH did not affect binding in vitro. TRH caused body turning to the lesioned side in unilateral 6-OHDA nigral-lesioned animals, and enhanced apomorphine- and L-DOPA-induced body turning in animals with unilateral caudate lesions (49). These findings could imply either a direct action of TRH on the intact nigrostriatal dopamine system or a secondary effect on that system via an effect of TRH on the nucleus accumbens, since the dopamine systems of accumbens and striatum are known to modify each other's activities. It is of interest that TRH also increased DA-stimulated-c-AMP formation in super-sensitized caudate but not in normal tissue. Thus, TRH could affect striatal dopamine functions in certain pathological conditions, such as Parkinson's disease and tardive dyskinesia, when the striatal dopamine system is super-sensitive.

OTHER EFFECTS   A number of other behavioral effects have been attributed to TRH, such as rearing (60), body shakes (61–63), head turning (64), stereotypy (65), and inhibition of feeding and drinking (66). Most of these responses appear to involve dopamine mechanisms, although other neurotransmitters may play secondary or indirect roles.

Analeptic Effect

Although many pharmacological properties have been ascribed to TRH, its analeptic action in shortening the duration of various depressant drugs remains one of its most intriguing effects. The recent review by Nemeroff et al (7) provides excellent background information on this property of TRH; therefore, only a brief summary of the literature through 1981 will be presented here, and more detailed attention will be given to subsequent publications.

The original observation of the analeptic effect of TRH was made by Breese et al (67) in mice and rats. Subsequently the effect was observed in several other species (67, 68). The suggestion of a cholinergic involvement in its mechanism of action was supported by the fact that it was antagonized by anticholinergic drugs (67, 69). The rat proved to be an exception in that atropine or scopolamine, even in high doses, did not block the analeptic effect (70), although Miyamoto et al (71) showed sensitivity to cholinergic blockade. Kalivas & Horita (72) localized the analeptic effect to several brain sites, with the greatest sensitivity being in the area of the medial septum and nucleus of the diagonal band of Broca (MS/DBB), areas that were subsequently shown to contain high densities of TRH receptors (27). It is of interest that whereas the analeptic effect of i.c.v.-administered TRH was resistant to cholinergic blockade, when TRH was injected into the medial septum it was readily blocked by atropine (73); it would thus appear that the septohippocampal cholinergic pathway was involved in part in the analeptic response. That TRH injected into the septum of animals anesthetized with pentobarbital activated hippocampal cholinergic innervation was subsequently demonstrated neurochemically (74). Miyamoto et al (71) also localized multiple brain sites mediating the analeptic effect in rats. They found that i.c.v. or intrahypothalamic injections of atropine methyl bromide blocked the analeptic effect of TRH administered i.p. or into the hypothalamus, but not when the peptide was administered into other brain sites.

It appears that in the rat the analeptic effect may be mediated by multiple neural substrates and, depending upon the route of administration, different systems are activated to arouse the animal. For instance, when the authors determined the diffusion of ^{14}C-DN-1417, a TRH analogue, after its injection i.c.v. or into lateral hypothalamus, they found different patterns of ^{14}C distribution. After i.c.v. injection the highest density of grains was found in periventricular structures, including the septal regions, hippocampus, central gray substance, etc. As expected, after injection into the lateral hypothalamus, the greatest density of radioactivity was retained at and near the site of injection.

Sharp et al (75) recently reported on the analeptic, respiratory, and shaking effects of TRH and several of its analogues. They selected the lateral septum, nucleus accumbens, and striatum of the rat as sites for microinjection because they contain TRH and its receptors. As reported by others, these investigators showed analeptic activity in pentobarbitalized rats when TRH was microinjected into the septum and nucleus accumbens, but not into the striatum. They also noted that whereas their data were qualitatively similar to those reported by Kalivas & Horita, it required some 200 times the dose of TRH microinjected into the septum to produce a similar analeptic response.

It should be pointed out that Kalivas & Horita found a marked difference in sensitivity to TRH between the medial and lateral septal areas. The MS/DBB exhibited far greater sensitivity than the lateral septum to TRH in evoking the analeptic response. According to the description of the stereotaxic coordinates and the diagrams presented in their article, Sharp et al did not microinject into the medial septum, and this may explain the apparent discrepancy in sensitivity to TRH.

These differences in results raise an interesting question regarding the neural substrate(s) mediating the analeptic effect of TRH. Several investigators have reported on the presence of high concentrations of TRH in the lateral, but not in the medial, septum. Recently, Ishikawa et al (76) demonstrated by immunohistochemical techniques the presence of large numbers of TRH-containing nerve terminals in the lateral septum, but not in the medial. In contrast, the density of TRH receptors is greater in the MS/DBB (27). A recent study clearly demonstrated that neurons of the MS/DBB were highly sensitive to TRH (77). Iontophoretic application of TRH onto these sites produced an atropine-insensitive excitatory response. Most of these same cells could be excited by cholinergic agonists. From these results Lamour et al (77) suggested that among the septohippocampal neurons examined the cholinergic neurons were the most sensitive to TRH. Their data also suggest that TRH exerts a direct effect on the cholinergic cell bodies of the septohippocampal neurons and not by a presynaptic release of acetylcholine.

The neurochemical evidence for a role of the cholinergic system in the analeptic effect was first suggested by Schmidt (78), who found that the reduction of sodium-dependent high affinity ^{3}H-choline uptake in hippocampus and cortex by pentobarbital anesthesia was attenuated or prevented by TRH and MK-771. Similar results with TRH and its analogue DN-1417 were also shown in rat brain slices (79). It is interesting to note that under in vitro conditions TRH (10^{-4} M) and DN-1417 (10^{-5} M) were also inactive in increasing ^{3}H-choline uptake in brain slices, but they attenuated or blocked pentobarbital's ability to lower ^{3}H-choline uptake. These peptides also increased O_2 consumption and cyclic AMP formation in brain slices and reversed the depression of these responses produced by pentobarbital.

From these results the authors suggested possible relationships between the biochemical effects in vitro and the analeptic effect produced by these agents in intact animals. It is important, however, to recall that the pentobarbital-induced reduction of choline uptake in the hippocampus in vivo was not produced by a direct action of the barbiturate at that brain site, but was initiated at some other site that sent projections to the hippocampus via the septum (80). Thus, the effects of pentobarbital on choline uptake in hippocampal or cortical slices in vitro may not represent the same mechanism affected by anesthesia in the intact animal. It is nevertheless important with respect to the TRH antagonism of pentobarbital effects that there is a biochemical correlate with the interaction in vivo.

The role of TRH in natural arousal (i.e. not from drug-induced CNS depression) is not known. The interesting work of Stanton et al (81) on the arousal of animals from hibernation supports the view that TRH may act as a natural arousal agent. Doses as low as 0.1 ng of TRH microinjected into the dorsal hippocampus of the hibernating ground squirrel *(Citellus lateralis)* not only aroused, but also reversed the depressed metabolism and temperature states associated with hibernation. In later studies they demonstrated that the TRH effect varied with the initial arousal state of the animal. In awake animals it produced effects opposite to those seen in the hibernating animals— hypothermia, behavioral quieting, and decreased metabolic and EMG activity. The magnitude of these responses was greater during periods when animals were behaviorally active (82). Regional brain levels of TRH in these animals varied during different seasons of euthermia and during hibernation. While several regions exhibited seasonal variations in brain TRH levels, the most pronounced change was seen in the pineal, in which TRH levels rose over threefold between the early and late hibernation periods. The authors suggested that the change in pineal TRH might be associated with the activation of neuronal mechanisms necessary for arousal (83).

Body Temperature Effects

Peripherally and centrally administered TRH has been reported to increase body temperature in different species of animals. However, negative results have also been reported in the rat. In conscious animals, the increase in body temperature may be a secondary effect of the increased locomotor activity and body shaking behavior induced by TRH. Thus far, no attempt has been made to isolate the influence of these factors on the temperature effects of TRH.

Effects of TRH on thermoregulation in the conscious rat have been studied by Lin et al (84). Intracerebroventricular TRH produced hypothermia at lower ambient temperatures from 8–20°C, but hyperthermia at an ambient temperature of 30°C. These data indicate a loss of thermoregulatory response after i.c.v. TRH injection. However, TRH injected into the preoptic-anterior hypothalamus (85) produced only hyperthermia at all ambient temperatures studied (8–30°C); thus a change of body temperature set point had been initiated by TRH. The hyperthermia caused by TRH injection into the preoptic-anterior hypothalamus was due either to cutaneous vasoconstriction or to an increase in metabolism, depending upon the ambient temperature, and was blocked by intrahypothalamic injections of yohimbine, phentolamine, or DL-propranolol; thus, involvement of adrenergic mechanisms is suggested (86).

Although many studies have been undertaken of the interaction of TRH with other drugs on body temperature, few have focused on the brain mechanisms of this response. Kalivas & Horita (61) investigated the brain loci of this thermal effect of TRH. In agreement with their finding that the anterior hypothalamus/ preoptic area of the rat was the most sensitive site for TRH in reversing pentobarbital-induced hypothermia, Salzman & Beckman (87) showed that the warm-sensitive cells in the anterior hypothalamus/preoptic area were inhibited by iontophoretically applied TRH, whereas cold-sensitive cells in that same area were relatively less sensitive. Thus, the effect of TRH on the warm-sensitive cells could conceivably lead to a hyperthermic response.

That the thermogenic effect of TRH has a specific brain locus of action is further confirmed by a recent multiple-dissociation study of Sharp et al (75) on TRH and its analogues RX 77368 and CG 3509. Pentobarbital-induced hypothermia was reversed after microinjection of these drugs into the nucleus accumbens and septum, but no significant effect was seen after intrastriatal injection. It was also interesting that the analeptic effect of these drugs seemed to correlate with the thermogenic effect, i.e. analeptic effect of TRH was seen after intra-accumbens and intraseptal injections but not with intrastriatal injection. It is possible that the analeptic and thermal effects of TRH could interact with each other.

Other recent studies have been devoted to the interactions of TRH and other peptides on body temperature. In conscious rats i.c.v. TRH (10 µg) antagonized hypothermia induced by naloxone and somatostatin, but not that produced by bombesin and neurotensin (88). However, in mice, hypothermia induced by intracisternally administered neurotensin was antagonized by TRH or its analogues (89). The discrepancy between the above two studies could reflect differences in animal species used or the routes of drug administration.

Effects on Autonomic Functions

The central administration of TRH in experimental animals produces effects associated with increased activity of the peripheral sympathetic and parasympathetic nervous systems. The sympathetic responses observed include vasopressor activity, increased heart rate, piloerection, pupillary dilation, hyperthermia, and hyperglycemia. Most of these effects are probably the consequence of catecholamine release from adrenal medulla and sympathetic nerve endings (90). Concomitantly, one observes increased gastrointestinal (GI) motor activity (91), intestinal transit and diarrhea (92), gastric acid secretion (93), pancreatic secretion (94), and activation of superior laryngeal nerve to the thyroid gland (95, 96). All of these responses were antagonized by atropine and/or vagal transection. These observations, together with the fact that TRH is found in high concentrations in several discrete areas in the medulla (dorsal motor nucleus of vagus, nucleus tractus solitarius, nucleus ambiguus) and preganglionic autonomic neurons in several species, strongly support the growing view that TRH serves as a central regulator of peripheral autonomic function (97, 98).

CARDIOVASCULAR EFFECTS   Prior to 1981 little attention was paid to the cardiovascular actions of TRH. Microinjections of TRH into cisterna magna or into the cerebral ventricle of rabbits and rats (99) produced pressor responses. In rabbits the response was not totally abolished by α-adrenergic or ganglionic blockers, nor by thoracic cord transection (100). These results prompted the search for other potential vasopressor agents released by TRH. Vasopressin was considered as a possible candidate when blood levels were found to be increased in animals after central administration of TRH (101). It may play a part in the TRH reversal of drug-induced hypotension. This was suggested by the finding that the pressor response of TRH in clonidine- or α-methyldopa–pretreated animals was blocked by a vasopressin antagonist, but not by prazosin or hexamethonium (102).

A most important discovery was the finding that TRH improved cardiovascular function and survival of animals exposed to experimental endotoxic or hemorrhagic shock (103, 104). This pressor effect of i.c.v. TRH was absent in endotoxic rats with demedullated adrenals, but the response persisted when TRH was given i.v. The TRH-induced respiratory stimulation persisted under all experimental conditions. The ability of TRH to reverse hypotension appears to be relatively nonspecific, for it is effective against hypotension produced by anaphylactic shock (105, 106), leukotriene (107), and platelet-activating factor (108), as well as endotoxin and hemorrhage.

Feuerstein et al (109) found that microinjection of 0.8–80 nM TRH into the medial preoptic nucleus (POM) of conscious rats elicited dose-related pressor and cardiac-stimulant responses accompanied by increased plasma levels of norepinephrine and epinephrine. These cardiovascular effects of TRH were also produced in adrenal demedullated animals, but were abolished in adrenal demedullated + bretylium-pretreated animals. These results suggested that the vasopressor effect of TRH injected into POM was largely mediated by catecholamine release, especially of norepinephrine, from sympathetic nerves. The injections of TRH (30–150 nM) into the nucleus tractus solitarius produced responses of lesser magnitude and duration.

Diz & Jacobowitz (110) further delineated the brain site(s) for the cardiovascular actions of TRH to specific preoptic and hypothalamic nuclei. Microinjection of doses as low as 1.4 pmol (0.5 ng) into medial and suprachiasmatic preoptic nuclei increased blood pressure and heart rate. Both responses were also seen with TRH injections into the posterior hypothalamic nucleus, but only tachycardia was seen after injection into anterior and dorsomedial hypothalamic nuclei. Changes in regional blood flow may also contribute to the TRH effect in experimental shock. Koskinen & Bill (111) demonstrated in rabbits that i.v. injections of 2 mg/kg of TRH produced approximately a 70% increase in cerebral blood flow. Mean arterial blood pressure and arterial $PaCO_2$ were also increased, but these effects could not account for the increases in cerebral blood flow. Peripheral organs showed mainly a reduced blood flow after TRH administration; in some the effect was blocked in sympathectomized animals. It would thus appear that the effect was mediated via sympathetic innervation.

It is clear from this discussion that TRH can produce dramatic improvement of cardiovascular function in animals exposed to various forms of shock and traumatic injury. The high sensitivity of the POM to TRH, and the known presence of TRH nerve cells in preoptic-hypothalamic areas, strongly suggest a role of this peptide in central control of the cardiovascular system. The current status of its possible mechanism of action has been discussed in recent reviews (112, 113).

GASTROINTESTINAL EFFECTS   One of the most profound autonomic effects of TRH is that produced on the GI tract in rabbits. Even in the intact anesthetized animal the GI response to TRH is recognizable as a massive vermiform movement of the abdominal region. In conscious animals a watery diarrhea is consistently observed, and with larger doses it is reminiscent of the diarrhea described after administration of cholera toxin. With the long-acting compounds, such as MK-771, the diarrhea lasts for over 24 hours. TRH, in doses as low as 0.1 μg i.c.v. to anesthetized rabbits, initiated increased smooth muscle contractions of the entire GI tract. It was evident that these effects were mediated via central vagal mechanisms, for they were completely blocked by bilateral vagotomy, hexamethonium, and atropine (91).

In other studies in which motility and rate of colonic transit were compared, it became clear that the two were unrelated and that only the latter was related to the development of the diarrhea. Atropine or bilateral vagotomy blocked the former, whereas only vagotomy attenuated the transit and diarrhea responses. Examination of the intestinal tract showed massive fluid accumulation, which fluidized the fecal material and enhanced its transit in an aboral direction. That serotonin release was involved was suggested by the findings that (a) anti-serotonin drugs blocked the colonic transit and diarrhea effects of TRH (but not the hypermotility), and (b) TRH administered centrally produced a dose-related increase in levels of portal blood serotonin. High doses of TRH (e.g. 100 μg i.c.v.) produced prolonged hyperserotonemia (>2 hr). Like the diarrhea response, the hyperserotonemia was attenuated by bilateral vagotomy but not by atropine (92). Therefore, centrally administered TRH produced not only a cholinergically mediated hypermotility, but also a vagally mediated release of intestinal serotonin; the latter was responsible for the production of diarrhea.

TRH effects on the GI system have been reported in other species, although they appear not to be identical with those in the rabbit. For instance, rats exhibit vagally mediated hypermotility (114), gastric acid secretion (95) leading to gastric erosion (115), hyperserotonemia, and intestinal fluid accumulation, but even with high doses there was no evidence of watery diarrhea as was seen in the rabbit (A. Horita and M. A. Carino, unpublished). In contrast, Metcalf & Myers (116) reported frequent salivation, vomiting, and defecation in cats given small quantities of TRH into the lateral ventricles. The response to TRH in mice and dogs represents a departure from that described in most other species in showing a decrease in GI transit (117) and acid secretion (118), respectively.

The GI effects produced by i.c.v. TRH in rabbits have shown some interesting drug interactions. Naloxone (2.5 mg/kg i.p.) or naltrexone (1.0 mg/kg i.p.) blocked the charcoal transit, fluid accumulation, and diarrhea formation induced by i.c.v. TRH, but not the cholinergically mediated hypermotility. The TRH-induced portal hyperserotonemia was also not affected by these antagonists (119). The authors suggested that this TRH-opiate antagonist interaction was probably not associated with specific blockade of mu-opiate receptors because of the large doses required. Some indirect evidence suggested that naloxone and naltrexone blocked serotonin on the secretory and/or smooth muscle receptors. In contrast, the TRH-mediated inhibition of GI transit in mice was blocked by 0.1 mg/kg of naloxone, which suggested that opiate receptors may be involved in this response in mice (117).

Other drug interactions of interest on the GI effects of TRH have been reported. Clonidine (120) or a combination of 6-hydroxydopamine (i.c.v.) and α-methyltyrosine (121) abolished TRH-induced acid secretion, as did dopamine agonists (122), and corticotropin-releasing factor (123). These interactions occurred centrally and add further evidence that central monoaminergic and peptidergic systems modulate vagal responses to the GI tract.

Effects on Spinocerebellar Functions

After having observed beneficial effects of TRH on hypotensive shock produced in animals with spinal cord injury, Faden et al (124, 125) examined its effects on the neurological symptoms produced by the injury. The neurologic function scores of TRH-treated animals were higher than those of dexamethasone- or saline-treated animals over the six-week period of the study. Whereas the latter animals displayed spasticity and/or ataxia, the TRH animals exhibited normal motor function. In addition, all six animals given TRH survived for six weeks, whereas four animals died in each of the dexamethasone and saline groups. Surprisingly, histopathologic evaluation of the area of injury showed no differences between treated and control animals; thus, other more specific histological methods are necessary in order to differentiate degrees of spinal cord injury. In subsequent studies, the authors found a dose-response relationship (0.02–2.0 mg/kg/hr i.v.) in which even the lowest dose produced better motor recovery than saline controls. An especially important finding was that the high dose of TRH given 1 or 24 hr after injury produced essentially the same degree of improvement of neurological function (126). This finding is of considerable clinical significance since it is generally assumed that 4–8 hr after spinal cord injury the neuropathological effects are irreversible.

Partly as a result of these successful animal studies, Engel et al (127) employed TRH and found its favorable effects in patients with amyotrophic lateral sclerosis (ALS). Large doses of TRH (up to 500 mg in 2–5 hr/day) were infused intravenously into twelve patients. Moderate to marked improvement of muscle weakness and spasticity were observed, although all affected muscle areas were not equally improved. Some of the improved responses included increased vital capacity, speech clarity and volume, and improved walking agility. All of the improvements persisted during the infusion and for 0.5–1 hr afterwards. Side effects included shivering, tachypnea, sweating, urinary urgency, and abdominal cramps. With higher doses increased blood pressure and heart rate were noted. The high doses used in these studies may be necessary to produce therapeutic effects since other workers using 4 mg i.m. for two weeks failed to demonstrate improved muscle strength in nine patients with ALS (128).

While Engel was the first to report on the efficacy of TRH in ALS, similar observations were made by Sobue et al (129), who employed the peptide in the treatment of ataxia of spinocerebellar degeneration (SCD). TRH was given i.m. in doses of 2 mg, 0.5 mg, or placebo once a day for two weeks. Global improvement and ataxia improvement ratings showed that both doses of TRH were significantly superior to placebo in patients with predominantly cerebellar forms of SCD, and this effect persisted for a week after cessation of treatment. The 2-mg dose was also more effective than placebo in improving standing, speech, and writing.

The mechanism of TRH activity in spinocerebellar injury is not known. It has been suggested that TRH might exert effects opposite to those produced by some of the endogenous opioids released after trauma (103). Numerous investigators have demonstrated not only pharmacologic activity, but also the localization and distribution of TRH and its receptors in spinal cord. More recent studies on the distribution of TRH in monkey (98) and human (130) spinal cord confirm earlier rat data that TRH is present in motoneurons and preganglionic autonomic neurons. ALS patients display lowered TRH levels in their anterior horn (131). Lesion studies indicate that the perikarya of TRH neurons in spinal cord originate in the ventral medulla, and that many of these also contain 5-hydroxytryptamine (5HT), suggesting that they are cotransmitters (132). Motoneuron damage induced by neurectomy or virus infection was associated with redistribution of fibers containing 5HT and TRH. Treatment with TRH normalized this redistribution response (133). TRH infusions also antagonized motor deficits produced by reserpine, but not those produced by strychnine; thus monoaminergic systems in descending motor pathways might be important for this TRH effect (134). TRH administered to chick embryo enhanced survival of spinal cord motoneurons that would normally have died during development. This effect may be mediated by c-GMP activation by TRH (135). Also, treatment of cultured spinal ventral horn neurons from rat embryos with TRH for 2–5 weeks enhanced growth of cells and produced a 16-fold increase over controls of choline acetyltransferase activity (136).

Alterations in TRH receptors may be involved in genetically or experimentally induced spinocerebellar dysfunctions. Administration of TRH to ataxic mice has been reported to cause instantaneous recovery from ataxia. In the ataxic mutant Rolling Mouse Nagoya, the number of TRH receptors was significantly lower in cerebellum and higher in spinal cord than in normal mice (137). Newborn mice showed decreased numbers of TRH receptors in spinal cord at 2 weeks, but not at 4 weeks, after inoculation with murine leukemia virus. The change in receptor density preceded the neurological signs, since motor dysfunction appeared 4–5 weeks after exposure to the virus (138). In contrast, Hawkins & Engel (139) hypothesize that the effects of TRH and its analogues on the spinal cord might be mediated via non-TRH receptors.

CONCLUSIONS

In this review we have discussed the current status of some aspects of the pharmacology of TRH. The presence of TRH and its receptors in various regions of brain and spinal cord and the many diverse effects associated with its administration into specific brain sites strongly support the growing contention that it serves as an endogenous regulator of neural function. It appears that many of the extrapituitary effects of TRH are mediated by other neurotransmitters, notably acetylcholine and the monoamines, so that this peptide is delegated the role of a neuromodulator of those systems.

Some important beginnings as to possible clinical utility of TRH have been made. In addition to its use in spinocerebellar disorders as discussed above, its potential application in some forms of cardiovascular shock seems imminent. Speculations and suggestions as to these and other possible clinical uses of TRH have also been made (140–142). If any of the pharmacological properties of TRH becomes important in clinical medicine, it is unlikely that TRH itself will be selected as the drug of choice. Because of its transient action due to rapid inactivation and the need for high doses in parenteral form, synthetic analogues with the appropriate potency, specificity, and pharmacokinetic properties will be sought. Indeed, several compounds with some of these attributes have been developed. TRH and its analogues are becoming a unique class of drugs that may be useful in certain clinical disorders previously treated with little or no success. Continued neuropsychopharmacological and neurochemical research of TRH mechanisms is necessary for a full understanding of the basis for its clinical efficacy.

ACKNOWLEDGMENT

The authors' research has been supported in part by a grant from the US Department of Health and Human Services, NS-19210.

Literature Cited

1. Miyamoto, M., Fukuda, N., Narumi, S., Nagai, Y., Saji, Y., Nagawa, Y. 1981. γ-Butyrolactone-γ-carbonyl-L-histidyl-L-prolinamide citrate (DN-1417): A novel TRH analog with potent effects on the central nervous system. *Life Sci.* 28:861–70

2. Kisfaludy, L., Mess, B., Palosi, E., Ruzzas, C., Szirtes, T., Szporny, L. 1983. Novel TRH analogs of low hormonal but increased activity on the central nervous system. In *Thyrotropin Releasing Hormone*, ed. E. C. Griffiths, G. W. Bennett, p. 379. New York: Raven

3. Yarbrough, G. G. 1979. On the neuropharmacology of thyrotropin releasing hormone (TRH). *Prog. Neurobiol.* 12:291–312

4. Morley, J. E. 1979. Extrahypothalamic thyrotropin releasing hormone (TRH)—its distribution and its functions. *Life Sci.* 25:1539–50

5. Breese, G. R., Mueller, R. A., Mailman, R. B., Frye, G. D. 1981. Effects of TRH on central nervous system function. In *The Role of Peptides and Amino Acids as Neurotransmitters*, ed. J. B. Lombardini, A. D. Kenny, pp. 99–116. New York: Liss

6. Horita, A., Kalivas, P. W., Simasko, S. M. 1983. Thyrotropin releasing hormone (TRH): Possible physiological functions not related to the neuroendocrine system. *Rev. Pure Appl. Pharmacol. Sci.* 4:111–37

7. Nemeroff, C. B., Kalivas, P. W., Golden, R. N., Prange, A. J. 1984. Behavioral effects of hypothalamic hypophysiotropic hormones, neurotensin, substance P and other neuropeptides. *Pharmacol. Ther.* 24:1–56

8. Burt, D. R., Snyder, S. H. 1975. Thyrotropin releasing hormone (TRH): Apparent receptor binding in rat brain membranes. *Brain Res.* 93:309–28

9. Taylor, R. L., Burt, D. R. 1982. Species differences in the brain regional distribution of receptor binding for thyrotropin-releasing hormone. *J. Neurochem.* 38:1649–56

10. Simasko, S. M., Horita, A. 1982. Characterization and distribution of ^{3}H-(3MeHis^2)thyrotropin releasing hormone in rat brain. *Life Sci.* 30:1793–99

11. Parker, C. R., Capdevila, A. 1984. Thyrotropin releasing hormone (TRH) binding sites in the adult human brain: localization and characterization. *Peptides* 5:701–6

12. Sharif, N. A., Burt, D. R. 1983. Receptors for thyrotropin-releasing hormone (TRH) in rabbit spinal cord. *Brain Res.* 270:259–63

13. Prasad, C., Edwards, R. M. 1984. Thyrotropin-releasing hormone (TRH): Apparent receptor binding in rat spinal cord. *Brain Res.* 311:1–6

14. Dettmar, P. W., Lynn, A. G., Metcalf, G., Morgan, B. A. 1983. Brain TRH receptors are the same as pituitary receptors. *J. Pharm. Pharmacol.* 35:399–400

15. Sharif, N. A., Burt, D. R. 1983. Biochemical similarity of rat pituitary and CNS TRH receptors. *Neurosci. Lett.* 39:57–63

16. Sharif, N. A., Burt, D. R. 1984. Modulation of receptors for thyrotropin-releasing hormone by benzodiazepines: Brain re-

gional differences. *J. Neurochem.* 43: 742–46

17. Ogawa, N. 1983. Biochemical properties of TRH receptors in the rat central nervous system. *Kurume Med. J.* 30:s51–s56

18. Sharif, N. A., Burt, D. R. 1984. Sulfhydryl groups in receptor binding of thyrotropin-releasing hormone to rat amygdala. *J. Neurochem.* 42:209–14

19. Ogawa, N., Mizuno, S., Mori, A., Kuroda, H. 1984. Chronic dihydroergotoxine administration sets on receptors for enkephalin and thyrotropin releasing hormone in the aged-rat brain. *Peptides* 5:53–56

20. Sharif, N. A., Zuhowski, E. G., Burt, D. R. 1983. Benzodiazepines compete for thyrotropin-releasing hormone receptor binding: Micromolar potency in rat pituitary, retina and amygdala. *Neurosci. Lett.* 41:301–6

21. Simasko, S. M., Horita, A. 1984. Chlordiazepoxide displaces thyrotropin releasing hormone (TRH) binding. *Eur. J. Pharmacol.* 98:419–23

22. Ogawa, N., Yamawaki, Y., Kuroda, H., Nukina, I., Ota, Z., et al. 1982. Characteristics of thyrotropin releasing hormone (TRH) receptors in rat brain. *Peptides* 3:669–77

23. Johnson, W. A., Nathanson, N. M., Horita, A. 1984. Solubilization and characterization of thyrotropin releasing hormone receptor from rat brain. *Proc. Natl. Acad. Sci. USA* 81:4227–31

24. Palacios, J. M. 1983. Autoradiographic visualization of receptor binding sites for thyrotropin-releasing hormone in the rodent brain. *Eur. J. Pharmacol.* 92:165–66

25. Rostene, W. H., Morgat, J.-L., Dussaillant, M., Rainbow, T. C., Sarrieau, A., et al. 1984. In vitro biochemical characterization and autoradiographic distribution of ³H-thyrotropin-releasing hormone binding sites in rat brain sections. *Neuroendocrinology* 39:81–86

26. Pilotte, N. S., Sharif, N. A., Burt, D. R. 1984. Characterization and autoradiographic localization of TRH receptors in sections of rat brain. *Brain Res.* 293:372–76

27. Manaker, S., Winokur, A., Rostene, W. H., Rainbow, T. C. 1985. Autoradiographic localization of thyrotropin releasing hormone (TRH) receptors in rat CNS. *J. Neurosci.* 5:167–74

28. Mantyh, P. W., Hunt, S. P. 1985. Thyrotropin-releasing hormone (TRH) receptors. *J. Neurosci.* 5:551–61

29. Sharif, N. A., Pilotte, N. S., Burt, D. R.

1983. Biochemical and autoradiographic studies of TRH receptors in sections of rabbit spinal cord. *Biochem. Biophys. Res. Commun.* 116:669–74

30. Manaker, S., Winokur, A., Rhodes, C. H., Rainbow, T. C. 1985. Autoradiographic localization of thyrotropin-releasing hormone (TRH) receptors in human spinal cord. *Neurology* 35:328–32

31. Ogawa, N., Mizuno, S., Nukina, I., Tsukamoto, S., Mori, A. 1983. Chronic thyrotropin releasing hormone (TRH) administration on TRH receptors and muscarinic cholinergic receptors in CNS. *Brain Res.* 263:348–50

32. Simasko, S. M., Horita, A. 1985. Treatment of rats with the TRH analog MK-771. *Neuropharmacology* 24:157–65

33. Simasko, S. M., Horita, A. 1984. Localization of thyrotropin releasing hormone (TRH) receptors in the septal nucleus of the rat brain. *Brain Res.* 296:393–95

34. Manaker, S., Winokur, A., Rainbow, T. C. 1984. Effects of 6-hydroxydopamine on the autoradiographic distribution of thyrotropin-releasing hormone (TRH) receptors in rat CNS. *Soc. Neurosci.* 10:377 (Abstr.)

35. Pirola, C. J., Balda, M. S., Finkielman, S., Nahmod, V. E. 1983. Thyrotropin-releasing hormone increases the number of muscarinic receptors in the lateral septal area of the rat brain. *Brain Res.* 273:387–91

36. Pirola, C. J., Balda, M. S., Finkielman, S., Nahmod, V. E. 1984. Increase in muscarinic receptors in rat intestine by thyrotropin releasing hormone (TRH). *Life Sci.* 34:1643–49

37. Barrett, J. E. 1983. Effects of thyrotropin-releasing hormone (TRH) and MK-771 on schedule-controlled behavior of squirrel monkeys, rabbits and pigeons. *Peptides* 4:177–81

38. Brady, L. S., Barrett, J. E. 1984. Effects of thyrotropin-releasing hormone (TRH) and MK-771 on behavior of squirrel monkey controlled by noxious stimuli. *Peptides* 5:783–87

39. Brady, L. S., Valentine, J. O., Barrett, J. E. 1984. Effects of thyrotropin-releasing hormone (TRH) and a TRH analogue, MK-771, on punished responding of squirrel monkey. *Psychopharmacology* 83:151–54

40. Witkin, J. M., Sickle, J. B., Barrett, J. E. 1984. Potentiation of the behavioral effects of pentobarbital, chlordiazepoxide and ethanol by thyrotropin-releasing hormone. *Peptides* 5:809–13

41. Tamaki, Y., Kameyama, Y. 1982. Effects of TRH on acquisition and extinction of shuttlebox-avoidance behavior in Fischer-344 rats. *Pharmacol. Biochem. Behav.* 16:943–47

42. Taukulis, H. K. 1983. Thyrotropin-releasing hormone (TRH) potentiates pentobarbital-based flavor aversion learning. *Behav. Neural Biol.* 39:135–39

43. Andrews, J. S., Sahgal, A. 1984. The effects of thyrotropin releasing hormone on a visual discrimination task in rats. *Pharmacol. Biochem. Behav.* 21:715–19

44. Segal, D. S., Mandell, A. J. 1974. Differential behavioral effects of hypothalamic polypeptides, In *The Thyroid Axis, Drugs, and Behavior*, ed. A. J. Prange Jr., pp. 129–33. New York: Raven

45. Miyamoto, M., Nagawa, Y. 1977. Mesolimbic involvement in the locomotor stimulant action of thyrotropin releasing hormone (TRH) in rats. *Eur. J. Pharmacol.* 44:143–53

46. Ushijima, I., Yamada, K., Noda, Y., Furukawa, T. 1984. Progressive augmentation of locomotor activity in mice by long-term treatment with thyrotropin releasing hormone. *Arch. Int. Pharmacodyn. Ther.* 270:29–37

47. Lin, M. T., Chan, H. K., Chen, C. F., Teh, G. W. 1983. Involvement of both opiate and catecholaminergic receptors in the behavioral excitation provoked by thyrotropin-releasing hormone: Comparisons with amphetamine. *Neuropharmacology* 22:463–69

48. Andrews, J. S., Sahgal, A. 1983. The effects of thyrotropin-releasing hormone, metabolites and analogues on locomotor activity in rats. *Reg. Peptides* 7:97–109

49. Narumi, S., Nagawa, Y. 1983. Modification of dopaminergic transmission by thyrotropin-releasing hormone, In *Molecular Pharmacology of Neurotransmitter Receptors*, ed. T. Segawa, H. I. Yamamura, K. Kuriyama, pp. 185–97. New York: Raven

50. Sharp, T., Bennett, G. W., Marsden, C. A., Tullock, I. F. 1984. A comparison of the locomotor effects induced by centrally injected TRH and TRH analogues. *Regul. Peptides* 9:305–15

51. Masserano, J. M., King, C. 1981. TRH increases locomotor activity in rats after injection into the hypothalamus. *Eur. J. Pharmacol.* 69:217–219

52. Breese, G. R., Frye, G. D., McCown, T. J., Mueller, R. A. 1984. Comparison of the CNS effects induced by TRH and bicuculline after microinjection into medial septum, substantia nigra and inferior colliculus: Absence of support for a GABA antagonist action of TRH. *Pharmacol. Biochem. Behav.* 21:145–49

53. Breese, G. R., Coyle, S., Towle, A. C., Mueller, R. A., McCown, T. J., Frye, G. D. 1984. Ethanol-induced locomotor stimulation in rats after thyrotropin-releasing hormone. *J. Pharmacol. Exp. Ther.* 229:731–37

54. Katsuura, G., Yoshikawa, K., Itoh, S., Hsiao, S. 1984. Behavioral effects of thyrotropin releasing hormone in decorticated rats. *Peptides* 5:899–903

55. Yamada, K., Demarest, K. T., Moore, K. E. 1984. Effects of behaviorally active doses of thyrotropin-releasing hormone and its analog MK-771 on dopaminergic neuronal systems in the brain of the rat. *Neuropharmacology* 23:735–39

56. Sharp, T., Brazell, M. P., Bennett, G. W., Marsden, C. A. 1984. The TRH analogue CG-3509 increases in vivo catechol/ascorbate oxidation in the nucleus accumbens but not in the striatum of the rat. *Neuropharmacology* 23:617–23

57. Pinnock, R. D., Woodruff, G. N., Turnbull, M. J. 1983. Actions of substance P, MIF, TRH and related peptides in the substantia nigra, caudate nucleus and nucleus accumbens. *Neuropharmacology* 22:687–96

58. Hashimoto, T., Fukuda, N., Saji, Y., Nagawa, Y. 1983. Effects of TRH and an analog, DN-1417 on the activities of single neurons in the nucleus accumbens, cerebral cortex and caudate-putamen of rats. *Kurume Med. J.* 30:S19–S27

59. Oki, K., Kinoshita, Y., Nomura, Y., Segawa, T. 1983. Influence of thyrotropin-releasing hormone on general behavior and striatal [^{3}H]spiperone binding in developing rats. *J. Pharmacodyn.* 6:507–12

60. Miyamoto, M., Narumi, S., Nagai, Y., Saji, Y., Nagawa, Y. 1984. A TRH analog (DN-1417): Motor stimulation with rearing related to catecholaminergic mechanisms in rats. *Neuropharmacology* 23:61–72

61. Kalivas, P. W., Horita, A. 1981. Neuroanatomical dissociation of thyrotropin releasing hormone–induced shaking behavior and thermogenic mechanisms. *Regul. Peptides* 1:335–45

62. Yamada, K., Matsuki, J., Ushijima, I., Inoue, T., Furukawa, T. 1983. Behavioral studies of shaking behavior induced by thyrotropin-releasing hormone and morphine withdrawal in rats. *Arch. Int. Pharmacodyn. Ther.* 262:24–33

63. Drust, E. G., Connor, J. D. 1983. Phar-

macological analysis of shaking behavior induced by enkephalins, thyrotropin-releasing hormone or serotonin in rats: Evidence for different mechanisms. *J. Pharmacol. Exp. Ther.* 224:148–54

64. Malouin, F., Bedard, P. J. 1982. Head turning induced by unilateral intracaudate thyrotropin-releasing hormone (TRH) injection in the cat. *Eur. J. Pharmacol.* 81:559–67

65. Ushijima, I., Yamada, K., Furukawa, T. 1984. Acute and long-term effects of thyrotropin releasing hormone on behavior mediated by dopaminergic and cholinergic activities in mice. *Psychopharmacology* 82:301–5

66. Suzuki, T., Kohno, H., Sakurada, T., Tadano, T., Kisara, K. 1982. Intracranial injection of thyrotropin releasing hormone (TRH) suppresses starvation-induced feeding and drinking in rats. *Pharmacol. Biochem. Behav.* 17:249–53

67. Breese, G. R., Cott, J. M., Cooper, B. R., Prange, A. J., Lipton, M. A., Plotnikoff, N. P. 1975. Effects of thyrotropin releasing hormone (TRH) on the actions of pentobarbital and other centrally acting drugs. *J. Pharmacol. Exp. Ther.* 193:11–22

68. Horita, A., Carino, M. A., Chesnut, R. M. 1976. Influence of thyrotropin releasing hormone (TRH) on drug-induced narcosis and hyperthermia in rabbits. *Psychopharmacology* 49:57–62

69. Horita, A., Carino, M. A., Smith, J. R. 1976. Effects of TRH on the CNS of the rabbit. *Pharmacol. Biochem. Behav.* 5(Suppl. 1):111–16

70. Santori, E. M., Schmidt, D. E., Kalivas, P. W., Horita, A. 1981. Failure of muscarinic blockade to antagonize TRH and MK-771-induced analepsis in the rat. *Psychopharmacology* 74:13–16

71. Miyamoto, M., Nagai, Y., Narumi, S., Saji, Y., Nagawa, Y. 1982. TRH and its novel analog (DN-1417): Antipentobarbital action and involvement of cholinergic mechanisms. *Pharmacol. Biochem. Behav.* 17:797–806

72. Kalivas, P. W., Horita, A. 1980. TRH: Neurogenesis of action in the pentobarbital narcotized rat. *J. Pharmacol. Exp. Ther.* 212:203–10

73. Kalivas, P. W., Horita, A. 1983. Involvement of the septohippocampal system in TRH antagonism of pentobarbital narcosis. See Ref. 2, pp. 283–90

74. Brunello, N., Cheney, D. L. 1981. The septal-hippocampal cholinergic pathway: Role in antagonism of pentobarbital anesthesia and regulation by various affe-

rents. *J. Pharmacol. Exp. Ther.* 219:489–95

75. Sharp, T., Tullock, I. F., Bennett, G. W., Marsden, C. A., Metcalf, G., Dettmar, P. W. 1984. Analeptic effects of centrally injected TRH and analogues of TRH in the pentobarbitone-anesthetized rat. *Neuropharmacology* 23:339–48

76. Ishikawa, K., Inoue, K., Tosaka, H., Shimada, O., Suzuki, M. 1984. Immunohistochemical characterization of thyrotropin-releasing hormone-containing neurons in rat septum. *Neuroendocrinology* 39:448–52

77. Lamour, Y., Dutar, P., Jobert, A. 1985. Effects of TRH, cyclo-(His-Pro) and (3-Me-His^2)TRH on identified septohippocampal neurons in the rat. *Brain Res.* 331:343–47

78. Schmidt, D. W. 1977. Effects of thyrotropin releasing hormone (TRH) on pentobarbital-induced decrease in cholinergic neuronal activity. *Psychopharmacol. Commun.* 1:469–73

79. Narumi, S., Nagai, Y., Miyamoto, M., Nagawa, Y. 1983. Thyrotropin-releasing hormone (TRH) and its analog (DN-1417): Interaction with pentobarbital in choline uptake and acetylcholine synthesis of rat brain slices. *Life Sci.* 32:1637–45

80. Richter, J. A., Gormley, J. M. 1982. Inhibition of high affinity choline uptake in the hippocampus: studies on the site of pentobarbital action. *J. Pharmacol. Exp. Ther.* 222:778–85

81. Stanton, T. L., Winokur, A., Beckman, A. L. 1980. Reversal of natural CNS depression by TRH action in the hippocampus. *Brain Res.* 181:470–75

82. Stanton, T. L., Beckman, A. L., Winokur, A. 1981. Thyrotropin-releasing hormone effects in the central nervous system: Dependence on arousal state. *Science* 214:678–91

83. Stanton, T., Winokur, A., Beckman, A. L. 1982. Seasonal variation in thyrotropin-releasing hormone (TRH) content of different brain regions and the pineal in the mammalian hibernator, *Citellus lateralis. Regul. Peptides* 3:135–44

84. Lin, M. T., Chandra, A., Chern, Y. F., Tsay, B. L. 1980. Effects of thyrotropin-releasing hormone (TRH) on thermoregulation in the rat. *Experientia* 36:1077–78

85. Lin, M. T. 1982. Metabolic, respiratory, vasomotor and body temperature responses to TRH, angiotensin II, substance P, neurotensin, somatostatin, LH-RH, beta-endorphin, oxytocin or vaso-

pressin in the rat, In *Current Status of Centrally Active Peptides*, ed. B. N. Dhawan, pp. 229–51. Oxford: Pergamon

86. Chi, M. C., Lin, M. T. 1984. Involvement of adrenergic receptor mechanisms within hypothalamus in the fever induced by amphetamine and thyrotropin-releasing hormone in the rat. *J. Neural Transm.* 58:213–22

87. Salzman, S. K., Beckman, A. L. 1981. Effects of thyrotropin releasing hormone on hypothalamic thermosensitive neurons of the rat. *Brain Res. Bull.* 7:325–32

88. Morley, J. E., Levine, A. S., Oken, M. M., Grace, M., Kneip, J. 1982. Neuropeptides and thermoregulation: The interactions of bombesin, neurotensin, TRH, somatostatin, naloxone and prostaglandins. *Peptides* 3:1–6

89. Hernandez, D. E., Nemeroff, C. B., Valderrama, M. H., Prange, A. J. Jr. 1984. Neurotensin-induced antinociception and hypothermia in mice: Antagonism by TRH and structural analogs of TRH. *Regul. Peptides* 8:41–49

90. Brown, M. B. 1981. Thyrotropin releasing factor: A putative CNS regulator of the autonomic nervous system. *Life Sci.* 28:1789–95

91. LaHann, T. R., Horita, A. 1982. Thyrotropin releasing hormone (TRH): Centrally mediated effects on gastrointestinal motor activity. *J. Pharmacol. Exp. Ther.* 222:66–70

92. Horita, A., Carino, M. A. 1982. Centrally administered thyrotropin releasing hormone (TRH) stimulates colonic transit and diarrhea production by a vagally mediated serotonergic mechanism in the rabbit. *J. Pharmacol. Exp. Ther.* 222: 367–71

93. Tache, Y., Vale, W., Brown, M. 1980. Thyrotropin releasing hormone–CNS action to stimulate gastric acid secretion. *Nature* 287:149–51

94. Kato, Y., Kanno, T. 1983. Thyrotropin-releasing hormone injected intracerebroventricularly in the rat stimulates exocrine pancreatic secretion via the vagus nerve. *Regul. Peptides* 7:347–56

95. Tonoue, T. 1982. Stimulation by thyrotropin-releasing hormone of vagal outflow to the thyroid gland. *Regul. Peptides* 3:29–39

96. Tonoue, T., Somiya, H., Matsumoto, H., Ogawa, N., Leppaluoto, J. 1982. Evidence that endogenous thyrotropin-releasing hormone (TRH) may control vagal efferents of thyroid gland: Neural

inhibition by central administration of TRH antiserum. *Regul. Peptides* 4:293–98

97. Kubek, M. J., Rea, M. A., Hodes, Z. I., Aprison, M. H. 1983. Quantitation and characterization of thyrotropin-releasing hormone in vagal nuclei and other regions of the medulla oblongata of the rat. *J. Neurochem.* 40:1307–13

98. Lechan, R. M., Snapper, S. B., Jacobson, S., Jackson, I. M. D. 1984. The distribution of thyrotropin-releasing hormone (TRH) in the rhesus monkey spinal cord. *Peptides* 5:185–94

99. Beale, J. S., White, R. P., Huang, S. 1977. EEG and blood pressure effects of TRH in rabbits. *Neuropharmacology* 16:499–506

100. Horita, A., Carino, M. A., Lai, H., LaHann, T. R. 1979. Behavioral and autonomic effects of TRH in animals, In *Central Nervous System Effects of Hypothalamic Hormones and Other Peptides*, ed. R. Collu, A. Barbeau, J. R. Ducharme, J.-G. Rochefort, pp. 65–74. New York: Raven

101. Horita, A., Carino, M. A., Weitzman, R. E. 1979. Role of catecholamines and vasopressin release in the TRH-induced vasopressor response, In *Catecholamines: Basic and Clinical Frontiers*, ed. E. Usdin, I. J. Kopin, J. Barchas, pp. 1140–42. New York: Pergamon

102. Kunos, G., Newman, F., Farsang, C., Ungar, W. 1984. Thyrotropin releasing hormone and naloxone attenuate the antihypertensive action of central α-adrenoceptor stimulation through different mechanisms. *Endocrinology* 115:2481–83

103. Holaday, J. W., D'Amato, R. J., Faden, A. I. 1981. Thyrotropin releasing hormone improves cardiovascular function in experimental endotoxic and hemorrhagic shock. *Science* 213:216–18

104. Holaday, J. W., Faden, A. I. 1983. Thyrotropin releasing hormone: Autonomic effects upon cardiorespiratory function in endotoxic shock. *Regul. Peptides* 7:111–25

105. Lux, W. E. Jr., Feuerstein, G., Faden, A. I. 1983. Thyrotropin-releasing hormone reverses experimental anaphylactic shock through non-endorphin-related mechanisms. *Eur. J. Pharmacol.* 90: 301–2

106. Amir, S., Harel, M., Schachar, A. 1984. Thyrotropin-releasing hormone (TRH) improves survival in anaphylactic shock: A central effect mediated by the sympatho-adrenomedullary β-adrenoceptive system. *Brain Res.* 298:219–24

107. Lux, W. E. Jr., Feuerstein, G., Faden,

A. I. 1983. Thyrotropin-releasing hormone reverses the hypotension and bradycardia produced by leukotriene D4 in unanesthetized guinea pigs. *Prost. Leuk. Med.* 10:301–7

108. Feuerstein, G., Lux, W. E., Snyder, F., Ezra, D., Faden, A. I. 1984. Hypotension produced by platelet-activating factor is reversed by thyrotropin-releasing hormone. *Circ. Shock* 13:255–60

109. Feuerstein, G., Hassen, A. H., Faden, A. I. 1983. TRH: Cardiovascular and sympathetic modulation in brain nuclei of the rat. *Peptides* 4:617–20

110. Diz, D. I., Jacobowitz, D. M. 1984. Cardiovascular effects produced by injections of thyrotropin-releasing hormone in specific preoptic and hypothalamic nuclei in the rat. *Peptides* 5:801–8

111. Koskinen, L., Bill, A. 1984. Thyrotropin-releasing hormone (TRH) causes sympathetic activation and cerebral vasodilation in the rabbit. *Acta Physiol. Scand.* 122:127–36

112. Holaday, J. W. 1984. Neuropeptides in shock and traumatic injury: sites and mechanisms of action, In *Neuroendocrine Perspectives*, ed. E. E. Muller, R. M. MacLeod, 1:161–99. New York: Elsevier

113. Bernton, E. W., Long, J. B., Holaday, J. W. 1985. Opioids and neuropeptides: Mechanisms in circulatory shock. *Fed. Proc.* 44:290–99

114. Tonoue, T., Nomoto, T. 1979. Effect of intracerebroventricular administration of thyrotropin releasing hormone upon electroenteromyogram of rat duodenum. *Eur. J. Pharmacol.* 58:369–77

115. Goto, Y., Tache, Y. 1985. Gastric erosions induced by intracisternal thyrotropin-releasing hormone (TRH) in rats. *Peptides* 6:153–56

116. Metcalf, G., Myers, R. D. 1976. A comparison between the hypothermia induced by intraventricular injections of thyrotropin releasing hormone, noradrenaline or calcium ions in unanaesthetized cats. *Br. J. Pharmacol.* 58:489–95

117. Pillai, N. P., Bhargava, H. N. 1984. The effect of thyrotropin releasing hormone and morphine on gastrointestinal transit. *Peptides* 5:1055–59

118. Soldani, G., Del Tacca, M., Martino, E., Bartelloni, A., Impicciatore, M. 1983. The involvement of the vagal pathway in the antisecretory effect of thyrotropin-releasing hormone on gastric secretion in the dog. *J. Pharm. Pharmacol.* 35:119–21

119. Horita, A., Carino, M. A., Pae, Y.-S.

1985. Blockade by naloxone and naltrexone of the TRH-induced stimulation of colonic transit in the rabbit. *Eur. J. Pharmacol.* 108:289–93

120. Maeda-Hagiwara, M., Watanabe, H., Watanabe, K. 1984. Inhibition by central alpha-2 adrenergic mechanism of thyrotropin-releasing hormone-induced gastric acid secretion in the rat. *Jpn. J. Pharmacol.* 36:131–36

121. Tache, Y., Lesiege, D., Bale, W., Collu, R. 1985. Gastric hypersecretion by intracisternal TRH: Dissociation from hypophysiotropic activity and role of central catecholamine. *Eur. J. Pharmacol.* 107:149–55

122. Maeda-Hagiwara, M., Watanabe, K. 1983. Influence of dopamine receptor agonists on gastric acid secretion induced by intraventricular administration of thyrotropin-releasing hormone in the perfused stomach of anaesthetized rats. *Br. J. Pharmacol.* 79:297–303

123. Tache, Y., Gunion, M. 1985. Corticotropin-releasing factor: Central action to influence gastric secretion. *Fed. Proc.* 44:255–58

124. Faden, A. I., Jacobs, T. P., Holaday, J. W. 1981. Thyrotropin-releasing hormone improves neurologic recovery after spinal trauma in cats. *N. Engl. J. Med.* 305:1063–67

125. Faden, A. I., Jacobs, T. P., Smith, M. T., Holaday, J. W. 1983. Comparison of thyrotropin-releasing hormone (TRH), naloxone, and dexamethasone treatments in experimental spinal injury. *Neurology* 33:673–78

126. Faden, A. I., Jacobs, T. P., Smith, M. T. 1984. Thyrotropin-releasing hormone in experimental spinal injury: Dose response and late treatment. *Neurology* 34:1280–84

127. Engel, W. K., Siddique, T., Nicoloff, J. T. 1983. Effect on weakness and spasticity in amyotrophic lateral sclerosis of thyrotropin-releasing hormone. *Lancet* 2:73–75

128. Imoto, K., Saida, K., Iwamura, K., Saida, T., Nishitani, H. 1984. Amyotrophic lateral sclerosis: A double-blind crossover trial of thyrotropin-releasing hormone. *J. Neurol. Neurosurg. Psychiatry* 47:1332–34

129. Sobue, I., Takayanagi, T., Nakanishi, T., Tsubaki, T., Uono, M., et al. 1983. Controlled trial of thyrotropin-releasing hormone tartrate in ataxia of spinocerebellar degenerations. *J. Neurol. Sci.* 61:235–48

130. Lechan, R. M., Adelman, L. S., Forte, S., Jackson, I. M. D. 1984. Organization

of thyrotropin-releasing hormone (TRH) immunoreactivity in the human spinal cord. *Soc. Neurosci.* 10:431 (Abstr.)

131. Mitsuma, T., Nogimori, T., Adachi, K., Mukoyama, M., Ando, K. 1984. Concentrations of immunoreactive thyrotropin-releasing hormone in spinal cord of patients with amyotropic lateral sclerosis. *Am. J. Med. Sci.* 287:34–36

132. Lechan, R. M., Jackson, I. M. D. 1985. Thyrotropin releasing hormone but not histidyl-proline diketopiperazine is depleted from rat spinal cord following 5,7-dihydroxytryptamine treatment. *Brain Res.* 326:152–55

133. Zimmermann, E. M., Coffield, J. A., Miletic, V., Hoffert, M. J., Brooks, B. R. 1984. Localization of substance P, 5HT and TRH-like immunoreactivity in mouse spinal cord following motor neuron damage. *Soc. Neurosci.* 10:891 (Abstr.)

134. Anderson, R. J., Campbell, G. W., Boyd, D. K. 1984. Possible sites of action of TRH as a modulator of motor control pathways. *Soc. Neurosci.* 10:852 (Abstr.)

135. Weill, C. L. 1984. The prevention of natural motoneuron cell death by thyrotropin releasing hormone (TRH). *Soc. Neurosci.* 10:641 (Abstr.)

136. Schmidt-Achert, K. M., Askanas, V., Engel, W. K. 1984. Thyrotropin releasing hormone enhances choline acetyltransferase and creatine kinase in cultured spinal ventral horn neurons. *J. Neurochem.* 43:586–89

137. Yamaguchi, T., Hayashi, K., Murakami, H., Maruyama, S., Yamaguchi, M. 1984. Distribution and characterization of the TRH receptors in the CNS of ataxic mutant mouse. *Neurochem. Res.* 9:477–505

138. Burt, D. R., Max, S. R., Hoffman, P. M. 1984. Decreases in spinal receptors for thyrotropin-releasing hormone precede symptom development in murine leukemia virus induced motor neuron disease. *Soc. Neurosci.* 10:1093 (Abstr.)

139. Hawkins, E. F., Engel, W. K. 1985. Analog specificity of the thyrotropin-releasing hormone receptor in the central nervous system: Possible clinical implications. *Life Sci.* 36:601–11

140. Metcalf, G. 1982. Regulatory peptides as a source of new drugs—the clinical prospects for analogues of TRH which are resistant to metabolic degradation. *Brain Res. Rev.* 4:389–408

141. Yarbrough, G. S. 1984. TRH interactions with cholinergic mechanisms and consequent therapeutic implications. In *Psychoneuroendocrine Dysfunction*, ed. N. S. Shag, A. G. Donald, pp. 73–81. New York: Plenum

142. Holaday, J. W., Bernton, E. W. 1984. Protirelin (TRH): A potent neuromodulator with therapeutic potential. *Arch. Int. Med.* 144:1138–40

Ann. Rev. Pharmacol. Toxicol. 1986. 26:333–69
Copyright © 1986 by Annual Reviews Inc. All rights reserved

THE REGULATION OF CYTOCHROME P-450 GENE EXPRESSION

James P. Whitlock, Jr.

Department of Pharmacology, Stanford University School of Medicine, Stanford, California 94305

INTRODUCTION

Scientific interest in cytochrome P-450 has increased dramatically since the unheralded discovery in 1958 of a hepatic microsomal carbon monoxide-binding pigment with an absorption maximum at 450 nm (1, 2). Omura & Sato subsequently showed that the pigment had the biochemical properties of a cytochrome and designated it "P-450" because of its unusual spectral characteristics (3–5). We now know that various forms of cytochrome P-450 exist in bacterial, plant, and animal organisms and that these hemoproteins catalyze the monoxygenation of a broad spectrum of lipophilic substrates. Biochemical analyses of cytochrome P-450 have revealed multiple isozymes, which often have broad and overlapping substrate specificities. We do not know how many forms of cytochrome P-450 exist; the data suggest that there may be between 30 and 100. In mammalian cells, cytochrome P-450-containing enzyme systems metabolize many different endogenous substances (e.g. steroids, fatty acids, prostaglandins), as well as exogenous compounds (e.g. drugs, dyes, pesticides, carcinogens).

The cytochrome P-450 apoproteins contain several regions of amino acid sequence homology. Presumably, these represent functionally similar domains among the different isozymes. Sequencing of cytochrome P-450 cDNAs and/or genes has revealed additional homology. Based on the degree of their relatedness in DNA sequence, the genes for cytochrome P-450 have been classified into different families, which together constitute a cytochrome P-450 multigene superfamily. These sequence analyses have generated a good deal of specula-

333

tion about the possible mechanisms involved in the evolution of the various cytochrome P-450 genes.

Specific chemicals induce one or more forms of cytochrome P-450. Inducibility may have evolved as a mechanism by which the cell can respond to specific chemical signals (e.g. hormonal or xenobiotic) by increasing the rate of specific cytochrome P-450-catalyzed reactions. In addition, the oxygenated product(s) of the cytochrome P-450-catalyzed reaction can be toxic, mutagenic, or carcinogenic. Therefore, some of the cytochromes P-450 also contribute to chemically induced toxicity or neoplasia. Enzyme induction also represents a potentially useful characteristic for studying changes in gene expression that occur in response to specific chemical signals, a topic that is the subject of this review. Because of space constraints, this chapter is limited to mammalian cytochrome P-450 gene expression. Other aspects of cytochrome P-450 biology have been reviewed in this series (6–9) and elsewhere (10–14). Additional reviews are cited in relevant areas of the text. Table 1 summarizes much of the data, which are discussed below.

GENES THAT RESPOND TO PHENOBARBITAL

About 25 years ago, three separate observations heightened scientific interest in cytochrome P-450. Studies of drug tolerance by Remmer revealed that chronic exposure to phenobarbital increased its rate of metabolism by the liver (15). Burns & Conney showed that barbiturates induced the hepatic metabolism of a carcinogenic azo dye (16). Cooper et al demonstrated the role of hepatic cytochrome P-450 in the metabolism of drugs and carcinogens (17). Because of the temporal association of these observations, phenobarbital has been known as an archetypal inducer of cytochrome P-450-catalyzed enzyme activities. The phenobarbital-inducible cytochromes P-450 oxygenate a number of lipophilic substrates, both exogenous (e.g. drugs) and endogenous (e.g. steroids) (18–21).

Early studies of cytochromes P-450 in rabbit (22) and rat (23) liver revealed three distinct forms (designated cytochrome P-450a, -b, and -c in the rat) and showed that phenobarbital induced the one designated cytochrome P-450b. Differences in the primary structures of the apoproteins indicated that each of the cytochromes P-450a, -b, and -c was encoded by a different gene (24). Later, Vlasuk et al (25) and Rampersaud & Walz (26) observed microheterogeneity within cytochrome P-450b; they identified at least six closely related forms of hepatic phenobarbital-inducible cytochrome P-450 polypeptides in different strains of rats. Analyses of the phenotypes of the F_1 progeny from inter-strain crosses suggested that the cytochrome P-450 apoproteins were encoded by two closely linked genetic loci, with (at least) four alleles at a locus designated *P-450b* and (at least) two alleles at a locus designated *P-450e* (26). By

Table 1 Summary of cytochrome P-450 gene expression[a]

Gene	Responds to[b]	Regulatory mechanism				Other properties[d]
		Direct vs. indirect[c]	↑mRNA Accumulation	↑Rate of transcription	Receptor	
P-450b,e	PB	Unknown	+	+	Unknown	1, 2
P-450b,e	DEX	Unknown	+	-	glucocorticoid?	
P-450c, P_1-450	PAHs	Direct	+	+	Ah	3
P-450d, P_3-450	ISF	Unknown	+	Unknown	Unknown	
P-450d, P_3-450	PAHs	Unknown	+	+	Ah	1
$P-450_{PCN}$	PCN	Unknown	+	Unknown	Unknown	4
$P-450_{scc}$	ACTH	Indirect	+	Unknown	ACTH?	1
$P-450_{11\beta}$	ACTH	Indirect	+	Unknown	ACTH?	1
$P-450_{17\alpha}$	ACTH	Unknown	+	Unknown	ACTH?	
$P-450_{C21}$	ACTH	Unknown	±	Unknown	ACTH?	
$P-450_{aromatase}$	ACTH	Unknown	Unknown	Unknown	ACTH?	

[a]See text for discussion of the regulatory mechanisms.
[b]Abbreviations used: PB, phenobarbital; DEX, dexamethasone; PAHs, polycyclic aromatic hydrocarbons; ISF, isosafrole; PCN, pregnenolone-16α-carbonitrile; ACTH, adrenocorticotrophic hormone.
[c]Direct: increases in mRNA accumulation and transcription rate do not require ongoing protein synthesis. Indirect: increases in mRNA accumulation and transcription rate require ongoing protein synthesis.
[d]1: Tissue-specific expression; 2: heme-dependent expression; 3: superinducible; 4: sex-dependent expression.

definition, forms b and e constitute the major phenobarbital-inducible species of cytochrome P-450 in the rat. An analogous situation apparently exists in other species, although the studies have been less extensive. Microheterogeneity analogous to that observed for the proteins also occurs at the nucleic acid level. Analyses of hepatic mRNA from different rat strains reveal several phenobarbital-inducible mRNAs that direct the in vitro synthesis of different, but antigenically-related, cytochrome P-450 apoproteins (27). Analyses of cloned cDNAs imply the existence of (at least) two related mRNAs for phenobarbital-inducible cytochrome P-450 (28). Use of these cDNAs to analyze restricted rat liver genomic DNA reveal (at least) six distinct genomic segments with substantial sequence homology (29, 30). Similar observations have been made in mice (31, 32), rabbits (33), and humans (34). These restriction analyses suggest that additional DNA sequences that are homologous to phenobarbital-responsive cytochrome P-450 genes remain to be cloned and characterized. It is possible that some of the DNA sequences do not represent functional genes (29, 30).

The analyses of restricted genomic DNA imply that variation at the genomic level accounts for the heterogeneity observed among the phenobarbital-inducible cytochrome P-450 apoproteins; however, the exact number of genes that encode these proteins is not yet known. Because of their sequence homology, these genes define a cytochrome P-450 multigene family. The designation of the gene family as "phenobarbital-responsive," while logical from an historical standpoint, is now somewhat misleading, because the members are related by DNA sequence and not necessarily by responsiveness to phenobarbital. For example, although they exhibit substantial (i.e. 60–70%) sequence homology to phenobarbital-responsive genes, the genes for cytochrome P-450 form 1 and form 3b are constitutively expressed in rabbit liver and do not respond to phenobarbital (35–37). The mechanism(s) that control the constitutive expression are unknown. Analyses of the genomic DNA from mouse-hamster somatic cell hybrids indicate that, in mice, the members of this gene family are clustered on chromosome 7, at the coumarin hydroxylase *(Coh)* locus (32, 38). In humans, this gene family maps to chromosome 19 (39).

Phenobarbital-responsive cytochrome P-450 genes apparently have a typical mammalian gene structure. Analysis of a functional cytochrome P-450e gene from rat liver reveals a total length of about 14 kilobases (kb), with nine exons and eight introns. The putative transcription start site is located 30 base pairs (bp) upstream of the ATG initiation codon, and a TATA-like sequence is present 27 bp farther 5'-ward. The 3' end contains a putative polyadenylation signal 25–26 bp upstream of the poly(A) attachment site. The exon/intron boundaries contain the appropriate consensus sequences (40).

Several investigators have studied the mechanism(s) by which phenobarbital alters the cytochrome P-450 content of the cell. In intact animals, phenobarbital stimulates the incorporation of amino acids into cytochrome P-450 protein (41). Phenobarbital produces an accumulation of cytochrome P-450-specific mRNA, measured either by in vitro translation (42–45, 48–51) or by hybridization to cDNA (46, 47, 50–52). The use of synthetic oligodeoxynucleotide probes specific for cytochrome P-450 b or e reveals that phenobarbital induces a marked accumulation of both mRNAs, from levels that are undetectable in livers of untreated rats (53). Nuclear transcription experiments indicate that, in rat liver, phenobarbital produces within three to four hours a 20- to 50-fold increase in the rate of transcription of the cytochrome P-450b (and, presumably, P-450e) gene (54–56). The transcription rate increases uniformly along the length of the cytochrome P-450 gene (M. Adesnik and E. Rivkin, unpublished observations). The increase in the rate of cytochrome P450 gene transcription is followed by the accumulation of polyadenylated cytoplasmic cytochrome P-450-specific mRNA (55). The increase in transcription rate is comparable to the 50-fold induction of cytochrome P-450b (and, presumably, P-450e) protein produced by phenobarbital under similar conditions (57). These data imply that phenobarbital induces the accumulation of cytochrome P-450 protein primarily by stimulating the rate of transcription of the corresponding cytochrome P-450 gene. Furthermore, phenobarbital apparently increases the rate of transcription initiation, because in uninduced liver there is no detectable transcription of the cytochrome P-450 gene in the region immediately downstream of the mRNA cap site (M. Adesnik and E. Rivkin, unpublished observations). The undetectable levels of mRNA for cytochrome P-450 b and e in uninduced animals (53) suggest that the presence of inducer may be absolutely required for the transcription of the cytochrome P-450 b and e genes.

The mechanism by which phenobarbital increases the rate of cytochrome P-450 gene transcription is unknown. The transcription rate begins to increase within an hour of phenobarbital administration (55), which suggests that induction does not involve many intermediary events. However, it is not known whether phenobarbital can stimulate the rate of cytochrome P-450 gene transcription directly (i.e. in the absence of ongoing protein synthesis).

The induction mechanism for polycyclic aromatic hydrocarbon-responsive forms of cytochrome P-450 involves the binding of the inducer to an intracellular protein receptor; the inducer-receptor complex then interacts with a genomic regulatory element to stimulate the transcription of the cytochrome P-450 gene (see next section). A similar mechanism governs the expression of steroid-responsive genes (58). By analogy, we might expect phenobarbital to act via a receptor-mediated mechanism. However, in contrast to compounds known to act at receptors, inducers of the phenobarbital-type are (a) effective only at high concentrations and (b) exhibit no obvious structural similarities (59); these properties are not suggestive of a receptor-mediated mechanism.

The development of more potent "phenobarbital-like" inducers has been modestly successful but has not yet helped to clarify the induction mechanism. For example, the compound TCPOBOP produces a phenobarbital type of response in mice, but not in rats; furthermore, TCPOBOP fails to antagonize the effects of phenobarbital in rats (60, 61). Thus, in rats, TCPOBOP does not seem to act at "phenobarbital receptors." The idea that phenobarbital-type inducers act via a nonreceptor mechanism and that induction reflects some physiochemical property that the compounds have in common (e.g. the ability to alter membrane structure) does not easily account for their ability to induce particular forms of cytochrome P-450 and not others. Thus, the data to date neither substantiate nor refute the idea that phenobarbital induces cytochrome P-450 gene expression by interacting with specific receptors. This is an area where additional research seems likely to generate useful information. For example, synthesis of more potent phenobarbital-type inducers may be useful in identifying specific receptors, if they exist. Mapping of nuclease-hypersensitive sites (62) in the vicinity of phenobarbital-responsive genes may help to identify genomic control elements that interact with regulatory proteins, including (hypothetical) inducer-receptor complexes. Construction of hybrid genes, combined with the use of gene transfer, may help to define the function of such genomic control elements (see next section for example). It is notable that genetic differences in responsiveness to phenobarbital exist among rats (63, 64) and mice (65) in the induction of hepatic aldehyde dehydrogenase. In mice, the genetic variation apparently occurs at a regulatory locus (65), which, therefore, might encode a phenobarbital-specific regulatory protein.

Heme may also regulate the level of cytochrome P-450 gene expression. Cobalt chloride and 3-amino-1,2,4-triazole, which are inhibitors of heme biosynthesis, also inhibit the synthesis of the apoprotein cytochrome P-450b (and, presumably, P-450e) (66). Using cDNA as a hybridization probe, Ravishankar & Padmanaban showed that both cobalt chloride and 3-amino-1,2,4-triazole inhibit the phenobarbital-induced accumulation of mRNA for cytochrome P-450b/e. Furthermore, nuclear transcription assays indicate that both compounds inhibit the phenobarbital-stimulated increase in the rate of cytochrome P-450b/e gene transcription (52). These results imply that the intracellular heme concentration influences cytochrome P-450 gene expression. Others have also observed a possible relationship between heme and cytochrome P-450 enzyme concentrations (67).

The mechanism(s) by which heme may regulate cytochrome P-450 gene transcription are unknown. However, an analogous system may function in S. cerevisiae, where heme regulates the transcription of the iso-1-cytochrome c (CYC1) gene. Heme-deficient cells transcribe the CYC1 gene at a low rate and contain undetectable levels of iso-1-cytochrome c apoprotein. Heme increases the rate of CYC1 gene transcription and acts at a genomic regulatory element (termed an "upstream activation site") located several hundred nucleotides 5'-ward of the *CYC1* gene (68). Furthermore, a *trans*-acting, recessive mutation at the *HAP1* ("heme activator protein") locus renders the upstream activation site uninducible by heme (69). Thus, the *HAP1* locus probably encodes a regulatory protein that binds heme and activates *CYC1* gene transcription by binding to the upstream activation site. It will be interesting to determine if a similar mechanism controls the expression of some cytochrome P-450 genes.

Decreases in cytochrome P-450 protein concentration produced by some inducers may be related to decreased availability of heme. Using immunological techniques to quantitate various cytochrome P-450 apoproteins, several investigators (18, 70–72) have reported that inducers may increase the concentration of one form(s) of cytochrome P-450 while simultaneously decreasing the concentration of another form(s). For example, phenobarbital (and other inducers) produces a decrease in a form of cytochrome P-450 that is "constitutive". Likewise, β-naphthoflavone and 3-methylcholanthrene, which induce the PAH-responsive subset of proteins, produce decreases in the subset that is phenobarbital-inducible. Other workers have observed that the β-naphthoflavone-induced decrease in a phenobarbital-inducible form of cytochrome P-450 is associated with a corresponding decrease in its mRNA (48, 49). Thus, the lower cytochrome P-450 content probably reflects decreased transcription of the corresponding gene(s). The mechanism by which these decreases occur is unknown. However, in view of the apparent ability of heme to regulate the transcription of (at least some) cytochrome P-450 genes, one possibility is that, as a result of increased transcription of some cytochrome P-450 genes, the availability of heme may become rate-limiting for the transcription of others. An alternative possibility is that some inducers have more than one primary effect and may stimulate the expression of one cytochrome P-450 gene(s) while inhibiting the expression of another (72). This is an area that seems worthy of future study.

Responsiveness to phenobarbital is also a function of the tissue in which the cytochrome P-450 gene is expressed. For example, using three different cDNAs to measure mRNA concentrations, Leighton & Kemper detected all three mRNA species in rabbit liver, only one in kidney, and none in lung. Furthermore, in liver, two mRNA species were phenobarbital-inducible, and one was expressed constitutively (37). Thus, three closely related genomic sequences are differentially responsive to phenobarbital and exhibit tissue-specific patterns of expression. Others have made related observations at the protein level. For example, one form of cytochrome P-450, which is phenobarbital-inducible in rabbit liver, is constitutively expressed in the lung (73, 74). Presumably, these findings reflect tissue-specific differences in the transcription rate, because transcriptional control probably determines the tissue-specific pattern of gene expression (75). Furthermore, it seems likely that *trans*-acting regulatory factors govern the tissue-specific transcription rate (76).

There is also evidence for posttranscriptional control of the cytochrome P-450b gene. In rat liver, phenobarbital induces a 20-fold increase in the rate of cytochrome P-450b gene transcription, which is followed by a corresponding increase in mRNA accumulation. In contrast, dexamethasone has no effect on the transcription rate, yet it produces a 10-fold increase in mRNA concentration (C. B. Kasper, personal communication). These findings suggest that dexamethasone may stabilize cytochrome P-450b mRNA. The mechanism by which dexamethasone produces this effect is unknown. Possibly, it activates the transcription of a gene(s) whose product selectively inhibits the degradation of particular mRNAs.

The findings outlined above imply the existence of several distinct mechanisms that regulate the transcription of phenobarbital-responsive cytochrome P450 genes. A working hypothesis might envision a hierarchy of *cis*-acting genomic control elements, each of which influences the rate of gene transcription upon its interaction with a specific *trans*-acting regulatory factor. One element would respond to phenobarbital, a second to heme, and a third to a tissue-specific factor(s). Additional elements might also exist. At any given time, the rate of cytochrome P-450 gene transcription would reflect the contribution of each component of the regulatory hierarchy.

GENES THAT RESPOND TO POLYCYCLIC AROMATIC HYDROCARBONS

During studies of the hepatic metabolism of chemical carcinogens, the Millers observed that ingestion of polycyclic aromatic hydrocarbons (PAHs) increased the rate of carcinogen metabolism in rats and mice (77). Subsequent experiments implied that PAHs induced the synthesis of carcinogen-metabolizing enzyme molecules (78). Shortly thereafter, Cooper et al implicated cytochrome P-450 in carcinogen metabolism (17). By virtue of these findings, 3-methylcholanthrene became the prototype of a class of inducers of cytochrome P-450-catalyzed enzyme activities. The PAH-inducible cytochromes P-450 metabolize a spectrum of lipophilic compounds that overlaps those of other forms of cytochrome P-450 (18). Studies of the metabolism of carcinogenic PAHs, such as benzo(a)pyrene, have revealed the major role of the PAH-inducible cytochromes P-450 in chemically induced neoplasia and toxicity (79–81).

Studies in rat liver implied that 3-methylcholanthrene induced a single form of cytochrome P-450 (designated P-450c), which was distinctly different from the two other known forms of cytochrome P-450 (23). Subsequently, Ryan et al observed that isosafrole preferentially induces a fourth form of cytochrome

P-450 (designated P-450d), which is immunologically related to cytochrome P-450c, but which has different catalytic activities and a different primary structure (82–84). PAHs induce cytochrome P-450d to a somewhat lesser extent than they induce cytochrome P-450c (85). By definition, forms c and d constitute the major PAH-inducible species of cytochrome P-450 in the rat. Similarly, PAHs induce two forms of cytochrome P-450 in rabbit liver (86).

In mice, 3-methylcholanthrene (and other PAHs) also induces two hepatic forms of cytochrome P-450, which differ in their catalytic activities and primary structures; isosafrole preferentially induces one of the forms (designated cytochrome P_3-450) (87). The isolation, characterization, and comparison of cDNA and genomic clones (see below) for the PAH-inducible cytochromes P-450 in rats and mice indicate that cytochrome P-450c (rat) is equivalent to cytochrome P_1-450 (mouse) and that cytochrome P-450d (rat) is equivalent to cytochrome P_3-450 (mouse). Analogous isozymes (form 6 and form 4) exist in rabbits (88). In addition, in a mouse strain (DBA/2N), which is "nonresponsive" to PAHs (see below), isosafrole induces an hepatic form that has been designated cytochrome P_2-450 (89). However, the mRNAs for cytochrome P_2-450 and cytochrome P_3-450 are both 20S (90, 91), and anti-cytochrome P_2-450 antibodies precipitate the protein translated in vitro from cytochrome P_3-450 mRNA (91). These findings imply the existence of substantial similarities between cytochrome P_2-450 and cytochrome P_3-450; whether they represent the products of different genes remains to be established.

Several investigators have isolated cDNAs for PAH-inducible forms of cytochrome P-450 (91–102). Analyses of the cDNAs for rat cytochrome P-450c (96) and cytochrome P-450d (98), for mouse cytochrome P_1-450 and cytochrome P_3-450 (101), and for the human equivalent of cytochrome P_1-450 (102) reveal that they contain substantial sequence homologies. There is notably less sequence homology between PAH-responsive cytochrome P-450 genes and phenobarbital-responsive cytochrome P-450 genes. Thus, the PAH-responsive cytochrome P-450 genes represent a distinct family within the larger superfamily of cytochrome P-450 genes. Analyses of restricted genomic DNA imply that the PAH-responsive cytochrome P-450 gene family is considerably smaller than the phenobarbital-responsive cytochrome P-450 gene family (99, 101, 102).

Analyses of the PAH-responsive cytochrome P-450 genes in the rat (103–105) and mouse (99, 106) reveal similar exon-intron arrangements, which differ substantially from the exon-intron organization of the phenobarbital-responsive cytochrome P-450e gene. Sequence analyses reveal putative TATA structures and polyadenylation signals at appropriate locations. The 5'-flanking regions contain sequences capable of forming Z-DNA and sequences with some homology to viral enhancers. The functional significance of these observations remains to be determined. It is notable that there is relatively little sequence homology between rat cytochromes P-450c and P-450d (and between mouse cytochromes P_1-450 and P_3-450) in the DNA flanking the 5' ends of the genes, despite the fact that each gene is PAH-responsive (103, 107). However, the genomic control element(s) that is recognized by the PAH-receptor complex may be located still farther 5'-ward of the regions that have been sequenced (see below).

Analyses of restricted genomic DNA from a panel of mouse × hamster somatic cell hybrids, using cytochrome P_1-450-specific and cytochrome P_3-450-specific DNA sequences as hybridization probes, reveal that both the cytochrome P_1-450 gene and the cytochrome P_3-450 gene are located on mouse chromosome 9 (107). Thus, the PAH-responsive cytochrome P-450 genes, the phenobarbital-responsive cytochrome P-450 genes, the PCN-responsive cytochrome P-450 genes, and the steroid 21-hydroxylase cytochrome P-450 genes (see following sections) are located on four different chromosomes in the mouse. Similar analyses of human × rodent somatic cell hybrids have localized the equivalent of the cytochrome P_1-450 gene to human chromosome 15 (108).

The induction mechanism for PAH-responsive cytochrome P-450 genes has been studied in some detail. PAHs induce the accumulation of mRNA specific for cytochrome P-450c and cytochrome P-450d in rat liver (109–114), for cytochrome P_1-450 and cytochrome P_3-450 in mouse liver (90, 91, 115–119), and for cytochrome P_1-450-specific mRNA in mouse hepatoma cells in culture (120). These findings suggest that PAHs may increase the rate of cytochrome P-450 gene transcription. However, rates of transcription were not measured in these studies. In rat liver, cytochrome P-450c mRNA and cytochrome P-450d mRNA accumulate at similar rates in response to 3-methylcholanthrene, and a measurable increase occurs relatively rapidly (within four hours). Furthermore, the induction mechanisms for both cytochrome P-450c and cytochrome P-450d exhibit similar sensitivities to PAH-type inducers. In contrast, in uninduced liver, the concentration of cytochrome P-450d mRNA is substantially higher than that of cytochrome P-450c mRNA. In addition, isosafrole preferentially induces the accumulation of cytochrome P-450d mRNA (113). Together, these findings imply that the regulatory mechanisms governing the expression of these two cytochrome P-450 genes may have a component (which controls PAH-responsiveness) that is similar, as well as components (which control "constitutive" expression and isosafrole-responsiveness) that are different.

In mouse liver, 3-methylcholanthrene increases the rate of synthesis of both cytochrome P_1-450 mRNA and cytochrome P_3-450 mRNA (119). Likewise, in mouse hepatoma cells, 2,3,7,8-tetrachlorodibenzo-p-dioxin (TCDD, the most potent known PAH-type inducer) induces a 20-fold increase in the rate of cytochrome P_1-450 mRNA synthesis. In the cells in culture, the effect is maximal within 30 min and does not require ongoing protein synthesis; thus, the increased cytochrome P_1-450 transcription rate is a primary response to the inducer (121). The simplest interpretation of all the data is that PAHs stimulate the rate of transcription of both PAH-responsive cytochrome P-450 genes. It remains to be determined whether (a) the elevated level of cytochrome P-450d (or cytochrome P_3-450) mRNA in uninduced cells and (b) the mRNA accumulation that occurs in response to isosafrole reflect corresponding increases in the rate of transcription of the cytochrome P-450d (or cytochrome P_3-450) gene. Furthermore, it is not known whether isosafrole acts via a receptor-mediated mechanism to induce the accumulation of cytochrome P-450 mRNA and protein (122). Thus, the mechanism(s) that governs the cellular response to isosafrole may be an area worthy of additional study.

More is known about the mechanism by which PAHs stimulate the expression of the mouse cytochrome P_1-450 gene. This knowledge stems in part from observations that, in certain inbred strains of mice, a single autosomal dominant gene apparently controls several responses to PAHs (123–128). For example, the induction of aryl hydrocarbon hydroxylase (AHH), a cytochrome P_1-450-catalyzed enzyme activity, is expressed as an autosomal dominant trait in crosses between the C57BL/6 and DBA/2 mouse strains (127, 128). In addition, other responses to PAHs segregate in the same pattern as AHH inducibility (129). Therefore, the genetic locus controlling the expression of these responses is thought to be regulatory, and has been designated *Ah*, for aromatic hydrocarbon responsiveness. The observations (a) that TCDD can induce AHH activity in mouse strains (e.g. DBA/2) that do not respond to other PAHs (130), (b) that the AHH induction mechanism in responsive mouse strains (e.g. C57BL/6) is 10- to 20-fold more sensitive to TCDD than the induction mechanism in nonresponsive strains (131), and (c) that the livers of responsive strains contain a protein that binds TCDD with high affinity and low capacity (132) led to the concept that the *Ah* locus encodes an intracellular "receptor" protein that is required for the induction response. Nonresponsive mouse strains contain a receptor that binds TCDD poorly (and less potent PAHs not at all) (133). The F_1 progeny of crosses between C57BL/6 (responsive) and DBA/2 (nonresponsive) mice exhibit the responsive phenotype for AHH induction, yet contain about one-half the number of *Ah* receptors as the C57BL/6 parent. This observation implies that, in the C57BL/6 mouse, the number of receptors is not rate limiting for the induction of AHH by PAHs. This and other aspects of *Ah* receptor biology have been reviewed recently (134).

The induction of AHH activity involves the formation of inducer-receptor complexes and the temperature-dependent accumulation of these complexes in the nucleus (135, 136). It is not yet clear whether, in the intact cell, unoccupied receptors are cytoplasmic (137) or nuclear (138). Furthermore, the related issue of whether the temperature-dependent step in enzyme induction is a "translocation" of the inducer-receptor complex from the cytoplasm to the nucleus (137) or some other event (e.g. enzymatic modification), which takes place in the nucleus (138), remains to be resolved. There is general agreement, however, that the inducer-receptor complex acts in the nucleus to stimulate the transcription of the cytochrome P_1-450 gene. In mouse hepatoma cells, the accumulation of inducer-receptor complexes in the nucleus correlates temporally with increases in the rate of cytochrome P_1-450 gene transcription (D. I. Israel and J. P. Whitlock, Jr., unpublished observations).

Studies of AHH induction in cells in culture have revealed additional aspects of the control of cytochrome P_1-450 gene expression. Hankinson devised a selection protocol, which takes advantage of the metabolic activation of PAHs by the AHH system (139), to isolate mutant mouse hepatoma cells defective in AHH activity (140). Using the same (Hepa 1c1c7) cells, Miller & Whitlock employed the fluorescence-activated cell sorter to isolate variants that either underproduce or overproduce AHH in response to PAHs (141). Both groups identified two complementation groups of receptor-defective variants with altered AHH induction mechanisms (142, 143). Variants that form few inducer-receptor complexes accumulate little cytochrome P_1-450 mRNA and AHH activity in response to TCDD (120, 144), and variants in which the inducer-receptor complex binds weakly to the nucleus (138) fail to transcribe the cytochrome P_1-450 gene in response to TCDD (121) and contain no detectable cytochrome P_1-450 mRNA or AHH activity (120, 144). These findings indicate that transcription of the cytochrome P_1-450 gene requires functional inducer-receptor complexes. Hankinson and co-workers have isolated additional classes of AHH-defective mutants; one class apparently contains a lesion(s) in the cytochrome P_1-450 structural gene (145); another class exhibits a dominant phenotype (146).

The existence of dominant, AHH-defective mutants (146), which also fail to accumulate cytochrome P_1-450 mRNA in response to TCDD (144), implies that a *trans*-acting inhibitory factor(s) may regulate cytochrome P_1-450 gene transcription. Studies of the "superinduction" of AHH activity support this hypothesis. In cells in culture, temporary exposure to cycloheximide (an inhibitor of protein synthesis) plus a PAH inducer is followed by an increase in AHH activity that is greater than the maximal increase produced by the PAH alone (147). Superinduction of enzyme activity is associated with the (super) accumulation of cytochrome P_1-450 mRNA (120), which is due to a (super) increased rate of cytochrome P_1-450 gene transcription (148). Cycloheximide produces no detectable effect on the properties of *Ah* receptors. The superinduction response indicates that functional inducer-receptor complexes are not sufficient for maximal transcription of the cytochrome P_1-450 gene. The observations suggest the existence of a labile repressor protein that inhibits the transcription of the cytochrome P_1-450 gene (148). The possible relationship between the negative regulatory factor implied by the dominant mutants and the labile repressor implied by the superinduction response remains to be determined. Together, the data imply that (at least) two *trans*-acting factors control cytochrome P_1-450 gene expression: the inducer-receptor complex stimulates, and a labile repressor inhibits, the transcription of the cytochrome P_1-450 gene. Therefore, expression of this gene reflects a balance between positive and negative control of transcription.

These *trans*-acting regulatory factors act via *cis*-acting genomic control elements located upstream (5'-ward) of the cytochrome P_1-450 gene. Jones et al have analyzed variant mouse hepatoma cells (high activity variant [HAV] cells) that overexpress AHH activity in response to TCDD. The HAV cells overtranscribe the cytochrome P_1-450 gene in response to TCDD, contain no detectable alteration in their TCDD receptors, and exhibit a phenotype that is co-dominant with wild type, suggesting that they contain a *cis*-acting regulatory alteration (149). Jones et al isolated a 2.6-kb DNA fragment located 5'-ward of the cytochrome P_1-450 gene in the HAV cells (150). In order to analyze the function of this DNA, they constructed a recombinant molecule that contained the 2.6-kb fragment situated immediately upstream of the bacterial chloramphenicol acetyltransferase (CAT) gene. Transfection experiments showed that, in this construct, the CAT gene was inducible by PAHs. Furthermore, deletion analyses revealed that the 2.6-kb DNA fragment contained three functional domains: a promoter, located immediately upstream of the transcription start site; an inhibitory domain (which presumably interacts with the labile repressor), located 700–1000 bp upstream of the promoter; and a PAH-responsive domain (which presumably interacts with the inducer-receptor complex), located 1300–1600 bp upstream of the promoter. The regulatory model is depicted schematically in Figure 1.

The data imply that two different regulatory proteins act via two distinct genomic elements to control cytochrome P_1-450 (and, by analogy, cytochrome P-450c) gene transcription. Whether similar components control the transcription of the cytochrome P_3-450 (and cytochrome P-450d) gene remains to be determined. The existence of tissue-specific differences (90, 151–153) and developmental differences (90, 154) in the expression of PAH-responsive cytochrome P-450 genes suggest that additional regulatory proteins and their affiliated genomic control elements remain to be characterized.

Genetic studies using inbred mice imply that the *Ah* regulatory system contains additional complexity. In crosses between the C3H/He (responsive) and DBA/2 (nonresponsive) strains, AHH inducibility segregates in co-dominant fashion (155, 156). This may indicate the existence of a third allele at the *Ah* locus. In crosses between the C57BL/6N (responsive) and AKR/N (nonresponsive) strains, the nonresponsive phenotype segregates in autosomal dominant fashion (156). As yet, there has been no published model that can account for all of these observations. It would seem worthwhile to follow-up these provocative findings (in particular, the unusual reversal of dominance) with more detailed studies of cytochrome P-450 gene expression in these

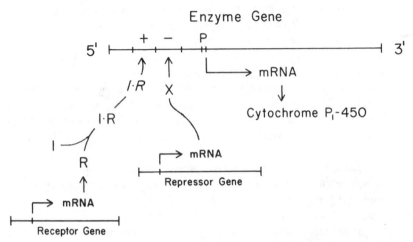

Figure 1   Regulation of cytochrome P_1-450 gene expression in HAV mouse hepatoma cells. The inducer (I) forms a complex (I·R) with an intracellular receptor (R), which (presumably) is encoded by a gene at the *Ah* locus. The inducer-receptor complex undergoes a temperature-dependent change to a form (*I·R*), which binds tightly to chromatin. The binding of the inducer-receptor complex to a genomic domain (+) upstream of the promoter (P) stimulates cytochrome P_1-450 gene transcription. A hypothetical, cycloheximide-sensitive labile repressor (×) binds to a second upstream genomic domain (−) and inhibits transcription. Therefore, cytochrome P_1-450 gene transcription represents a balance between positive and negative control. See Ref. 150 for experimental data. It is possible that additional regulatory factors and genomic control elements also exist for the cytochrome P_1-450 gene (see text).

animals. Likewise, the existence of a mouse fibroblast cell line in which some, but not all, PAHs induce AHH activity (157, 157a) raises the question of heterogeneity of the *Ah* receptor. This observation also seems worthy of additional study.

The chromosomal location of the *Ah* locus is unknown. Although studies in somatic cell hybrids suggest that a gene that regulates AHH inducibility is located on mouse chromosome 17, there is no direct evidence that it encodes the receptor protein (158). Furthermore, the organization and structure of the *Ah* locus is unknown. To describe it as the "*Ah* complex" is misleading, in that there is no evidence that the locus encodes more than one protein. Similarly, designation of the cytochrome P_1-450 and cytochrome P_3-450 apoproteins as "structural products of the *Ah* locus" is not justified, in the absence of any evidence that the gene(s) that encodes the receptor is linked to the genes that encode the enzymes. Although these issues may seem semantic, the failure to use precise terminology adds needless confusion to an area of study that is already complicated.

Several investigators have described other proteins that saturably bind 3-

methylcholanthrene, benzo(a)pyrene, and/or other PAHs with high affinity (159–162). These proteins differ from the receptor encoded by the *Ah* locus with respect to their PAH binding and/or physical characteristics. Although their properties are consistent with those expected for PAH "receptors", their function(s) remains unknown.

In summary, the data imply that PAHs induce cytochrome P-450-catalyzed enzyme activity by activating the rate of transcription of the corresponding gene. The inducer forms a complex with an intracellular regulatory protein (encoded by the *Ah* locus in mice); the complex binds to a *cis*-acting genomic control element upstream of the cytochrome P-450 gene. The ability of the genomic control element to activate transcription from a distance suggests that it may be a PAH-responsive enhancer (163). (At least) one additional regulatory component (an inhibitory one) modulates the response of the cytochrome P_1-450 gene to PAHs. Additional control elements may also exist: those mediating tissue-specific expression, temporal (developmental) expression, and, possibly, responsiveness to heme. The instantaneous rate of cytochrome P-450 gene transcription presumably reflects the contribution of each component of this putative regulatory hierarchy.

GENES THAT RESPOND TO STEROIDS

Inducers of cytochrome P-450 were originally classified as either "phenobarbital-type" or "3-methylcholanthrene-type," based upon the profile of microsomal enzyme activities that each compound induced. In the early 1970s, Selye (164) studied in rats a class of "catatoxic" steroids that conferred protection against toxic chemicals by increasing their rate of metabolism. The most potent, pregnenolone-16α-carbonitrile (PCN), caused proliferation of hepatic endoplasmic reticulum and an increase in hepatic cytochrome P-450 content. In addition, PCN induced a profile of cytochrome P-450-catalyzed enzyme activities different from those induced by either phenobarbital or 3-methylcholanthrene (165). The latter observation suggested that PCN might induce a unique form(s) of cytochrome P-450 and, thus, would represent a third class of inducer. Subsequently, Elshourbagy & Guzelian purified from rat liver a PCN-inducible form of cytochrome P-450. The enzyme had distinctive biochemical, immunologic, and catalytic properties, implying that it was encoded by a unique cytochrome P-450 gene (166). The physiological substrate(s) for this form of cytochrome P-450 is unknown. However, its high constitutive expression in male rats suggests its possible involvement in androgen metabolism.

Hardwick et al constructed a cDNA library using immunoenriched mRNA from male rats and identified a cDNA for cytochrome P-450$_{PCN}$ (167). Analysis of restricted genomic DNA using the cDNA as a hybridization probe reveals multiple bands containing 50 to 60 kb of DNA (167, 168). This finding implies either that the cytochrome P-450$_{PCN}$ gene is large and contains much more intron DNA than exon DNA or, more likely, that the rat genome contains additional elements with sequence homology to the cytochrome P-450$_{PCN}$ gene. Together, the elements may constitute a distinct cytochrome P-450 gene family (169). It is unknown whether these additional DNA elements are either functional or PCN-responsive.

Simmons et al used the rat cytochrome P-450$_{PCN}$ cDNA to analyze restricted genomic DNA isolated from a panel of mouse-hamster somatic cell hybrids, containing different combinations of mouse chromosomes. All the mouse sequences hybridizable to the cDNA mapped to chromosome 6, implying that the cytochrome P-450$_{PCN}$ gene(s) is located on this chromosome in the mouse, at a locus tentatively termed *Pcn* (168).

Because PCN was ineffective as an inducer in several established cell lines, Guzelian et al utilized primary cultures of female rat hepatocytes to study the mechanism of cytochrome P-450$_{PCN}$ induction. Immunoprecipitation experiments indicate that PCN increases both the rate of synthesis of the cytochrome P-450$_{PCN}$ protein and the accumulation of translatable cytochrome P-450$_{PCN}$ mRNA (170). These findings imply the existence of a transcriptional step in the induction mechanism.

In male rats, PCN induces within 12 hours a 6-fold increase in the hepatic content of cytochrome P-450$_{PCN}$-specific mRNA (167). Phenobarbital also induces a 4-fold increase in cytochrome P-450$_{PCN}$ mRNA accumulation. However, the response to phenobarbital is considerably slower than the response to PCN, suggesting that, in this system, the two inducers might act via different mechanisms. Experiments to determine whether phenobarbital and PCN have an additive (or synergistic) effect on cytochrome P-450$_{PCN}$ mRNA accumulation have not been reported.

The mechanism by which PCN induces the accumulation of cytochrome P-450$_{PCN}$ mRNA is not known. It is unknown whether PCN-induced mRNA accumulates in the absence of ongoing protein synthesis. Furthermore, we do not know if PCN acts to increase the rate of transcription of the cytochrome P-450$_{PCN}$ gene, although this seems likely, given what we know about the mechanism of cytochrome P-450 enzyme induction by phenobarbital and PAHs.

Other steroid hormones, such as dexamethasone, act via intracellular protein receptors to activate the transcription of specific genes (58). By analogy, we might expect PCN action to be receptor-mediated. In intact rat liver and in primary rat hepatocyte cultures, dexamethasone induces cytochrome P-450$_{PCN}$; in fact, some glucocorticoids are more effective inducers than PCN itself (171–173). However, the mechanism by which dexamethasone induces cytochrome P-450$_{PCN}$ does not exhibit characteristics typical of other glucocorticoid-induced responses. For example, in cultured hepatocytes, (a) maximal induction of cytochrome P-450$_{PCN}$ requires a dexamethasone concentration that is at least two orders of magnitude higher than that required to maximally induce tyrosine aminotransferase (TAT); (b) PCN and spironolactone induce cytochrome P-450$_{PCN}$ but do not induce TAT; (c) the kinetics of induction of cytochrome P-450$_{PCN}$ and TAT by dexamethasone are different; (d) the rank order of potency of various steroids as inducers of TAT is different from their rank order as inducers of cytochrome P-450$_{PCN}$; (e) glucocorticoid antagonists inhibit induction of TAT but enhance induction of cytochrome P-450$_{PCN}$ (173). Thus, the induction of cytochrome P-450$_{PCN}$ by steroids apparently involves a mechanism distinct from those described for other systems in which classical glucocorticoid receptors mediate the induction response (58). Whether the response to PCN is receptor-mediated remains to be determined. The identification of more potent inducers of the PCN-type, the identification of PCN antagonists, and the synthesis of PCN-type inducers that can be used as photoaffinity reagents should facilitate the study of this system in the future.

In addition to its control by steroids, the cytochrome P-450$_{PCN}$ gene also exhibits sex-dependent expression. Uninduced male rats contain a substantial amount of hepatic cytochrome P-450$_{PCN}$ mRNA and protein (18, 167, 174). In fact, in untreated male rats, cytochrome P-450$_{PCN}$ constitutes about 15% of the total cytochrome P-450. In contrast, untreated females contain very little cytochrome P-450$_{PCN}$. Presumably, these sex-dependent differences reflect an increased "constitutive" rate of cytochrome P-450$_{PCN}$ gene transcription in the male. The mechanism that governs the increased expression in the male is not well understood. It might be similar to the mechanism(s) that controls the sex-dependent expression of other cytochrome P-450 genes (see section on sexual dimorphism).

Thus, the cytochrome P-450$_{PCN}$ gene apparently exhibits (at least) two distinct control mechanisms: one is steroid-dependent, the other is sex-dependent. Both presumably operate at the transcriptional level. Each control mechanism apparently functions relatively independently, because even in males the gene responds to PCN.

GENES THAT RESPOND TO PITUITARY HORMONES

Studies of steroid biosynthesis in the adrenal cortex led to the discovery of the physiological function of cytochrome P-450. Using Warburg's photochemical action spectrum technique, Estabrook et al demonstrated that the microsomal hemoprotein functioned as an oxygenase in the C_{21}-hydroxylation of steroids (175). Subsequently, several additional steroidogenic reactions were found to be catalyzed by various forms of cytochrome P-450. Two forms (cytochrome P-450$_{scc}$ and cytochrome P-450$_{11\beta}$) are integral components of the inner mitochondrial membrane and are synthesized as larger precursor molecules. The mitochondrial electron transport system consists of both a flavoprotein (NADPH-adrenodoxin reductase) and an iron-sulfur protein (adrenodoxin), analogous to the situation in bacteria. Other forms (cytochrome $P-450_{17\alpha}$, cytochrome $P-450_{C21}$, and cytochrome $P-450_{aromatase}$) are microsomal, are synthesized as the mature protein, and utilize an electron transport system consisting of only a flavoprotein (NADPH-cytochrome P-450 reductase). [For review, see (176, 177).]

Cytochrome $P-450_{scc}$

This enzyme catalyzes the conversion of cholesterol to pregnenolone (a reaction termed cholesterol side-chain cleavage), which is the rate-limiting step in the biosynthetic pathway leading from cholesterol to steroid hormones. Bovine adrenal cytochrome $P-450_{scc}$ cDNA has been cloned by several groups (178–180). Analyses of restricted bovine adrenocortical genomic DNA using a partial-length cDNA as a hybridization probe reveal a relatively simple pattern, suggesting that the genome does not contain multiple elements homologous to the cytochrome $P-450_{scc}$ gene (179). This observation awaits confirmation in studies using full-length cDNA. The cytochrome $P-450_{scc}$ cDNA hybridizes to a 2-kb polyadenylated RNA species, which is present in bovine adrenal cortex and corpus luteum but not in liver, heart, or kidney. Thus, the cytochrome $P-450_{scc}$ gene exhibits tissue-specific expression appropriate to its function.

In the intact rat, endocrine ablation and hormone replacement experiments suggest that ACTH contributes to the maintenance of cytochrome P-450-catalyzed enzyme activities in the adrenal cortex (181). Using a bovine adrenocortical cell culture system, DuBois et al found that ACTH produces, over 36 hr, an increased rate of synthesis of cytochrome $P-450_{scc}$, which is accompanied by a comparable increase in the amount of translatable cytochrome $P-450_{scc}$ mRNA (182). In this system, ACTH stimulates the formation of cyclic AMP, which apparently is responsible for producing the accumulation of cytochrome $P-450_{scc}$ protein and translatable mRNA (183). The rate of ACTH-induced cytochrome $P-450_{scc}$ mRNA accumulation is relatively slow (179). Furthermore, ACTH does not induce cytochrome $P-450_{scc}$ mRNA accumulation in the presence of cycloheximide, indicating that mRNA accumulation requires ongoing protein synthesis [unpublished observations, cited in (184)].

One interpretation of these findings is that ACTH (presumably via membrane receptors) increases the intracellular concentration of cAMP. Cyclic AMP then may induce the synthesis of a "steroid hydroxylase-inducing protein" (184), which subsequently induces the accumulation of cytochrome $P-450_{scc}$ mRNA, either by increasing its rate of synthesis or by performing a processing or stabilizing function at posttranscriptional level [see, for example, (185)].

Measurements of nuclear transcription rates would help to distinguish between these possibilities.

In primary cultures of bovine granulosa cells, follicle-stimulating hormone (FSH) and analogs of cyclic AMP increase the rate of synthesis of cytochrome P-450$_{scc}$ about 4-fold (186, 187). By analogy with the findings for ACTH-stimulated adrenocortical cells, the interaction of FSH with its membrane receptor presumably stimulates the intracellular production of cyclic AMP, which subsequently leads to the accumulation of cytochrome P-450$_{scc}$ mRNA. However, studies of mRNA synthesis and accumulation have not yet been described in this system. In addition, low density lipoprotein stimulates the rate of synthesis of cytochrome P-450$_{scc}$ in granulosa cells, although the effect is less than 2-fold. This increase may reflect the increased availability of the substrate, cholesterol, in the presence of LDL; however, the mechanism by which cholesterol would increase the rate of enzyme synthesis is not clear.

Both cytochrome P-450$_{scc}$ protein (in adrenocortical cells and in granulosa cells) and P-450$_{scc}$ mRNA (in adrenocortical cells) are detectable in uninduced cells (179, 183, 187). This could reflect residual hormonal stimulation of the primary cultures; however, the lack of detectable cytochrome P-450$_{17\alpha}$ under similar conditions argues against this possibility. On the other hand, these findings may reflect the constitutive expression of the cytochrome P-450$_{scc}$ gene. If so, the control mechanism(s) that permits constitutive expression remains to be determined. The data also indicate that, in (at least some) nonsteroidogenic tissues, P-450$_{scc}$ mRNA is undetectable. Thus, a tissue-specific mechanism for the control of cytochrome P-450$_{scc}$ gene expression presumably also exists.

Cytochrome P-450$_{11\beta}$

This enzyme catalyzes the 11β hydroxylation of 11-deoxycortisol to form cortisol. The enzyme is present in the adrenal cortex but not in the testis, ovary, or placenta (176, 177). John et al have isolated two overlapping partial-length adrenocortical cDNA clones for cytochrome P-450$_{11\beta}$ (184). Filter hybridization analyses of adrenocortical RNA reveal three distinct species of polyadenylated RNA, each of which directs the in vitro synthesis of immunoprecipitable cytochrome P-450$_{11\beta}$. These RNA species are detectable in the adrenal cortex but not in the corpus luteum, liver, heart, or kidney. It is not yet clear whether the presence of multiple mRNAs reflects the expression of more than one cytochrome P-450$_{11\beta}$ gene or whether the mRNAs are generated by the differential processing of a single transcript. Filter hybridization analyses reveal that, over a 24 hr period, ACTH and dibutyryl cyclic AMP each induce in adrenocortical cell cultures a 4- to 8-fold accumulation of P-450$_{11\beta}$ RNA; the data do not reveal whether each of the three RNA species is induced equally. Cycloheximide inhibits the ACTH or dibutyryl cyclic AMP-induced RNA accumulation; thus, mRNA induction requires ongoing protein synthesis. Uninduced cells contain a substantial amount of cytochrome P-450$_{11\beta}$ mRNA. Again, this could reflect residual hormonal stimulation or constitutive expression of the cytochrome P-450$_{11\beta}$ gene.

ACTH and dibutyryl cyclic AMP induce the accumulation of mRNA for both cytochrome P-450$_{11\beta}$ and cytochrome P-450$_{scc}$. For each enzyme, the kinetics of mRNA accumulation are similar, and cycloheximide inhibits mRNA accumulation. These observations suggest that, in the adrenal cortex, the mitochondrial steroidogenic cytochromes P-450 may be regulated coordinately at the transcriptional level (176). On the other hand, the tissue-specific expression of the two enzymes is different, which implies that the control mechanisms governing the expression of these two genes are not identical.

Cytochrome P-450$_{17\alpha}$

This enzyme catalyzes the hydroxylation of progestins at the 17α position, a step in the pathway of androgen biosynthesis. The enzyme is present in the adrenal cortex, the gonads, and the placenta (176, 177). Experiments in intact animals suggest that the enzyme in the adrenal cortex is under pituitary control (181). In cultured bovine adrenocortical cells, ACTH induces a marked increase both in the rate of synthesis of cytochrome P-450$_{17\alpha}$ protein and in the accumulation of translatable cytochrome P-450$_{17\alpha}$ mRNA. Dibutyryl cyclic AMP produces similar effects (188). Likewise, luteinizing hormone or 8-bromo-cyclic AMP induce cytochrome P-450$_{17\alpha}$ enzyme activity in primary cultures of mouse Leydig cells (189). The time course of cytochrome P-450$_{17\alpha}$ enzyme induction is relatively slow and resembles those for cytochrome P-450$_{scc}$ and cytochrome P-450$_{11\beta}$. This similarity in induction kinetics plus the similarity in hormone responsiveness suggests that a "steroid hydroxylase-inducing protein" (184) may also regulate the expression of the cytochrome P-450$_{17\alpha}$ gene. On the other hand, uninduced cells synthesize no detectable translatable cytochrome P-450$_{17\alpha}$ RNA, a finding that differs from those for the two mitochondrial cytochromes. This apparent lack of constitutive expression may reflect a regulatory difference between cytochrome P-450$_{17\alpha}$, on the one hand, and cytochrome P-450$_{scc}$ and cytochrome P-450$_{11\beta}$ on the other. A cDNA clone for cytochrome P-450$_{17\alpha}$ has recently been isolated (M. X. Zuber, personal communication). This will allow more detailed studies of cytochrome P-450$_{17\alpha}$ gene regulation in the future.

Cytochrome P-450$_{C21}$

This enzyme catalyzes the 21-hydroxylation of progestins, a step in the biosynthesis of glucocorticoids and mineralocorticoids. The enzyme is present in the adrenal cortex, but not in the gonads or placenta (176, 177). Hereditary deficiency of the enzyme is the most common cause of the syndrome of congenital adrenal hyperplasia (190). Studies in intact animals suggest that the enzyme is under pituitary control (181).

In the bovine adrenocortical cell system, ACTH induces after 24 hr about a 15-fold increase in the rate of cytochrome P-450$_{C21}$ synthesis, but only a 2- to 3-fold increase in the amount of translatable cytochrome P-450$_{C21}$ RNA (191). The reason(s) for this apparent discrepancy is not known. Cyclic AMP may mediate the cytochrome P-450$_{C21}$ induction response (192).

Two groups have isolated partial-length cDNA clones specific for bovine adrenal cytochrome P-450$_{C21}$ (193, 194). Using cDNA as a hybridization probe, White et al identified two cytochrome P-450$_{C21}$ genes in the vicinity of the H-2 major histocompatibility complex on chromosome 17 in the mouse (195). Similarly, two groups have found that the human cytochrome P-450$_{C21}$ gene maps within the HLA complex, adjacent to the locus encoding the C4A component of complement (196, 197). Two copies of the cytochrome P-450$_{C21}$ gene are present in the human genome. However, it is possible that only one copy is functional, since one form of congenital adrenal hyperplasia apparently results from the deletion of only one of the two genes (196). Furthermore, individuals who do not carry the other copy of the gene are, nevertheless, hormonally normal (197a).

Cytochrome P-450$_{aromatase}$

This enzyme catalyzes the aromatization of androgens in the pathway of estrogen biosynthesis. The biochemical properties of the enzyme have been studied primarily in the placenta; it has not yet been purified, and antibodies are not available. Therefore, conclusions about the regulation of the cytochrome P-450$_{aromatase}$ gene(s) must be inferred from measurements of enzyme activity. In rat granulosa cells, FSH (via formation of cyclic AMP) induces aromatase activity; the time course of induction is relatively long (176, 177, 198). By analogy with the regulation of other steroidogenic cytochromes P-450, the increased enzyme activity presumably reflects increased transcription of the cytochrome P-450$_{aromatase}$ gene.

Cytochrome P-450$_{aromatase}$ is present in many tissues including skin, muscle, fat, and nerve, where it may contribute to sex-specific differences in cellular metabolism (177, 198, 199). In particular, cytochrome P-450$_{aromatase}$ in certain regions of the brain may play an important role in the irreversible neonatal "imprinting" of sex-specific differences in cytochrome P-450-catalyzed enzyme activities in adult rat liver (199, 200) (see next section).

In summary, the data imply that each gene encoding a steroidogenic form of cytochrome P-450 is responsive to ACTH or FSH, depending upon the cell type. The hormonal signal is transduced from the plasma membrane to the nucleus via cAMP, which, in other systems, is known to activate the transcription of specific genes (201, 202). Because the accumulation of cytochrome P-450-specific mRNA requires ongoing protein synthesis, cAMP apparently does not stimulate cytochrome P-450 gene transcription directly; instead, it (presumably) activates the transcription of a gene(s) that encodes a hypothetical steroid hydroxylase-inducing protein (SHIP). The SHIP would then regulate transcription by binding to a specific *cis*-acting genomic control element for the appropriate cytochrome P-450 gene(s). In addition, (at least some of) the steroidogenic cytochrome P-450 genes exhibit tissue-specific expression. Because this phenomenon probably reflects control at the level of transcription (75, 76), each steroidogenic cytochrome P-450 gene presumably has a second regulatory component responsible for tissue-specific control.

SEXUAL DIMORPHISM IN CYTOCHROME P-450 GENE EXPRESSION

A variety of biochemical reactions in the liver exhibit sexual dimorphism (203). For example, gender influences the pattern of cytochrome P-450-catalyzed hepatic metabolism of some steroids and drugs (204, 205). The sex-related differences are substantial in the rat; however, in other species the differences may be less marked. The clinical importance of such differences in humans is not known. Studies of sex-dependent differences in the hepatic metabolism of steroids have revealed an interesting neuro-hepatic-endocrine axis in rats (206).

Testosterone 16α-hydroxylase of rats has been the most thoroughly studied hepatic cytochrome P-450-dependent enzyme activity that exhibits sex-dependent expression. Enzyme activity is high in males and is virtually absent in females (207). The same rat enzyme apparently has been purified by several groups, although each has given the enzyme a different name (71, 208–212). Harada & Negishi have purified an analogous cytochrome P-450 from mice (213) and have used a cDNA clone to show that the high enzyme activity in males is associated with a high hepatic content of the corresponding mRNA (214). Thus, the sex-related difference in testosterone 16α-hydroxylase activity presumably reflects different rates of transcription of the corresponding cytochrome P-450 gene. Cytochrome P-450$_{PCN}$ also exhibits high constitutive activity in male rats. These animals contain a high hepatic concentration of translatable cytochrome P-450$_{PCN}$ mRNA (174). However, the mechanism of the sex-dependent expression of the cytochrome P-450$_{PCN}$ gene has not been studied in detail.

MacGeoch et al (215) have studied the regulation of a cytochrome P-450 steroid 15β-hydroxylase that is present at a high level in the livers of female rats and is undetectable in males (210, 211). The evidence implies that the mechanisms governing the expression of this female-specific enzyme are similar to those regulating the male-specific testosterone 16α-hydroxylase, described below.

In rats, sex-related differences in drug and steroid metabolism do not appear until puberty. Furthermore, castration of post-pubertal males reduces some steroid-metabolizing enzyme activities to levels near those of females, an effect that is reversible by administration of testosterone (216, 217). These findings implicate circulating androgens in the maintenance of male-female differences in some cytochrome P-450-catalyzed enzyme activities. However, androgen administration fails to induce a male pattern of steroid metabolism in females that are castrated after puberty (216). Furthermore, the failure of females to respond to androgens apparently is not due to a lack of androgen receptors (218). These findings suggest that the mechanism by which androgens control sex-related differences in hepatic drug and steroid metabolism does not operate primarily at the level of the liver.

The male pattern of metabolism never develops in adult rats that are castrated at birth. However, a single administration of testosterone during the neonatal period reverses the effect of castration and allows the male pattern to develop at puberty (207, 217, 219–221). Similarly, a single dose of testosterone administered during the neonatal period to ovariectomized females establishes a male pattern of steroid metabolism (222). These observations imply that the presence of testosterone (or a metabolite) during a critical neonatal period irreversibly programs the animal to develop the male pattern of hepatic metabolism as an adult.

The mechanism by which this irreversible "imprinting" occurs apparently involves the pituitary and hypothalamus. Hypophysectomy, in females, establishes a male pattern of hepatic metabolism (223, 224) and, in males, abolishes the response to androgens (225). Implantation of a pituitary gland ectopically into hypophysectomized males or females produces a female pattern of metabolism (223, 225). In males, lesions in particular regions of the hypothalamus generate a female pattern of metabolism (226). These observations imply (a) that an intact pituitary is required to establish male-female differences in metabolism, (b) that the pituitary secretes a factor that produces a feminine pattern of metabolism, and (c) that, in males, the hypothalamus inhibits the pituitary-controlled development of a female pattern of metabolism. Presumably, an area in the supraoptic region of the hypothalamus (227) undergoes neonatal imprinting and programs the adult male pattern of metabolism. In cases of other imprinted sexual phenotypes, the evidence suggests that, during the critical neonatal period, cytochrome $P-450_{aromatase}$ in the hypothalamus converts testosterone (secreted by the developing testis) to estradiol, which mediates the imprinting action via an estrogen receptor-mediated mechanism (200). This may involve the altered growth and/or differentiation of specific neurons in the hypothalamus (228). However, the mechanism that governs the imprinting of hepatic cytochrome P-450-catalyzed enzyme activities may not be identical (229).

Imprinting in the hypothalamus apparently produces a sex-specific difference in the temporal pattern of growth hormone (GH) release by the pituitary. Males exhibit a more episodic pattern of GH secretion than do females (230). Continuous (as opposed to intermittent) infusion of GH into male rats markedly decreases the level of testosterone 16α-hydroxylase activity (231). Furthermore, GH is apparently the feminizing factor that is responsible for establishing the female pattern of hepatic steroid metabolism (232). Because two other hormones, growth hormone releasing factor and somatostatin, control the secretion of GH, imprinting may alter the development of cells that synthesize these hypothalamic hormones. Indeed, antibodies to somatostatin partially feminize the pattern of hepatic steroid metabolism in male rats (233).

The mechanism by which the episodic vs continuous release of GH may differentially alter the expression of specific genes is unknown. It is possible that some of the actions of GH are direct, whereas others are mediated secondarily by other effectors; in addition, the secretory rhythm may influence the sensitivity of the effector cell as a result of the up or down regulation of membrane receptors (234). The possible changes in chromatin structure and/or DNA modification (e.g. methylation) that might accompany the imprinting of cytochrome P-450 gene expression are unknown.

The data to date imply that a neuro-hepatic-endocrine axis programs the sexual dimorphism observed in the expression of (at least some of) the cytochrome P-450 genes that encode steroid-metabolizing enzymes. It is not yet clear whether the same regulatory axis controls the expression of other cytochrome P-450 genes, which encode drug-metabolizing enzymes. There is evidence for the gonadal and pituitary control of drug-metabolizing enzyme activities (reviewed in Ref. 206). However, at least some of these activities (eg. ethylmorphine N-demethylation) may be catalyzed by a steroid-metabolizing form(s) of cytochrome P-450 (18) that is already known to exhibit sexual dimorphism.

Finally, Faris & Campbell have made the provocative observation that neonatal exposure to phenobarbital, an inducer of some forms of cytochrome P-450, may irreversibly alter the pattern of cytochrome P-450-catalyzed enzyme activities in adult male rats (235, 236). The mechanism by which this apparent imprinting occurs, and whether it influences the susceptibility of the host to chemically induced toxicity or neoplasia, remains to be determined.

FUTURE PROSPECTS

Control of the transcription rate plays a major role in the regulation of phenobarbital-responsive and PAH-responsive cytochrome P-450 genes. Presumably, future experiments will show that the other cytochrome P-450 genes are also primarily under transcriptional control. Thus, studies of the selective modulation of cytochrome P-450 gene transcription in response to specific chemical signals should continue to be an interesting area of research in the future. The cytochromes P-450 offer a variety of experimental systems that should be useful in studying the mechanisms by which mammalian cells transduce extracellular chemical signals into alterations in the expression of specific genes. Experiments in yeast and *Drosophila* also may be productive, because these systems are particularly amenable to genetic manipulation.

The development of techniques that permit cells in culture to retain a differentiated phenotype (e.g. 237, 238) could make an important contribution to a better understanding of cytochrome P-450 gene expression (239–241). For example, many established cell lines respond poorly to phenobarbital. The availability of a phenobarbital-responsive cell line would simplify the functional analyses of putative phenobarbital-responsive genomic control elements. In addition, the selection of variant cells from such a phenobarbital-responsive cell line would allow genetic experiments to complement the biochemical studies of cytochrome P-450 gene regulation. Similarly, the availability of appropriately responsive cell lines should facilitate analyses of the mechanisms by which other cytochrome P-450 genes are regulated.

The contribution that chromatin structure makes to the control of cytochrome P-450 gene expression is virtually unknown; this may be a potentially fruitful area for future research. Changes in chromatin structure may be particularly important in the imprinting and tissue-specific expression of cytochrome P-450 genes. Differences in nuclease sensitivity may be useful in identifying genomic regions potentially involved in transcriptional regulation. Isolation of cytochrome P-450 genes in minichromosome form may facilitate the study of protein-DNA interactions in the cytochrome P-450 genes and might be a prerequisite for establishing studies of regulated transcription in vitro.

The techniques of mutagenesis and gene transfer have the potential to reveal functional aspects of *cis*-acting genomic elements involved in the control of cytochrome P-450 gene transcription. The structural and functional analyses of such elements should provide insights into the mechanisms of signal transduction from the extracellular environment to the genome. Presumably, both stimulatory and inhibitory genomic control elements exist. Whether they can function relatively independently of each other, whether their effects are synergistic, additive, or antagonistic when several elements are linked, whether its position in a hierarchy influences the function of an element, and whether other position or orientation effects occur are interesting problems for the future. Similarly, the structures of the binding sites for *trans*-acting regulatory factors remain to be determined.

The properties of the *trans*-acting regulators that interact with the genomic control elements remain largely unknown. First of all, a number of hypothetical regulatory factors have not been characterized at the biochemical level at all (e.g. tissue-specific regulators, phenobarbital receptors, cycloheximide-sensitive repressors, etc). Even for *Ah* receptors, little is known of possible functional domains (e.g. inducer binding, chromatin binding), subunit structure, and overall receptor heterogeneity. In addition, the receptor-mediated, temperature-dependent step in enzyme induction remains to be analyzed. The isolation and characterization of additional regulatory variants, and attempts to complement defective variants using gene transfer methodology, may be productive experimental approaches for studying these regulatory factors in the future. The general question of how the binding of a regulatory factor to its cognate control element results in the modulation of gene transcription will not be easy to answer. However, the various cytochrome P-450 genes, with their selective responsiveness to different chemical stimuli, comprise an experimental system with unusual potential for addressing this question in the future.

Finally, the chaotic cytochrome P-450 nomenclature that has evolved over the past 20 years is unusually complicated and confusing. Future agreement on a coherent terminology (if possible) would increase everyone's understanding and appreciation of this interesting and important class of enzymes.

ACKNOWLEDGMENTS

I thank numerous colleagues for the sharing of information, fruitful discussion, and constructive criticism. I thank Karen Benight for expert secretarial assistance. The work in my laboratory has been supported by grants from the American Cancer Society and the National Institutes of Health.

Literature Cited

1. Klingenberg, M. 1958. Pigments of rat liver microsomes. *Arch. Biochem. Biophys.* 75:376–86
2. Garfinkel, D. 1958. Studies on pig liver microsomes. 1. Enzymic and pigment composition of different microsomal fractions. *Arch. Biochem. Biophys.* 77:493–509
3. Omura, T., Sato, R. 1962. A new cytochrome in liver microsomes. *J. Biol. Chem.* 237:1375–76
4. Omura, T., Sato, R. 1964. The carbon monoxide-binding pigment of liver microsomes. 1. Evidence for its hemoprotein nature. *J. Biol. Chem.* 239:2370–78
5. Omura, T., Sato, R. 1964. The carbon monoxide-binding pigment of liver microsomes. 2. Solubilization, purification, and properties. *J. Biol. Chem.* 239:2379–85
6. White, R. E., Coon, M. J. 1980. Oxygen activation by cytochrome P-450. *Ann. Rev. Biochem.* 49:315–56
7. Nebert, D. W., Eisen, H. J., Negishi, M., Lang, M. A., Hjelmeland, L. M., Okey, A. B. 1981. Genetic mechanisms controlling the induction of polysubstrate monooxygenase (P-450) activities. *Ann. Rev. Pharmacol. Toxicol.* 21:431–62
8. Ortiz de Montellano, P. R., Correia, M. A. 1983. Suicidal destruction of cytochrome P-450 during oxidative drug metabolism. *Ann. Rev. Pharmacol. Toxicol.* 23:481–503
9. Terriere, L. C. 1984. Induction of detoxification enzymes in insects. *Ann. Rev. Entomol.* 29:71–88
10. Sato, R., Omura, T., eds. 1978. *Cytochrome P-450.* New York: Academic. 233 pp.
11. Gunsalus, I. C., Sligar, S. G. 1978. Oxygen reduction by the P-450 monooxygenase systems. *Adv. Enzymol.* 47:1–44
12. Lu, A. Y. H., West, S. B. 1979. Multiplicity of mammalian microsomal cytochromes P-450. *Pharmacol. Rev.* 31:277–95

13. Waterman, M. R., Estabrook, R. W. 1983. The induction of microsomal electron transport enzymes. *Mol. Cell. Biochem.* 53/54:267–78

14. Adesnik, M., Atchison, M. 1985. Genes for cytochrome P-450 and their regulation. *CRC Crit. Rev. Biochem.* In press

15. Remmer, H. 1961. Drug tolerance. In *CIBA Foundation Symposium on Enzymes and Drug Action*, ed. J. L. Mongar, A. V. S. de Reuck, pp. 276–98. London: Churchill

16. Conney, A. H., Burns, J. J. 1959. Stimulatory effect of foreign compounds on ascorbic acid biosynthesis and on drug-metabolizing enzymes. *Nature* 184:363–64

17. Cooper, D. Y., Levin, S. S., Narasimhulu, S., Rosenthal, O., Estabrook, R. W. 1965. Photochemical action spectrum of the terminal oxidase of mixed-function oxidase systems. *Science* 147:400–2

18. Guengerich, F. P., Dannan, G. A., Wright, S. T., Martin, M. V., Kaminsky, L. S. 1982. Purification and characterization of liver microsomal cytochromes P-450: Electrophoretic, spectral, catalytic, and immunochemical properties and inducibility of eight isozymes isolated from rats treated with phenobarbital or β-naphthoflavone. *Biochemistry* 21:6019–30

19. Waxman, D. J., Walsh, C. 1982. Phenobarbital-induced rat liver cytochrome P-450. Purification and characterization of two closely related isozymic forms. *J. Biol. Chem.* 257:10446–57

20. Waxman, D. J., Ko, A., Walsh, C. 1983. Regioselectivity and stereoselectivity of androgen hydroxylations catalyzed by cytochrome P-450 isozymes purified from phenobarbital-induced rat liver. *J. Biol. Chem.* 258:11937–47

21. Ryan, D. E., Iida, S., Wood, A. W., Thomas, P. E., Lieber, C. S., Levin, W. 1984. Characterization of three highly purified cytochromes P-450 from hepatic microsomes of adult male rats. *J. Biol. Chem.* 259:1239–50

22. Haugen, D. A., van der Hoeven, T. A., Coon, M. J. 1975. Purified liver microsomal cytochrome P-450. Separation and characterization of multiple forms. *J. Biol. Chem.* 250:3567–70

23. Ryan, D. E., Thomas, P. E., Korzeniowski, D., Levin, W. 1979. Separation and characterization of highly purified forms of liver microsomal cytochrome P-450 from rats treated with polychlorinated biphenyls, phenobarbital, and 3-

methylcholanthrene. *J. Biol. Chem.* 254:1365–74

24. Botelho, L. H., Ryan, D. E., Levin, W. 1979. Amino acid compositions and partial amino acid sequences of three highly purified forms of liver microsomal cytochrome P-450 from rats treated with polychlorinated biphenyls, phenobarbital, or 3-methylcholanthrene. *J. Biol. Chem.* 254:5635–40

25. Vlasuk, G. P., Ghraybs, J., Ryan, D. E., Reik, L., Thomas, P. E., et al. 1982. Multiplicity, strain differences, and topology of phenobarbital-induced cytochromes P-450 in rat liver microsomes. *Biochemistry* 21:789–98

26. Rampersaud, A., Walz, F. G. Jr. 1983. At least six forms of extremely homologous cytochromes P-450 in rat liver are encoded at two closely linked genetic loci. *Proc. Natl. Acad. Sci. USA* 80:6542–46

27. Kumar, A., Raphael, C., Adesnik, M. 1983. Cloned cytochrome P-450 cDNA. Nucleotide sequence and homology to multiple phenobarbital-induced mRNA species. *J. Biol. Chem.* 258:11280–84

28. Fujii-Kuriyama, Y., Mizukami, Y., Kawajiri, K., Sogawa, K., Muramatsu, M. 1982. Primary structure of a cytochrome P-450: Coding nucleotide sequence of phenobarbital-inducible cytochrome P-450 cDNA from rat liver. *Proc. Natl. Acad. Sci. USA* 79:2793–97

29. Mizukami, Y., Fujii-Kuriyama, Y., Muramatsu, M. 1983. Multiplicity of deoxyribonucleic acid coding for rat phenobarbital-inducible cytochrome P-450. *Biochemistry* 22:1223–29

30. Atchison, M., Adesnik, M. 1983. A cytochrome P-450 multigene family. Characterization of a gene activated by phenobarbital administration. *J. Biol. Chem.* 258:11285–95

31. Simmons, D. L., Kasper, C. B. 1983. Genetic polymorphisms for a phenobarbital-inducible cytochrome P-450 map to the *Coh* locus in mice. *J. Biol. Chem.* 258:9585–88

32. Simmons, D. L., Lalley, P. A., Kasper, C. B. 1985. Chromosomal assignments of genes coding for components of the mixed-function oxidase system in mice. *J. Biol. Chem.* 260:515–21

33. Leighton, J. K., DeBrunner-Vossbrinck, B. A., Kemper, B. 1984. Isolation and sequence analysis of three cloned cDNAs for rabbit liver proteins that are related to rabbit cytochrome P-450 (form 2), the major phenobarbital-inducible form. *Biochemistry* 23:204–10

34. Phillips, I. R., Shephard, E. A., Ash-

worth, A., Rabin, B. R. 1985. Isolation and sequences of a human cytochrome P-450 cDNA clone. *Proc. Natl. Acad. Sci. USA* 82:983–87

35. Tukey, R. H., Okino, S. T., Barnes, H. J., Griffin, K. J., Johnson, E. F. 1985. Multiple gene-like sequences related to the rabbit hepatic progesterone 21-hydroxylase cytochrome P-450 1. *J. Biol. Chem.* 260: In press

36. Ozols, J., Heinemann, F. S., Johnson, E. F. 1985. The complete amino acid sequence of a constitutive form of liver microsomal cytochrome P-450. *J. Biol. Chem.* 260:5427–34

37. Leighton, J. K., Kemper, B. 1984. Differential induction and tissue-specific expression of closely related members of the phenobarbital-inducible rabbit cytochrome P-450 gene family. *J. Biol. Chem.* 259:11165–68

38. Wood, A. W., Taylor, B. 1979. Genetic regulation of coumarin hydroxylase activity in mice. Evidence for single locus control on chromosome 7. *J. Biol. Chem.* 254:5647–51

39. Phillips, I. R., Shephard, E. A., Povey, S., Davis, M. B., Kelsey, G., et al. 1985. A cytochrome P-450 gene family mapped to human chromosome 19. *Ann. Hum. Genet.* 49: In press

40. Mizukami, Y., Sogawa, K., Suwa, Y., Muramatsu, M., Fujii-Kuriyama, Y. 1983. Gene structure of a phenobarbital-inducible cytochrome P-450 in rat liver. *Proc. Natl. Acad. Sci. USA* 80:3958–62

41. Bhat, K. S., Padmanabau, G. 1980. Studies on the synthesis of cytochrome P-450 and cytochrome P-448 in rat liver. *J. Biol. Chem.* 255:522–25

42. DuBois, R. N., Waterman, M. R. 1979. Effect of phenobarbital administration to rats on the level of the *in vitro* synthesis of cytochrome P-450 directed by total rat liver RNA. *Biochem. Biophys. Res. Commun.* 90:150–57

43. Colbert, R. A., Bresnick, E., Levin, W., Ryan, D. E., Thomas, P. E. 1979. Synthesis of liver cytochrome P-450b in a cell-free protein synthesizing system. *Biochem. Biophys. Res. Commun.* 91: 886–91

44. Bar-Nun, S., Kreibich, G., Adesnik, M., Alterman, L., Negishi, M., Sabatini, D. D. 1980. Synthesis and insertion of cytochrome P-450 into endoplasmic reticulum membranes. *Proc. Natl. Acad. Sci. USA* 77:965–69

45. Phillips, I. R., Shephard, E. A., Mitani, F., Rabin, B. R. 1981. Induction by phenobarbital of the mRNA for a specific variant of rat liver microsomal cyto-chrome P-450. *Biochem. J.* 196:839–51

46. Adesnik, M., Bar-Nun, S., Maschio, F., Zunich, M., Lippman, A., Bard, E. 1981. Mechanism of induction of cytochrome P-450 by phenobarbital. *J. Biol. Chem.* 256:10340–45

47. Gonzalez, F. J., Kasper, C. B. 1982. Cloning of DNA complementary to rat liver NADPH-cytochrome c (P-450) oxidoreductase and cytochrome P-450b mRNAs. *J. Biol. Chem.* 257:5962–68

48. Shephard, E. A., Phillips, I. R., Pike, S. F., Ashworth, A., Rabin, B. R. 1982. Differential effect of phenobarbital and β-naphthoflavone on the mRNAs coding for cytochrome P-450 and NADPH cytochrome P-450 reductase. *FEBS Lett.* 150:375–80

49. Phillips, I. R., Shephard, E. A., Ashworth, A., Rabin, B. R. 1983. Cloning and sequence analysis of a rat liver cDNA coding for a phenobarbital-inducible microheterogeneous cytochrome P-450 variant: Regulation of its messenger level by xenobiotics. *Gene* 24:41–52

50. Morohashi, K., Yoshioka, H., Sogawa, K., Fujii-Kuriyama, Y., Omura, T. 1984. Induction of mRNA coding for phenobarbital-inducible form of microsomal cytochrome P-450 in rat liver by administration of 1,1-di(p-chorophenyl)-2,2-dichloroethylene and phenobarbital. *J. Biochem.* 95:949–57

51. Stupans, I., Ikeda, T., Kessler, D. J., Nebert, D. W. 1984. Characterization of a cDNA clone for mouse phenobarbital-inducible cytochrome P-450b. *DNA* 3: 129–37

52. Ravishankar, H., Padmanaban, G. 1985. Regulation of cytochrome P-450 gene expression. Studies with a cloned probe. *J. Biol. Chem.* 260:1588–92

53. Omiecinski, C. J., Walz, F. G. Jr., Vlasuk, G. P. 1985. Phenobarbital induction of rat liver cytochromes P-450b and P-450e. Quantitation of specific RNAs by hybridization to synthetic oligodeoxyribonucleotide probes. *J. Biol. Chem.* 260:3247–50

54. Adesnik, M., Rivkin, E., Kumar, A., Lippman, A., Raphael, C., Atchison, M. 1982. Genes for cytochrome P-450 and their regulation. In *Cytochrome P-450, Biochemistry, Biophysics, and Environmental Implications,* ed. E. Hietanen, M. Laitinen, O. Hanninen, pp. 143–48. New York: Elsevier

55. Hardwick, J. P., Gonzalez, F. J., Kasper, C. B. 1983. Transcriptional regulation of rat liver epoxide hydratase,

NADPH-cytochrome P-450 oxidoreductase, and cytochrome P-450b genes by phenobarbital. *J. Biol. Chem.* 258:8081–85

56. Pike, S. F., Shephard, E. A., Rabin, B. R., Phillips, I. R. 1985. Induction of cytochrome P-450 by phenobarbital is mediated at the level of transcription. *Biochem. Pharmacol.* 34:2489–94

57. Thomas, P. E., Reik, L. M., Ryan, D. E., Levin, W. 1981. Regulation of three forms of cytochrome P-450 and epoxide hydrolase in rat liver microsomes. *J. Biol. Chem.* 256:1044–52

58. Ringold, G. M. 1985. Steroid hormone regulation of gene expression. *Ann. Rev. Pharmacol. Toxicol.* 25:529–66

59. Snyder, R., Remmer, H. 1979. Classes of hepatic microsomal mixed function oxidase inducers. *Pharmacol. Ther.* 7:203–44

60. Poland, A., Mak, I., Glover, E., Boatman, R. J., Ebetino, F. H., Kende, A. S. 1980. 1,4-Bis[2-(3,5-dichloropyridyloxy)]benzene, a potent phenobarbital-like inducer of microsomal monooxygenase activity. *Mol. Pharmacol.* 18:571–80

61. Poland, A., Mak, I., Glover, E. 1981. Species differences in responsiveness to 1,4 - bis[2 - (3,5 - dichloropyridyloxy)]-benzene, a potent phenobarbital-like inducer of microsomal monooxygenase activity. *Mol. Pharmacol.* 20:442–50

62. Elgin, S. C. R. 1984. Anatomy of hypersensitive sites. *Nature* 309:213–14

63. Deitrich, R. A. 1971. Genetic aspects of increase in rat liver aldehyde dehydrogenase induced by phenobarbital. *Science* 173:334–36

64. Deitrich, R. A., Collins, A. C., Erwin, V. G. 1972. Genetic influence upon phenobarbital-induced increase in rat liver supernatant aldehyde dehydrogenase activity. *J. Biol. Chem.* 247:7232–36

65. Timms, G. P., Holmes, R. S. 1981. Genetics and ontogeny of aldehyde dehydrogenase isozymes in the mouse: Evidence for a locus controlling inducibility. *Biochem. Genet.* 19:1223–36

66. Ravishankar, H., Padmanaban, G. 1983. Effect of cobalt chloride and 3-amino-1,2,4-triazole on the induction of cytochrome P-450 synthesis by phenobarbitone in rat liver. *Arch. Biochem. Biophys.* 225:16–24

67. Guzelian, P. S., Diegelmann, R. F., Lamb, R. G., Fallon, H. J. 1979. Effects of hormones on changes in cytochrome P-450, prolyl hydroxylase, and glycerol phosphate acyltransferase in primary monolayer cultures of parenchymal cells from adult rat liver. *Yale J. Biol. Med.* 52:5–12

68. Guarente, L., Mason, T. 1983. Heme regulates transcription of the *CYC* gene of *S. cervisiae* via an upstream activation site. *Cell* 32:1279–86

69. Guarente, L., Lalonde, B., Gifford, P., Alani, E. 1984. Distinctly regulated tandem upstream activation sites mediate catabolite repression of the *CYC* gene of *S. cervisiae*. *Cell* 36:503–11

70. Dannan, G. A., Guengerich, F. P., Kaminsky, L. S., Aust, S. D. 1983. Regulation of cytochrome P-450. Immunochemical quantitation of eight isozymes in liver microsomes of rats treated with polybrominated biphenyl congeners. *J. Biol. Chem.* 258:1282–88

71. Waxman, D. J. 1984. Rat hepatic cytochrome P-450 isoenzyme 2c. Identification as a male-specific, developmentally-induced steroid 16α-hydroxylase and comparison to a female-specific cytochrome P-450 isoenzyme. *J. Biol. Chem.* 259:15481–90

72. Serabjit-Singh, C. J., Albro, P. W., Robertson, I. G. C., Philpot, R. M. 1983. Interactions between xenobiotics that increase or decrease the levels of cytochrome P-450 isozymes in rabbit lung and liver. *J. Biol. Chem.* 258:12827–34

73. Serabjit-Singh, C. J., Wolf, C. R., Philpot, R. M. 1979. The rabbit pulmonary monooxygenase system. Immunochemical and biochemical characterization of enzyme components. *J. Biol. Chem.* 254:9901–7

74. Dees, J. H., Masters, B. S. S., Muller-Eberhard, U., Johnson, E. F. 1982. Effect of 2,3,7,8-tetrachlorodibenzo-p-dioxin and phenobarbital on the occurrence and distribution of four cytochrome P-450 isozymes in rabbit kidney, lung, and liver. *Cancer Res.* 42:1423–32

75. Derman, E., Krauter, K., Walling, L., Weniberger, C., Ray, M., Darnell, J. E. Jr. 1981. Transcriptional control in the production of liver specific mRNAs. *Cell* 23:731–39

76. Killary, A. M., Fournier, R. E. K. 1984. A genetic analysis of extinction: Trans-dominant loci regulate expression of liver-specific traits in hepatoma hybrid cells. *Cell* 38:523–34

77. Brown, R. R., Miller, J. A., Miller, E. G. 1954. The metabolism of methylated aminoazo dyes. 4. Dietary factors enhancing demethylation *in vitro*. *J. Biol. Chem.* 209:211–22

78. Conney, A. H., Miller, E. C., Miller, J.

A. 1956. The metabolism of methylated aminoazo dyes. 5. Evidence for induction of enzyme synthesis in the rat by 3-methylcholanthrene. *Cancer Res.* 16: 450–59

79. Miller, J. A. 1970. Carcinogenesis by chemicals: an overview. G. H. A. Clowes Memorial Lecture. *Cancer Res.* 30:559–76

80. Gelboin, H. V. 1980. Benzo(a)pyrene metabolism, activation, and carcinogenesis: Role and regulation of mixed-function oxidases and related enzymes. *Physiol. Rev.* 60:1107–66

81. Conney, A. H. 1982. Induction of microsomal enzymes by foreign chemicals and carcinogenesis by polycyclic aromatic hydrocarbons: G. H. A. Clowes Memorial Lecture. *Cancer Res.* 42:4875–4917

82. Ryan, D. E., Thomas, P. E., Levin, W. 1980. Hepatic microsomal cytochrome P-450 from rats treated with isosafrole. *J. Biol. Chem.* 255:7941–55

83. Reik, L. M., Levin, W., Ryan, D. E., Thomas, P. E. 1982. Immunochemical relatedness of rat hepatic microsomal cytochromes P-450c and P-450d. *J. Biol. Chem.* 257:3950–57

84. Botelho, L. H., Ryan, D. E., Yuan, P. M., Kutney, R., Shively, J. E., Levin, W. 1982. Amino-terminal and carboxy-terminal sequence of hepatic microsomal cytochrome P-450d, a unique hemoprotein from rats treated with isosafrole. *Biochemistry* 21:1152–55

85. Thomas, P. E., Reik, L. M., Ryan, D. E., Levin, W. 1983. Induction of two immunochemically related rat liver cytochrome P-450 isozymes, cytochromes P-450c and P-450d, by structurally diverse xenobiotics. *J. Biol. Chem.* 258:4590–98

86. Johnson, E. F., Muller-Eberhard, U. 1977. Resolution of two forms of cytochrome P-450 from liver microsomes of rabbits treated with 2,3,7,8-tetrachlorodibenzo-p-dioxin. *J. Biol. Chem.* 252:2839–45

87. Negishi, M., Nebert, D. W. 1979. Structural gene products of the *Ah* locus: Genetic and immunochemical evidence for two forms of mouse liver cytochrome P-450 induced by 3-methylcholanthrene. *J. Biol. Chem.* 254:11015–23

88. Okino, S. T., Quattrochi, L. C., Barnes, H. J., Osanto, S., Griffin, K. J., et al. 1985. Cloning and characterization of cDNAs encoding 2,3,7,8-tetrachlorodibenzo-p-dioxin-mRNAs for cytochrome P-450 isozymes 4 and 6. *Proc. Natl. Sci. USA* 82:5310–14

89. Ohyama, T., Nebert, D. W., Negishi,

M. 1984. Isosafrole-induced cytochrome P₂-450 in DBA/2N mouse liver: Characterization and genetic control of induction. *J. Biol. Chem.* 259:2675–82

90. Ikeda, T., Altievi, M., Chen, Y. T., Nakamura, M., Tukey, R. H., et al. 1983. Characterization of cytochrome P₂-450 (20S) mRNA, association with the P₁-450 genomic gene and differential response to the inducers 3-methylcholanthrene and isosafrole. *Eur. J. Biochem.* 134:13–18

91. Tukey, R. H., Nebert, D. W. 1984. Regulation of mouse cytochrome P₃-450 by the *Ah* receptor. Studies with a P₃-450 cDNA clone. *Biochemistry* 23:6003–8

92. Bresnick, E., Levy, J., Hines, R., Levin, W., Thomas, P. E. 1981. The molecular cloning of cytochrome P-450c information. *Arch. Biochem. Biophys.* 212:501–7

93. Negishi, M., Swan, D. C., Enquist, L. W., Nebert, D. W. 1981. Isolation and characterization of a cloned DNA sequence associated with the murine *Ah* locus and 3-methylcholanthrene-induced form of cytochrome P-450. *Proc. Natl. Acad. Sci. USA* 78:800–4

94. Fagan, J. B., Pastewka, J. V., Park, S. S., Guengerich, F. P., Gelboin, H. V. 1982. Identification and quantitation of a 2.0-kilobase messenger ribonucleic acid coding for 3-methylcholanthrene-induced cytochrome P-450 using cloned cytochrome P-450 complementary deoxyribonucleic acid. *Biochemistry* 21: 6574–80

95. Kawajiri, K., Sogawa, K., Gotch, O., Tagashira, Y., Muramatsu, M., Fujii-Kuriyama, Y. 1983. Molecular cloning of a complementary DNA to 3-methylcholanthrene-inducible cytochrome P-450 mRNA from rat liver. *J. Biochem.* 94:1465–73

96. Yabusaki, Y., Shimizu, M., Murakami, H., Nakamura, K., Oeda, K., Ohkawa, H. 1984. Nucleotide sequence of a full-length cDNA coding for 3-methylcholanthrene-induced rat liver cytochrome P-450MC. *Nucleic Acids Res.* 12:2929–38

97. Yabusaki, Y., Murakami, H., Nakamura, K., Nomura, N., Shimizu, M., et al. 1984. Characterization of complementary DNA clones coding for two forms of 3-methylcholanthrene-inducible rat liver cytochrome P-450. *J. Biochem.* 96:793–804

98. Kawajiri, K., Gotoh, O., Sogawa, K., Tagashira, Y., Muramatsu, M., Fujii-Kuriyama, Y. 1984. Coding nucleotide sequence of 3-methylcholanthrene-in-

ducible cytochrome P-450d cDNA from rat liver. *Proc. Natl. Acad. Sci. USA* 81:1649–53

99. Gonzalez, F. J., Mackenzie, P. I., Kimura, S., Nebert, D. W. 1984. Isolation and characterization of full-length mouse cDNA and genomic clones of 3-methylcholanthrene-inducible cytochrome P₁-450 and P₃-450. *Gene* 29:281–92

100. Kimura, S., Gonzalez, F. J., Nebert, D. W. 1984. Mouse cytochrome P₃-450: Complete cDNA and amino acid sequence. *Nucleic Acids Res.* 12:2917–28

101. Kimura, S., Gonzalez, F. J., Nebert, D. W. 1984. The murine *Ah* locus. Comparison of the complete cytochrome P₁-450 and P₃-450 cDNA nucleotide and amino acid sequences. *J. Biol. Chem.* 259:10705–13

102. Jaiswal, A. K., Gonzalez, F. J., Nebert, D. W. 1985. Human dioxin-inducible cytochrome P₁-450: Complementary DNA and amino acid sequence. *Science* 228:80–83

103. Sogawa, K., Gotoh, O., Kawajiri, K., Harada, T., Fujii-Kuriyama, Y. 1985. Complete nucleotide sequence of a methylcholanthrene-inducible cytochrome P-450 (P-450d) gene in the rat. *J. Biol. Chem.* 260:5026–32

104. Sogawa, K., Gotoh, O., Kawajari, K., Fujii-Kuriyama, Y. 1984. Distinct organization of methylcholanthrene- and phenobarbital-inducible cytochrome P-450 genes in the rat. *Proc. Natl. Acad. Sci. USA* 81:5066–70

105. Hines, R. N., Levy, J. B., Conrad, R. D., Iverson, P. L., Shen, M. L., et al. 1985. Gene structure and nucleotide sequence for rat cytochrome P-450c. *Arch. Biochem. Biophys.* 237:465–76

106. Gonzalez, F. J., Kimura, S., Nebert, D. W. 1985. Comparison of the flanking regions and introns of the mouse 2,3,7,-8-tetrachloro-p-dioxin-inducible cytochrome P₁-450 and P₃-450 genes. *J. Biol. Chem.* 260:5040–49

107. Tukey, R. H., Lalley, P. A., Nebert, D. W. 1984. Localization of cytochrome P₁-450 and P₃-450 genes to mouse chromosome 9. *Proc. Natl. Acad. Sci. USA* 81:3163–66

108. Hildebrand, C. E., Gonzalez, F. J., McBride, O. W., Nebert, D. W. 1985. Assignment of the human 2,3,7,8-tetrachlorodibenzo - p - dioxin - inducible cytochrome P₁-450 gene to chromosome 15. *Nucleic Acids. Res.* 13:2009–16

109. Bresnick, E., Brosseau, M., Levin, W., Reik, L., Ryan, D. E., Thomas, P. E.

1981. Administration of 3-methylcholanthrene to rats increases the specific hybridizable mRNA coding for cytochrome P-450c. *Proc. Natl. Acad. Sci. USA* 78:4083–87

110. Pickett, C. B., Talakowski-Hopins, C. A., Donohue, A. M., Lu, A. Y. H., Hales, B. F. 1982. Differential induction of rat hepatic cytochrome P-448 and glutathione S-transferase B messenger RNAs by 3-methylcholanthrene. *Biochem. Biophys. Res. Commun.* 104:611–19

111. Morville, A. L., Thomas, P., Levin, W., Reik, L., Ryan, D. E., et al. 1983. The accumulation of mRNAs for the immunochemically related cytochromes P-450c and P-450d in rat liver following 3-methylcholanthrene treatment. *J. Biol. Chem.* 258:3901–6

112. Gozukara, E. M., Fagan, J., Pastewka, J. V., Guengerich, F. P., Gelboin, H. V. 1984. Induction of cytochrome P-450 mRNAs quantitated by *in vitro* translation and immunoprecipitation. *Arch. Biochem. Biophys.* 232:660–69

113. Kawajiri, K., Gotoh, O., Tagashira, Y., Sogawa, K., Fujii-Kuriyama, Y. 1984. Titration of mRNAs for cytochrome P-450c and P-450d under drug-inductive conditions in rat livers by their specific probes of cloned DNAs. *J. Biol. Chem.* 259:10145–49

114. Hardwick, J. P., Linko, P., Goldstein, J. A. 1985. Dose response for induction of two cytochrome P-450 isozymes and their mRNAs by 3,4,5,3',4',5'-hexachlorobiphenyl indicating coordinate regulation in rat liver. *Mol. Pharmacol.* 27:676–82

115. Negishi, M., Nebert, D. W. 1981. Structural gene products of the *Ah* complex. Increases in large mRNAs from mouse liver associated with cytochrome P₁-450 induction by 3-methylcholanthrene. *J. Biol. Chem.* 256:3085–91

116. Tukey, R. H., Nebert, D. W., Negishi, M. 1981. Structural gene product of the [Ah] complex. Evidence for transcriptional control of cytochrome P₁-450 induction by use of a cloned DNA sequence. *J. Biol. Chem.* 256:6969–74

117. Tukey, R. H., Negishi, M., Nebert, D. W. 1982. Quantitation of cytochrome P₁-450 mRNA with the use of a cloned DNA probe: Effects of various inducers in C57BL/6N and DBA/2N mice. *Mol. Pharmacol.* 22:779–86

118. Tukey, R. H., Hannah, R. R., Negishi, M., Nebert, D. W., Eisen, H. J. 1982. The *Ah* locus: Correlation of intranuclear appearance of inducer-receptor complex

with induction of cytochrome P_1-450 mRNA. *Cell* 31:275–84

119. Gonzalez, F. J., Tukey, R. H., Nebert, D. W. 1984. Structural gene products of the *Ah* locus. Transcriptional regulation of cytochrome P_1-450 and P_3-450 mRNA levels by 3-methylcholanthrene. *Mol. Pharmacol.* 26:117–21

120. Israel, D. I., Whitlock, J. P. Jr. 1983. Induction of mRNA specific for cytochrome P_1-450 in wild type and variant mouse hepatoma cells. *J. Biol. Chem.* 258:10390–94

121. Israel, D. I., Whitlock, J. P. Jr. 1984. Regulation of cytochrome P_1-450 gene transcription by 2,3,7,8-tetrachlorodibenzo-p-dioxin in wild type and variant mouse hepatoma cells. *J. Biol. Chem.* 259:5400–2

122. Cook, J. C., Hodgson, E. 1985. The induction of cytochrome P-450 by isosafrole and related methylenedioxyphenyl compounds. *Chem. Biol. Interact.* In press

123. Schmid, F. A., Elmer, I., Tarnowski, G. S. 1969. Genetic determination of differential inflammatory reactivity and subcutaneous tumor susceptibility of AKR/J and C57BL/6J mice to 7,12-dimethylbenz(a)anthracene. *Cancer Res.* 29:1585–89

124. Nebert, D. W., Gelboin, H. V. 1969. The *in vivo* and *in vitro* induction of aryl hydrocarbon hydroxylase in mammalian cells of different species, tissues, strains, and developmental and hormonal states. *Arch. Biochem. Biophys.* 134:76–89

125. Nebert, D. W., Bausserman, L. L. 1970. Genetic differences in the extent of aryl hydrocarbon hydroxylase induction in mouse fetal cell cultures. *J. Biol. Chem.* 245:6373–82

126. Kodama, Y., Bock, F. G. 1970. Benzo(a)pyrene metabolizing activity of livers of various strains of mice. *Cancer Res.* 30:1846–49

127. Nebert, D. W., Goujon, F. M., Gielen, J. E. 1972. Aryl hydrocarbon hydroxylase induction by polycyclic hydrocarbons: Simple autosomal dominant trait in the mouse. *Nature New Biol.* 236:107–10

128. Thomas, P. E., Kouri, R. E., Hutton, J. J. 1972. The genetics of aryl hydrocarbon hydroxylase induction in mice: A single gene difference between C57BL/6J and DBA/2J. *Biochem. Genet.* 6:157–68

129. Nebert, D. W., Jensen, N. M. 1979. The *Ah* locus: Genetic regulation of the metabolism of carcinogens, drugs, and other environmental chemicals by cytochrome P-450-mediated monooxy-

genases. *CRC Crit. Rev. Biochem.* 6:401–37

130. Poland, A. P., Glover, E., Robinson, J. R., Nebert, D. W. 1974. Genetic expression of aryl hydrocarbon hydroxylase activity. Induction of monooxygenase activities and cytochrome P_1-450 formation by 2,3,7,8-tetrachlorodibenzo-p-dioxin in mice genetically "nonresponsive" to other aromatic hydrocarbons. *J. Biol. Chem.* 249:5599–5606

131. Poland, A., Glover, E. 1975. Genetic expression of aryl hydrocarbon hydroxylase by 2,3,7,8-tetrachlorodibenzo-p-dioxin: evidence for a receptor mutation in genetically non-responsive mice. *Mol. Pharmacol.* 11:389–98

132. Poland, A. P., Glover, E., Kende, A. S. 1976. Stereospecific, high affinity binding of 2,3,7,8-tetrachlorodibenzo-p-dioxin by hepatic cytosol: Evidence that the binding species is the receptor for the induction of aryl hydrocarbon hydroxylase. *J. Biol. Chem.* 251:4936–46

133. Hannah, R. R., Nebert, D. W., Eisen, H. J. 1981. Regulatory gene product of the *Ah* complex. Comparison of 2,3,7,8-tetrachlorodibenzo-p-dioxin and 3-methylcholanthrene binding to several moieties in mouse liver cytosol. *J. Biol. Chem.* 256:4584–90

134. Greenlee, W. F., Neal, R. A. 1985. The *Ah* receptor: A biochemical and biological perspective. In *The Receptors*, ed. M. Conn, 2:89–129. New York: Academic. In press

135. Greenlee, W. F., Poland, A. 1979. Nuclear uptake of 2,3,7,8-tetrachlorodibenzo-p-dioxin in C57BL/6J and DBA/2J mice. Role of the hepatic cytosol receptor protein. *J. Biol. Chem.* 254:9814–21

136. Okey, A. B., Bondy, G. P., Mason, M. E., Kahl, G. F., Eisen, H. J., et al. 1979. Regulatory gene product of the *Ah* locus. Characterization of the cytosolic inducer-receptor complex and evidence for its nuclear translocation. *J. Biol. Chem.* 254:11636–48

137. Okey, A. B., Bondy, G. P., Mason, M. E., Nebert, D. W., Forster-Gibson, C. J., et al. 1980. Temperature-dependent cytosol-to-nucleus translocation of the Ah receptor for 2,3,7,8-tetrachlorodibenzo-p-dioxin in continuous cell culture lines. *J. Biol. Chem.* 255:11415–22

138. Whitlock, J. P. Jr., Galeazzi, D. R. 1984. 2,3,7,8-Tetrachlorodibenzo-p-dioxin receptors in wild type and variant mouse hepatoma cells. Nuclear location and strength of nuclear binding. *J. Biol. Chem.* 259:980–85

139. Gelboin, H. V., Huberman, E., Sachs, L. 1969. Enzymatic hydroxylation of benzopyrene and its relationship to cytotoxicity. *Proc. Natl. Acad. Sci. USA* 64:1188–94

140. Hankinson, O. 1979. Single-step selection of clones of a mouse hepatoma line deficient in aryl hydrocarbon hydroxylase. *Proc. Natl. Acad. Sci. USA* 76:373–76

141. Miller, A. G., Whitlock, J. P. Jr. 1981. Novel variants in benzo(a)pyrene metabolism. Isolation by fluorescence-activated cell sorting. *J. Biol. Chem.* 256:2433–37

142. Legraverend, C., Hannah, R. R., Eisen, H. J., Owens, I. S., Nebert, D. W., Hankinson, O. 1982. Regulatory gene product of the *Ah* locus. Characterization of receptor mutants among mouse hepatoma clones. *J. Biol. Chem.* 257:6402–7

143. Miller, A. G., Israel, D., Whitlock, J. P. Jr. 1983. Biochemical and genetic analysis of variant mouse hepatoma cells defective in the induction of benzo(a)-pyrene-metabolizing enzyme activity. *J. Biol. Chem.* 258:3523–27

144. Hankinson, O., Anderson, R. D., Birren, B. W., Sander, F., Negishi, M., Nebert, D. W. 1985. Mutations affecting the regulation of transcription of the cytochrome P_1-450 gene in the mouse Hepa-1 cell line. *J. Biol. Chem.* 260: 1790–95

145. Montisano, D. F., Hankinson, O. 1985. Transfection by genomic DNA of cytochrome P_1-450 enzymatic activity and inducibility. *Mol. Cell. Biol.* 5:698–704

146. Hankinson, O. 1983. Dominant and recessive aryl hydrocarbon hydroxylase-deficient mutants of mouse hepatoma line, Hepa-1, and assignment of recessive mutants to three complementation groups. *Somatic Cell Genet.* 9:497–514

147. Whitlock, J. P. Jr., Gelboin, H. V. 1973. Induction of aryl hydrocarbon [benzo(a)pyrene] hydroxylase in liver cell culture by temporary inhibition of protein synthesis. *J. Biol. Chem.* 248:6114–21

148. Israel, D. I., Estolano, M. G., Galeazzi, D. R., Whitlock, J. P. Jr. 1985. Superinduction of cytochrome P_1-450 gene transcription by inhibition of protein synthesis in wild type and variant mouse hepatoma cells. *J. Biol. Chem.* 260: 5648–53

149. Jones, P. B. C., Miller, A. G., Israel, D. I., Galeazzi, D. R., Whitlock, J. P. Jr. 1984. Biochemical and genetic analysis of variant mouse hepatoma cells which overtranscribe the cytochrome P_1-450

gene in response to 2,3,7,8-tetrachlorodibenzo-*p*-dioxin. *J. Biol. Chem.* 259: 12357–363

150. Jones, P. B. C., Galeazzi, D. R., Fisher, J. M., Whitlock, J. P. Jr. 1985. Control of cytochrome P_1-450 gene expression by dioxin. *Science* 227:1499–1502

151. Liem, H. H., Muller-Eberhard, U., Johnson, E. F. 1980. Differential induction by 2,3,7,8-tetrachlorodibenzo-p-dioxin of multiple forms of rabbit microsomal cytochrome P-450: Evidence for tissue specificity. *Mol. Pharmacol.* 18: 565–70

152. Goldstein, J. A., Linko, P. 1984. Differential induction of two 2,3,7,8-tetrachlorodibenzo-*p*-dioxin-inducible forms of cytochrome P-450 in extrahepatic versus hepatic tissues. *Mol. Pharmacol.* 25:185–91

153. Jaiswal, A. K., Nebert, D. W., Eisen, H. W. 1985. Comparison of aryl hydrocarbon hydroxylase and acetanilide 4-hydroxylase induction by polycyclic aromatic compounds in human and mouse cell lines. *Biochem. Pharmacol.* 34:2721–31

154. Guenthner, T. M., Nebert, D. W. 1978. Evidence in rat and mouse liver for temporal control of two forms of cytochrome P-450 inducible by 2,3,7,8-tetrachlorodibenzo-p-dioxin. *Eur. J. Biochem.* 91: 449–56

155. Thomas, P. E., Hutton, J. J. 1973. Genetics of aryl hydrocarbon hydroxylase induction in mice: Additive inheritance in crosses between C3H/HeJ and DBA/2J. *Biochem. Genet.* 8:249–57

156. Robinson, J. R., Considine, N., Nebert, D. W. 1974. Genetic expression of aryl hydrocarbon hydroxylase induction. Evidence for the involvement of other genetic loci. *J. Biol. Chem.* 249:5851–59

157. Gehly, E. B., Fahl, W. E., Jefcoate, C. R., Heidelberger, C. 1979. The metabolism of benzo(a)pyrene by cytochrome P-450 in transformable and non-transformable C3H mouse fibroblasts. *J. Biol. Chem.* 254:5041–48

157a. Okey, A. B., Mason, M. E., Gehley, E. B., Heidelberger, C., Muncan, J., Dufrense, M. J. 1983. Defective binding of 3-methylcholanthrene to the Ah receptor within C3H/10T1/2 clone 8 mouse fibroblasts in culture. *Eur. J. Biochem.* 132:219–27

158. Legraverend, C., Karenlampi, S. O., Bigelow, S. W., Lalley, P. A., Kozak, C. A., et al. 1984. Aryl hydrocarbon hydroxylase induction by benzo(a)-anthracene: Regulatory gene local-

ized to the distal portion of mouse chromosome 17. *Genetics* 107:447–61

159. Tierney, B., Weaver, D., Heintz, N. H., Schaffer, W. I., Bresnick, E. 1980. The identity and nuclear uptake of a cytosolic binding protein for 3-methylcholanthrene. *Arch. Biochem. Biophys.* 200:513–23

160. Holder, G. M., Tierney, B., Bresnick, E. 1981. Nuclear uptake and subsequent nuclear metabolism of benzo(a)pyrene complexed to cytosolic proteins. *Cancer Res.* 41:4408–14

161. Zytkovicz, T. H. 1982. Identification and characterization of a high-affinity saturable binding protein for the carcinogen benzo(a)pyrene. *Cancer Res.* 42:4387–93

162. Collins, S., Marletta, M. A. 1984. Carcinogen-binding proteins. High-affinity binding sites for benzo(a)pyrene in mouse liver distinct from the *Ah* receptor. *Mol. Pharmacol.* 26:353–59

163. Gruss, P. 1984. Magic enhancers? *DNA* 3:1–5

164. Selye, H. 1971. Hormones and resistance. *J. Pharm. Sci.* 60:1–28

165. Lu, A. Y. H., Somogyi, A., West, S., Kuntzman, R., Conney, A. H. 1972. Pregneneolone-16α-carbonitrile: A new type of inducer of drug metabolizing enzymes. *Arch. Biochem. Biophys.* 152:457–62

166. Elshourbagy, N. A., Guzelian, P. S. 1980. Separation, purification, and characterization of a novel form of hepatic cytochrome P-450 from rats treated with pregnenolone-16α-carbonitrile. *J. Biol. Chem.* 255:1279–85

167. Hardwick, J. P., Gonzalez, F. J., Kasper, C. B. 1983. Cloning of DNA complementary to cytochrome P-450 induced by pregnenolone-16α-carbonitrile. *J. Biol. Chem.* 258:10182–86

168. Simmons, D. L., Lalley, P. A., Kasper, C. B. 1985. Chromosomal assignments of genes coding for components of the mixed-function oxidase system in mice. *J. Biol. Chem.* 260:515–21

169. Gonzalez, F. J., Nebert, D. W., Hardwick, J. P., Kasper, C. B. 1985. Complete cDNA and protein sequence of a pregnenolone 16α-carbonitrile-induced cytochrome P-450. A representative of a new gene family. *J. Biol. Chem.* 260:7435–41

170. Elshourbagy, N. A., Barwick, J. L., Guzelian, P. S. 1981. Induction of cytochrome P-450 by pregnenolone-16α-carbonitrile in primary monolayer cultures of adult rat hepatocytes and in a cell-free translation system. *J. Biol. Chem.* 256:6060–68

171. Heuman, D. M., Gallagher, E. J., Barwick, J. L., Elshourbagy, N. A., Guzelian, P. S. 1982. Immunochemical evidence for induction of a common form of hepatic cytochrome P-450 in rats treated with pregnenolone-16α-carbonitrile or other steroidal or non-steroidal agents. *Mol. Pharmacol.* 21:753–60

172. Schuetz, E. G., Wrighton, S. A., Barwick, J. L., Guzelian, P. S. 1984. Induction of cytochrome P-450 by glucocorticoids in rat liver. I. Evidence that glucocorticoids and pregnenolone 16α-carbonitrile regulate de novo synthesis of a common form of cytochrome P-450 in cultures of adult rat hepatocytes and in the liver *in vivo*. *J. Biol. Chem.* 259:1999–2006

173. Schuetz, E. G., Guzelian, P. S. 1984. Induction of cytochrome P-450 by glucocorticoids in rat liver. 2. Evidence that glucocorticoids regulate induction of cytochrome P-450 by a nonclassical receptor mechanism. *J. Biol. Chem.* 259:2007–12

174. Gozukara, E. M., Fagan, J., Pastewka, J. V., Guengerich, F. P., Gelboin, H. V. 1984. Induction of cytochrome P-450 mRNAs quantitated by *in vitro* translation and immunoprecipitation. *Arch. Biochem. Biophys.* 232:660–69

175. Estabrook, R. W., Cooper, D. Y., Rosenthal, O. 1963. The light-reversible carbon monoxide inhibition of the steroid C-21 hydroxylation system of the adrenal cortex. *Biochem. Z.* 338:741–55

176. Waterman, M. R., Simpson, E. R. 1985. Regulation of the biosynthesis of cytochromes P-450 involved in steroid hormone synthesis. *Mol. Cell. Endocrinol.* 39:81–89

177. Fevold, H. R. 1983. Regulation of the adrenal and gonadal microsomal mixed-function oxygenases of steroid hormone biosynthesis. *Ann. Rev. Physiol.* 45:19–36

178. Morohashi, K., Fujii-Kuriyama, Y., Okada, Y., Sogawa, K., Hirose, T., Inayama, S., Omura, T. 1984. Molecular cloning and nucleotide sequence of cDNA for mRNA of mitochondral cytochrome P-450(scc) of bovine adrenal cortex. *Proc. Natl. Acad. Sci. USA* 81:4647–51

179. John, M. E., John, M. C., Ashley, P., MacDonald, R. J., Simpson, E. R., Waterman, M. R. 1984. Identification and characterization of cDNA clones specific for cholesterol side-chain cleav-

age cytochrome P-450. *Proc. Natl. Acad. Sci. USA* 81:5628–32

180. Matteson, K. J., Chung, B., Miller, W. L. 1984. Molecular cloning of DNA complementary to bovine adrenal P-450$_{scc}$ mRNA. *Biochem. Biophys. Res. Commun.* 120:264–70

181. Purvis, J. L., Canick, J. A., Mason, J. I., Estabrook, R. W., McCarthy, J. L. 1973. Lifetime of adrenal cytochrome P-450 as influenced by ACTH. *Ann. NY Acad. Sci.* 212:319–43

182. DuBois, R. N., Simpson, E. R., Kramer, R. E., Waterman, M. R. 1981. Induction of synthesis of cholesterol side chain cleavage cytochrome P-450 by adrenocorticotropin in cultured bovine adrenocortical cells. *J. Biol. Chem.* 256:7000–5

183. Kramer, R. E., Rainey, W. E., Funkenstein, B., Dee, A., Simpson, E. R., Waterman, M. R. 1984. Induction of synthesis of mitochondrial steroidogenic enzymes of bovine adrenocortical cells by analogs of cyclic AMP. *J. Biol. Chem.* 259:707–13

184. John, M. E., John, M. A., Simpson, E. R., Waterman, M. R. 1985. Regulation of cytochrome P-450$_{11\beta}$ gene expression by adrenocorticotropin. *J. Biol. Chem.* 260:5760–67

185. Vannice, J. L., Taylor, J. M., Ringold, G. M. 1984. Glucocorticod-mediated induction of α_1-acid glycoprotein: Evidence for hormone-regulated RNA processing. *Proc. Natl. Acad. Sci. USA* 81:4241–45

186. Funkenstein, B., Waterman, M. R., Masters, B. S. S., Simpson, E. R. 1983. Evidence for the presence of cholesterol side chain cleavage cytochrome P-450 and adrenodoxin in fresh granulosa cells. *J. Biol. Chem.* 258:10187–91

187. Funkenstein, B., Waterman, M. R., Simpson, E. R. 1984. Induction of synthesis of cholesterol side chain cleavage cytochrome P-450 and adrenodoxin by follicle-stimulating hormone, 8-bromocyclic AMP, and low density lipoprotein in cultured bovine granulosa cells. *J. Biol. Chem.* 259:8572–77

188. Zuber, M. X., Simpson, E. R., Hall, P. F., Waterman, M. R. 1985. Effects of adrenocorticotropin on 17_α-hydroxylase activity and cytochrome P-450$_{17\alpha}$ synthesis in bovine adrenocortical cells. *J. Biol. Chem.* 260:1842–48

189. Malaska, T., Payne, A. H. 1984. Luteinizing hormone and cyclic AMP-mediated induction of microsomal cytochrome P-450 enzymes in cultured mouse Leydig cells. *J. Biol. Chem.* 259:11654–57

190. New, M. I., Levine, L. S. 1984. Recent advances in 21-hydroxylase deficiency. *Ann. Rev. Med.* 35:649–63

191. Funkenstein, B., McCarthy, J. L., Dus, K. M., Simpson, E. R., Waterman, M. R. 1983. Effect of adrenocorticotropin on steroid 21-hydroxylase synthesis and activity in cultured bovine adrenocortical cells. *J. Biol. Chem.* 258:9398–9405

192. Boggaram, V., Simpson, E. R., Waterman, M. R. 1984. Induction of synthesis of bovine adrenocorticol cytochromes P-450$_{scc}$, P-450$_{11\beta}$, P-450$_{c21}$, and adrenodoxin by prostaglandins E$_2$ and F$_{2\alpha}$ and cholera toxin. *Arch. Biochem. Biophys.* 231:271–79

193. White, P. C., New, M. I., DuPont, B. 1984. Cloning and expression of cDNA encoding a bovine adrenal cytochrome P-450 specific for steroid 21-hydroxylation. *Proc. Natl. Acad. Sci. USA* 81:1986–90

194. Chung, B. C., Matteson, K. J., Miller, W. L. 1985. Cloning and characterization of the bovine gene for steroid 21-hydroxylase (P-450$_{C21}$). *DNA* 4:211–19

195. White, P. C., Chaplin, D. D., Weis, J. H., Dupont, B., New, M. I., Seidman, J. G. 1984. Two steroid 21-hydroxylase genes are located in the murine S region. *Nature* 312:465–67

196. White, P. C., New, M. I., DuPont, B. 1984. HLA-linked congenital adrenal hyperplasia results from a defective gene encoding a cytochrome P-450 specific for steroid 21-hydroxylation. *Proc. Natl. Acad. Sci. USA* 81:7505–9

197. Carroll, M. C., Campbell, R. D., Porter, R. R. 1985. Mapping of steroid 21-hydroxylase genes adjacent to complement component C4 genes in *HLA*, the major histocompatibility complex in man. *Proc. Natl. Acad. Sci. USA* 82:521–25

197a. White, P. C., Grossberger, D., Onufer, B. J., Chaplin, D. D., New, M. I., et al. 1985. Two genes encoding steroid 21-hydroxylase are located near the genes encoding the fourth component of complement in man. *Proc. Natl. Acad. Sci. USA* 82:1089–93

198. Erickson, G. F. 1983. Primary cultures of ovarian cells in serum-free medium as models of hormone-dependent differentiation. *Mol. Cell. Endocrinol.* 29:21–49

199. Bardin, C. W., Catterall, J. F. 1981. Testosterone: A major determinant of ex-

tragenital sexual dimorphism. *Science* 211:1285–94

200. MacLusky, N. J., Naftolin, F. 1981. Sexual differentiation of the central nervous system. *Science* 211:1294–1303

201. Wynshaw-Boris, A., Lugo, T. G., Short, J. M., Fournier, R. E. K., Hanson, R. W. 1984. Identification of a cAMP regulatory region in the gene for rat cytosolic phosphoenolpyruvate carboxykinase (GTP). *J. Biol. Chem.* 259:12161–69

202. Hashimoto, S., Schmid, W., Schutz, G. 1984. Transcriptional activation of the rat liver tyrosine aminotransferase gene by cAMP. *Proc. Natl. Acad. Sci. USA* 81:6637–41

203. Roy, A. K., Chatterjee, B. 1983. Sexual dimorphism in the liver. *Ann. Rev. Physiol.* 45:37–50

204. Kato, R. 1974. Sex-related differences in drug metabolism. *Drug Metab. Rev.* 3:1–32

205. Colby, H. D. 1980. Regulation of drug and steroid metabolism by androgens and estrogens. *Adv. Sex Horm. Res.* 4:27–71

206. Gustafsson, J. A., Mode, A., Norstedt, G., Skett, P. 1983. Sex steroid induced changes in hepatic enzymes. *Ann. Rev. Physiol.* 45:51–60

207. Einarsson, K., Gustafsson, J. A., Stenberg, A. 1973. Neonatal imprinting of liver microsomal hydroxylation and reduction of steroids. *J. Biol. Chem.* 248:4987–97

208. Cheng, K. C., Schenkman, J. B. 1982. Purification and characterization of two constitutive forms of rat liver microsomal cytochrome P-450. *J. Biol. Chem.* 257:2378–85

209. Chao, H., Chung, L. W. K. 1982. Neonatal imprinting and hepatic cytochrome P-450: Immunochemical evidence for the presence of a sex-dependent and neonatally-imprinted form(s) of hepatic cytochrome P-450. *Mol. Pharmacol.* 21:744–52

210. Kamataki, T., Maeda, Y., Yamazoe, T., Nagai, T., Kato, R. 1983. Sex difference in cytochrome P-450 in the rat: purification, characterization, and quantitation of constitutive forms of cytochrome P-450 from liver microsomes of male and female rats. *Arch. Biochem. Biophys.* 225:758–70

211. Ryan, D. E., Iida, S., Wood, A. W., Thomas, P. E., Lieber, C. S., Levin, W. 1984. Characterization of three highly purified cytochromes P-450 from hepatic microsomes of adult male rats. *J. Biol. Chem.* 259:1239–50

212. Morgan, E. T., MacGoech, C., Gustafsson, J. A. 1985. Sexual differentiation of cytochrome P-450 in rat liver: Evidence for a constitutive isozyme as the male-specific 16α-hydroxylase. *Mol. Pharmacol.* 27:471–79

213. Harada, N., Negishi, M. 1984. Mouse liver testosterone 16α-hydroxylase (cytochrome P-$450_{16\alpha}$). Purification, regioselectivity, stereospecificity, and immunochemical characterization. *J. Biol. Chem.* 259:12285–90

214. Harada, N., Negishi, M. 1985. Sexual-dependent expression of mouse testosterone 16α-hydroxylase (cytochrome P-$450_{16\alpha}$): cDNA cloning and pretranslational regulation. *Proc. Natl. Acad. Sci. USA* 82:2024–28

215. MacGeoch, C., Morgan, E. T., Halpert, J., Gustafsson, J. A. 1984. Purification, characterization, and pituitary regulation of the sex-specific cytochrome P-450 15β-hydroxylase from liver microsomes of untreated female rats. *J. Biol. Chem.* 259:15433–39

216. Berg, A., Gustafsson, J. A. 1973. Regulation of hydroxylation of 5α-androstane-3a, 17β-diol in liver microsomes from male and female rats. *J. Biol. Chem.* 248:6559–67

217. Gustafsson, J. A., Stenberg, A. 1974. Neonatal programming of androgen responsiveness of liver of adult rats. *J. Biol. Chem.* 249:719–23

218. Gustafsson, J. A., Pousette, A., Stenberg, A., Wrange, O. 1975. High-affinity binding of 4-androstenene-3,17-dione in rat liver. *Biochemistry* 14:3942–48

219. Gustafsson, J. A. Stenberg, A. 1974. Irreversible androgenic programming at birth of microsomal and soluble rat liver enzymes active on 4-androstene-3, 17-dione and 5α-androstane-3α, 17β-diol. *J. Biol. Chem.* 249:711–18

220. DeNoor, P., Denef, C. 1968. The "puberty" of the rat liver. Feminine pattern of cortisol metabolism in male rats castrated at birth. *Endocrinology* 82:480–92

221. Denef, C., DeNoor, P. 1968. The "puberty" of the rat liver. 2. Permanent changes in steroid metabolizing enzymes after treatment with a single injection of testosterone propionate at birth. *Endocrinology* 83:791–98

222. Stenberg, A. 1975. On the modulating effects of ovaries on neonatal androgen programming of rat liver enzymes. *Acta Endocrinol.* 78:294–301

223. Denef, C. 1974. Effect of hypophysectomy and pituitary implants at puberty on the sexual differentiation of testosterone metabolism in rat liver. *Endocrinology* 94:1577–82

224. Gustafsson, J. A., Stenberg, A. 1974. Masculinization of rat liver enzyme activities following hypophysectomy. *Endocrinology* 95:891–96
225. Gustafsson, J. A., Stenberg, A. 1976. On the obligatory role of the hypophysis in sexual differentiation of hepatic metabolism in rats. *Proc. Natl. Acad. Sci. USA* 73:1462–65
226. Gustafsson, J. A., Ingelman-Sundberg, M., Stenberg, A., Hokfelt, T. 1976. Feminization of hepatic steroid metabolism in male rats following electrothermic lesion of the hypothalamus. *Endocrinology* 98:922–26
227. Gustafsson, J. A., Eneroth, P., Hokfelt, T., Skett, P. 1978. Central control of hepatic steroid metabolism. Effect of discrete hypothalamic lesions. *Endocrinology* 103:141–51
228. Toran-Allerand, C. D. 1984. Gonadal hormones and brain development: Implications for the genesis of sexual differentiation. *Ann. NY Acad. Sci.* 435:101–10
229. Gustafsson, J. A., Stenberg, A. 1976. Specificity of neonatal, androgen-induced imprinting of hepatic steroid metabolism in rats. *Science* 191:203–4
230. Eden, S. 1979. Age- and sex-related differences in episodic growth hormone secretion in the rat. *Endocrinology* 105:555–60
231. Mode, A., Norstedt, G., Simic, B., Eneroth, P., Gustafsson, J. A. 1981. Continuous infusion of growth hormone feminizes hepatic steroid metabolism in the rat. *Endocrinology* 108:2103–8
232. Mode, A., Norstedt, G., Eneroth, P., Gustafsson, J. A. 1983. Purification of liver feminizing factor from rat pituitaries and demonstration of its identity with growth hormone. *Endocrinology* 113:1250–60
233. Norstedt, G., Mode, A., Hokfelt, T., Eneroth, P., Ferland, L., et al. 1983. Possible role of somatostatin in the regulation of the sexually differentiated steroid metabolism and prolactin receptor in rat liver. *Endocrinology* 112:1076–90
234. Norstedt, G., Palmiter, R. 1984. Secretory rhythm of growth hormone regulates sexual differentiation of mouse liver. *Cell* 36:805–12
235. Faris, R. A., Campbell, T. C. 1981. Exposure of newborn rats to pharmacologically active compounds may permanently alter carcinogen metabolism. *Science* 211:719–21
236. Faris, R. A., Campbell, T. C. 1983. Long-term effects of neonatal phenobarbital exposure on aflatoxin B_1 disposition in adult rats. *Cancer Res.* 43:2576–83
237. Enat, R., Jefferson, D. M., Ruiz-Opazo, N., Gatmaitan, Z., Leinwand, L. A., Reid, L. M. 1984. Hepatocyte proliferation in vitro: Its dependence on the use of serum-free hormonally defined medium and substrata of extracellular matrix. *Proc. Natl. Acad. Sci. USA* 81:1411–15
238. Isom, H. C., Secott, T., Georgoff, I., Woodworth, C., Mummaw, J. 1985. Maintenance of differentiated rat hepatocytes in primary culture. *Proc. Natl. Acad. Sci. USA* 82:3252–56
239. Newman, S., Guzelian, P. S. 1982. Stimulation of de novo synthesis of cytochrome P-450 by phenobarbital in primary non-proliferating cultures of adult rat hepatocytes. *Proc. Natl. Acad. Sci. USA* 79:2922–26
240. Frey, A. B., Rosenfeld, M. G., Dolan, W. J., Adesnik, M., Kreibich, G. 1984. Induction of cytochrome P-450 isozymes in rat hepatoma-derived cell cultures. *J. Cell. Physiol.* 120:169–80
241. Wiebel, F. J., Park, S. S., Kiefer, F., Gelboin, H. V. 1984. Expression of cytochromes P-450 in rat hepatoma cells. Analysis of monoclonal antibodies specific for cytochromes P-450 from rat liver induced by 3-methylcholanthrene or phenobarbital. *Eur. J. Biochem.* 145:455–62

Ann. Rev. Pharmacol. Toxicol. 1986. 26:371–99

COMPARATIVE TOXICOLOGY AND MECHANISM OF ACTION OF POLYCHLORINATED DIBENZO-P-DIOXINS AND DIBENZOFURANS

S. H. Safe

Department of Physiology and Pharmacology, College of Veterinary Medicine, Texas A&M University, College Station, Texas 77843

INTRODUCTION

Polychlorinated dibenzo-p-dioxins (Pcdds) and polychlorinated di-benzofurans (PCDFs) are members of a chemical family (polyhalogenated aromatics) that also includes the polychlorinated biphenyls, naphthalenes, azobenzenes, and azoxybenzenes, and the polybrominated biphenyls. In contrast to the polychlorinated biphenyls and naphthalenes and the polybrominated biphenyls, the PCDDs and PCDFs are not primary industrial products. PCDFs are found as by-products ($<$ 1 ppm) in commercial polychlorinated biphenyls and naphthalenes and are probably derived from dibenzofuran impurities in the industrial hydrocarbons that are subsequently chlorinated (1–3). There is also circumstantial evidence that the effects of heat or arcing may produce PCDFs from polychlorinated biphenyls during use (4). This is evidenced by the relatively high levels of PCDFs (ca 100 ppm) detected in the polychlorinated biphenyl–containing heat transfer fluids that were the toxic agents in the Yusho disasters in Japan and Taiwan (3, 5, 6). PCDDs and PCDFs are also found as impurities in chlorinated phenols and their derived products (3, 7, 8), and it is apparent that the combustion of chlorinated aromatics and diverse types of chemical, industrial, and municipal waste results in the formation and release of these toxic chemicals into the environment (9–14). The potential for the

371

0362-1642/86/0415-0371$02.00

formation of PCDDs and PCDFs from nonindustrial sources, i.e. energy-derived combustion and forest fires, led to the "trace chemistries of fire" hypothesis, which speculated that the origins of PCDDs and PCDFs in the environment were nonanthropogenic (15, 16). However, analysis of aquatic sediment cores from the Saginaw River and Bay and from Lake Huron does not support the trace chemistries of fire hypothesis (17, 18). The PCDD and PCDF congener composition of dated sediment cores demonstrates that the concentrations of these compounds in sediments have greatly increased since the 1940s and that "this historical increase is similar to trends for the production, use, and disposal of chlorinated organic compounds" (17, 18).

Human exposure to PCDDs and PCDFs has occurred via three major pathways: occupational, accidental, and environmental. Industrial workers engaged in the manufacture or use of polychlorinated biphenyls, chlorinated phenols, and their derived products are exposed to PCDDs and/or PCDFs in combination with their associated major commercial product (19–21). Accidents in which PCDDs have been released into the workplace or into the environment (e. g. the Seveso accident in Italy) have also resulted in human exposure to mixtures of the industrial chemicals and their PCDD/PCDF toxic contaminants (22–24). The Yusho poisoning in Japan and Taiwan involved the exposure of several thousand individuals to PCBs and their PCDF contaminants (5, 6, 25–27). The uptake of environmental residues of PCDDs and PCDFs into higher trophic levels of the food chain is only now being investigated, and trace levels (parts per trillion) have been detected in fish, wildlife, and human tissues (19, 28–32). In common with accidental and industrial exposures to PCDDs and PCDFs, exposure levels to these toxins represent only a small fraction of the total bioavailable lipophilic environmental pollutants. 2,3,7,8-Tetrachlorodibenzo-p-dioxin (TCDD) is the major by-product formed from 2,4,5-trichlorophenol and its derived products; this highly toxic compound has been the focus of most biologic and toxic studies on the PCDDs. However, all other human and environmental exposures to PCDDs and PCDFs involve a complex mixture of isomers and congeners in combination with other chemicals.

The scientific, regulatory, and media attention focused on PCDDs, PCDFs, and particularly 2,3,7,8-TCDD has continued unabated; moreover, with the recent identification of trace levels of these toxins in human tissue, domestic animals, the environment, and toxic chemical waste dumpsites, the scientific and societal concern about this class of compounds will no doubt continue. It is apparent from the scientific literature that one member of this class of compounds, namely 2,3,7,8-TCDD, ranks with benzo[a]pyrene as one of the most thoroughly studied toxins. Unfortunately, the biologic and toxic effects of the remaining 74 PCDD and 135 PCDF congeners have not been thoroughly investigated, and the interactive effects of these compounds or their activities in combination with polychlorinated biphenyls and chlorinated phenols have also not been addressed. This article (*a*) briefly reviews the species-dependent toxic and biologic effects of PCDDs and PCDFs, (*b*) demonstrates the parallel modes of action of PCDDs and PCDFs and endogenous cellular hormones, (*c*) summarizes the data that support the proposed receptor-mediated mechanism of action, including the structure-activity relationships (SARs) that have been developed for both PCDD and PCDF congeners, and (*d*) discusses the few interactive studies published.

TOXIC AND BIOLOGIC EFFECTS OF PCDDs AND PCDFs

Several review articles (33–45) have summarized the toxic and biologic effects elicited by PCDDs, PCDFs, and related toxic halogenated aryl hydrocarbons. The toxic effects resulting from exposure to this group of chemicals are dependent on a number of factors which include the dose of the toxin, and the age, strain, species, and sex of the animals used. The complete spectrum of toxicity is not usually observed in any single animal species; however, the limited data available indicate that the toxic PCDDs, PCDFs, and related compounds elicit the same qualitative pattern of responses within each species. The differences in species susceptibility to this group of chemicals are illustrated by the LD_{50} values for 2,3,7,8-TCDD, which vary over 5000-fold (33, 34) from the highly sensitive guinea pig to the resistant hamster [LD_{50}s (μg/kg): guinea pig (0.6–2.0), rat (22–45), chicken (25–50), monkey (70), rabbit (115), dog (100–200), mouse (114–284), bullfrog (>1000), hamster (1157–5051)]. The quantitative differences in the toxicity of PCDF congeners have recently been demonstrated (47) for a series of ten congeners (see structure-activity section, below). The 2,3,4,7,8-pentachlorodibenzofuran (PeCDF) ED_{50} values for thymic atrophy and body weight loss in the rat were 0.21 and 1.04 μmol/kg; the 1,2,4,7,8-PeCDF isomer elicited the same toxic effects, but the ED_{50} values were 220 and 47 times higher, respectively (47). The toxic responses observed in several animal species by PCDDs and PCDFs include dermal toxicity, teratogenicity, reproductive problems, body weight loss, hepatotoxicity, gastric lesions, lymphoid involution, immunotoxicity, and carcinogenicity. The two most characteristic toxic effects observed in all laboratory animals are lymphoid involution and/or immunotoxicity and body weight loss. Chloracne and related dermal lesions are the most frequently noted signs of PCDD and PCDF toxicosis in humans; dermal lesions are also observed in rhesus monkeys, hairless mice, and rabbits that have been exposed to this group of toxins. In contrast, rats, most strains of mice, guinea pigs, and hamsters do not develop chloracne and related dermal toxic lesions after

Figure 1   Structure of the polychlorinated dibenzofurans and dibenzo-p-dioxins.

exposure to 2,3,7,8-TCDD. Poland & Knutson (38) have noted that many of the observed toxic lesions are either hyperplastic/metaplastic or hypoplastic, and primarily affect epithelial tissues. The mechanisms by which PCDDs and PCDFs elicit this diverse group of species-dependent toxicities remain unexplained although several hypotheses have been advanced and are discussed in this review.

PCDDs and PCDFs cause diverse biological responses in mammals and mammalian cells in culture including the highly characteristic induction of microsomal benzo[a]pyrene hydroxylase (aryl hydrocarbon hydroxylase, AHH) and several related cytochrome P-450-dependent monooxygenases (37, 38, 44, 47–53). In the rat, these activities are associated with the preferential induction of cytochrome P-450c, P-450d, and P-450a, with the former isozyme responsible for most of the induced monooxygenase enzyme activities (54). In the mouse, 2,3,7,8-TCDD induces cytochromes P_1-450 and P_3-450 (55–57), and the former isozyme exhibits antigenic and enzymatic similarities with the rat cytochrome P-450c (58). 2,3,7,8-TCDD induces two cytochrome P-450 isozymes (forms 4 and 6) in the rabbit, and their inducibility is highly tissue-specific (59, 60). 2,3,7,8-TCDD and related compounds also induce glutathione S-transferases (61) and glucuronosyl transferase (62, 63) and several other enzymes including DT-diaphorase (64), ornithine decarboxylase (65), δ-aminolevulinic acid synthetase (48), epidermal transglutaminase (66), and hepatic DNA polymerase B (67). Detailed summaries of these and other biochemical effects of 2,3,7,8-TCDD have recently been reviewed (38, 42).

The remarkably broad spectrum of biologic and toxic responses observed in animals exposed to 2,3,7,8-TCDD and related toxic halogenated aromatics has stimulated research on the mechanism or mechanisms of action of these chemicals. Unlike many toxins, the most active halogenated aryl hydrocarbons do not appear to require metabolic activation into presumed "toxic" intermediates that alkylate specific cellular acceptors (e. g. DNA, RNA, and protein) or initiate cellular lipoperoxidation. On the contrary, the most toxic halogenated aryl hydrocarbons are highly resistant to oxidative metabolic degradation and exhibit minimal metabolically mediated alkylation of cellular macromolecules (68–70); moreover limited data suggest that PCDD and PCDF metabolites are much less toxic than their parent hydrocarbons (71). Many of the effects of this class of environmental toxins are comparable to those associated with modulation of several hormone-mediated responses. For example, there are many similarities between animals that exhibit thyroid dysfunction and those treated with toxic halogenated aryl hydrocarbons. Daily injections of the active thyroid hormone, triiodothyronine (T_3) to male mice treated with a lethal dose (200 μg/kg) of 2,3,7,8-TCDD did increase their mean surival times; however, all the animals in the 2,3,7,8-TCDD and 2,3,7,8-TCDD + T_3-treated groups died (43). More recent studies (71, 72) have demonstrated that thyroid hormones may play a more important role in modulating the toxicity of 2,3,7,8-TCDD; radiothyroidectomy protected rats against 2,3,7,8-TCDD-mediated T-cell immunotoxicity (as measured by the spleen anti-SRBC plaque-forming cell assay), mortality, and body weight loss (73). Like the glucocorticoids, PCDDs, PCDFs, and related toxic halogenated aryl hydrocarbons cause lymphoid involution (33, 34, 37, 38, 40, 41, 74, 75), are teratogens in mice (76–80), and induce cytochrome P-450-dependent monooxygenases (37, 38, 44, 46–54). However the mechanisms of action of glucocorticoids and 2,3,7,8-TCDD are not directly linked since the latter compound is toxic to adrenalectomized rats, does not bind to the glucocorticoid receptor, and does not induce tyrosine aminotransferase (43) or the dexamethasone-induced cytochrome P-450 isozyme (81). Other adrenal steroids resemble the toxic halogenated aryl hydrocarbons since they also induce several hepatic drug-metabolizing enzymes, including monooxygenases and glucuronosyl transferases (81–84).

It has been proposed that 2,3,7,8-TCDD and related toxic isostereomers, like the steroid hormones, elicit their responses via the initial noncovalent interaction with a cytosolic receptor protein in target tissues (37, 38, 75). The synthesis of radiolabelled [^{3}H]-2,3,7,8-TCDD with high specific activity (52.5 Ci/mmol) resulted in the identification of a specific binding protein in hepatic cytosol of responsive C57BL/6J mice, whereas minimal binding activity was observed in nonresponsive DBA/2J hepatic cytosol (85). The role of this Ah receptor protein in the mechanism of action of toxic halogenated aryl hydrocarbon has been thoroughly investigated and satisfies most of the specific criteria that support a receptor mediated cellular process. These criteria include: (a) the existence of a finite number of binding or receptor sites and therefore saturable binding, (b) high affinity ligand binding that is commensurate with the usually low levels of circulating hormones, (c) stereoselective binding capacity for the receptor, (d) tissue or organ response specificity for the receptor ligand, and (e) a correlation between binding affinities, receptor occupancy, and the magnitude of the response. This review focuses on research that supports the role of the Ah receptor in the mechanism of action of PCDDs and PCDFs and highlights the detailed structure activity relationships (SARs) that have been developed for this group of environmental and industrial toxins.

PCDD AND PCDF ACTIVITIES: EVIDENCE THAT SUPPORTS THE ROLE OF THE CYTOSOLIC Ah RECEPTOR PROTEIN

High Affinity Saturable Binding

The saturable binding of [^{3}H]-2,3,7,8-TCDD with hepatic and extrahepatic cytosolic receptor protein from several species has been demonstrated using the following receptor assay procedures: charcoal/dextran absorption, protamine sulfate precipitation, hydroxylapatite absorption, isoelectric focusing in polyacrylamide gels, gel permeation chromatography, sucrose density gradient centrifugation, and gel permeation high performance liquid chromatography (85–110). Scatchard plot analysis of [^{3}H]-2,3,7,8-TCDD specific binding to hepatic cytosolic receptor protin gives dissociation consants (K_D) that are dependent on a number of factors including the animal species and strain, the receptor binding assay used, and the age of the animal. The K_D values for responsive C57BL/6 mice and rats vary from 0.27–3.0 nM (85, 95) and 0.13–1.2 nM (91, 95, 102), respectively, and the value for cynomolgus monkeys was approximately 3 nM (108). The concentration of hepatic cytosolic receptor was also highly variable, but the upper limit for most studies was less than 110 fmol/mg cytosolic protein (85, 91, 95). One study demonstrated that hepatic receptor levels in the rat varied with age and that these levels were endocrine independent since hepatic receptor levels were virtually unaltered by orchiectomy, ovariectomy, adrenalectomy, or hyposectomy (106). This observation was consistent with the inactivity of several steroid hormones as competitive ligands for this receptor protein (85, 86, 89, 99, 102).

Since certain polycyclic aromatic hydrocarbons resemble 2,3,7,8-TCDD in their mode of induction of AHH and related cytochrome P-450 isozymes in responsive strains of mice and mammalian cells in cultures, it is not surprising that many of these compounds competitively displace [^{3}H]-2,3,7,8-TCDD from the receptor protein. Moreover, [^{3}H]-3-methylcholanthrene, benzo[a]pyrene, and dibenzo[a,h]anthracene, three active AHH inducers, exhibit saturable binding with the rat hepatic receptor protein and the ligand-receptor complex sediments at 8-9 S under low ionic strength conditions using the sucrose density gradient technique (97, 105). The radioactive binding peaks were eliminated after competition with a 200-fold molar excess of 2,3,7,8-TCDD. Similar results were also observed with responsive C57BL/6 mouse hepatic cytosol. However, [^{3}H]-benzo[a]pyrene unexpectedly does not yield a radiolabelled ligand-receptor binding peak that is eliminated after competition with a 200-fold molar excess of unlabelled 2,3,7,8-TCDD.

Tissue/Organ, Strain, and Cell Culture Response Specificity

The 2,3,7,8-TCDD receptor levels in several organs and tissues in Sprague-Dawley rats, C57BL/6J and DBA/2J mice have been reported (96, 103, 104,

106). The cytosolic Ah receptor concentrations (fmol/mg cytosolic protein) in the C57BL/6J mice and Sprague-Dawley rat organs and tissues were: liver, 32 ± 1.5 and 39 ± 1.9; lung, 23 ± 6.4 and 47 ± 4.3; kidney, 10 ± 0.4 and 1.2 ± 0.9; intestine, 8 ± 2.3 and 15 ± 1.7; thymus, 8 ± 2.2 and 54 ± 3.9 (The Ah receptor was not detectable in the adrenals, heart, brain, skeletal muscle, and testis). Although the Ah receptor was not detected in the cytosol of DBA/2J mice, 18 hr after administration of [^{3}H]-2,3,7,8-TCDD to these animals levels of the receptor-ligand complex could be measured in nuclear protein extracts from liver (5.4 ± 0.3 fmol/mg), lung (7.4 ± 0.3 fmol/mg), and kidney (4.7 ± 0.1 fmol/mg). The appearance of hepatic nuclear radiolabeled ligand-receptor protein complexes and the elimination of this radioactivity by preinjection with a large excess of unlabeled 2,3,7,8-TCDD has been reported by several groups (89, 91, 96, 99, 102, 106); however, Mason & Okey (96) demonstrated that lung, liver, and kidney nuclear Ah receptor levels were higher in the responsive C57BL/6J mice than in the nonresponsive DBA/2J strain. This observation is consistent with the fact that 2,3,7,8-TCDD and other toxic halogenated aryl hydrocarbons elicit biologic and toxic responses in both strains of mice but at different dose levels. Unfortunately there are insufficient data available to correlate tissue/organ receptor levels with the magnitude of specific responses in these target sites.

The criteria for receptor response specificity are supported by numerous studies with genetically inbred responsive and nonresponsive strains of mice and with some mammalian cells in culture. For example, there is an excellent rank order correlation between the maximum AHH inducibility in several inbred strains of mice and F$_1$ hybrids and the number of Ah receptor molecules per liver cell (109). Nebert and co-workers have also shown a linear correlation ($r = 0.99$) between the amount of 2,3,7,8-TCDD-receptor complex appearing in hepatic nuclei of C57BL/6 and DBA/2 mice and the percentage of maximally induced cytochrome P$_1$-450 mRNA (104). Hudson and co-workers have demonstrated that for several human squamous cell carcinoma lines, the relative amount of receptor measured in each cell line correlated well with the 7-ethoxycoumarin 0-deethylase inducibility in these cells by 2,3,7,8-TCDD (110).

These data that support the receptor-mediated response specificity are in contrast to data in several other studies with animals and cell cultures. Hepatic 2,3,7,8-TCDD receptor levels in guinea pigs, rats, mice, hamsters, and nonhuman primates vary less than tenfold (10–100 fmol/mg cytosolic protein) and exhibit comparable K$_D$ values for [^{3}H]-2,3,7,8-TCDD binding (93); these levels show no correlation between their maximal hepatic AHH inducibility or susceptibility to the toxic effects of 2,3,7,8-TCDD and related halogenated aryl hydrocarbons (93, 97, 108). For several mammalian cells in culture there is no correlation between receptor levels and their AHH inducibility (98, 99, 111–113). Recent studies by Whitlock and co-workers indicate "that transcription of the cytochrome P_1-450 gene is under both positive and negative control by at least two trans-acting regulatory factors" (113). The factors that control cytochrome P_1-450 in variant mouse heptoma cells may also play a role in some animal species and requires further investigation. It is apparent that response specificity to Ah receptor ligands is a highly complex process that depends not only on receptor levels but also on many other factors, an observation not unique to the Ah receptor protein (113, 114).

Structure-Activity Relationships

RECEPTOR BINDING AFFINITIES OF PCDDs AND PCDFs: SUBSTITUTION EFFECTS   Poland, Glover & Kende first reported the relative binding affinities of 23 halogenated dibenzo-p-dioxins and dibenzofurans using the dextran charcoal receptor assay and [³H]-2,3,7,8-TCDD as the competing radioligand (85). This study included 10 PCDD congeners and 7 PCDF congeners that differed only with respect to their degree of chlorination and substitution pattern. Table 1 summarizes results from a more recent study of the effects of structure on the receptor binding affinities of 14 PCDDs and 14 PCDFs using rat hepatic cytosol and the sucrose density gradient assay procedure (47, 51; G. Mason, J. Pikorska-Pilszczynska, B. Keys & S. Safe, unpublished results). 2,3,7,8-TCDD and 1,2,3,7,8-pentachlorodibenzo-p-dioxin were the most avid PCDD competitive binding ligands for displacement of [³H]-2,3,7,8-TCDD from the receptor protein, and their EC_{50} values were 1.0×10^{-8} and 7.9×10^{-8} M, respectively. Inspection of these data clearly demonstrated the importance of the lateral Cl substituents in facilitating the interaction between the PCDD ligands and the cytosolic receptor protein. The relative receptor binding EC_{50} values for a series of tetrachloro isomers were 2,3,7,8- > 2,3,6,7- > 1,3,7,8- > 1,2,3,4-, in the order of decreasing number of lateral substituents. The fivefold difference in the receptor binding activities of the 2,3,6,7- and 1,3,7,8-TCDD isomers illustrates a more subtle structural feature that affects binding. The increased affinity of the former compound must be due to the receptor binding site preference for a vicinal 6,7- (or, 1,2) group over a meta 1,3-dichloro functionality. The data also illustrate that the degree of chlorination of non-lateral sites is an important structural determinant for interaction with the receptor protein. The 2,3,7,8-tetra-, 1,2,3,7,8-penta-, 1,2,3,4,7,8-hexa-, and 1,2,3,4,6,7,8,9-octachlorodibenzo-p-dioxins all contain four lateral Cl substituents; however, there is a marked decrease in their receptor binding avidities with increasing Cl substitution at the nonlateral 1, 4, 6, and 9 positions. The stepwise addition of Cl groups at 1, 4, 6, and 9 would result in several structural changes in the more highly chlorinated PCDDs including increased molecular size and volume, increased lipophilicity, a possible decrease in PCDD coplanarity associated with steric crowding, and decreased

Table 1 The effects of structure on the rat hepatic cytosolic receptor binding affinities and AHH/EROD induction potencies of PCDDs and PCDFs

PCDD	In Vitro EC$_{50}$ (M)			PCDF	In Vitro EC$_{50}$ (M)		
	Receptor Binding	AHH	EROD		Receptor Binding	AHH	EROD
2,3,7,8-	1.0×10^{-8}	7.2×10^{-11}	1.9×10^{-10}	2,3,4,7,8-	1.5×10^{-8}	2.6×10^{-10}	1.3×10^{-10}
1,2,3,7,8-	7.9×10^{-8}	1.1×10^{-8}	1.7×10^{-8}	2,3,4,7-	2.5×10^{-8}	1.8×10^{-8}	1.5×10^{-8}
2,3,6,7-	1.6×10^{-7}	6.1×10^{-8}	1.1×10^{-8}	2,3,7,8-	4.1×10^{-8}	3.9×10^{-10}	2.0×10^{-10}
2,3,6-	2.2×10^{-7}	—	—	2,3,4,6,7,8-	4.7×10^{-8}	6.9×10^{-10}	5.8×10^{-10}
1,2,3,4,7,8-	2.8×10^{-7}	2.1×10^{-9}	4.1×10^{-9}	1,2,3,7,8-	7.5×10^{-8}	2.5×10^{-9}	3.1×10^{-8}
1,3,7,8-	7.9×10^{-7}	5.9×10^{-7}	3.2×10^{-7}	1,2,3,7-	1.1×10^{-7}	2.7×10^{-5}	6.3×10^{-5}
1,2,4,7,8-	1.1×10^{-6}	2.1×10^{-8}	1.1×10^{-8}	1,3,4,7,8-	2.0×10^{-7}	1.6×10^{-9}	1.4×10^{-9}
1,2,3,4-	1.3×10^{-6}	3.7×10^{-6}	2.4×10^{-6}	2,3,4,7,9-	2.0×10^{-7}	7.9×10^{-9}	5.8×10^{-9}
2,3,7-	7.1×10^{-6}	3.6×10^{-7}	1.4×10^{-7}	2,3,4,8-	2.0×10^{-7}	4.1×10^{-8}	3.8×10^{-8}
2,8-	3.2×10^{-6}	$>1.0 \times 10^{-4}$	$>1.0 \times 10^{-4}$	1,2,3,4,7,8-	2.3×10^{-7}	3.6×10^{-10}	3.8×10^{-10}
1,2,3,4,7-	6.4×10^{-6}	6.6×10^{-7}	8.2×10^{-7}	1,2,3,6,7,8-	2.7×10^{-7}	1.5×10^{-9}	1.2×10^{-9}
1,2,4-	1.3×10^{-5}	4.8×10^{-5}	2.2×10^{-6}	1,2,3,7,9-	4.0×10^{-7}	8.6×10^{-8}	8.6×10^{-8}
OCDD	$>1.0 \times 10^{-5}$	3.1×10^{-7}	7.0×10^{-7}	1,2,4,7,8-	1.3×10^{-6}	1.1×10^{-7}	1.5×10^{-7}
1-	$>1.0 \times 10^{-4}$	$>1.0 \times 10^{-4}$	$>1.0 \times 10^{-4}$	1,2,4,6,8-	3.1×10^{-6}	1.0×10^{-5}	1.2×10^{-5}

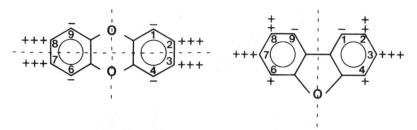

Figure 2   The differential effects of chlorine substituents at different positions in the dibenzo-p-dioxin and dibenzofuran rings on the relative receptor binding affinities of PCDD and PCDF congeners.

aromatic ring electron density (due to the additional electronegative Cl groups). One or more of these changes may be related to the decrease in binding affinities of the more highly chlorinated 2,3,7,8-substituted PCDDs. Figure 2 summarizes the differential effects of Cl substituents on the affinities of PCDDs for the cytosolic receptor protein and illustrates the importance of lateral chloro groups. It has also been suggested that the other critical structural factors that contribute to the high binding affinities of 2,3,7,8-TCDD include the planar ring structure and an ideal ligand area, 3×10 Å (37, 38).

The direct binding of radiolabelled 2,3,7,8-tetrachlorodibenzofuran (TCDF) and other PCDFs to the Ah receptor protein has not been demonstrated. However, the competitive binding affinities of three 2,3,7,8-substituted compounds demonstrated their relatively high binding affinities for the receptor protein (85). The development of new procedures for the synthesis of PCDFs (115) has resulted in the preparation of over 40 congeners that have been used to develop detailed SARs for this series of halogenated aryl hydrocarbons (47, 51). The dibenzofuran ring system possesses a single axis of symmetry (Figure 2); therefore there are four geometrically different positions on each aromatic ring, namely C-1 (or C-9), C-2 (or C-8), C-3 (or C-7), and C-4 (or C-6). A complete SAR for PCDFs as ligands for the receptor protein must distinguish between the differential contributions of all four positions on the dibenzofuran ring. (See Table 1 for compounds selected for this study.) Inspection of these data confirms that the most active congeners, 2,3,4,7,8-penta-chlorodibenzofuran (PeCDF, 1.5×10^{-8} M), 2,3,7,8-TCDF (4.1×10^{-8} M), 2,3,4,6,7,8-hexachlorodibenzofuran (HCDF, 4.7×10^{-8} M), and 1,2,3,7,8-PeCDF (7.5×10^{-8} M) were all fully substituted in their lateral 2, 3, 7, and 8 positions. Moreover, a comparison of the receptor binding EC_{50} values for the 2,3,4,7,8-, 1,2,4,7,8-, and 1,2,4,6,8-PeCDF isomers demonstrates the importance of lateral chloro substituents since there is a decrease in receptor binding affinities with decreasing lateral substitution. Two pairs of PCDF isomers, namely 1,3,4,7,8- and 1,2,4,7,8-PeCDF, 2,3,4,7- and 2,3,4,8-TCDF, differ only with respect to their substitution of C-2 (or C-8) and C-3 (or

C-7). In both cases the C-3 (or C-7) substituted compounds were 6.5–8 times more active than the corresponding C-2 (or C-8) isomers as competitive ligands for the rat hepatic cytosolic receptor protein. A comparison of the relative binding affinities of a series of C-1 (or C-9) and C-4 (or C-6) isomer pairs illustrates the higher binding activities of the isomer that retains the C-4 (or C-6) substituent. For example the EC_{50} values for the 2,3,4,7-, 2,3,4,7,8-, 2,3,4,7,9-, and 2,3,4,6,7,8-substituted PCDFs were 2.5×10^{-8} M, 1.5×10^{-8} M, 2.0×10^{-7}, and 4.7×10^{-8} M whereas the values for the corresponding C-1 (or C-9) isomers (i.e. 1,2,3,7-TCDF, 1,2,3,7,8-, and 1,2,3,7,9-PeCDF, and 1,2,3,6,7,8-HCDF) were 1.1×10^{-7} M, 7.5×10^{-8} M, 3.4×10^{-7} M, and 2.7×10^{-7} M, respectively.

Figure 3 illustrates an overlay of 2,3,7,8-TCDD and 2,3,4,7,8-PeCDF, the two most active PCDD and PCDF ligands for the Ah receptor. The molecular areas and volumes of the dibenzofuran and dibenzo-p-dioxin ring systems are similar, but the spatial orientations of their substituents exhibit marked differences. The C-3 (or C-7) substituents occupy a position between the lateral 2,3 (or 7,8) groups in 2,3,7,8-TCDD and clearly occupy the dominant lateral position in the dibenzofuran ring system. The spatial orientations of the C-4 (and C-6) and C-2 (and C-8) substituents are comparable and exhibit less overlap with the lateral positions of 2,3,7,8-TCDD; the C-1 (or C-9) PCDF-substituents exhibit the least overlap with the lateral positions of 2,3,7,8-TCDD. These observations on the molecular orientations of the dibenzofuran Cl substituents are consistent with the observed SARs for PCDF receptor binding affinities and illustrate the stereospecific nature of the receptor protein-ligand interactions.

RECEPTOR BINDING AFFINITIES OF PCDDs AND PCDFs: A QSAR ANALYSIS   The receptor binding avidities of PCDDs and PCDFs summarized in Table 1 and in other studies (37, 38, 47, 51) not only demonstrate the importance of Cl substitution patterns on ligand-receptor protein complex formation but also show that substituents are important structural determinants for these interactions. For example, the receptor binding EC_{50} values for 2,3,7-trichlorodibenzo-p-dioxin is 7.1×10^{-8} M; replacement of the 7-Cl substituent with H gives 2,3-dichlorodibenzo-p-dioxin, which exhibits a greatly diminished receptor binding EC_{50} value ($> 10^{-5}$ M). It is clear that these substituent effects at this lateral C-7 position must be related to differences in their physicochemical characteristics which in turn influence ligand-receptor avidities. A series of substituted PCDD, PCDF, and polychlorinated biphenyl analogs have been synthesized (Figure 4) as probes for delineating the effects of substituent structure on ligand-receptor binding affinities (116–118). Each series of analogs contains a variable substituent group at a single lateral position, and it is apparent that substituent structure has a remarkable effect on

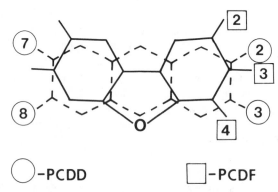

$\bigcirc$-PCDD $\square$-PCDF

Figure 3   Overlay of 2,3,7,8-TCDD and 2,3,4,7,8-PeCDF structures.

the receptor binding avidities of these compounds. For example the EC_{50} value for 7-trifluoromethyl-2,3-dichlorodibenzo-p-dioxin (1.95×10^{-8} M) was 1000 times lower than the value for 7-amino-2,3-dichlorodibenzo-p-dioxin (2.88×10^{-5} M). The effects of different substituents on the activity of a series of analogs can be analyzed quantitatively by correlating the differences in a biological effect (e.g. receptor binding) with known substituent physicochemical parameters (116–119), such as lipophilicity (π), electronegativity (σ), hydrogen bonding capacity (HB), and substituent width (ΔB_5). Multiparameter linear regression analysis of the receptor binding data for sixteen 7-substituted-2,3-dichlorodibenzo-p-dioxins gave the following equation (1):

$$\log (1/EC_{50}) = 1.24\pi + 6.11 \qquad 1.$$

$(n = 14, s = 0.29, r = 0.950),$

where π is the substituent lipophilicity, s is the standard deviation, and r is the correlation coefficient. The only substituents treated as outliers for the derivation of this equation were the bulky C_6H_5 and t-C_4H_9 groups, which possess van der Waals volumes of 48.5 and 41.8 cm^3/mol, respectively. This suggests that substituent molecular volumes are also important structural determinants for determining ligand affinities for the receptor protein binding site. Previous studies with the 4'-substituted-2,3,4,5-tetrachlorobiphenyls indicated that the maximum molecular volume for lateral substituents was < 35 cm^3/mol (118). However it is apparent that if substituent molecular volume requirements are satisfied, the the receptor binding affinities of these analogs are directly related to the lipophilicity of the 7-substituents.

The competitive receptor binding affinities of a series of thirteen 8-substituted-2,3,4-trichlorodibenzofurans and ten 8-substituted-2,3-dichlorodibenzofurans (Figure 4) have also been determined, and the competi-

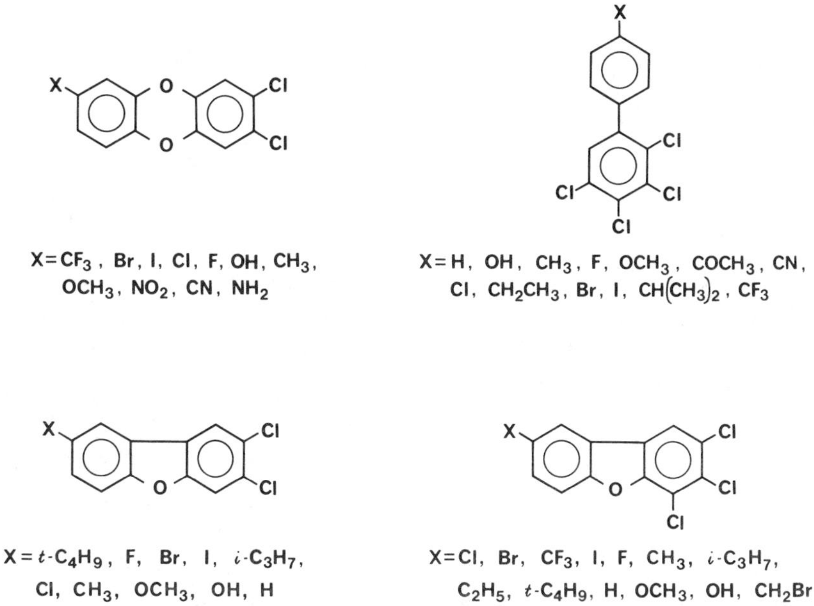

X = CF$_3$, Br, I, Cl, F, OH, CH$_3$,
OCH$_3$, NO$_2$, CN, NH$_2$

X = H, OH, CH$_3$, F, OCH$_3$, COCH$_3$, CN,
Cl, CH$_2$CH$_3$, Br, I, CH(CH$_3$)$_2$, CF$_3$

X = t-C$_4$H$_9$, F, Br, I, i-C$_3$H$_7$,
Cl, CH$_3$, OCH$_3$, OH, H

X = Cl, Br, CF$_3$, I, F, CH$_3$, i-C$_3$H$_7$,
C$_2$H$_5$, t-C$_4$H$_9$, H, OCH$_3$, OH, CH$_2$Br

Figure 4 Structures of substituted PCDDS, PCDFs, and polychlorinated biphenyls used for QSAR studies.

tive displacement binding data results have been analyzed by multiparameter linear regression analysis to give Equations 2 and 3, respectively.

$$\log (1/EC_{50}) = 1.09\pi + 5.77 \qquad\qquad 2.$$

$$\log (1/EC_{50}) = 1.10\pi + 5.19 \qquad\qquad 3.$$

For the 8-substituted-2,3,4-trichlorodibenzofurans, both the t-C$_4$H$_9$ and i-C$_3$H$_7$ were outliers, whereas only the t-C$_4$H$_9$ substituent was not included in the derivation of Equation 3. Analysis of the collective data for 33 substituted polychlorinated dibenzofurans and dibenzo-p-dioxins (Figure 5) has demonstrated the excellent linear correlation between the log (1/EC$_{50}$) receptor binding data and lipophilicity (π). Moreover the slopes and intercepts for Equations 1–3 were not significantly different. These data are consistent with a receptor protein that binds the PCDDs and PCDFs at a common binding site(s) on the protein; this site must accommodate the molecular area and volume encumbered by these ligands, and the QSAR results are consistent with a binding site that is highly hydrophobic.

The effects of substituent structure on the rat hepatic cytosolic receptor binding affinities of 4-substituted-2,3,4,5-tetrachlorobiphenyls have also been

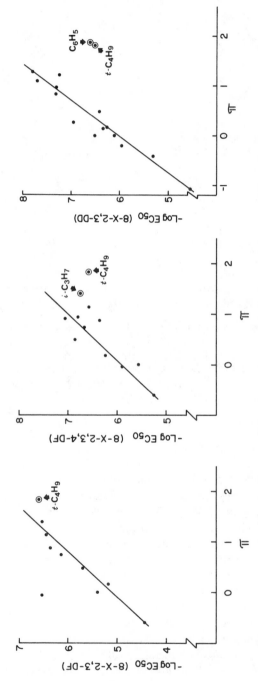

Figure 5   Correlation between receptor binding avidities for the substituted PCDDs and PCDFs vs the substituent lipophilicity (π) values.

reported (118). Multiparameter linear regression analysis of the results of these analogs gave Equation 4, which suggests that substituent lipophilicity, electronegativity (σ) and hydrogen bonding capacity (HB) are factors that influence receptor-ligand affinities:

$$\log (1/EC_{50}) = 1.39 \, \sigma + 1.31\pi + 1.12 \, HB + 4.20 \qquad 4.$$

The bulky t-C_4H_9 and C_6H_5 substituents were also treated as outliers for the derivation of Equation 4. These results demonstrate that substituent molecular volumes play a role in ligand-receptor interactions for the substituted PCBs, PCDDs, and PCDFs. However, the data analysis for the former group of analogs suggests that the critical 4'-substituent for the PCBs interacts with both polar and hydrophobic regions of the receptor binding site. The differences between Equations 1–3 and Equation 4 are somewhat paradoxical since molecular overlap of the four sets of substituted ligands does not indicate that there are major differences in their spatial orientation (Figure 4). Therefore it is likely that the differences observed for the substituted PCBs are due to the free rotation about the Ph-Ph bond and a limited population of the coplanar conformers. Chlorinated biphenylenes that possess a fixed coplanar ring structure exhibit binding affinities comparable to those of 2,3,7,8-TCDD and related isostereomers; this emphasizes the importance of a planar ring system. It is also possible that the receptor binding sites for the substituted PCBs and PCDDs/ PCDF are not identical, a problem currently being investigated in my laboratory.

AHH INDUCTION ACTIVITIES OF PCDDs AND PCDFs   The in vivo and in vitro SARs for PCDDs and PCDFs as inducers of hepatic and extrahepatic AHH have been reported by several groups (37, 38, 47–49, 51–53). The most active PCDDs were substituted in their 2,3,7, and 8 position; inspection of the data in Table 1 indicates that there were comparable SARs for PCDDs as ligands for the receptor protein and as AHH inducers; however, there is not a linear correlation between these two bioassays. SARs for several PCDF congeners as in vitro AHH inducers were comparable to those already discussed for receptor binding. Moreover, for the PCDFs summarized in Table 1 a comparison of in vitro EC_{50} values for AHH induction in rat hepatoma H-4-II E cells and in vivo ED_{50}s for AHH induction in male Wistar rats showed a linear correlation between these two values. Like the PCDD congeners, however, there was not a strong correlation between AHH induction potencies and receptor binding avidities for the PCDF congeners. A comparison of the AHH and EROD induction potencies of the 7-substituted-2,3-dichlorodibenzo-p-dioxins with their rat hepatic cytosolic receptor binding avidities also showed that there was not a linear correlation between the two in vitro activities for this series of analogs (116). Multiple parameter linear regression analysis of the AHH induction results for these compounds gave the following equation:

$$\log (1/EC_{50})_{AHH} = 1.60 \, \pi - 0.33(\Delta B_5)^2 + 5.85 \qquad 5.$$

Like the receptor binding avidities for these substituted PCDDs, their AHH induction potencies were dependent on substituent lipophilicity; however, a second parameter, STERIMOL (ΔB_5) has also been included in the derivation of this equation. The STERIMOL parameter (119) is a measure of the maximum width of the substituents (compared to H) from the axis connecting the 7-substituent to the rest of the molecule and has previously been used in QSAR studies that involve the interaction of substituted organic ligands and macromolecules. The dependence of AHH induction activities by the substituted PCDDs on both ΔB_5 and π suggests that substituent-dependent effects such as conformational changes in the ligand-receptor complex occur after the initial receptor-ligand binding process.

The AHH and EROD induction EC_{50} values for the 8-substituted-2,3-di- and 2,3,4-trichlorodibenzofurans in rat hepatoma H-4-II E cells were also subjected to multiple parameter linear regression analysis to give Equations 6 and 7, respectively (117).

$$\log (1/EC_{50})_{AHH} = 0.80\pi + 0.87\Delta B_5 - 0.35(\Delta B_5)^2 + 4.63 \qquad 6.$$

$$\log (1/EC_{50})_{AHH} = 0.76\pi + 1.11\Delta B_5 + 2.23 \, \sigma_p + 6.78 \qquad 7.$$

Both Equations 5 and 6 showed that AHH induction potencies for the 8-substituted-2,3-dichlorobenzofurans and 2,3-dichlorodibenzo-p-dioxins were dependent on substituent and ΔB_5 parameters. The correlation for the more highly chlorinated set of analogs, the 8-substituted-2,3,4-trichlorodibenzofurans, also includes a Hammett substituent parameter (σ_p); presumably the requirement for σ_p must be due to the effects of the C-4 chlorine group, which constitutes the only structural difference between the two sets of substituted PCDF analogs.

Equations 8–10 were developed from the AHH and EROD induction data for the 8-substituted-2,3-dichlorodibenzo-p-dioxins, -2,3-dichlorodibenzofurans, and -2,3,4-trichlorodibenzofurans, respectively.

$$\log (1/EC_{50})_{EROD} = 0.99 \log (1/EC_{50})_{AHH} - 0.07 \qquad 8.$$

$$\log (1/EC_{50})_{EROD} = 0.90 \log (1/EC_{50})_{AHH} + 0.83 \qquad 9.$$

$$\log (1/EC_{50})_{EROD} = 0.92 \log (1/EC_{50})_{AHH} + 0.28\pi + 0.27 \qquad 10.$$

For a total of twenty-five 7-substituted-2,3-dichlorodibenzo-p-dioxins and 8-substituted-2,3-dichlorodibenzofurans and fifteen 4'-substituted-2,3,4,5-tetrachlorobiphenyls there was a linear correlation between the EC_{50} values for AHH and EROD induction, and the slopes for these equations were not significantly different from that of equation one. These data suggest that both ethoxyresorufin and benzo[a]pyrene are catalyzed by the same cytochrome P-450 isozyme(s). In contrast, Equation 10 required a π term to correlate the effects of the substituted 2,3,4-trichlorodibenzofurans; the rationale for these differences between the two sets of substituted PCDF analogs is unknown.

OTHER BIOLOGIC EFFECTS OF Pcdds AND Pcdfs: STRUCTURE-ACTIVITY RELATIONSHIPS   PCDDs and PCDFs elicit a broad spectrum of species-dependent biologic effects, but because pure standards have been unavailable few studies report qualitative or quantitative SARs for these compounds. The SARs for PCDDs as inducers of ALA synthetase were comparable to the effects of structure on their activities as AHH inducers (48). Knutson & Poland have used cultured XB cells derived from a mouse teratoma as an in vitro model for halogenated aryl hydrocarbon toxicity (120). 2,3,7,8-TCDD and related toxic isostereomers produce a dose-dependent keratinization response which in part resembles the in vivo dermal toxicity that develops in some animals after exposure to these toxins. The most active PCDD congeners in this in vitro assay possessed three or four lateral substituents, and the SARs were similar to those reported for their receptor binding affinities. 2,3,7,8-TCDD causes comparable dermal toxicity in cultures of newborn foreskin keratinocytes (121).

Several human squamous cell carcinoma (SCC) lines have been utilized as model systems for investigating the mechanism of action of toxic halogenated aryl hydrocarbons (110, 122). SCC cells possess variable Ah receptor levels, and the relative amount of receptor in several cell lines correlates with the maximal 7-ethoxycoumarin 0-deethylase inducibility in these cell lines. 2,3,7,8-TCDD causes down-regulation of the epidermal growth factor (EGF) receptor in the SCC-12F cell line, and this effect is dose- and structure-dependent. Both 2,3,7,8-TCDD and 2,3,7,8-tetrabromodibenzofuran, which exhibit a high affinity for the Ah receptor, decrease EGF receptor binding, whereas 2,7-dichlorodibenzo-p-dioxin is inactive (123). Comparable results have been observed in keratinocyte strains derived from normal neonatal foreskin; the authors report that 2,3,7,8-TCDD acts (in part) through the Ah receptor in epidermal basal cells to enhance terminal differentiation (123). 2,3,7,8-TCDD also down-regulates EGF receptor activity in hepatic plasma membranes in several animal species and cultured mouse hepatoma cells (124, 125); however, structure-activity effects in the rat do not necessarily support the role of the Ah receptor in mediating this process (125).

TOXICOLOGY OF PCDDs AND PCDFs: STRUCTURE-ACTIVITY RELATIONSHIPS
The dose-response acute toxicities of nine PCDD isomers and congeners in the
guinea pig and responsive mouse have been reported (33, 34, 126). The
relative LD_{50} values in both species were highly dependent on the number of
lateral Cl substituents and the degree of substitution; their rank order of toxic
potencies was similar to their in vitro receptor binding and AHH induction
activities as discussed above. A comparative study (127) of the toxicity of
2,3,7,8-TCDF, 2,3,7,8-tetrabromodibenzofuran, and 2,3,4,7,8-penta-
chlorodibenzofuran in guinea pigs, mice, and rhesus monkeys confirms that
these compounds elicit the characteristic broad spectrum of toxic effects
observed for 2,3,7,8-TCDD and related isostereomers.

Poland & Glover (75) reported the effects of several PCDD congeners and
other toxic halogenated aryl hydrocarbons on genetically inbred strains of mice.
Although dose-response studies were carried out only with 2,3,7,8-TCDD, the
relative toxicities (i. e. thymic atrophy) of these compounds correlated with
their in vitro binding and induction activities. The dose-response toxicities
(thymic atrophy and body weight loss) of the PCDFs listed in Table 1 have been
determined in the immature male Wistar rat (47). Inspection of the ED_{50} data
for the toxic effects showed that the potencies of these congeners were structure-dependent and that the in vivo SARs for toxicity were identical to those
observed for their in vitro AHH induction potencies. Figure 6 summarizes a plot
of the $-\log ED_{50}$ values for thymic atrophy and body weight loss in immature
male Wistar rats vs their in vitro AHH induction activities. The linear correlation constant (r) and slope for the plots of the reciprocal log values for AHH
induction vs body weight loss were 0.96 and 1.30 (slope), respectively, and
values of 0.88 (r) and 1.16 (slope) were obtained for the comparable plot of the
reciprocal log values for AHH induction vs thymic atrophy. The linear correlation was observed only for those compounds that do not contain vicinal
unsubstituted carbon atoms and are not significantly metabolized. For example,
the toxicity of 1,2,3,7- or 2,3,4,8-TCDF in the rat was lower than predicted by
the in vitro AHH (or EROD) induction data (not shown) owing to in vivo
metabolism. Current research in my laboratory (S. H. Safe, unpublished
results) indicates that for several PCDD isomers and congeners there is a linear
correlation between $-\log EC_{50}$ (AHH induction) and $-\log ED_{50}$ (thymic
atrophy and body weight loss in the rat). These results suggest that the rat
hepatoma cell monooxygenase induction bioassay may serve as a short-term
test system for predicting the toxicities of PCDDs, PCDFs, and related halogenated aryl hydrocarbons.

Poland and co-workers have investigated the effects of 2,3,7,8-TCDD,
several PCDD congeners, and related halogenated aryl hydrocarbons in the skin
of inbred HRS/J hairless mice segregating for the *hr* locus (128, 129). The
homozygous *hr/hr* hairless and heterozygous *hr/+* haired mice exhibit identical

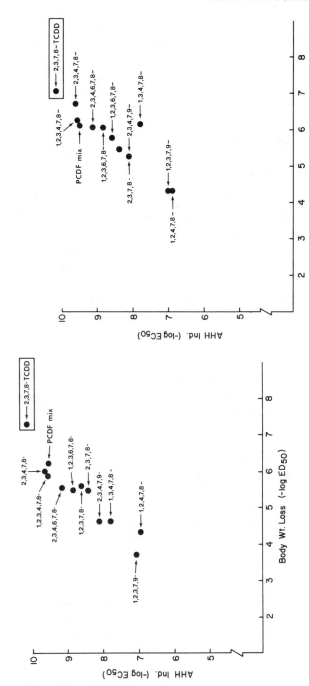

Figure 6 A plot of the −log EC₅₀ values for in vitro AHH induction vs the −log ED₅₀ values for thymic atrophy (right) and body weight loss (left) in the male Wistar rat for several PCDF congeners and 2,3,7,8-TCDD.

genetics except for one allele at the *hr* locus. Topical application of 2,3,7,8-TCDD to the dorsal skin of hairless mice resulted in epidermal hyperplasia, sebaceous gland metaplsia, and hyperkeratosis, but these histological lesions are not observed in *hr/+* haired mice. The development of a graded epidermal response by several PCDD congeners, 2,3,7,8-TCDF, and related toxic aryl hydrocarbons was structure-dependent and correlated with rank order of receptor binding affinities for these compounds (128). For example, the total dose (nmol/mouse) required to produce a 2^+ response was 0.36, 1.76, 1.2 > 360 and > 360 for 2,3,7,8-TCDD, 1,2,3,6,7,8-HCDF, 2,3,7,8-TCDD, 1,3,6,8-TCDD, and 2,7-DCDD, respectively. These results are consistent with the involvement of both the *Ah* and *hr* loci in the development of murine epidermal lesions after exposure to PCDDs, PCDFs, and related toxins. 2,3,7,8-TCDD can also act as a potent tumor promoter in HRS/J mice, and the results of this study confirm the segregation of the activity with the *Ah* and *hr* loci. A qualitative structure-activity study also suggests a possible role for the Ah receptor in mediating the tumor promotion activities of the toxic halogenated aryl hydrocarbons (130).

The SARs for PCDDs and PCDFs clearly support an Ah receptor-mediated mechanism of action for these compounds; comparable studies have been reported for other classes of halogenated aryl hydrocarbons. It is assumed that the persistent effects elicited by these toxins are related to a sustained receptor-ligand occupancy of nuclear binding sites, but this has not yet been demonstrated experimentally. The identity and role of any endogenous ligand(s) for the Ah receptor have not been determined; however, lumichrome, a riboflavin metabolite, does bind to the receptor (131).

Genetic Evidence

Pharmacogenetic studies with genetically inbred strains of mice typefied by the Ah-responsive C57BL/6 and nonresponsive DBA/2 mice have provided strong evidence in support of the role of the Ah receptor in mediating the biologic and toxic effects of toxic halogenated aryl hydrocarbons. Nonresponsive DBA/2 mice contain relatively low levels of hepatic or extrahepatic cytosolic or nuclear Ah receptor (< 1 fmol/mg cytosolic protein), whereas much higher levels of the receptor are detected in responsive strains of mice. The ED_{50} for 2,3,7,8-TCDD mediated hepatic microsomal AHH induction in C57B1/6J mice was 1 nmol/kg whereas this value is at least tenfold higher in DBA/2J mice. In genetic crosses and backcrosses between C57BL/6J and DBA/2J mice the trait or responsiveness to AHH induction is inherited in a simple autosomal mode (50, 132–134). The responsive backcross animals also had detectable hepatic receptor levels (85, 89, 97, 103, 109). The segregation of the toxicity of PCDDs and PCDFs with the Ah locus has been determined primarily with 2,3,7,8-TCDD using both responsive and nonresponsive genetically inbred mice and their crosses and backcrosses. The results illustrate that several toxic effects including teratogenicity, porphyria and hepatotoxicity, immunotoxicity, and body weight loss segregate with the Ah locus (75–80, 135–139). Dermal toxic lesions appear to be dependent on the interaction between the Ah and hr locus as previously noted (128–130). It has also been suggested that additional genetic loci may also be involved in the hepatotoxic effects of 2,3,7,8-TCDD, however this observation requires further substantiation (140).

PCDDs, PCDFs, AND RELATED COMPOUNDS—INTERACTIVE EFFECTS

Although the SARs and toxicology of PCDDs and PCDFs have been extensively studied the interactive effects of PCDD/PCDF mixtures and related compounds are not well understood. 2,3,7,8-TCDD can act as a tumor promoter for several initiators in the rodent liver (141), mouse skin (130), and C3H/10T1/2 cells (142), and as a cocarcinogen causing 3-methylcholanthrene-initiated subcutaneous tumors in nonresponsive DBA/2 mice (143). In contrast, 2,3,7,8-TCDD exhibits anticarcinogen activity in female CD-1 mice (144). These effects are related to the agent's induction of drug-metabolizing enzymes that alter rates of metabolic activation of polynuclear aromatic hydrocarbon initiators. Several studies (51, 53, 120, 145, 146) report the application of in vitro bioassays as short-term tests for assessing the potential toxicity of PCDD/PCDF mixtures; a comparison of the in vitro AHH induction activity of a reconstituted mixture of PCDFs identified in Yusho patients (147) and the toxicity of this mixture (Figure 6) suggest that the effects of the individual PCDFs in this mixture are additive (148). In contrast, the immunotoxicity and AHH induction activity of 2,3,7,8-TCDD in C57BL/6 mice were decreased by coadministering a nontoxic or noninducing dose of 2,3,7,8-TCDF (10 μg/kg) (149). A rational explanation for the antagonistic effects of 2,3,7,8-TCDF is not apparent.

Birnbaum and co-workers (77) have reported that treatment of pregnant mice with a combination of 2,3,7,8-TCDD (3 μg/kg) and a nontoxic dose of 2,3,3',4,4',5-hexachlorobiphenyl (20 μg/kg) resulted in a tenfold increase in incidence in cleft palate compared to those animals receiving only 2,3,7,8-TCDD. A second PCB congener, 2,2',4,4',5,5'-hexachlorobiphenyl, at dose levels of 50 or 25 mg/kg in combination with 2,3,7,8-TCDD (3μg/kg), did not effect the teratogenic potency of the latter compound. Although 2,3,3',4,4',5-hexachlorbiphenyl is less toxic than 2,3,7,8-TCDD, this monortho coplanar PCB congener elicits several receptor-mediated biologic and toxic effects (74). It is conceivable that the interactive effects of 2,3,3',4,4',5-hexachlorobiphenyl and 2,3,7,8-TCDD may be additive if the dose-response curve for the former compound is steep and if the 20 mg/kg dose level is just below the minimum observable teratogenic dose. Current research in my laboratory has demonstrated that administration of several compounds, including several polychlorinated biphenyl congeners, increase hepatic 2,3,7,8-TCDD receptor levels in rats and C57BL/6 mice. Pretreatment of rats and mice with these receptor modulators followed by administration of 2,3,7,8-TCDD results in markedly increased hepatic AHH and EROD induction activities. Both positive and negative modulators and antagonists of the hepatic and extrahepatic cytosolic receptor protein are currently being investigated as probes for delineating the mechanism of action of PCDDs and PCDFs and the role of the receptor protein in mediating these effects. These interactive studies will also be important for assessing the effects of polyhalogenated aromatic environmental pollutant mixtures and their potential human health impact.

ACKNOWLEDGMENTS

The author gratefully acknowledges the financial assistance of the National Institutes of Health (EC-03554), the Environmental Protection Agency, and the Texas Agricultural Experiment Station. The collaboration of G. Mason, M. A. Denomme, K. Homonko, L. Safe, B. Keys, S. Bandiera, T. Sawyer, M. Romkes, J. Piskorska-Pliszczynska, B. Zmudzka, and T. Fujita are gratefully acknowledged.

Literature Cited

1. Bowes, G. W., Mulvihill, M. J., Simoneit, B. R. T., Burlingame, A. L., Risebrough, R. W. 1975. Identification of chlorinated dibenzofurans in American polychlorinated biphenyls. *Nature* 256:305–7

2. Vos, J. G., Koeman, J. H., Van der Maas, H. L., Ten Noever de Brauw, M. C., de Vos, R. H. 1970. Identification and toxicological evaluation of chlorinated dibenzofuran and chlorinated napthalene in two commercial polychlorinated biphenyls. *Food Cosmet. Toxicol.* 8:625–33.

3. Rappe, C., Buser, H. R. 1980. Chemical properties and analytical methods. In *Halogenated Biphenyls, Terphenyls, Napthalenes, Dibenzodioxins and Related Products*, ed. R. D. Kimbrough, pp. 41–76. Amsterdam: Elsevier. 406 pp.

4. Morita, M., Nakagawa, J., Rappe, C. 1978. Polychlorinated dibenzofuran (PCDF) formation from PCB mixture by heat and oxygen. *Bull. Environ. Contam. Toxicol.* 19:665–70

5. Kunita, N., Kashimoto, T., Miyata, H., Fukushima, S., Hori, S., Obana, H.

1984. Causal agents of Yusho. *Am. J. Ind. Med.* 5:45–58

6. Masuda, Y., Yoshimura, H. 1984. Polychlorinated biphenyls and dibenzofurans in patients with Yusho and their toxicological significance. *Am. J. Ind. Med.* 5:31–44

7. National Research Council of Canada. 1978a. *Phenoxy Herbicides—Their Effects on Environmental Quality*, Ottawa NRCC Publication No. 16075, 440 pp.

8. Firestone, D. 1977. Determination of polychlorodibenzo-p-dioxins and polychlorodibenzofurans in commercial gelatins by gas liquid chromatography. *J. Agric. Food. Chem.* 25:1274–80

9. Rappe, C., Marklund, S., Buser, H. R., Bosshardt, H. P. 1978. Formation of polychlorinated dibenzo-p-dioxins heating chlorophenates. *Chemosphere* 7: 269–81

10. Ballschmiter, K., Zoller, W., Scholz, C. H., Nottrodt, A. 1983. Occurrence and absence of polychlorodibenzofurans and polychlorodibenzodioxins in fly ash from municipal incinerators. *Chemosphere* 12: 585–94

11. Buser, H. R., Bosshardt, H. P., Rappe, C. 1978. Identification of polychlorinated dibenzo-p-dioxin isomers found in fly ash. *Chemosphere.* 7:165–72

12. Buser, H. R. 1979. Formation of polychlorinated dibenzofurans (PCDFs) and dibenzo-p-dioxins (PCDDs) from the pyrolysis of chlorobenzenes. *Chemosphere* 8:415–24

13. Olie, K., Vermeulen, P. L., Hutzinger, O. 1977. Chlorodibenzo-p-dioxins and chlorodibenzofurans are trace components of fly ash and flue gas of some municipal incinerators in The Netherlands. *Chemosphere* 6:455–59.

14. Rappe, C., Marklund, S., Bergqvist, P. A., Hansson, M. 1983. Polychlorinated dioxins, dibenzofurans and other polynuclear aromatics formed during incineration and PCB fires. In *Chlorinated Dioxins and Dibenzofurans in the Total Environment,* ed. G. Choudhary, L. H. Keith, C. Rappe, pp. 99–124. Boston: Butterworth

15. Bumb, R. R., Crummett, W. B., Cutie, S. S., Gledhill, J. R., Hummel, R. H., et al. 1980. Trace chemistries of fire: A source of chlorinated dioxins. *Science* 210:385–90

16. Crummett, W. B., Townsend, D. I. 1984. The trace chemistries of fire: review and update. *Chemosphere* 13:777–88

17. Czuczwa, J. M., McVeety, B. D., Hites, R. A. 1984. Environmental fate of combustion-generated polychlorinated dioxins and furans. *Environ. Sci. Technol.* 18:444–50

18. Czuczwa, J. M., McVeety, B. D., Hites, R. A. 1984. Polychlorinated dibenzo-p-dioxins and dibenzofurans in sediments from Siskiwit Lake, Isle Royale. *Science* 226:568–69

19. Rappe, C., Bergquist, P. A., Hansson, M., Kjeller, L-O., Lindstrom, G., et al. 1984. In *Biological Mechanisms of Dioxin Action,* ed. A. Poland, R. D. Kimbrough, pp. 17–25. Banbury Report 18, Cold Spring Harbor Laboratory. 500 pp.

20. Lathrop, G. D., Wolfe, W. D., Albanese, R. A., Moynahan, P. 1984. An epidemiologic investigation of health effects in Air Force personnel following exposure to herbicides. In *Mechanisms of Dioxin Action,* ed. A. Poland, R. D. Kimbrough, pp. 471–74. Banbury Report 18, Cold Spring Harbor Laboratory. 500 pp.

21. Fingerhut, M. A., Halperin, W. E., Honchar, P. A., Smith, A. B., Groth, D. H., Russell, W. O. 1984. An evaluation of reports of dioxin exposure and soft tissue

sarcoma pathology in U.S. chemical workers. In *Biological Mechanisms of Dioxin Action,* ed. A. Poland, R. D. Kimbrough, pp. 461–70. Banbury Report 18, Cold Spring Harbor Laboratory. 500 pp.

22. Fara, G., Del Corono, G., Bonetti, F., Caramaschi, F., Dardanoni, L., et al. Chloracne after release of TCDD at Sevesco, Italy. In *Chlorinated Dioxins and Related Compounds: Impact on the Environment,* ed. O. Hutzinger, R. Frei, E. Merian, F. Pocchiari, pp. 545–59. Oxford: Pergamon 658 pp.

23. Kimbrough, R. D., Falk, H., Stehr, P., Fries, G. 1984. Health implications of 2,3,7,8-tetrachlorodibenzo-p-dioxin (TCDD) contamination of residential soil. *J. Toxicol. Environ. Health* 14:47–93

24. Zack, J., Gaffey, W. 1983. A mortality study of workers employed at the Monsanto Company plant in Nitro, West Virginia. In *Human and Environmental Risks of Chlorinated Dioxins and Related Compounds,* ed. R. Tucker, A. Young, A. Gray, pp. 575–91. New York: Plenum. 823 pp.

25. Masuda, Y., Kuroki, H., Yamaryo, T., Haraguchi, K., Kuratsune, M., Hsu, S-T. 1982. Comparison of causal agents in Taiwan and Fukuoka Japan polychlorinated biphenyl poisoning. *Chemosphere* 2:199–206

26. Hsu, S-T., Ma, C-I., Kwo-Hsiung, S., Wu, S-S., Hsu, N. H-M., Yeh, C-C. 1984. Discovery and epidemiology of PCB poisoning in Taiwan. *Amer. J. Ind. Med.* 5:71–79

27. Kashimoto, T., Miyata, H., Shiriji, K., Tung, T., Hsu, S-T., et al. 1981. Role of polychlorinated dibenzofuran in Yusho (PCB Poisoning). *Arch. Environ. Health* 36:321–26

28. Norstrom, R. J., Hallet, D. J., Simon, M., Mulvihill, M. J. 1982. Analysis of great lakes herring gull eggs for tetrachlorodibenzo-p-dioxins. In *Chlorinated Dioxins and Related Compounds. Impact on the Environment,* ed. O. Hutzinger, R. W. Frei, E. Merian, F. Pocchiari, pp. 173–81. Oxford: Pergamon 658 pp.

29. Van Den Berg, M., Olie, K., Hutzinger, O. 1985. Polychlorinated dibenzofurans (PCDFs): environmental occurrence, physical, chemical and biological properties. *Toxicol. Environ. Chem.* 9:171–217

30. Rappe, C., Buser, H. R., Stalling, D. L., Smith, L. M., Dougherty, R. C. 1981. Identification of polychlorinated dibenzofurans in environmental samples. *Nature* 292:524–26

31. Tiernan, T. O., Taylor, M. L., Garrett, J. H., Van Ness, G. F., Solch, J. G., et al. 1985. Sources and fate of polychlorinated dibenzo-p-dioxins, dibenzofurans and related compounds in human environments. *Environ. Health Persp.* 59:145–158

32. Stalling, D. L., Smith, L. M., Petty, J. D., Hogan, J. W., Johnson, J. L., et al. 1983. Residues of polychlorinated dibenzo-p-dioxins and dibenzofurans in Laurentian Great Lakes fish. In *Human and Environmental Risks of Chlorinated Dioxins and Related Compounds,* ed. R. E. Tucker, A. L. Young, Λ. P. Gray, pp. 221–40. New York: Plenum. 823 pp.

33. Kociba, R. J., Schwetz, B. A. 1982. Toxicity of 2,3,7,8-tetrachlorodibenzo-p-dioxin (TCDD). *Drug Metabolism Reviews* 13:387–406

34. Kociba, R. J., Schwetz, B. A. 1982. A review of the toxicity of 2,3,7,-8-tetrachlorodibenzo-p-dioxin (TCDD) with a comparison of the toxicity of other chlorinated dioxin isomers. *Assoc. Food Drug Officials Quart. Bull.* 46:168–88

35. Lowrance, W. W., ed. 1984. *Public Health Risks of the Dioxins.* New York: Rockefeller University Press. 389 pp.

36. National Research Council of Canada. 1981. *Polychlorinated dibenzo-p-dioxins: Criteria for Their Effects on Man and his Environment.* NRCC Publication No. 18574. 251 pp.

37. Poland, A., Greenlee, W. F., Kende, A. S. 1979. Studies on the mechanism of action of the chlorinated dibenzo-p-dioxins and relted compounds. *Ann. N.Y. Acad. Sci.* 30:214–30

38. Poland, A., Knutson, J. C. 1982. 2,3,7,8-Tetrachlorodibenzo-p-dioxin and related halogenated aromatic hydrocarbons: examination of the mechanisms of toxicity. *Ann. Rev. Pharmacol. Toxicol.* 22:517–24

39. Reggiani, G. 1983. Toxicology of TCDD and related compounds: Observations in man. *Chemosphere* 12:463–75

40. Poiger, H., Schlatter, C. 1983. Animal toxicology of chlorinated dibenzo-p-dioxins. *Chemosphere* 12:453–62

41. McConnell, E. E. 1980. Acute and chronic toxicity, carcinogenesis, reproduction teratogenesis and mutagenesis in animals. In *Halogenated Biphenyls, Terphenyls, Naphthalenes, Dibenzodioxins and Related Products,* ed. R. D. Kimbrough, pp. 109–50. Amsterdam: Elsevier. 406 pp.

42. Matsumura, F. 1983. Biochemical aspects of action mechanisms of 2,3,7,-8-tetrachlorodibenzo-p-dioxin (TCDD)

43. Neal, R. A., Beatty, P. W., Gasiewicz, T. A. 1979. Studies on the mechanisms of toxicity of 2,3,7,8-tetrachlorodibenzo-p-dioxin (TCDD). *Ann. N. Y. Acad. Sci.* 320:204–13

44. Poland, A. 1984. Reflections on the mechanism of action of halogenated aromatic hydrocarbons. In *Biological Mechanisms of Dioxin Action,* ed. A. Poland, R. D. Kimbrough, pp. 109–17. Banbury Report 18, Cold Spring Harbor Laboratory. 450 pp.

45. McConnell, E. E. 1984. Clinicopathologic concepts of dibenzo-p-dioxin intoxication. In *Biological Mechanisms of Dioxin Action,* ed. A. Poland, R. D. Kimbrough, pp. 27–37. Banbury Report 18, Cold Spring Harbor Laboratory. 450 pp.

46. Kociba, R. 1984. Evaluation of the carcinogenic and mutagenic potential of 2,3,7,8-TCDD and other chlorinated dioxins. In *Biological Mechanisms of Dioxin Action,* ed. A. Poland, R. D. Kimbrough, pp. 73–84. Banbury Report 18, Cold Spring Harbor Laboratory. 450 pp.

47. Mason, G., Sawyer, T., Keys, B., Bandiera, S., Romkes, M., et al. 1985. Polychlorinated dibenzofurans (PCDFs): in vivo and in vitro quantitative structure-activity relationships (QSAR). *Toxicol.* 37:1–12

48. Poland, A., Glover, E. 1973. Chlorinated dibenzo-p-dioxins: Potent inducers of δ-aminolevulinic acid synthetase and aryl hydrocarbon hydroxylase II. A study of the structure activity relationship. *Mol. Pharmacol.* 9:737–47

49. Yoshihara, S., Nagata, K., Yoshimura, H., Kuroki, H., Masuda, Y. 1981. Inductive effect on hepatic enzymes and acute toxicity of individual polychlorinated dibenzofuran congeners in rats. *Toxicol. Appl. Pharmacol.* 59:580–88

50. Poland, A. P., Glover, E., Robinson, J. R., Nebert, D. W. 1974. Genetic expression of aryl hydrocarbon hydroxylase activity. Induction of monooxygenase activities and cytochrome P-450 formation by 2,3,7,8-tetrachlorodibenzo-p-dioxin in mice generally "nonresponsive" to other aromatic hydrocarbons. *J. Biol. Chem.* 249:5599–606

51. Bandiera, S., Sawyer, T., Romkes, M., Zmudzka, B., Safe, L., et al. 1984. Polychlorinated dibenzofurans (PCDFs): effects of structure on binding to the 2,3,7,8-TCDD cytosolic receptor protein, AHH induction and toxicity. *Toxicol.* 32:131–44

52. Nagayama, J., Kuroki, H., Masuda, Y., Kuratsune, M. 1983. A comparative study of polychlorinated dibenzofurans, polychlorinated biphenyls and 2,3,7,8-tetrachlorodibenzo-p-dioxin on aryl hydrocarbon hydroxylase inducing potency in rats. *Arch. Toxicol.* 53:177–84

53. Bradlaw, J. A., Casterline, J. L. 1979. Induction of enzyme activity in cell culture: a rapid screen for detection of planar polychlorinated organic compounds. *J. Assoc. Off. Anal. Chem.* 62:904–16

54. Goldstein, J. A., Linko, P. 1984. Differential induction of 2,3,7,8-tetrachlorodibenzo-p-dioxin-inducible forms of cytochrome P-450 in extrahepatic versus hepatic tissues. *Mol. Pharmacol.* 25: 185–91

55. Tukey, R. H., Negishi, M., Nebert, D. W. 1982. Quantitation of hepatic cytochrome P_1-450 mRNA with the use of cloned DNA probe: effects of various P-450 inducers in C57BL/6N and DBA/2N mice. *Mol. Pharmacol.* 22:779–86

56. Tukey, R. H., Nebert, D. W. 1984. Regulation of mouse cytochrome P_3-450 by the Ah receptor studies with P_3-450 DNA clone. *Biochem.* 23:6003–8

57. Kimura, S., Gonzalez, F. J., Nebert, D. W. 1984. The murine Ah locus. Comparison of the complete cytochrome P_1-450 and P_3-450 DNA nucleotide and amino acid sequences. *J. Biol. Chem.* 259:10705–13

58. Thomas, P. E., Reedy, J., Reik, L. M., Ryan, D. E., Koop, D. R., Levin, W. 1984. Use of monoclonal antibodies probes against rat hepatic cytochromes P-450c and P-450d to detected immunochemically related isozymes in liver microsomes from different species. *Arch. Biochem. Biophys.* 235:239–53

59. Serabjit-Singh, C. J., Albro, P. W., Robertson, I. G. C., Philpot, R. M. 1983. Interaction between xenobiotics that increase or decrease the levels of cytochrome P-450 isozymes in rabbit lung and liver. *J. Biol. Chem.* 258: 12827–34

60. Liem, H. H., Muller-Eberhard, U., Johnson, E. F. 1980. Differential induction of 2,3,7,8-tetrachlorodibenzo-p-dioxin of multiple-forms of rabbit microsomal cytochrome P-450: evidence or tissue specificity. *Mol. Pharmacol.* 18: 565–70

61. Baars, A. J., Jansen, M., Breimer, D. D. 1978. The influence of phenobarbital, 3-methylcholanthrene and 2,3,7,8-tetrachlorodibenzo-p-dioxin on glutathione S-transferase activity of rat liver cytosol. *Biochem. Pharmacol.* 27:2487–94

62. Owens, I. S. 1977. Genetic regulation of UDP-glucuronosyltransferase induction by polycyclic aromatic hydrocarbons in mice. *J. Biol. Chem.* 252:2827–33

63. Thunberg, T., Ahlborg, U. G., Wahlstrom, B. 1984. Comparison between the effects of 2,3,7,8-tetrachlorodibenzo-p-dioxin and six other compounds on vitamin A storage, the UDP-glucuronosyl transferase and the aryl hydrocarbon hydroxylase activity in the rat liver. *Arch. Toxicol.* 55:16–19

64. Beatty, P. W., Neal, R. A. 1976. Induction of DT-diaphorase by 2,3,7,8-tetrachlorodibenzo-p-dioxin (TCDD). *Biochem. Biophys. Res. Commun.* 68:197–204

65. Nebert, D. W., Jensen, N., Perry, J., Oka, T. 1980. Associations between ornithine decarboxylase E.C.-4.1.1.17 induction and the Ah locus in mice treated with polycyclic aromatic compounds. *J. Biol. Chem.* 255:6836–42

66. Puhvel, S. M., Ertl, D. C., Lynberg, C. A. 1984. Increased epidermal transglutaminase activity following 2,3,7,8-tetrachlorodibenzo-p-dioxin: *In vivo* and *in vitro* studies in mouse skin. *Toxicol. Appl. Pharmacol.* 73:42–47

67. Kurl, R. N., Lund, J., Poellinger, L., Gustafsson, J-A. 1982. Differential effects of 2,3,7,8-tetrachlorodibenzo-p-dioxin on nuclear RNA polymerase activity in the rat liver and thymus. *Biochem. Pharmacol.* 31:2459–62

68. Sawahata, T., Olson, J. R., Neal, R. A. 1982. Identification of metabolites of 2,3,7,8-tetrachlorodibenzo-p-dioxin (TCDD) formed on incubation with isolated rat hepatocytes. *Biochem. Biophys. Res. Commun.* 105:341–46

69. Poland, A., Glover, E. 1979. An estimate of the maximum in vivo covalent binding of 2,3,7,8-tetrachlorodibenzo-p-dioxin to rat liver protein, ribosomal RNA and DNA. *Cancer Res.* 39:3341–44

70. Weber, H., Poiger, H., Schlatter, C. 1982. Fate of 2,3,7,8-tetrachlorodibenzo-p-dioxin metabolites from dogs and rats. *Xenobiotica* 12:353–57

71. Weber, H., Poiger, H., Schlatter, C. 1982. Acute oral toxicity of TCDD metabolites in male guinea pigs. *Toxicol. Lett.* 14:177–82

72. Rozman, K., Rozman, T., Greim, H. 1984. Effect of thyroidectomy and thyroxine on 2,3,7,8-tetrachlorodibenzo-p-dioxin (TCDD) induced toxicity. *Toxicol. Appl. Pharmacol.* 72:372–76

73. Pazdernik, T. L., Rozman, K. L. Effect of thyroidectomy and thyroxine on

2,3,7,8-tetrachlorodibenzo-p-dioxin - induced immunotoxicity. *Life Sci.* 36: 695–703

74. Safe, S. 1984. Polychlorinated biphenyls (PCBs) and polybrominated biphenyls (PBBs): biochemistry, toxicology and mechanism of action. *CRC Crit. Rev. Toxicol.* 13:319–95

75. Poland, A., Glover, E. 1980. 2,3,7,8-Tetrachlorodibenzo-p-dioxin: Segregation of toxicity with the Ah locus. *Mol. Pharmacol.* 17:86–94

76. Pratt, R. M., Dencker, L., Diewert, V. M. 1984. 2,3,7,8-Tetrachlorodibenzo-p-dioxin-induced cleft palate in the mouse: evidence for alterations in palatal shelf fusion. *Teratogenesis Carcin. and Mutagen* 4:427–36

77. Birnbaum, L. S., Weber, H., Harris, M. W., Lamb, J. C., McKinney, J. D. 1985. Toxic interaction of specific polychlorinated biphenyls and 2,3,7,8-tetrachlorodibenzo-p-dioxin: increased incidence of cleft palate in mice. *Toxicol. Appl. Pharmacol.* 77:292–302

78. Weber, H., Lamb, J. C., Harris, M. W., Moore, J. A. 1984. Teratogenicity of 2,3,7,8-tetrachlorodibenzofuran (TCDF) in mice. *Toxicol. Lett.* 20:183–88

79. Hassoun, E., d'Argy, R., Dencker, L. 1984. Teratogenicity of 2,3,7,8-tetrachlorodibenzofuran in the mouse. *J. Toxicol. Environ. Health* 14:337–51

80. Hassoun, E., d'Argy, R., Dencker, L., Lundin, L. G., Borwell, P. 1984. Teratogenicity of 2,3,7,8-tetrachlorodibenzofuran in BXD recombinant inbred strains. *Toxicol. Lett.* 23:37–42

81. Scheutz, E. G., Wrighton, S. A., Barwick, J. L., Guzelian, P. S. 1984. Induction of cytochrome P-450 in rat liver. *J. Biol. Chem.* 259: 1999–2006

82. Lax, R. E., Baumann, P., Schriefers, H. 1984. Changes in the activities of microsomal enzymes involved in hepatic steroid metabolism in the rat after administration of androgenic, estrogenic and progestational anabolic and catatoxic steroids. *Biochem. J.* 33:1235–41

83. Rumbaugh, R. C., McCoy, Z., Lucier, G. W. 1984. Correlation of hepatic cytosolic androgen binding proteins with androgen induction of hepatic microsomal ethylmorphine N-demethylase in the rat. *J. Steroid Biochem.* 21:243–54

84. Leakey, J. A., Althaus, Z. R., Bailey, J. R., Slikker, W. 1985. Dexamethasone increased UDP-glucuronosyl transferase activity towards bilirubin, oestradiol and testosterone in foetal liver from rhesus monkey during late gestation. *Biochem. J.* 225:183–88

85. Poland, A. P., Glover, E., Kende, A. S. 1976. Stereospecific, high affinity binding of 2,3,7,8-tetrachlorodibenzo-p-dioxin by hepatic cytosol. Evidence that the binding species is the receptor for the induction of aryl hydrocarbon hydroxylase. *J. Biol. Chem.* 251:4936–46

86. Greenlee, W. F., Poland, A. P. 1979. Nuclear uptake of 2,3,7,8-tetrachlorodibenzo-p-dioxin in C57BL/6J and DBA/2J mice. *J. Biol. Chem.* 254:9814–21

87. Carlstedt-Duke, J., Elfstrom, G., Snochowski, M., Hogberg, B., Gustafsson, J-A. 1978. Detection of the 2,3,7,8-tetrachlorodibenzo-p-dioxin (TCDD) receptor in rat liver by isoelectric focusing in polyacrylamide gels *Toxicol. Lett.* 2:365–73

88. Hannah, R. R., Nebert, D. W., Eisen, H. J. 1981. Regulatory gene product of the Ah complex. Comparison of 2,3,7,8-tetrachlorodibenzo-p-dioxin and 3-methylcholanthrene binding to several moieties in mouse liver cytocol. *J. Biol. Chem.* 256:4584–90

89. Okey, A. B., Bondy, G. P., Mason, M. E., Kahl, G. F., Eisen, H. J., et al. 1979. Regulatory gene products of the Ah receptor complex and evidence for its nuclear translocation. *J. Biol. Chem.* 254:11636–48

90. Gasiewicz, T. A., Neal, R. A. 1982. The examination and quantitation of tissue cytosolic receptors for 2,3,7,8-tetrachlorodibenzo-p-dioxin using hydroxyapatite. *Anal. Biochem.,* 124:1–11

91. Gasiewicz, T. A., Rucci, G. 1984. Examination and rapid analysis of hepatic cytosolic receptors for 2,3,7,8-tetrachlorodibenzo-p-dioxin using gel permeation high performance liquid chromatography. *Biochem. Biophys. Acta* 798:37–45

92. Carlstedt-Duke, J. M. B. 1979. Tissue distribution of the receptor for 2,3,7,8-tetrachlorodibenzo-p-dioxin in the rat. *Cancer Res.* 39:3172–76

93. Gasiewicz, T. A. Evidence for a homologous nature of Ah receptors among mammalian species 1984. In *Mechanisms of Dioxin Action,* ed. A. Poland, R. D. Kimbrough, pp. 161–75. Banbury Report 18, Cold Spring Harbor Laboratory. 500 pp.

94. Kahl, G. F., Friederici, D. E., Bigelow, S. W., Okey, A. B., Nebert, D. W. Ontogenetic expression of regulatory and structural gene products associated with the Ah locus. Comparison of rat, mouse,

rabbit and *Sigmoden hispedies. Devel. Pharmacol. Ther.* 1:137–52

95. Okey, A. B., Vella, L. M. 1982. Binding of 3-methylcholanthrene and 2,3,7,8-tetrachlorodibenzo-p-dioxin to a common Ah receptor site in mouse and rat hepatic cytosols. *Eur. J. Biochem.* 127:39–47

96. Mason, M. E., Okey, A. B. 1982. Cytosolic and nuclear binding of 2,3,7,8-tetrachlorodibenzo-p-dioxin to the Ah receptor in extrahepatic tissues of rats and mice. *Eur. J. Biochem.* 123:209–15

97. Okey, A. B., Mason, M. E., Vella, L. M. 1983. The Ah receptor: species and tissue variation in binding of 2,3,7,8-tetrachlorodibenzo-p-dioxin and carcinogenic aromatic hydrocarbons. In *Extrahepatic Drug Metabolism and Chemical Carcinogenesis*, ed. J. Rydstrom, J. Bengtsson, pp. 389–93. Amsterdam: Elsevier

98. Miller, A. G., Israel, D., Whitlock, J. P. 1983. Biochemical and genetic analysis of variant mouse hepatoma cells defective in the induction of benzo[a]pyrene metabolizing enzyme activity. *J. Biol. Chem.* 258:3523–27

99. Okey, A. B., Bondy, G. P., Mason, M. E., Nebert, D. W., Forster-Gibson, C. J., et al. 1980. Temperature-dependent cytosol-to-nucleus translocation of the Ah receptor for 2,3,7,8-tetrachlorodibenzo-p-dioxin in continuous cell culture lines. *J. Biol. Chem.* 255:11415–22

100. Carlstedt-Duke, J. M. B., Harnemu, U. B., Hogbert, B., Gustafsson, J. A. 1981. Interaction of hepatic receptor protein for 2,3,7,8-tetrachlorodibenzo-p-dioxin with DNA. *Biochem. Biophys. Acta* 672:131–41

101. Whitlock, J. P., Galeazzi, R. 1984. 2,3,7,8-Tetrachlorodibenzo-p-dioxin receptors in wild type and variant mouse hepatoma cells; nuclear location and strength of nuclear binding. *J. Biol. Chem.* 259:980–85

102. Poellinger, L., Kurl, R. N., Lund, J., Gillner, M., Carlstedt-Duke, J. M. B., et al. 1982. High affinity binding of 2,3,7,8-tetrachlorodibenzo-p-dioxin in cell nuclei from rat liver. *Biochem. Biophys. Acta* 714:516–23

103. Gasiewicz, T. A. and Rucci, G. 1984. Cytosolic receptor for 2,3,7,8-tetrachlorodibenzo-p-dioxin. *Mol. Pharmacol.* 26:90–98

104. Gasiewicz, T. A., Ness, W. C., Rucci, G. 1984. Ontogeny of the cytosolic receptor for 2,3,7,8-tetrachlorodibenzo-p-dioxin in rat liver, lung and thymus.

105. Okey, A. B., Dube, A. W., Vella, L. M. 1984. Binding of benzo[a]pyrene and dibenz[a,h]anthracene to the Ah receptor in mouse and rat hepatic cytosols. *Cancer Res.* 44:1426–32

106. Carlstedt-Duke, J. M. B., Elfstrom, G., Hogberg, B., Gustafsson, J. A. 1979. Ontogeny of the rat hepatic receptor for 2,3,7,8-tetrachlorodibenzo-p-dioxin and its endocrine independence. *Cancer Res.* 39:4653–56

107. Poellinger, L., Lund, J., Gillner, M., Hansson, L. A., Gustaffson, J. A. 1984. Physiochemical characterization of specific and nonspecific polyaromatic hydrocarbon binders in rat and mouse liver cytosol. *J. Biol. Chem.* 258:13535–42

108. Okey, A. B., Vella, L. M., Iverson, F. 1984. Ah receptor in primate liver: binding of 2,3,7,8-tetrachlorodibenzo-p-dioxin and carcinogenic polycyclic aromatic hydrocarbons. *Can. J. Physiol. Pharmacol.* 62:1292–95

109. Nebert, D. W., Eisen, H. J., Hankinson, O. 1984. The Ah receptor: binding specificity only for foreign chemicals. *Biochem. Pharmacol.* 33:917–24

110. Hudson, L. G., Shaikh, R., Toscano, W. A., Greenlee, W. F. 1983. Induction of 7-ethoxycoumarin 0-deethylase activity in cultured human epithelial cells by 2,3,7,8 - tetrachlorodibenzo - p - dioxin (TCDD): evidence for a TCDD receptor. *Biochem. Biophys. Res. Commun.* 115:611–17

111. Jones, P. B. C., Miller, A. G., Israel, D. I., Galeazzi, D. R., Whitlock, J. P. 1984. Biochemical and genetic analysis of variant mouse hepatoma cells which overtranscribe the cytochrome P_1-450 gene in response to 2,3,7,8-tetrachlorodibenzo-p-dioxin. *J. Biol. Chem.* 259:12357–63

112. Israel, D. I., Whitlock, J. P. 1984. Regulation of cytochrome P_1-450 gene transcription by 2,3,7,8-tetrachlorodibenzo-p-dioxin in wild type and variant mouse hepatoma cells. *J. Biol. Chem.* 254:5400–2

113. Jones, P. B. C., Galeazzi, D. R., Fisher, J. M., Whitlock, J. P. 1985. The control of cytochrome P_1-450 gene expression by dioxin. *Science* 227:1499–1502

114. Ringold, G. M. 1985. Steroid hormone regulation of gene expression. *Ann. Rev. Pharmacol. Toxicol.* 25:529–66

115. Safe, S., Safe, L. 1984. Synthesis and characterization of twenty-two poly-

chlorinated dibenzofurans. *J. Agric. Food Chem.* 32:68–72

116. Denomme, M. A., Homonko, K., Fujita, T., Sawyer, T., Safe, S. 1985. The effects of substituents on the cytosolic receptor binding avidities and AHH induction potencies of 7-substituted-2,3-dichlorodibenzo-p-dioxins-QSAR analysis. *Mol. Pharmacol.* 27:656–61

117. Denomme, M. A., Homonko, K., Fujita, T., Sawyer, T., Safe, S. 1986. Substituted polychlorinated dibenzofuran receptor binding affinities and AHH induction potencies—a QSAR analysis. *Chem. Biol. Interact.* In press

118. Bandiera, S., Sawyer, T., Campbell, M. A., Fujita, T., Safe, S. 1983. Competitive binding to the cytosolic 2,3,7,8-TCDD receptor: effects of structure on the affinities of substituted halogenated biphenyls—a QSAR approach. *Biochem. Pharmacol.* 32:3803–13

119. Verloop, A. 1983. The STERIMOL approach: further development of the method and new applications. In *Pesticide Chemistry, Human Welfare and the Environment,* ed. J. Miyamoto, P. C. Kearney, pp. 334–44. Oxford: Pergamon

120. Knutson, J. C., Poland, A. 1980. Keratinization of mouse teratoma cell line XB produced by 2,3,7,8-tetrachlorodibenzo-p-dioxin: an in vitro model of toxicity. *Cell* 22:27–36

121. Milstone, L. M., LaVigne, J. F. 1984. 2,3,7,8-Tetrachlorodibenzo-p-dioxin inducers hyperplasia in confluent cultures of keratoinocytes. *J. Invest. Dermatol.* 82:532–34

122. Hudson, L. G., Toscano, W. A., Greenlee, W. F. 1985. Regulation of epidermal growth factor binding in a human keratinocyte cell line by 2,3,7,8-tetrachlorodibenzo-p-dioxin. *Toxicol. Appl. Phrmacol.* 77:251–59

123. Osborne, R., Greenlee, W. F. 1985. 2,3,7,8-Tetrachlorodibenzo-p-dioxin (TCDD) enhances terminal differentiation of cultured human epidermal cells. *Toxicol. Appl. Pharmacol.* 77:434–43

124. Karenlampi, S. O., Eisen, H. J., Hankinson, O., Nebert, D. W. 1983. Effects of cytochrome P_1-450 inducers on the cell-surface receptors for epidermal growth factor, phorbol 12,13-dibutyrate or insulin of cultured mouse hepatoma cells. *J. Biol. Chem.* 258:10378–83

125. Madhukar, B. V., Brewster, D. W., Matsumura, F. 1984. Effects of in vivo administered 2,3,7,8-tetrachlorodibenzo-p-dioxin on receptor binding of epidermal growth factor in the hepatic plasma membrane of rat, guinea

pig, mouse and hamster. *Proc. Natl. Acad. Sci. U.S.A.* 81:7407–11

126. McConnell, E. E., Moore, J. A., Haseman, J. K., Harris, M. W. 1978. The comparative toxicity of chlorinated dibenzo-p-dioxin in mice and guinea pigs. *Toxicol. Appl. Pharmacol.* 44:335–56

127. Moore, J. A., McConnell, E. E., Dalgard, D. N., Harris, M. W. 1979. Comparative toxicity of three halogenated dibenzofurans in guinea pigs, mice and rhesus monkeys. *Ann. N. Y. Acad. Sci.* 30:151–63

128. Knutson, J. C., Poland, A. 1982. Response of murine epidermis to 2,3,7,8-tetrachlorodibenzo-p-dioxin. Interaction of *Ah* and *hr* loci. *Cell* 30:225–234

129. Poland, A., Knutson, J. C., Glover, E. 1984. Histologic changes produced by 2,3,7,8-tetrachlorodibenzo-p-dioxin in the skin of mice carrying mutations that affect integument. *J. Invest. Derm.* 83:454–59

130. Poland, A., Palen, D., Glover. 1982. Tumour promotion by TCDD in skin of HRS/J hairless mice. *Nature* 300:271–73

131. Kurl, R. N. and Villee, C. A. 1985. A metabolite of riboflavin binds to the 2,3,7,8 - tetrachlorodibenzo - p - dioxin (TCDD) receptor. *Pharmacol.* 30:241–44

132. Poland, A., Glover, E. 1975. Genetic expression of aryl hydrocarbon hydroxylase by 2,3,7,8-tetrachlorodibenzo-p-dioxin: Evidence for a receptor mutation in genetically non-responsive mice. *Mol. Pharmacol.* 11:389–98

133. Nebert, D. W., Robinson, J. R., Niwa, A., Kumaki, K., Poland, A. P. 1975. Genetic expression of aryl hydrocarbon hydroxylase activity in the mouse. *J. Cell. Physiol.* 85:393–14

134. Niwa, A., Kumaki, K., Nebert, D. W. 1975. Induction of aryl hydrocarbon hydroxylase in various cell cultures by 2,3,7,8 - tetrachlorodibenzo - p - dioxin. *Mol. Pharmacol.* 11:399–08

135. Jones, K. G., Sweeney, G. D. 1980. Dependence of the porphyrogenic effect of 2,3,7,8-tetrachlorodibenzo-p-dioxin upon inheritance of aryl hydrocarbon hydroxylase responsiveness. *Toxicol. Appl. Pharmacol.* 53:42–49

136. Nagarkatti, P., Sweeney, G. D., Gauldie, J., Clark, D. A. 1984. Sensitivity to suppression of cytotoxic T cell generation by 2,3,7,8-tetrachlorodibenzo-p-dioxin (TCDD) is dependent on the Ah genotype of the murine host. *Toxicol. Appl. Pharmacol.* 72:169–76

137. Clark, D. A., Sweeney, G. D., Safe, S., Hancock, E., Kilburn, D. G., Gauldie, J.

1983. Cellular and genetic basis for suppression of cytotoxic T cell generation by haloaromatic hydrocarbons. *Immunopharmacol.* 6:143–53

138. Vecchi, A., Sironi, M., Canegrati, M. A., Recchia, M., Garattini, S. 1983. Immunosuppressive effects of 2,3,7,8-tetrachlorodibenzo-p-dioxin in strains of mice with different susceptibility to induction of aryl hydrocarbon hydroxylase. *Toxicol. Appl. Pharmacol.* 68:434–41

139. Vecchi, A., Mantovani, A., Sironi, M., Luini, W., Spreafico, F., Garattini, S. 1980. The effect of acute administration of 2,3,7,8-tetrachlorodibenzo-p-dioxin (TCDD) on humoral antibody production and cell-mediated activities in mice. *Arch. Toxicol.* 4:163–65

140. Greig, J. B., Francis, J. E., Kay, S. J. E., Lovell, D. P., Smith, A. G. 1984. Incomplete correlation of 2,3,7,8-tetrachlorodibenzo-p-dioxin hepatotoxicity with Ah phenotype in mice. *Toxicol.Appl. Pharmacol.* 74:17–25

141. Pitot, H. C., Goldsworthy, T., Campbell, H. A., Poland, A. 1980. Quantitative evaluation of the promotion of 2,3,7,8-tetrachlorodibenzo-p-dioxin of hepatocarcinogenesis from diethylnitrosamine. *Cancer Res.* 40:3616–20

142. Abernethy, D. J., Greenlee, W. F., Huband, J. C., Boreiko, C. J. 1985. 2,3,7,8 - Tetrachlorodibenzo - p - dioxin (TCDD) promotes the transformation of C3H/10T1/2 cells. *Carcin.* 6:651–53

143. Kouri, R. E., Rude, T. H., Joglekar, R., Dansette, P. M., Jerina, D. M., et al.

1978. 2,3,7,8-Tetrachlorodibenzo-p-dioxin as cocarcinogen causing 3-methylcholanthrene-initiated subcutaneous tumors in mice genetically nonresponsive at Ah locus. *Cancer Res.* 38: 2777–83

144. DiGiovanni, J., Berry, D. L., Gleason, G. L., Kishore, G. S., Slaga, T. J. 1980. Time-dependent inhibition by 2,3,7,-8-tetrachlorodibenzo-p-dioxin of skin tumorigenesis with polycyclic hydrocarbons. *Cancer Res.* 40:1580–87

145. Sawyer, T., Bandiera, S., Safe, S., Hutzinger, O., Olie, K. 1983. Bioanalysis of polychlorinated dibenzofuran and dibenzo-p-dioxin mixtures in fly ash. *Chemosphere* 12:529–35

146. Gierthy, J. F., Crane, D., Frenkel, G. D. 1984. Application of an in vitro keratinization assay to extracts of soot from a fire in a polychlorinated biphenyl-containing transformer. *Fund. Appl. Toxicol.* 4:1036–41

147. Bandiera, S., Farrell, K., Mason, G., Kelley, M., Romkes, M., et al. 1984. Comparative toxicities of the polychlorinated dibenzofuran (PCDF) and biphenyl (PCB) mixtures in Yusho victims. *Chemosphere* 13:507–12

148. Sawyer, T., Safe, S. 1985. In vitro AHH induction by polychlorinated biphenyl and dibenzofuran mixtures: additive effects. *Chemosphere* 14:79–84

149. Rizzardini, M., Romano, M., Tursi, F., Salmona, M., Vecchi, A., et al. 1983. Toxicological evaluation of urban waste emissions. *Chemosphere* 12:559–64

Ann. Rev. Pharmacol. Toxicol. 1986. 26:401–26

OBSERVATIONS ON THE PHARMACOLOGY OF GLAUCOMA

Irving H. Leopold and Efraim Duzman

Department of Ophthalmology, University of California, Irvine, California 92717

CLASSIFICATION OF GLAUCOMA

Glaucoma is a term frequently used to describe a group of diseases character-ized by progressive atrophy of the optic nerve head (evidenced by cupping of the optic disc) accompanied by a gradual loss of the field of vision. The intraocular pressure (IOP) is usually elevated and if left untreated can cause further optic nerve damage and irreversible visual loss. In its early stages, cupping of the disc can be recognized as an extension of the central physiologic cup toward the superior or inferior pole of the disc. Recent histopathologic studies show that up to 35% of the axones in the optic nerve can be lost prior to the detection of a visual field abnormality (1). Since cupping can occur prior to loss of vision, the astute physician might be able to detect glaucoma in its very early stages by learning to recognize this diagnostic feature.

When glaucoma is diagnosed, a procedure called gonioscopy of the anterior chamber angle helps to differentiate between the two principal groups of glaucoma, namely open-angle and closed-angle. The most common type is open-angle glaucoma. In this condition, the aqueous humor has free access to the trabecular meshwork in the anterior chamber angle. If the trabecular meshwork in the angle is physically occluded by the bulging of the peripheral iris, the angle is considered closed and the patient is diagnosed as having closed-angle glaucoma. Many subclassifications of these two principal groups of glaucoma exist, as well as other types of glaucoma secondary to inflamma-tion, hemorrhage, trauma, cellular or pigmentary deposits, medication, or fibrovascular membranes.

Much has been written about the etiology of glaucoma. The immediately recognizable causal factor is insufficient drainage of aqueous humor leading to elevated IOP. Most of the therapy in the past has been directed toward correc-tion of this factor. It is now evident that elevated IOP is a secondary phenom-

401

0362-1642/86/0415-0401$02.00

enon and not the specific etiology. However, therapy directed to correct the basic abnormalities producing glaucoma is not yet available. Reduction of elevated IOP by various means is currently the only clinically acceptable treatment for glaucoma.

AQUEOUS HUMOR PATHWAYS

Trabecular Route

Aqueous humor enters the posterior chamber from the ciliary processes as a consequence of (a) hydrostatic and osmotic gradients between the ciliary process vasculature and stroma and the posterior chamber and (b) active ion transport across the ciliary epithelium (2–5). The aqueous humor then flows around the lens, through the pupil into the anterior chamber, and leaves the eye by passive bulk flow by way of two pathways in the anterior chamber angle. One pathway runs through the trabecular meshwork across the inner wall of Schlemm's canal and then into collector channels, aqueous veins, and the general venous circulation. This is called the trabecular or usual route.

Uveoscleral Pathway

The second pathway by which aqueous humor leaves the eye is the uveoscleral pathway. Aqueous humor flows across the iris and the anterior face of the ciliary muscle, through the connective tissue between the muscle bundles of the ciliary body, into the suprachoroidal space, and out through the sclera (5). The bulk of the outflow in experimental species would seem to be by the trabecular route (between 45 and 70%), and the uveoscleral pathway accounts for the remainder (6). However, in human eyes the uveoscleral outflow may account for about 5 to 20% of total aqueous drainage (7).

PHARMACOLOGIC AGENTS USED IN GLAUCOMA THERAPY

Drugs for the control of glaucoma can be divided into at least five subgroups: (a) parasympathomimetic agents, including the cholinergic and anticholinesterase drugs, which act primarily on the musculature of the iris and ciliary body; (b) sympathomimetic agents, which appear to increase the facility of outflow and may also alter aqueous humor formation; (c) sympathomimetic blocking agents, which appear to work mostly by reduction of aqueous humor formation; (d) drugs, such as carbonic anhydrase inhibitors and cardiac glycosides, that diminish the formation of aqueous humor by enzyme inhibition; and (e) osmotic agents, which raise the osmolarity of the plasma and thus extract fluid from the eye.

CHOLINERGIC AGENTS

It has been well known ever since the original observations of Weber regarding pilocarpine (8) and Laqueur regarding eserine (9) that the cholinergic and anticholinesterase agents lower IOP in experimental and in human eyes. Over the years many cholinergic and anticholinesterase agents have been investigated. Cholinergic agonists have been shown to decrease resistance to aqueous humor outflow (10), whereas ganglionic blocking agents and cholinergic antagonists increase resistance (10–13).

Most of the evidence suggests that iris sphincter and/or ciliary muscle contraction physically alters the meshwork configuration so as to decrease resistance; however, not all of the experimental evidence supports this strictly mechanical view of cholinergic and anticholinergic effects on meshwork function. There is the possibility of a resistance-decreasing pharmacologic effect directly on the endothelium of the trabecular meshwork or Schlemm's canal (14–15). This suggests that cholinergics have a direct cytologic effect that produces a decrease in vacuoles in the endothelial cells of the trabecular meshwork. Nomura & Smelser (16) have reported on the identification of cholinergic and adrenergic nerve endings in the trabecular meshwork. Their studies reveal a 6-to-1 proportion of cholinergic to adrenergic nerve terminals located in the posterior part of the trabecular meshwork just anterior to the insertion of the longitudinal ciliary muscle.

Topically applied acetylcholine is rapidly hydrolyzed to inactive choline; its action is too fleeting for therapeutic use as a miotic unless it is given by subconjunctival or intracameral application. When introduced into the anterior chamber during or after surgery, it brings about a marked miosis that lasts about 10 min, and it is effective even after the ciliary ganglion has been blocked by procaine. The vasodilatory action of acetylcholine is considerable, producing a marked congestion after instillation in the conjunctival sac. This is true for cholinergic drugs in general (17–20).

All of the cholinergic agents and particularly the anticholinesterase drugs cause an alteration of the blood-aqueous barrier, which leads to increased protein and cells in the aqueous humor as seen by biomicroscopy. It has been suggested that cholinergic drugs increase blood-aqueous permeability as a result of vasodilation that leads to disruption of the tight junctions in the anterior uveal blood vessels (21).

Anatomically, the longitudinal fibers of the ciliary muscle attach directly to the trabecular meshwork and to the scleral spur. It is postulated that the contractions of these muscle bundles open the trabecular meshwork and thereby enhance aqueous outflow (22). The iris itself is not directly attached to the scleral spur or to the trabecular meshwork, so that its state of contraction or relaxation does not necessarily affect outflow facility (23). Extreme miosis, however, may alter this situation by creating a physiological iris bombé. Ordinarily, minor forward displacement of the iris is more than compensated for by ciliary muscle contraction. But if the chamber angle is very narrow, as in some cases of closed-angle glaucoma, its closure may result from the physiologic iris bombé and miosis. Parasympatholytic drugs like homatropine block contraction of the ciliary muscle and decrease outflow, as the pupil becomes coincidentally mydriatic.

Vacuoles have been demonstrated by electronmicroscopy in the endothelium of the inner wall of Schlemm's canal. In monkey eyes, pilocarpine treatment reduced the number of vacuoles by half. It was hypothesized that, by pulling and stretching of trabeculum, pilocarpine straightens and shortens the channels by which these vacuoles move through the wall of Schlemm's canal, and thus it reduces the chance of their existing in ultrathin sections (24). Studies of the trabecular meshwork and Schlemm's canal have also demonstrated pilocarpine-induced alterations in the size and shape of the intertrabecular spaces and in various characteristics including vacuolization of the inner canal wall endothelium (22, 24–26). At the present time, we do not understand what structure alterations in the meshwork account for the decrease in resistance to bulk outflow caused by ciliary muscle contraction (27). It is still not known whether the cholinergics open entirely new channels, decrease the resistance of some or all of the existing channels, widen Schlemm's canal, or produce some other critical alteration.

Cholinergic Effect on IOP

Krill & Newell (28) reported that a 2% solution of pilocarpine caused a decrease in IOP in both normal and glaucomatous eyes. The drop in IOP in normal eyes was between 8 and 38% and in glaucomatous eyes between 12 and 40%. Diurnal fluctuations in IOP were reduced. The onset of the fall in IOP was seen in 60 min and reached a maximum in 75 min after topical application in both normal and glaucomatous eyes. Very little difference in the drop in IOP was found after instillation of a single drop of either 1 or 10% pilocarpine solution (29–30). This suggests that 1% pilocarpine produces close to the maximal ocular hypotensive effect and that the higher concentration does not provide a greater response. However, the duration of response was greater with 4% than with 1% pilocarpine. There was not much difference between 8 and 4% pilocarpine in duration of response. There appears to be a reduced cholinergic effect in eyes with pigmented irides (31).

Studies have been conducted in which the iris in monkey eyes was totally removed at its root and the ciliary muscle was disinserted at the anterior end, where it normally is attached to the scleral spur (32–33). In these studies, the ciliary muscle retained its normal morphology and its contractability in response to pilocarpine, and the meshwork exhibited its normal light and electronmicroscopic appearance (34).

In these experiments, aniridia has no effect on IOP, resting outflow resistance, or resistance to intravenous or intracameral pilocarpine (27). After total iris removal and ciliary muscle disinsertion, however, there is virtually no acute resistance response to either intravenous or intracameral pilocarpine (33). It seems, therefore, that the acute resistance-decreasing action of pilocarpine and presumably of other cholinomimetics is mediated entirely by drug-induced ciliary muscle contraction with no direct pharmacologic effect on the meshwork itself.

Cholinergic Effect on the Trabecular and Uveoscleral Routes

When perfused through the anterior chamber, radio-tagged albumin or I125 leaves the anterior chamber essentially by bulk outflow through the trabecular and uveoscleral drainage routes. In the eye that has received pilocarpine, radioactive material from the anterior chamber will also be present in the iris stroma, the iris root, the area of Schlemm's canal and the surrounding sclera, and the most anterior portion of the ciliary muscle. In the eye treated with atropine, radioactive material is found in all these tissues but, additionally, is found throughout the entire ciliary muscle and further into the choroid and sclera.

It would appear from these findings that pilocarpine and presumably other cholinergic agonists augment aqueous humor drainage through the trabecular route and diminish drainage through the uveoscleral route. This finding may be explained by the fact that when the ciliary muscle contracts in response to exogenously applied pilocarpine the spaces between the muscle bundles are essentially obliterated, resulting in a reduction in uveoscleral outflow (35). When atropine is instilled, the ciliary muscle relaxes and the spaces are widened; this will usually increase uveoscleral outflow (36).

The drainage through the trabecular route exceeds that through the uveoscleral route. Therefore, when pilocarpine is used, the net result is enhanced aqueous drainage and decreased IOP. In the monkey eye where the drainage through the trabecular and uveoscleral routes is approximately equal, pilocarpine may induce a slight rise in IOP, perhaps by inhibiting uveoscleral drainage more than by increasing trabecular drainage (37).

Cholinergic Effect on Pseudofacility

Pseudofacility is defined as the ultrafiltration component of aqueous humor formation; it is pressure sensitive and decreases with increasing IOP. The term "pseudofacility" is used because a pressure-sensitive decrease in inflow will appear as an increase in outflow when techniques such as tonography and constant pressure profusion are used to measure outflow (4, 6). Researchers have pointed out that pilocarpine may occasionally increase pseudofacility (4, 38).

Cholinergic Effect on Aqueous Humor Formation

How cholinergic agents influence aqueous humor formation is not yet clear. Some results show an increase in aqueous humor formation, others show a decrease, and still others show no alteration at all. It appears that the effects of cholinergic drugs on aqueous humor depend on many factors, but all of the data indicate that these effects are not important in determining the drug-induced decrease in IOP.

Cholinergic Effect on Ciliary Muscle Action

The insertion of the ciliary muscle in the scleral spur provides the outflow channels with the cholinergic smooth muscle that can generate tension on the spur and thereby influence IOP. In addition, the ciliary muscle places tension on the lens zonules, which results in accommodation of the lens. These two physiological responses, even though related, are not always associated. Dissociation has been demonstrated, for example, with the use of ocuserts, by Brown et al (39), who point out that this means of administering a low but constant dose of pilocarpine produces a pronounced decrease in IOP but insignificant refractive changes. It would appear, then, that the energy exerted by the multilayered ciliary muscle in the direction of the lens is not necessarily the same degree of energy exerted in the direction of the scleral spur. Armaly (40) has shown that cholinergic action on pupil size and outflow facility cannot be dissociated.

Subsensitivity to Cholinergic Agents

Sometimes the cholinergic agent that initially was sufficient fails to control IOP in an eye with glaucoma. Loss of responsiveness in these cases may be explained by progression of the glaucoma or by the ciliary muscle becoming subsensitive to stimulation because of the chronic use of cholinergics.

In several studies it has been shown that even after long-term use of pilocarpine the ciliary muscle is still able to contract. For example, Abramson et al (41) examined presbyopic patients with glaucoma, who were on pilocarpine therapy for 1 to 14 years, and presbyopic patients without glaucoma. They were able to demonstrate that a similar increase in lens thickness in response to pilocarpine occurred in both groups.

Similar findings have been reported by Brown et al (39) who found that most glaucomatous patients had refractive changes in response to topical pilocarpine after 1 to 23 months of treatment. It would appear that the ciliary muscle still responds to pilocarpine applications over a long period of time. However, there is no question that IOP may not respond that well in all patients.

There are somewhat different results with strong anticholinesterase agents. Investigations have demonstrated the development of cholinergic subsensitivity in the iris sphincter and in the ciliary muscle with prolonged topical use of cholinesterase inhibitors like phospholine iodide (42, 43). It has been reported that repeated topical treatment with phospholine iodide in monkeys leads to subsensitive responses of accommodation and outflow facility when the animals are later challenged with pilocarpine. The recovery phase to normal sensitivity requires more than one month without drug therapy (44).

Continuous exposure to high levels of any potent cholinergic agonists induces a subsensitivity to all agonists, but subsensitivity to some agonists is more profound than others. Closer analysis of both in vivo physiological and in vitro receptor binding data suggests that differential partial agonism alone may not explain differing agonist potencies in the subsensitive eye. This might be explained by the presence of two or more distinct populations of relevant muscarinic receptors in the iris sphincter and ciliary muscles of cynomolgus monkeys (45).

Anticholinesterase Agents

Isofluorophate-induced miosis is of rapid onset and prolonged duration. In the normal human eye, miosis begins within 5 to 10 min and is maximal within 15 to 20 min. The duration of miosis is from one to four weeks. The maximal miosis appears to be brought about by a solution of 0.05%. A suitable concentration of diisopropyl fluorophosphate (DFP) or isofluorophate eyedrops for therapeutic purposes is 0.01%. The watery drops are unstable, but oily drops of 0.025 to 0.1% in anhydrous peanut oil retain their activity for almost two months.

Topically applied DFP or isofluorophate reduces the IOP of the normal eye with maximal hypotensive effect within 24 hr. The return to normal IOP requires about one week. Ciliary spasm caused by isofluorophate treatment results in myopia that is maximal and lasts for three to seven days (46–47).

Topically applied anticholinesterase agents may be absorbed systemically and may produce depression of serum and red cell cholinesterase. The fewest systemic effects are seen with echothiophate (48).

ADRENERGIC AGENTS

Adrenergic Receptors in the Eye

After adrenergic receptors were classified into α- and β-receptors and then further classified into α_1, α_2, β_1, and β_2, most of these receptor types were found to be present in eye tissues. Even though the full distribution of these receptor subpopulations in eye tissues has not yet been clearly delineated, data exist to indicate that the receptors on the iris dilator muscle are mainly of the α_1

type, and the receptors populating the ciliary body stroma and epithelium and the ciliary blood vessels are mainly of the β_2 type. Both β_2- and α_1-receptors are believed to be present in the trabecular meshwork. The receptors in the retina are believed to be mainly of the α_2 type.

Many agents have been developed that affect one or more subpopulations of receptors. This work has led to the discovery of a number of adrenergic drugs that lower IOP. Most of these agents are able to markedly reduce IOP without the side effects typically associated with parasympathomimetic drugs, but they do have other undesirable features.

Mechanism of Action of Adrenergic Agents

The mechanism of action by which adrenergic agents lower IOP has not been completely elucidated. The present state of knowledge suggests that their action is related to their effects on the various α- and β-receptors located either in the outflow channels or in the inflow apparatus of the ciliary body epithelium and blood vessels. There is also evidence indicating that stimulation of the α-receptors in the outflow channels results in an increase in the facility of aqueous outflow (49–52).

It has been suggested that sympathomimetic drugs reduce the rate of aqueous secretion by stimulating β-receptors (50, 53). A reduction in aqueous secretion could result from a reduced blood flow to the ciliary processes, which has been shown to occur with sympathetic stimulation, but it could also result from direct action on the ciliary epithelium (54). An excellent attempt has been made to review the body of data and analyze the many differences in findings, particularly the small effects seen after pharmacologic doses in several species (55, 56).

Epinephrine

Epinephrine (adrenaline) has been used for many years to reduce IOP in patients with simple glaucoma. Its action in reducing IOP appears to result from a combination of many factors, none of which are absolutely established.

Glaucoma patients differ in their responses to epinephrine treatment. Some patients respond within hours, others respond only after continued use for weeks or months, and some do not respond at all to topically administered epinephrine. Differences in response may reflect the extent of the disease, the damage to the anterior chamber angle, the amount of pigment in the eye, or other factors presently unknown. In some patients, epinephrine initially reduces IOP but later becomes ineffective. This type of reduced response might be due to loss of adrenergic receptors with continued epinephrine treatment, as has been recently demonstrated in the cornea (57). Age may also play an important role in the response of the human eye to epinephrine (58).

Neufeld (59) has pointed out that topically administered epinephrine may have an influence on the ciliary processes and the formation of aqueous humor. It influences aqueous secretion associated with active transport of ions by stimulating a cyclic adenosine monophosphate (AMP) mediated pathway in the nonpigmented epithelium. In addition, it probably influences ultrafiltration that is due to pressure-dependent flow by ordering the profusion pressure in the vascular bed. However in what direction, that of increased or decreased inflow, is the net effect of epinephrine? The observations of Macri (60) suggest that epinephrine decreases ultrafiltration. Recent aqueous fluorophotometric measurements, however, suggest that topical epinephrine increases inflow (61).

Early tonographic studies led to the conclusion that topical epinephrine acts primarily by decreasing the rate of aqueous humor production (62–65). Many subsequent clinical studies have demonstrated improvement in outflow facility with topical epinephrine treatment. Ballintine & Garner (66) found that outflow facility improved by 50% in almost half their patients within one month after the addition of epinephrine to the treatment regimen. Becker et al (67) also reported significant increases in outflow facility three to six months after initiation of epinephrine treatment. In a more recent study (68), it was confirmed that after several weeks of epinephrine therapy outflow facility was improved by 30%.

Yablonski (69) has pointed out that since epinephrine is an α-, β_1, and β_2-agonist, it is not surprising that its effect on IOP is the result of several independent alterations in the aqueous humor dynamics of the eye. The study concluded that IOP is determined by the interaction of four independent factors: (a) the rate of aqueous humor formation, (b) the outflow facility, (c) uveoscleral flow, and (d) episcleral venous pressure. All but the last—episcleral venous pressure—are affected by topical epinephrine.

CLINICAL USE OF EPINEPHRINE   Topical administration of epinephrine reduces IOP in patients with open-angle glaucoma but has only a slight effect in normal eyes (70). Although concentrations as low as 0.125% do have some ocular hypotensive effect, a 1% concentration is substantially more effective (71). Epinephrine constricts conjunctival vessels, contracts the pupil dilator muscle, and may dilate the pupil after topical application. It relaxes the ciliary muscle only slightly, so cycloplegia does not occur.

Topical application of epinephrine often results in ocular discomfort and conjunctival irritation with transient burning or stinging, lacrimation, and pain around or in the eye. Occasionally, conjunctival allergy will occur. Adverse corneal effects include epithelial edema, endothelial cell toxicity, and adrenochrome deposits (72). Visual haze and, rarely, central scotoma can occur but are reversible when epinephrine therapy is discontinued. Dramatic visual acuity decreases have been reported occasionally, especially in aphakic patients (72).

In 20 to 30% of aphakic patients, macular edema occurs but, again, usually disappears when epinephrine treatment is discontinued (73).

The following systemic effects have been associated with topical application of epinephrine: palpitations, faintness, tachycardia, extrasystoles, cardiac arrhythmia, hypertension, anxiety, trembling, sweating, and pallor. Many of these systemic side effects can be avoided by punctal occlusion for 15 to 30 sec after application of the drug. Punctal occlusion prevents drainage of the drug into the nasopharynx, where it may be systemically absorbed (72).

Dipivefrin (Propine®)

Dipivalyl epinephrine (dipivefrin) is a prodrug formed by diesterification of epinephrine. It has been shown to lower IOP when given in concentrations approximately one-tenth of those used for epinephrine (74). Most glaucoma patients respond well to dipivefrin treatment (75, 76). Dipivefrin was developed because of concern about the side effects of epinephrine.

Epinephrine has been established as a valuable drug for glaucoma therapy. However, its use is often limited by a high incidence of adverse reactions. Some of these reactions, such as reactive hyperemia, blepharitis, and localized pain and itching, may be related to the local concentration of epinephrine or its degradation products in the conjunctival sac. The fact that the maximum effect of dipivefrin on IOP occurs with a concentration one-tenth (0.1%) of that required for epinephrine (1%) and the fact that dipivefrin must be activated by an esterase indicate that it can be used to avoid the side effects of epinephrine on the conjunctiva and lids. Dipivefrin resides in the conjunctival sac in a molecular form other than epinephrine, thus decreasing the likelihood of a conjunctival or allergic reaction to epinephrine. In a 0.1% concentration, dipivefrin has demonstrated ocular hypotensive effectiveness and good tolerance in patients who have displayed intolerance to epinephrine (77).

It would also seem that systemic reactions to epinephrine, such as cardiac arrythmias and elevated systemic blood pressure, are less likely to occur with dipivefrin, since these reactions relate to the total amount of epinephrine administered. As similar intraocular concentrations of epinephrine are thought to result with topical administration of both dipivefrin and epinephrine, one would not anticipate any significant difference between dipivefrin and epinephrine in the incidence of aphakic epinephrine-induced maculopathy.

α-Adrenergic Agents

α-ADRENERGIC AGONISTS   Drugs with agonistic effects on either the α_1- or α_2-receptors are currently not being used for the treatment of glaucoma, mainly because the efficacy of available α-agonists has not been proven. Topically applied phenylephrine produces a small reduction in IOP, but it is much less effective than topical epinephrine. Phenylephrine pivalate penetrates the eye much better than phenylephrine, but its effect on IOP is still minimal. Naphazoline, tetrahydrozaline, and oxymetazoline are used clinically as vasoconstrictors and also have limited effects on IOP. Topically applied to rabbit eyes, methoxamine produced a dose-related early rise in IOP followed by a reduction that lasted six to eight hours.

Selective α-adrenergic agents may have value in the management of glaucoma, but we are just beginning to understand their actions in the eye. Increased understanding should aid in the selection of drugs to treat elevated IOP.

Clonidine   Clonidine is a relatively specific α_2-adrenergic agonist used clinically as a potent systemic antihypertensive drug (78). Topically applied in normal and glaucomatous human eyes, clonidine causes a significant decrease in IOP (79–84). In one study clonidine had no effect on the tonographic facility of outflow (82), but in another study clonidine caused a 5 to 15% improvement in outflow facility (84).

Topically applied clonidine has both local and systemic circulatory effects. It decreased episcleral venous pressure in both treated and untreated fellow eyes of normal and glaucomatous human subjects (81–83). In concentrations of 0.25 and 0.5%, clonidine caused a dose-dependent decrease in the diastolic and systolic ophthalmic arterial pressures in patients with open-angle glaucoma (85–86), but in a 0.125% concentration it caused little or no decrease in systemic blood pressure (79, 80, 83–85). Clonidine has been shown not to affect pupil size (79–80) or visual acuity (80).

In one study by Allen & Langham (87), topically applied 0.125% clonidine caused a significant decrease in the IOP of treated eyes and a small but significant decrease in untreated fellow eyes. Aqueous humor flow was significantly lower (by 21%) in clonidine-treated eyes than in untreated fellow eyes. The decreases in IOP and aqueous humor flow were associated with decreases in pupil size in both eyes (although greater in the clonidine-treated eyes) and in systolic blood pressure. It appears from these findings that topically administered clonidine has both local and systemic effects.

The mechanism for the decrease in aqueous humor flow is unclear. Clonidine may decrease flow by reducing ciliary blood circulation. Local and systemic effects could be involved in the reduction of ciliary blood flow. Clonidine may also decrease aqueous flow through its effect on α-adrenergic receptors in the ciliary body, but other studies of α-adrenergic agents have demonstrated very small and usually insignificant effects on flow (61, 88–91).

The possibility remains that the effect of clonidine on aqueous humor flow may be independent of and unrelated to its α-adrenergic actions. Future study of other relatively specific α-adrenergic drugs should help to better define the effects of these drugs on aqueous humor flow in the human eye.

α-ADRENERGIC ANTAGONISTS   A number of α-adrenergic blocking agents given systemically or topically have been shown to lower IOP in experimentally ocular hypertensive rabbits (92–94).

Dibenamine has to be administered intravenously and lowers IOP by reducing the secretion of aqueous humor (95). Phenoxybenzamine, or dibenyline, has an action similar to that of dibenamine, i.e. the blockade of α-receptors. It reduces IOP in acute angle-closure glaucoma but appears to have no effect on IOP in simple glaucoma (96).

Phenoxybenzamine, a noncompetitive long-acting antagonist, has been shown to lower IOP in normotensive and in experimentally ocular hypertensive rabbits when given systemically or topically (92, 97). Yohimbine, an indolealkylamine alkaloid with chemical similarity to reserpine, is a selective α_2-blocker. In rabbits, yohimbine lowers IOP (98), but its ocular hypotensive effect in higher mammals has not been demonstrated.

Prazosin   In 1979, Smith et al (94) reported that topical application of concentrations of 0.0001 to 0.1% of the α-adrenergic antagonist prazosin reduced IOP in normotensive rabbits. The maximum effect of 0.1% prazosin occurred at two hours and lasted for almost eight hours; the drop was about 6 to 7 mm Hg. Sympathectomy did not eliminate the ocular hypotensive action of prazosin, however, and reduced it only slightly. It appears that prazosin may not lower IOP by blocking endogenous catecholamine activity. In the studies of Smith et al, the drop in IOP was not associated with a fall in systemic blood pressure.

Krupin et al (99) confirmed the observation that the effect of prazosin on IOP in rabbits was not due to a systemic effect on blood pressure. They also demonstrated a decrease in the rate of aqueous humor formation and showed that prazosin-induced reductions in IOP could be prevented by systemic pretreatment with the α-adrenergic blocker phentolamine, but not with propranolol or atropine.

β-*Adrenergic Agents*

β-ADRENERGIC AGONISTS   At the molecular level, stimulation of β-adrenergic receptors leads to activation of membrane-bound adenyl cyclase and an accelerated rate of production of intracellular cyclic AMP. The ciliary processes contain predominantly β_2-receptors (100); β_2 stimulation is an especially effective way to lower IOP (101). However, as has been pointed out by many researchers (55, 102–106), the use of β_2-agonists is often accompanied by disappointing results, including rapid loss of ocular hypotensive effect, ocular hyperemia, and tachycardia.

Reviews by Mishima (55) and Potter (56) suggest that α-adrenoreceptors mediate increases in true outflow while β-adrenoreceptors mediate changes in inflow. The site of action for the effects of α-reception on outflow is probably trabecular, and the effects are modest in comparison with increases produced by the action of cholinergics on the ciliary muscle. The site of action for the β-agonist-induced reduction in inflow is in some part of the ciliary epithelium, possibly the nonpigmented epithelium. Uveoscleral flow is also increased by adrenergic agonists (6, 107–109).

Isoproterenol, a β-adrenergic agonist, has been found to lower IOP (102); however, its clinical usefulness is limited by erratic results and consistent production of tachycardia in elderly patients (102, 103). The results of several studies (50, 103, 110) suggest that isoproterenol reduces aqueous humor formation, but the studies of Bill (108) suggest that the drug increases aqueous humor formation. Two other β-adrenergic agonists, salbutamol and metaproterenol, have been found to increase aqueous formation (111–113).

Brubaker & Gaasterland (113) were unable to demonstrate either a lowering of IOP with isoproterenol or an effect of isoproterenol on the flow of aqueous humor in the normal eye. It may be that the effect on flow in their studies was too small or too transient to be detected with their study methods or at the time period they chose to measure IOP. The effect of isoproterenol on IOP might, of course, be due to other factors that were not measured, such as uveoscleral flow.

Selective β₂-agonists   Several β-agonists (salbutamol, terbutaline, soterenol) that have greater affinity for β_2-receptors than for β_1-receptors are being used systemically to treat asthma. These drugs have also been shown to lower IOP in monkeys (104) and humans (114–115). Topical application of 4% salbutamol significantly lowers IOP in human eyes. The reduction in IOP seems to be mainly a result of reduction in aqueous humor production; however, an increase in both trabecular and uveoscleral outflow may also play an important role (116). Substantial conjunctival injection and eye pain experienced by patients using the drug, as well as rapid tachyphylaxis developing within a few weeks, limit the usefulness of this drug for the treatment of glaucoma.

Nonselective β-agonists   Isoxuprine and nylidrine are nonselective β-agonists. They are phenylisopropylamines, very similar to ephedrine, and they act indirectly by increasing the β-vascular effect of endogenous catecholamines. Topical isoxuprine and nylidrine in 1% solution have been shown effective in lowering IOP in glaucomatous eyes but have also been associated with miosis and conjunctival hyperemia (117).

β-ADRENERGIC ANTAGONISTS   A variety of β-adrenergic antagonists have been reported to lower IOP when administered topically or systemically to normal volunteers or glaucomatous patients (118). Topical β-blockers have become the most popular agents for the medical management of glaucoma.

Many clinical trials and several years of clinical experience with thousands of patients receiving these drugs strongly support excellent long-term ocular hypotensive efficacy.

Mechanism of action of β-adrenergic antagonists   Most of the data for experimental animals, particularly for those with artificially elevated IOP, suggest that the reduction of aqueous humor inflow is a local action of the drug upon the eye. The decrease in IOP sometimes seen in the untreated contralateral eye after topical administration of a β-adrenergic antagonist in the treated eye is usually less than the decrease in the treated eye. It has been suggested that the effect in the treated eye is a local phenomenon and that the effect in the contralateral eye is a result of systemic absorption.

Although the existing data support a local action of the β-adrenergic antagonist timolol, there still remains a question as to whether the ocular hypotensive activity is related directly to an ability to block β-adrenergic receptors. Schmitt et al (119) could find little relationship between the ability of timolol, propranolol, alprenolol, oxprenolol, and practolol to antagonize the IOP lowering effect of isoproterenol in water-loaded rabbits and the ability of these agents to lower IOP. The ability of these β-adrenergic blocking agents to antagonize isoproterenol-induced elevation of aqueous humor cyclic AMP was also not correlated with their ocular hypotensive activity.

Alprenolol effectively lowered IOP but exhibited little or no activity in antagonizing either the effects of isoproterenol on IOP or cyclic AMP. Oxprenolol, on the other hand, had little or no ocular hypotensive activity but was very active in antagonizing both actions of isoproterenol. All of these agents penetrated the anterior chamber readily. At this point, there is no explanation for the fact that both β-adrenergic antagonists and agonists lower IOP and reduce aqueous flow in humans and animals. There may be an as yet undefined mechanism unrelated to classical β-adrenergic blockade that accounts for the hypotensive action of these agents.

The formation of aqueous humor appears to decrease after topical treatment with timolol (120–121), while the outflow facility seems to remain unchanged (68, 122). The ability to decrease the formation of aqueous humor implies that timolol is active in the ciliary processes and affects secretion or ultrafiltration or both.

The exact mechanism by which topical β-blocking agents affect the formation of aqueous humor is not known. Perhaps timolol and other β-blocking agents are interfering with the normal β-adrenergic stimulation of the ciliary processes that promotes the everyday production of aqueous humor. There is some evidence that agents such as epinephrine or isoproterenol may transiently increase the formation of aqueous humor in rabbits, monkeys, and humans (61, 108, 123). Whether the primary influence of the topical β-blockers is exerted on the vascular smooth muscle or on the epithelium of the ciliary processes is not known (124).

It is also possible that the β-adrenergic antagonism of the vascular smooth muscle receptors may block vasodilation, promote vasoconstriction in the anterior ciliary arterioles, and thus reduce ultrafiltration by decreasing the capillary perfusion pressure. This reduction in blood flow would also indirectly decrease secretion. As Bartels & Neufeld (124) have pointed out, the β-blocking agent may directly block tonic stimulation to secretory epithelium. Such a mechanism mediated by cyclic AMP has been found in many transporting epithelia and has been suggested but not demonstrated in the ciliary processes.

In summary, the mechanism of action of the β-blocking agents in lowering IOP has not been fully established. It has been shown that β-blockers substantially reduce aqueous humor formation, and it has been suggested that they may do this independent of their interaction with β-adrenergic receptors of the ciliary processes. Recently, Liu & Chiou (125) have shown that the *dextro*-isomer of timolol, which has low affinity for β-receptors, may be as effective in decreasing aqueous flow as the *levo*-isomer of timolol. This may support the idea of some other mechanism being responsible for the decrease in IOP.

Agents that Affect Both α- and β-Receptors: Labetalol

Labetalol is a unique compound with both α- and β-blocking activity. The drug has been used for the treatment of patients with systemic hypertension resulting from a variety of etiologies (126). In rabbit eyes, topically applied labetalol in concentrations ranging from 0.01 to 1% was shown to reduce IOP (127). The mechanism by which this pressure reduction occurs is unclear. It seems that some mechanism other than α- and β-blockade is involved (128). The ocular hypotensive effect of labetalol in humans is negligible (129–130).

Agents that Affect Postganglionic Neuron Function

GUANETHIDINE   The effect of guanethidine on the sympathetic nervous system might continue through several phases, depending on the frequency and the duration of therapy. Initially, guanethidine interferes with norepinephrine released from postganglionic sympathetic nerves on stimulation. It also interferes with the re-uptake of norepinephrine from the synapse into the sympathetic nerve terminals (131). Long-term guanethidine therapy leads to depletion of norepinephrine in nerve terminals (chemical sympathectomy). This reaction is reversible within a week or two after discontinuation of guanethidine therapy (132).

Topically administered guanethidine in concentrations ranging from 1 to 10% significantly reduces IOP in humans; some tachyphylaxis has been reported with long-term therapy. The mechanism of action is presumed to be through amplification of intrinsic adrenergic mediators. Early mydriasis, conjunctival injection, and corneal epithelial toxicity evidenced by punctate keratitis have been reported with topical guanethidine treatment. With chronic therapy, when partial adrenergic denervation develops, miosis and ptosis may occur.

Medications combining guanethidine and epinephrine in a variety of concentrations have been found to be clinically useful; guanethidine seems to potentiate the ocular hypotensive effect of epinephrine (133–134).

Two other drugs that may affect postganglionic function are 6-hydroxydopamine and pargyline. 6-Hydroxydopamine completely and selectively destroys peripheral sympathetic nerve terminals in the anterior segment of the eye. This reversible chemical sympathectomy causes a supersensitivity to exogenously administered catecholamines (135). 6-Hydroxydopamine induces supersensitivity to topically applied epinephrine in patients with open-angle glaucoma (136). Pargyline is a monoamine oxidase (MAO) inhibitor; its application to the eye may activate intrinsically present as well as extrinsically administered epinephrine to cause a reduction in IOP (137–138).

Agents that Stimulate Adenylate Cyclase Directly: Forskolin

Forskolin is a dipertene that acts directly on the enzyme adenylate cyclase without cell surface mediation to increase intracellular levels of cyclic adenosine monophosphate. Forskolin has been shown to lower IOP in experimental animals and in humans (139–142).

Cannabinoids

Cannabinoid drugs—Δ9-tetrahydrocannabinol (THC), SP-1, and SP-106—have been shown to decrease IOP in intact, normal eyes and in ganglionectomized eyes (143), which indicates that these drugs may have ocular and extraocular sites of action. The direct effect of THC on IOP in the ganglionectomized eye could be inhibited in part by phenoxybenzamine and sotalol, which suggests that THC has local α- and β-adrenoceptor activity. Cannabinoids also seem to have an effect on the central nervous system, evidenced by the observation that in rabbits ganglionectomy and preganglionectomy partially inhibit the fall in IOP produced by these drugs.

Drugs that Affect Sodium/Potassium ATPase

SODIUM VANADATE   Vanadate given either as sodium metavanadate (NAVO-3) or sodium orthovanadate (NAVO-4) lowers IOP in rabbits (144). The fall in IOP is not associated with significant changes in outflow facility or episcleral venous pressure. It is possible that this drug may reduce the rate of aqueous humor formation as a result of inhibition of ciliary epithelium sodium/

potassium ATPase. In rabbits, chronographic studies have shown an aqueous humor flow decrease of approximately 30% two hours after topical administration of 1% vanadate (144, 145).

Using fluorometric techniques and agents to enhance penetration (DMSO and Tween-80), Podos et al (146) studied the effects of topically applied 1% sodium vanadate (NAVO-3) on IOP, outflow facility, and aqueous humor flow in cynomolgus monkeys. In this study, vanadate significantly reduced IOP. No alteration in outflow facility was demonstrated, and the reduction in IOP was associated with a 30% reduction in aqueous humor flow as measured by fluorophotometry.

Vanadate has been shown to stimulate adenylate cyclase activity in isolated membrane preparations (147). There is also evidence that vanadate stimulates monkey ciliary body, iris, and adenylate cyclase in vitro. Cyclic AMP and its analogs are reported to increase outflow facility (64). Another report (140) indicates that forskolin lowers IOP in rabbits, monkeys, and humans when topically applied. The effect was shown to be a result of a reduction in aqueous flow.

CARDIAC GLYCOSIDES   Cardiac glycosides, such as systemically administered ouabain, have also been shown to lower IOP. These drugs are presumed to act by interfering with the sodium/potassium pump, located in the nonpigmented ciliary epithelium, and by reducing aqueous formation.

Prostaglandins and Corticosteroids

In addition to the well-known ability of prostaglandins to raise IOP in rabbit eyes, it has been reported recently that moderately low doses of PGE-2 and PGF-2a significantly reduce IOP in a variety of experimental animals. These studies suggest that prostaglandins may serve as an endogenous regulator of outflow facility in the trabecular meshwork if these autocoids were produced and secreted by human trabecular cells (148). Physiological levels of glucocorticoids may regulate prostaglandin production within the trabecular meshwork. Therefore, studies of endogenous prostaglandin production by trabecular cells could provide new clues to the pathogenesis of a number of glaucoma syndromes including primary open-angle glaucoma and steroid-induced glaucoma (148).

It has also been suggested that epinephrine stimulates the formation and release of prostaglandins, and perhaps that is one of the mechanisms by which epinephrine lowers IOP (149). This would suggest that agents inhibiting the release of prostaglandins, such as nonsteroidal anti-inflammatory drugs like aspirin and indomethacin, could reduce the effectiveness of topically applied epinephrine or perhaps even of β-blocking agents such as timolol.

Dopamine in the Eye

Until recently, investigations into the role of dopamine (DA) in the eye have focused mainly on its function as a neurotransmitter in the retina. In contrast to extensive studies on retinal DA, only a few studies dealing with DA in the anterior segment of the eye have been published.

In an early study of DA in nonretinal ocular tissues, it was reported that DA given either topically or intravitreally lowered IOP in rabbits with α-chymotrypsin-induced ocular hypertension (150). Furthermore, at doses of 10 μg and 100 μg, DA decreased IOP without concurrent mydriasis, which suggests a dissociation of ocular hypotension from α-adrenergically mediated mydriatic response. DA-induced ocular hypotension was abolished by intramuscular haloperidol but not by intravenous propranolol. Cervical gangli-onectomy had no effect on the hypotensive response to DA. Thus, it was concluded that (a) DA is capable of lowering rabbit IOP by activating specific DA receptors, and (b) this action is independent of the ocular sympathetic system. In another study in which a higher topical dose of DA was administered, a rise in IOP was reported (105). Thus, DA may elicit different IOP responses, depending on the dose.

Investigation into the mechanisms underlying the ocular action of DA indicates that this agent can influence aqueous humor formation. Topical administration of DA has been reported to increase aqueous humor formation in rabbits (151). These DA-induced increases in aqueous formation and in permeability were blocked by the nonselective α-adrenoceptor antagonist phentolamine, but DA antagonists such as butaclamol and chlorpromazine were relatively ineffective. This finding implicates the activation of the adrenergic receptors rather than specific DA receptors as a mechanism of action.

Other investigators have reported that DA reduces aqueous humor formation. In the enucleated perfused cat eye, arterial infusion of DA produced immediate vasoconstriction and a 55% reduction in the rate of aqueous humor formation (152). Since phenoxybenzamine blocked both of these effects, it is likely that the activation of α-adrenergic receptors was involved in this action. When these findings are taken together, they indicate that DA can alter the rate of aqueous humor formation through its actions on the vasculature and/or secretory processes. However, there is no evidence for the involvement of specific DA receptors in these actions at this time.

One of the problems in using DA as an agonist to study the DA system is its relative lack of specificity. It is well known that DA is capable of activating α- and β-receptors as well as DA receptors (153). Furthermore, DA receptors themselves are classified into at least two subtypes (154). The activation of Type 1 DA receptors (DA-1) is linked to renal vasodilation and stimulation of adenylate cyclase. The activation of Type 2 DA receptors (DA-2) is associated with such responses as inhibition of both prolactin release and neurotransmission. Unlike DA-1 responses, DA-2 responses are not mediated by stimulation of adenylate cyclase. Clearly, there is a need to use more selective DA agonists and antagonists in order to investigate further the role of a DA system in regulating IOP. Although no systematic evaluation of the selective DA agonists and antagonists has been published, there are several reports indicating that these agents may possess ocular hypotensive activity.

A rigid analog of DA, 6,7-dihydroxy-2-aminotetralin (6,7-ADTN) is a DA-1 agonist. The topical administration of 6,7-ADTN has been shown to lower IOP in albino New Zealand rabbits and to suppress ocular hypertension after water loading (155). Since superior cervical ganglionectomy attenuated the ocular hypotension induced by 6,7-ADTN, the mechanism of this hypotensive action appears to involve the modulation of ocular sympathetic nervous activity.

LY 141865 is a potent and selective DA-2 agonist that produced a bilateral decrease in IOP when administered topically to albino New Zealand rabbits (155). It also suppressed IOP recovery rate after intravenous infusion of hypertonic saline in rabbits. As with 6,7-ADTN, the ocular hypotension produced by LY 141865 was attenuated by surgical sympathectomy.

Pretreatment with domperidone, a DA-2 antagonist, has been reported to inhibit the ocular hypotensive effects of bromocriptine and pergolide, two ergot derivatives (156). Furthermore, the ergot derivatives were shown to depress the rate of IOP recovery but had a minimal effect on outflow facility. It was concluded that the most probable site of action is the inflow site via the activation of DA-2 receptors.

Topical administration of both pergolide and lergotrile also significantly decreased IOP in the Cebus monkey (157). Interestingly, oral administration of bromocriptine has been reported to reduce IOP in normal human volunteers without changing heart rate or blood pressure (158). Moreover, a recent report (159) indicates that topical administration of bromocriptine is also effective in unilaterally lowering IOP in normal human volunteers.

In terms of DA antagonists, only the ocular effects of the butyrophenones and phenothiazines have been reported. Using the cat constant pressure perfusion model, Chiou (160) reported that the topical administration of haloperidol produced an initial increase in aqueous humor outflow followed by a decrease in inflow. Haloperidol and several other butyrophenones were also reported to suppress IOP recovery rate after intravenous infusion of hypertonic saline in rabbits. Chiou concluded that in rabbits this class of DA antagonists may have ocular hypotensive activity by inhibiting aqueous humor formation.

Chlorpromazine, a DA antagonist belonging to the phenothiazine class, has been reported to decrease IOP in rabbits and cats when administered intramuscularly (161, 162). When topically administered, however, it was irritating and failed to lower IOP. Since a study to identify the specificity of action has not been performed, it is not known if the ocular effects of the butyrophenones and phenothiazines are related to a blockade of the DA system. In summary, the role of DA in the anterior portion of the eye is not clear. Nevertheless, there are several reports indicating that agents known to influence the DA system can lower IOP in vivo. Further investigations in this area of research should (*a*) identify which subclass of DA receptors, if any, is involved in regulating IOP, and (*b*) determine the mechanism of action.

Literature Cited

1. Quigley, H. A. 1982. Glaucomas—optic nerve damage. Changing clinical perspectives. *Ann. Ophthalmol.* 14:611–12
2. Kinsey, V. E. 1971. Ion movement in ciliary processes. In *Membrane and Ion Transports*, Vol. 3, ed. E. E. Bittar. New York: Wiley
3. Marin, T. H. 1974. Bicarbonate formation in aqueous humor: mechanism and relation to the treatment of glaucoma. *Invest. Ophthalmol.* 13:179–483
4. Barany, E. H. 1963. A mathematical formulation of intraocular pressure as dependent on secretion, ultra filtration, bulk outflow and osmotic reabsorption of fluid. *Invest. Ophthalmol.* 2:584–90
5. Bill, A. 1975. Blood circulation and fluid dynamics in the eye. *Pharm. Rev.* 55:383–417
6. Bill, A. 1971. Aqueous humor dynamics in monkeys. *Exp. Eye Res.* 911:195–206
7. Bill, A., Phillips, C. I. 1971. Uveal scleral drainage of aqueous humor in human eyes. *Exp. Eye Res.* 12:275–81
8. Weber, A. 1877. Korresp. *Zentralbl. Med. Wiss.* 14:986
9. Laqueur, L. 1876. Uber Eine Neue Therapeutische Verwendung Des Physostigmin. *Zentralbl. Med. Wiss.* 14:421–22
10. Barany, E. H. 1965. Relative importance of autonomic nervous tone and structure as determinants of outflow resistance in normal monkey eyes. In *The Structure of the Eye, 2nd Symposium*, ed. J. W. Rohen, pp. 223–36. Stuttgart: Schattauer
11. Harris, L. S. 1968. Cycloplegic-induced intraocular pressure elevations. *Arch. Ophthalmol.* 79:242–46
12. Schimick, R., Lieberman, W. J. 1961. The influence of cyclogyl and neosynephrine on tonographic studies of miotic control and open-angle glaucoma. *Am. J. Ophthalmol.* 51:781–84
13. Barany, E. H., Christensen, R. E. 1967. Cycloplegics and outflow resistance. *Arch. Ophthalmol.* 77:757–60
14. Barany, E. H. 1962. The mode of action of pilocarpine on outflow resistance in

the eye of a primate. *Invest. Ophthalmol.* 1:712–27
15. Barany, E. H. 1966. The mode of action of miotics on outflow resistance; the study of pilocarpine in the vervet monkey. *Trans. Ophthalmol. Soc. UK* 86:539–78
16. Nomura, T., Smelser, G. K. 1974. The identification of adrenergic and cholinergic nerve endings in the trabecular meshwork. *Invest. Ophthalmol.* 13:525–32
17. Gartner, S. 1944. Blood vessels of the conjunctiva. *Arch. Ophthalmol.* 32:464–76
18. Wilke, K. 1974. Early effects of epinephrine and pilocarpine on the intraocular pressure and the episcleral venous pressure in the normal human eye. *Acta Ophthalmol.* 52:231
19. Alm, A., Bill, A., Young, F. A. 1973. The effects of pilocarpine and neostigmine on blood flow throuigh the anterior uvea in monkeys; a study with radioactively labeled microspheres. *Exp. Eye Res.* 15:31–36
20. James, R. G., Calkins, J. 1957. The effects of certain drugs on iris vessels. *Arch. Ophthalmol.* 57:414–17
21. Szabo, A. L., Maxwell, D. S., Krieger, A. E. 1976. Structural alterations in the ciliary process and the blood aqueous barrier of the monkey after systemic urea injections. *Am. J. Ophthalmol.* 81:162–72
22. Flocks, M., Zweng, H. C. 1957. Studies on the mode of action of pilocarpine on aqueous outflow. *Am. J. Ophthalmol.* 44:380
23. Havener, W. H. 1978. *Ocular Pharmacology*, p. 274. St. Louis: C. V. Mosby. 4th ed.
24. Holmberg, A., Barany, E. H. 1966. The effect of pilocarpine on the endothelium formed on the inner wall of Schlemm's Canal; Schlemm's Canal, an electronmicroscopic study in the monkey. *Invest. Ophthalmol.* 5:53–58

25. Allan, L., Burin, H. M. 1965. The valve action of the trabecular meshwork; studies with silicone models. *Am. J. Ophthalmol.* 59:382–89

26. Fortin, E. P. 1925. Canal de Schlemm y ligamento pectineo. *Arch. Ophthalmol.* 4:454–59

27. Kaufman, P. L. 1979. Aqueous humor dynamics following total iridectomy in the cynomolgus monkey. *Invest. Ophthalmol. Visual Sci.* 18:870–75

28. Krill, A. E., Newell, F. W. 1964. Effects of pilocarpine on ocular tension dynamics. *Am. J. Ophthalmol.* 57:34

29. Fenton, R., Schwartz, B. 1963. The effect of 2% pilocarpine in normal and glaucomatous eyes; the time response of pressure. *Invest. Ophthalmol.* 2:289

30. Harris, L. S., Galin, M. A. 1970. Dose response analysis of pilocarpine induced hypotension. *Arch. Ophthalmol.* 84:605–8

31. Harris, L. S., Galin, M. A. 1971. Effect of ocular pigmentation on hypotensive response to pilocarpine. *Am. J. Ophthalmol.* 72:923

32. Kaufman, P. L., Lutjen-Drecol, E. 1975. Total iridectomy of the primate in vivo; surgical technique and post-operative anatomy. *Invest. Ophthalmol.* 14:766–71

33. Kaufman, P. L., Barany, E. H. 1976. Loss of acute pilocarpine effect on outflow facility following surgical disinsertion and retrodisplacement of the ciliary muscle from the scleral spur in the cynomolgus monkey. *Invest. Ophthalmol.* 15:793–807

34. Lutjen-Drecol, E., Kaufman, P. L., Barany, E. H. 1977. Light and electronmicroscopy in the anterior chamber: angle structures following surgical disinsertion of the ciliary muscle in the cynomolgus monkey. *Invest. Ophthalmol. Visual Sci.* 16:218–25

35. Rohen, J. W., Lutjen-Drecol, E., Barany, E. H. 1967. The relation between the ciliary muscle and the trabecular meshwork and its importance for the effect of miotics on aqueous outflow resistance. *Albrecht von Graefes, Arch. Klin. Exp. Ophthalmol.* 172:23–47

36. Barany, E. H., Rohen, J. W. 1965. Localized contraction and relaxation within the ciliary muscle of the vervet monkey. See Ref. 10, pp. 287–311

37. Bill, A. 1967. Effects of atropine and pilocarpine on aqueous humor dynamics in cynomolgus monkeys. *Exp. Eye Res.* 6:120–25

38. Gaasterland, D., Kupfer, C., Ross, K. 1975. Studies of aqueous humor dynamics in man. 4. Effects of pilocarpine upon measurements in young, normal volunteers. *Invest. Ophthalmol.* 14:848–53

39. Brown, H. S., Meltzer, G., Merrill, R. C., Fisher, M., Ferré, C., Place, V. A. 1976. Visual effect of pilocarpine in glaucoma; comparative study of administration by eyedrops or by ocular therapeutic systems. *Arch. Ophthalmol.* 94:1716

40. Armaly, M. F. 1959. Studies on intraocular effects of the orbital parasympathetic pathway. 3. Effect on steady state dynamics. *AMA Arch. Ophthalmol.* 62:817

41. Abramson, D. H., Chang, S., Coleman, D. J. 1976. Pilocarpine therapy in glaucoma; effects on anterior chamber depth and lens thickness in patients receiving long-term therapy. *Arch. Ophthalmol.* 94:914

42. Bito, L. Z., Dawson, M. J. 1970. The site and mechanism of the control of cholinergic sensitivity. *J. Pharmacol. Exp. Ther.* 175:673

43. Bito, L. Z., Dawson, M. J., Petrinovic, L. 1971. Cholinergic sensitivity; normal variability as a function of stimulus background. *Science* 172:583–85

44. Kaufman, P. L., Barany, E. H. 1976. Subsensitivity to pilocarpine in the aqueous outflow system in monkeys after topical anticholinesterase treatment. *Am. J. Ophthalmol.* 82:883

45. Kaufman, P. L., Wiedman, T., Robinson, J. R. 1984. Cholinergics. In *Pharmacology of the Eye*, ed. M. L. Sears, pp. 149–91. Berlin: Springer Verlag

46. Leopold, I. H., Comroe, J. H. 1946. Effect of diisopropyl fluorophosphate (DFP) on the normal eye. *Arch. Ophthalmol.* 36:17

47. DeRoetth, A. 1951. Further studies on cholinesterase activities in ocular tissues. *Am. J. Ophthalmol.* 34:120

48. Leopold, I. H., Krishna, N., Lehman, R. A. 1959. Effects of anticholinesterase agents and the blood cholinesterase level on normal and glaucoma subjects. *Trans. Am. Ophthalmol. Soc.* 57:63

49. Sears, M. L., Barany, E. H. 1960. Outflow resistance and adrenergic mechanisms. *Arch. Ophthalmol.* 64:839

50. Eakins, K. 1963. Effect of intravitreous injections of norepinephrine, epinephrine and isoproterenol on intraocular pressure and aqueous humor dynamics of rabbit eyes. *J. Pharmacol. Exp. Ther.* 140:79

51. Eakins, K., Eakins, H. 1964. Adrenergic mechanisms and the outflow of aqueous

humor from the rabbit eye. *J. Pharmacol. Exp. Ther.* 144:60–65

52. Sears, M. L. 1966. The mechanism of action of adrenergic drugs in glaucoma. *Invest. Ophthalmol.* 5:115–19

53. Langham, M. E. 1965. The response of the pupil and intraocular pressure of conscious rabbits to adrenergic drugs following unilateral superior cervical ganglionectomy. *Exp. Eye Res.* 4:381

54. Weekers, R., Collignon-Brach, J., Grieten, J. 1966. Contribution to the study of ocular hypotension caused by various sympathomimetic amines. In *Drug Mechanisms in Glaucoma*, ed. G. Paterson, S. J. H. Miller, G. D. Paterson, pp. 51–65. Boston: Little, Brown

55. Mishima, S. 1982. Ocular effects of beta-adrenergic agents. *Surv. Ophthalmol.* 27:187–208

56. Potter, D. E. 1981. Adrenergic pharmacology; aqueous humor dynamics. *Pharmacol. Rev.* 33:133–53

57. Neufeld, A. H., Zawistouski, K. A., Page, E. D., Bromberg, B. B. 1978. Influences on the density of beta adrenergic receptors in the cornea and iris/ciliary body of the rabbit. *Invest. Ophthalmol. Visual Sci.* 17:1069

58. Kupfer, C., Gaasterland, D., Ross, K. 1977. Studies of aqueous humor dynamics in man. Effects of acetazolamide and isoproterenol in young and normal volunteers. *Invest. Ophthalmol.* 15:349

59. Neufeld, A. 1981. Epinephrine and timolol: how do these drugs lower intraocular pressure? *Ann. Ophthalmol.* 13:1109–11

60. Macri, F. J. 1964. The constrictor action of various antiglaucoma drugs on the iris artery of the cat. *Int. J. Neuropharmacol.* 3:205

61. Townsend, D. J., Brubaker, R. F. 1980. Immediate effect of epinephrine on aqueous formation in the normal human eye as measured by fluorophotometry. *Invest. Ophthalmol. Visual Sci.* 19:256–66

62. Weekers, R., Prijot, E., Gustin, J. 1954. Recent advances and the future prospects of the medical treatment of ocular hypertension. *Br. J. Ophthalmol.* 38:742–46

63. Becker, B., Ley, A. P. 1958. Epinephrine and acetazolamide in the treatment of chronic glaucoma. *Am. J. Ophthalmol.* 45:639–43

64. Neufeld, A. H. 1978. Influence of cyclic nucleotides on outflow facility in the vervet monkey. *Exp. Eye Res.* 27:387

65. Neufeld, A. H., Dueker, D. K., Vegge, T., Sears, M. L. 1975. Adenosine 3', 5' monophosphate increases the outflow of

aqueous humor from the rabbit eye. *Invest. Ophthalmol.* 14:40

66. Ballintine, E. J., Garner, L. L. 1961. Improvement of the coefficient of outflow in glaucomatous eyes. *Arch. Ophthalmol.* 66:314–17

67. Becker, B., Pettit, T. H., Gay, A. J. 1969. Topical epinephrine therapy of open-angle glaucoma. *Arch. Ophthalmol.* 66:219

68. Sonntag, J. R., Brindley, G. D., Shields, M. B., Arafat, N. T., Phelps, C. D. 1979. Timolol and epinephrine; comparison of efficacy and side effects. *Arch. Ophthalmol.* 97:273

69. Yablonski, M. E. 1984. Mechanism of action of topical epinephrine. Editorial. *Ann. Ophthalmol.* 307–8

70. Becker, B., Montgomery, S. W., Kass, M. A., Shin, D. H. 1977. Increased ocular and systemic responsiveness to epinephrine in primary open-angle glaucoma. *Arch. Ophthalmol.* 95:789–90

71. Ostbaum, S. A., Kolker, A. E., Phelps, C. D. 1974. Low-dose epinephrine. *Arch. Ophthalmol.* 92:118

72. Kolker, A. E., Hetherington, J. 1983. Adrenergic agents. In *Becker-Shaffer's Diagnosis and Therapy of the Glaucomas*, p. 393. St. Louis: C. V. Mosby. 5th ed.

73. Havener, W. H. 1983. Autonomic drugs. In *Ocular Pharmacology*. St. Louis: C. V. Mosby. 5th ed.

74. Kaback, M. D., Pados, S. M., Harbin, T. S., Mandell, A., Becker, B. 1976. The effects of dipivalyl epinephrine on the eye. *Am. J. Ophthalmol.* 81:768–72

75. Kass, M. A., Mandell, A., Goldberg, I., Paine, J. M., Becker, B. 1979. Dipivefrin and epinephrine treatment of elevated intraocular pressure; a comparative study. *Arch. Ophthalmol.* 97L:1865–66

76. Cohn, A. N., Moss, A. P., Hargett, N. A., Ritch, R., Smith, H., et al. 1979. Clinical comparison of dipivalyl epinephrine and epinephrine in the treatment of glaucoma. *Am. J. Ophthalmol.* 87: 196–201

77. Yablonski, M. E., Gray, J. R. 1983. Use of the Flurotron master to measure aqueous flow. *Invest. Ophthalmol. Visual Sci.* 24:88 (Suppl.)

78. Kobinger, W. 1978. Central α-adrenergic systems as targets for hypotensive drugs. *Rev. Physiol. Biochem. Pharmacol.* 81:39–100

79. Harrison, R., Kaufmann, C. S. 1977. Clonidine, effects of a topically administered solution on intraocular pressure and

blood pressure in open-angle glaucoma. *Arch. Ophthalmol.* 95:1368–73

80. Hodapp, E., Kolker, A. E., Kass, M. A., Goldberg, I., Becker, B., Gordon, M. 1981. The effect of topical clonidine on intraocular pressure. *Arch. Ophthalmol.* 99:1208–11

81. Kaskel, D., Becker, B., Rudolf, H. 1980. Early effects of clonidine, epinephrine, and pilocarpine on the intraocular pressure and the episcleral venous pressure in normal volunteers. *Albrecht von Graefes Arch. Klin. Exp. Ophthalmol.* 213:251–59

82. Krieglstein, G. K., Langham, M. E., Leydhecker, W. 1978. The peripheral and central neural actions of clonidine in normal and glaucomatous eyes. *Invest. Ophthalmol.* 17:149–58

83. Krieglstein, G. K., Leydhecker, W. 1977. The effect of topically applied clonidine on the episcleral and conjunctival venous pressure in glaucomatous eyes. *Bibl. Anat.* 16:89–91

84. Ralli, R. 1975. Clonidine effect on the intraocular pressure and eye circulation. *Acta Ophthalmol.* 125:37

85. Heilmann, K. 1973. Intraocular pressure, blood pressure and the optic nerve. *Exp. Eye Res.* 7:392–93

86. Krieglstein, G. K., Cramer, E. 1978. The response of ophthalmic arterial pressure to topically applied clonidine. *Albrecht von Graefes Arch. Klin. Exp. Ophthalmol.* 207:1–5

87. Allen, R., Langham, M. E. 1976. The intraocular pressure response of conscious rabbits to clonidine. *Invest. Ophthalmol. Visual Sci.* 18:815–23

88. Higgins, R. G., Brubaker, R. F. 1980. Acute effect of epinephrine on aqueous humor formation in the timolol-treated normal eye as measured by fluorophotometry. *Invest. Ophthalmol. Visual Sci.* 19:420–23

89. Lee, D. A., Brubaker, R. F., Nagataki, S. 1981. Effect of thymoxamine on aqueous humor formation in the normal human eye as measured by fluorophotometry. *Invest. Ophthalmol. Visual Sci.* 21:805–11

90. Lee, D. A., Rinele, T. J., Brubaker, R. F. 1983. Effect of thymoxamine on the human pupil. *Exp. Eye Res.* 36:655–62

91. Lee, D. A., Brubaker, R. F. 1982. Effect of phenylephrine on aqueous humor flow. *Curr. Eye Res.* 2:89–92

92. Langham, M. E., Sinjle, A., Josephs, S., Nagataki, S., Vanhoutte, P. M. 1973. The alpha- and beta-adrenergic responses to epinephrine in the rabbit eye. *Exp. Eye Res.* 15:75–84

93. Bonomi, L., Tomazzoli, L. 1977. Thimixamine and intraocular pressure. *Albrecht von Graefes Arch. Klin. Exp. Ophthalmol.* 204:95–100

94. Smith, B. R., 1979. Influence of topically applied prazosin on the intraocular pressure of experimental animals. *Arch. Ophthalmol.* 97:1133–36

95. Delongs, S., Scheie, H. 1953. Dibenamine—an experimental and clinical study. *Arch. Ophthalmol.* 50:289

96. Primrose, J. 1955. Dibenzyline in glaucoma. *Br. J. Ophthalmol.* 39:307–11

97. Green, K., Kim, K. 1976. Mediation of ocular tetrahydrocannabinol effects by the adrenergic system. *Exp. Eye Res.* 23:443–48

98. Murray, D. L., Leopold, I. H. 1980. Evidence for more than one type of alpha-adrenergic receptor in rabbit eyes. *Invest. Ophthalmol. Visual Sci.* 19:66 (Suppl.)

99. Krupin, T., Feitel, M., Becker, B. 1980. Effect of prazosin on aqueous humor dynamics in rabbits. *Arch. Ophthalmol.* 98:1639–42

100. Nathanson, J. A. 1980. Adrenergic regulation of intraocular pressure; identification of beta$_2$ adrenergic-stimulated adenylate cyclase in the ciliary process epithelium. *Proc. Natl. Acad. Sci. USA* 77:7420–24

101. Colasanti, B. K., Trotter, R. R. 1981. Effects of selective beta$_1$ and beta$_2$ adrenoceptor agonists and antagonists on intraocular pressure in the cat. *Invest. Ophthalmol. Visual Sci.* 20:69–76

102. Weekers, R., Delmarcelle, Y., Gustin, J. 1955. Treatment of ocular hypertension by adrenalin and diverse sympathomimetic amines. *Am. J. Ophthalmol.* 40:666–72

103. Ross, R. A., Drance, S. M. 1970. Effects of topically applied isoproterenol on aqueous humor dynamics in man. *Arch. Ophthalmol.* 83:39

104. Langham, M. E., Biggs, E. 1974. Beta adrenergic responses in the eyes of rabbits, primates and man. *Exp. Eye Res.* 19:281–95

105. Potter, D. E., Rowland, J. M. 1978. Adrenergic drugs in intraocular pressure; effects of selective beta-adrenergic agonists. *Exp. Eye Res.* 27:615–25

106. Miichi, H., Nagataki, S. 1982. The effects of cholinergic drugs and adrenergic drugs on aqueous humor formation in the rabbit eye. *Jpn. J. Ophthalmol.* 26:425–36

107. Bill, A. 1969. Early effects of epinephrine on the aqueous humor dynam-

ics in vervet monkeys. *Exp. Eye Res.* 83:35–43

108. Bill, A. 1970. Effects of norepinephrine, isoproterenol and sympathetic stimulation on aqueous humor dynamics in vervet monkeys. *Exp. Eye Res.* 10:31–46

109. Schenker, H. I., Yablonski, M., Pados, S. M., Linder, L. 1981. Fluorophotometric study of epinephrine and timolol in human subjects. *Arch. Ophthalmol.* 99:1212–16

110. Gaasterland, D., Kupfer, C., Ross, K., Gabelnick, H. L. 1973. Studies of aqueous humor dynamics in man. 3. Measurements in young, normal subjects using norepinephrine and isoproterenol. *Invest. Ophthalmol.* 12:267

111. Coakes, R. L., Siah, P. B. 1982. The effects of topical salbutamol on aqueous humor dynamics in the normal human eye. *Invest. Ophthalmol. Visual Sci.* 22:40 (Suppl.)

112. Araie, M., Takase, M. 1981. Effects of various drugs on aqueous humor dynamics in man. *Jpn. J. Ophthalmol.* 25:91

113. Brubaker, R. F., Gaasterland, D. 1984. The effect of isoproterenol on aqueous humor formation in humans. *Invest. Ophthalmol Visual Sci.* 25:357

114. Paterson, G. D., Paterson, G. 1972. Drug therapy of glaucoma. *Br. J. Ophthalmol.* 56:288–318

115. Wettrell, K., Wilke, K., Pandolfi, M. 1977. Effect of beta-adrenergic agonists and antagonists on repeated tonometry and episcleral venous pressure. *Exp. Eye Res.* 24:613–19

116. Kaham, A. 1981. Miscellaneous effects of adrenergic activators and inhibitors on the eye. In *Adrenergic Activators and Inhibitors,* Part 2, ed. L. Szederes, pp. 319–44. Berlin: Springer-Verlag

117. Bucci, M. G. 1977. Effects of new topical β-mimetic (isoxuprine and nylidrine) and β-lytic (oxprenolol) agents on the ocular pressure in glaucomatous eyes. *Ophthalmol. Res.* 9:238–46

118. Boger, W. P. 1979. The treatment of glaucoma; role of beta blocking agents. *Drugs* 18:25–32

119. Schmitt, C., Lott, V. J., Vareilles, P., LeDovarec, J. C. 1981. Beta-adrenergic blockers: lack of relationship between antagonism of isoproterenol and lowering of intraocular pressure. In *New Directions in Ophthalmic Research,* ed. M. L. Sears, pp. 147–62. New Haven: Yale Univ. Press

120. Coakes, R. L., Brubaker, R. S. 1978. The mechanism of timolol in lowering intraocular pressure. *Arch. Ophthalmol.* 96:2045

121. Yablonski, M. E., Zimmerman, T. J., Waltman, S. R., Becker, B. 1978. A fluorometric study of the effect of topical timolol on aqueous humor dynamics. *Exp. Eye Res.* 27:135

122. Zimmerman, T., Harbin, R., Pett, M., Kaufman, H. E. 1977. Timolol and facility of outflow. *Invest. Ophthalmol. Visual Sci.* 16:623

123. Green, K., Padget, B. 1979. The effect of various drugs on pseudofacility and aqueous humor formation in the rabbit eye. *Exp. Eye Res.* 28:239

124. Bartels, S. P., Neufeld, A. H. 1980. Mechanisms of topical drugs used in the control of open-angle glaucoma; clinical pharmacology of the anterior segment. In *International Ophthalmology Clinics,* ed. F. Holly, pp. 111–14. Boston: Little, Brown

125. Liu, H. K., Chiou, G. C. Y. 1981. Continuous, simultaneous and instant display of aqueous humor dynamics with a micro-spectrophotometer and a sensitive drop counter. *Exp. Eye Res.* 32:583–92

126. Frishman, W. H., MacCarthy, E. P., Kimmel, B., Lazar, E., Michelson, E. L., Bloomfield, S. S. 1984. Labetalol: a new β-adrenergic blocker vasodilator. In *Clinical Pharmacology of the β-Adrenoceptor Blocking Drugs,* ed. W. H. Frishman, p. 205. New York: Appleton-Century Crofts. 2nd ed.

127. Murray, D. L., Podos, S. M., Wei, C. P., Leopold, I. H. 1979. Ocular effects in normal rabbits of topically applied labetalol, a combined α- and β-adrenergic receptor antagonist. *Arch. Ophthalmol.* 97:723–26

128. Leopold, I. H., Murray, D. L. 1979. Ocular hypotensive action of labetalol. *Am. J. Ophthalmol.* 88:427–31

129. Bonomi, L., Perfetti, S., Bellucci, R., Massa, F., Noya, E. 1981. Ocular hypotensive action of labetalol in rabbit and human eyes. *Albrecht von Graefes Archiv. Für Ophthalmologie* 217:175–81

130. Krieglstein, G. K., Kontic, D. 1981. Nadolol and labetalol: comparative efficacy of two beta-blocking agents in glaucoma. *Albrecht von Graefes Archiv Für Ophthalmologie* 216:313–17

131. Weiner, N. 1980. Drugs that inhibit adrenergic nerves and block adrenergic receptors. In *The Pharmacological Basis of Therapeutics,* ed. A. G. Gilman, L. S. Goodman, A. Gilman, p. 138. New York: MacMillan. 6th ed.

132. Riley, F. C., Moyer, N. J. 1970. Experimental Horner's syndrome: a pupillographic evaluation of guanethi-

dine-induced adrenergic blockade in humans. *Am. J. Ophthalmol.* 69:442

133. Romano, J., Nogasubramanian, S., Poinoosawny, D. 1981. Double-masked cross-over comparison of guanethidine 1% and adrenaline 0.2% with adrenaline 1% and with pilocarpine 1%. *Br. J. Ophthalmol.* 65:50–52

134. Murray, A., Glover, D., Hitchings, R. 1981. Low-dose-combined guanethidine 1% and adrenaline 0.5% in the treatment of chronic simple glaucoma: a prospective study. *Br. J. Ophthalmol.* 65:533–35

135. Holland, M. G., Mims, J. L. 1971. Anterior segment chemical sympathectomy with 6-hydroxydopamine. *Invest. Ophthalmol.* 10:120–43

136. Holland, M. G. 1972. Treatment of glaucoma by chemical sympathectomy with 6-hydroxydopamine. *Trans. Am. Acad. Ophthalmol. Otolaryngol.* 76:437–49

137. Zeller, E. A., Knepper, P. A., Shoch, D. 1975. Differential effects of inhibitors of monoamine oxidase types A and B on the adrenergic system of the rabbit iris. *Invest. Ophthalmol.* 14:155–59

138. Mehra, K. S., Roy, P. N., Singh, R. 1974. Pargyline drops in glaucoma. *Arch. Ophthalmol.* 92:453–54

139. Smith, B. R., Gaster, R. N., Leopold, I. H., Zeleznick, L. D. 1983. Forskolin, a potent adenylate cyclase activator that lowers rabbit IOP. *Invest. Ophthalmol.* 24:4 (Suppl.)

140. Caprioli, J., Sears, M. 1983. Forskolin lowers intraocular pressure in rabbits, monkeys and man. *Lancet* 19:58

141. Bausher, L. P., Gregory, D. S., Sears, M. L. 1983. Forskolin and adenylate cyclase in ciliary processes. *Invest. Ophthalmol.* 24:4 (Suppl.)

142. Neufeld, A. 1983. Forskolin stimulates cyclic AMP synthesis and lowers intraocular pressure and increases outflow facility in albino rabbits. *Invest. Ophthalmol.* 24:4 (Suppl.)

143. Green, K., Bigger, J. F., Kim, K., Bowman, K. 1977. Cannabinoid action on the eye as mediated through the central nervous system and local adrenergic activity. *Exp. Eye Res.* 24:189–96

144. Krupin, T., Becker, B., Podos, S. 1980. Topical vanadate lowers intraocular pressure in rabbits. *Invest. Ophthalmol. Visual Sci.* 19:1360–63

145. Krupin, Podos, S. M., Becker, B. 1983. Ocular effects of vanadate. Proceedings of the International Glaucoma Symposium. In *Glaucoma Update 11*, ed. G.

K. Krieglstein, W. Leydhecker, p. 2529. Berlin: Springer Verlag

146. Podos, S. M., Lee, P. Y., Severin, C., Mittag, T. 1984. The effect of vanadate on aqueous humor dynamics in cynomolgus monkeys. *Invest. Ophthalmol. Visual Sci.* 25:359

147. Schwabe, E., Puchstein, C., Hannemann, H., Söchtig, E. 1979. Activation of adenylate cyclase by vanadate. *Nature* 277:143

148. Weinreb, R. N., Mitchell, M. D., Polansky, J. R. 1983. Prostaglandin production by human trabecular cells *in vitro* inhibition by dexamethasone. *Invest. Ophthalmol. Visual Sci.* 24:1541–45

149. Yousufzai, A.-L. 1983. Effect of norepinephrine and other pharmacological agents on prostaglandin E_2 release by rabbit and bovine irides. *Exp. Eye Res.* 37:279–92

150. Shannon, R. P., Mead, A., Sears, M. L. 1976. The effect of dopamine on the intraocular pressure and pupil of the rabbit eye. *Invest. Ophthalmol.* 15:371–80

151. Chiou, G. C. Y., Chiou, F. Y. 1983. Dopaminergic involvement in intraocular pressure in the rabbit eye. *Ophthalmic Res.* 15:131–35

152. Macri, F. J., Cevario, S. J. 1976. The inhibitory actions of dopamine, hydroxyamphetamine and phenylephrine on aqueous humor formation. *Exp. Eye Res.* 26:85–89

153. Goldberg, L. I. 1972. Cardiovascular and renal actions of dopamine: potential clinical applications. *Pharmacol. Rev.* 24:1–29

154. Kaiser, C., Kebabian, J. W., eds. 1983. Dopamine Receptors. *ACS Symp. Ser.* 224:

155. Potter, D. E., Burke, J. A. 1983. Alteration in intraocular pressure (IOP) and pupillary function by dopamine agonists: lisuride, apomorphine, 6,7-ADTN and n-methyl dopamine. Dopamine Receptor Agonists Symp. sponsored by Smith-Kline & French Lab., Philadelphia, Feb. 1983. Abstr. 13

156. Potter, D. E., Burke, J. A., Chang, F. W. 1984. Ocular hypotensive action of ergoline derivatives in rabbits: effects of sympathectomy and domperidone pretreatment. *Curr. Eye Res.* 3:307–14

157. Potter, D. E., Burke, J. A. 1982. Effects of ergoline derivatives on intraocular pressure and iris function in rabbits and monkeys. *Curr. Eye Res.* 2:281–88

158. Mekki, Q. A., Hassan, S. M., Turner, P.

1983. Bromocriptine lowers intraocular pressure without affecting blood pressure. *Lancet* 2:1250–51

159. Mekki, Q. A., Pinsky, M., Summer, W., Hassan, S. M., Turner, P. 1984. Bromocriptine eyedrops lower intraocular pressure without affecting prolactin levels. *Lancet* 1:287–88

160. Chiou, G. C. Y. 1984. Ocular hypotensive actions of haloperidol, a dopa-minergic antagonist. *Arch. Ophthalmol.* 102:143–45

161. Constant, M. A., Becker, B. 1956. The effects of vasopressin, chlorpromazine, and phetolamine methanesulfonate. *AMA Arch. Ophthalmol.* 56:19–25

162. Paul, S. D., Leopold, I. H. 1956. The effect of chlorpromazine upon the intraocular pressure of experimental animals. *Am. J. Ophthalmol.* 41:318

Ann. Rev. Pharmacol. Toxicol. 1986. 26:427–53

MOLECULAR PHARMACOLOGY OF BOTULINUM TOXIN AND TETANUS TOXIN

Lance L. Simpson

Departments of Medicine and Pharmacology and Division of Environmental Medicine and Toxicology, Jefferson Medical College, 1025 Walnut Street, Philadelphia, Pennsylvania 19107

INTRODUCTION

Botulinum toxin is a term that has been used to describe eight different substances designated types A, B, C_1, C_2, D, E, F, and G. For many years it was assumed that these eight substances acted at the neuromuscular junction to block acetylcholine release. It is now known that this assumption is not entirely correct. Seven of the substances do act at cholinergic junctions (types A, B, C_1, D, E, F, and G), and they are properly referred to as botulinum neurotoxins. The eighth substance (type C_2) is unique in its structure and pharmacological actions. It is called the botulinum binary toxin.

Tetanus toxin is a term that has been used to describe a single substance that acts mainly in the central nervous system to block inhibitory transmission. There are many similarities between tetanus toxin and botulinum neurotoxin, including a common origin, a closely related structure, and perhaps the same subcellular mechanism of action. The similarities between tetanus toxin and the botulinum binary toxin are less clear.

The purpose of the present review is to discuss the proposed mechanism(s) of action of the three groups of clostridial toxins. Recent findings suggest that research is moving quickly toward a full determination of the cellular and subcellular actions of these substances. This is an encouraging turn of events, because the clostridial toxins are generally regarded as the most poisonous substances known to mankind.

427

0362-1642/86/0415-0427$02.00

MECHANISM OF ACTION

In 1980, the author proposed a three-step model to account for the neuromuscular blocking actions of botulinum neurotoxin (1). This model has been expanded in recent years (2), and it can be summarized in the following way. The neurotoxin binds to receptors on the external surface of the plasma membrane. The binding step is essential for development of paralysis, but it does not produce any adverse effect on nerve cell function.

The binding step is followed by an internalization step, which is itself a sequence of events. The toxin enters the cell by the process of receptor-mediated endocytosis. This allows the toxin to cross the plasma membrane but leaves it within an endocytic vesicle. The toxin enters the cytoplasm by a mechanism that has not been fully clarified but that may involve formation of channels.

The final step produces nerve cell dysfunction. The toxin acts in the cytoplasm or at the internal face of the plasma membrane to alter a molecule involved in exocytosis. The precise nature of this poisoning event has not been established. However, to the extent that botulinum neurotoxin mimics the intracellular actions of other potent protein toxins, one can reasonably propose a catalytic mechanism. Botulinum neurotoxin may block transmitter release by enzymatically modifying a subtrate involved in excitation-secretion coupling.

The model for toxin action can be closely linked to the structure of the toxin molecule. Botulinum neurotoxin is produced by an anaerobic organism, *Clostridium botulinum* (3). The molecule is synthesized as a single chain polypeptide having a molecular weight of $M_r \sim 150,000$ (Figure 1). This molecule undergoes proteolytic cleavage to yield a dichain polypeptide composed of a heavy chain ($M_r \sim 100,000$) and a light chain ($M_r \sim 50,000$). The single chain polypeptide is only weakly active, but the dichain molecule is fully active (4).

When the molecule is exposed to additional proteolytic cleavage with papain, the heavy chain is split into two components roughly equivalent in molecular weight. The free portion of the heavy chain is the carboxyterminus, and the bound portion covalently linked to the light chain is the aminoterminus. Reduction of the disulfide bond or proteolytic cleavage of the heavy chain produces loss of toxicity (4).

The structure of the molecule can be related to the proposed model for toxin action. It is envisioned that the carboxyterminus of the heavy chain possesses a binding domain, the aminoterminus of the heavy chain possesses a channel-forming domain, and the light chain possesses a poisoning domain. None of the domains alone is neurotoxic; only the holotoxin can block transmitter release.

Tetanus toxin is also produced by an anaerobic organism, *Clostridium tetani* (5–7). The synthesis and proteolytic processing of tetanus toxin is virtually identical to that of botulinum neurotoxin (8). Thus, the molecule is synthesized

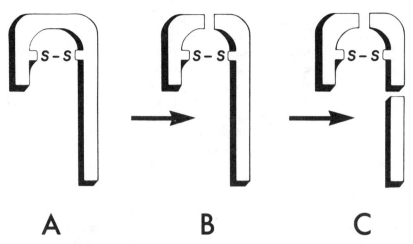

A   B   C

Figure 1   Botulinum neurotoxin is synthesized as a relatively inactive, single chain polypeptide that has a molecular weight of approximately 150,000 daltons (*A*). The single chain molecule possesses at least one intrachain disulfide bond. When exposed to trypsin or trypsin-like enzymes, the neurotoxin is nicked to yield an active dichain molecule with an interchain disulfide bond (*B*). The two chains are referred to as light (ca 50,000 daltons) and heavy (ca 100,000 daltons). When exposed to additional proteolytic cleavage with papain, the heavy chain is cleaved again (*C*). The result is two nontoxic polypeptides. The free portion of the heavy chain is the carboxyterminus, and it has a molecular weight of approximately 50,000 daltons. The bound portion of the heavy chain is the aminoterminus, and it remains covalently linked to the light chain.

The synthesis and proteolytic processing of tetanus toxin is identical to that of botulinum neurotoxin. The synthesis of the botulinum binary toxin is different. The binary toxin is synthesized as two polypeptide chains that have no disulfide bonds. There is a heavy chain (ca 100,000) and a light chain (ca 50,000), which mimics the status of botulinum neurotoxin and tetanus toxin. In addition, there is proteolytic processing. When the heavy chain is exposed to trypsin, it is converted from an inactive to an active form.

as an inactive, single chain polypeptide ($M_r \sim 150,000$) that is converted to an active, dichain molecule ($M_r \sim 100,000$ and $50,000$). Tetanus toxin is known for its effects on inhibitory interneurons, but it too can block neuromuscular transmission (9–12). In fact, the general features of its actions are very similar to those of botulinum neurotoxin (13–15). The data suggest that the molecule proceeds through a sequence of steps, including an extracellular binding step, a membrane penetration step, and an intracellular poisoning step (14). The data also suggest that the tetanus toxin molecule has three functional domains. As with botulinum neurotoxin, the carboxyterminus of the heavy chain mediates binding (16, 17), the aminoterminus of the heavy chain mediates internalization (18, 19), and the light chain is assumed to be responsible for poisoning nerve cell function.

The botulinum binary toxin is produced by *Clostridium botulinum* (3). There are some organisms that simultaneously produce both botulinum neurotoxin and the binary toxin. The structure of the latter is somewhat different from that of the botulinum and tetanus neurotoxins. It is synthesized as two separate polypeptide chains ($M_r \sim$ 100,000 and 50,000) that have no interchain covalent bonds (20, 21). Neither chain alone is very active, but the combination of chains is extremely toxic (20–22). Hence, it has been called a binary toxin (22).

The details of the mechanism of action of the binary toxin are in some respects less well understood and in other respects better understood than the details of neurotoxin action. The heavy chain of the binary toxin plays a key role in cell surface binding (22, 23); the light chain is an enzyme whose catalytic effects have been partially characterized (S. Leppla, personal communication; 24). The sequence of events that brings the toxin from an extracellular binding site to a supposed intracellular poisoning site has not been described.

When the general features of botulinum neurotoxin action were first proposed, the model was met by two sharply contrasting responses. Investigators in neuromuscular pharmacology tended to view it with skepticism, whereas investigators in microbiology and cell biology readily adopted it, in some cases viewing it as "intuitively obvious." There is an easily identifiable explanation for these dissimilar responses. The proposed model for botulinum neurotoxin action is seemingly complex and certainly different from models used to explain the mechanism of action of other neuromuscular blocking agents. However, the proposed action of botulinum neurotoxin shares many features with the known actions of potent protein toxins commonly studied by microbiologists and cell biologists (25). Examples of the latter include diphtheria toxin, which is microbial in origin, and abrin and ricin, which are plant lectins.

The trend during the past five years has been for an increasing number of pharmacologists to accept the model for botulinum neurotoxin action. This trend has been hastened by two discoveries: (a) the finding that the model is generalizable and appears to apply to tetanus toxin (14), and (b) the finding that the botulinum binary toxin possesses enzymatic activity similar to that of other potent protein toxins (S. Leppla, personal communication; 24). The current state of affairs is that most investigators now agree that the proposed model has merit and is worthy of experimental testing.

EVIDENCE TO SUPPORT THE MODEL

Binding Step

In 1949, Burgen and his associates published a manuscript that is regarded as one of the most important contributions to the botulinum neurotoxin literature (26). Their report introduced the isolated neuromuscular junction (phrenic nerve-hemidiaphragm) as a preparation on which to analyze toxin action. The phrenic nerve-hemidiaphragm preparation continues to be the mainstay of research on botulinum neurotoxin. In the recent past, Habermann and his associates have shown that tetanus toxin also blocks transmission at the phrenic nerve-hemidiaphragm (13). This was a particularly noteworthy finding, because it showed that a single tissue could be used to compare the actions of the two most potent neurotoxins.

Among the data reported in the paper by Burgen et al was the discovery that botulinum neurotoxin "fixed" to tissues very rapidly. Neuromuscular preparations that were exposed to toxin for short periods of time and then washed extensively continued to become paralyzed. Although the data were not discussed as such, the discovery of rapid fixation was the first indication that toxin action could be divided into at least two phases: an initial binding step and a later paralytic step. The fact that binding is rapid and that it is a separate event from paralysis has been confirmed by virtually every worker in the field.

Ideally, these suggestive findings on binding should be complemented by four specific types of research: (a) histological studies to demonstrate binding at the cholinergic nerve terminal, (b) radioligand studies to show selective and saturable binding at nerve endings, (c) peptide chemistry studies to show that fractionation of the toxin molecule will yield a nontoxic component with binding activity, and (d) isolation studies to extract an authentic receptor from nerve tissue. Varying degrees of success have been achieved in these four areas.

Hirokawa & Kitamura have shown binding of botulinum neurotoxin to the mouse phrenic nerve-hemidiaphragm (27). Using iodine-labeled toxin and light microscopic resolution, they obtained autoradiograms in which binding of neurotoxin was coincident with areas of acetylcholinesterase staining, which along with other evidence suggested localization at endplates. Dolly et al similarly showed binding of iodine-labeled toxin at the neuromuscular junction, but the work was more refined (28). They used a highly purified preparation of toxin, they exposed tissues to a much smaller amount of toxin (2.5×10^3 mouse LD_{50} versus 1.3×10^6 LD_{50}), and they provided evidence for selectivity and saturability of binding. Subsequent studies by the same group have localized the binding of iodine-labeled neurotoxin at the electron microscopic level (29, 30). Binding sites were found on nerve terminals of motoneurons, where there were approximately 150 to 500 binding sites per micrometer of membrane.

No one has reported radioligand binding studies to characterize the interaction between botulinum neurotoxin and its receptor in peripheral nerves. Because of the presumably small number or receptors in peripheral tissue, such work may require a toxin preparation that is labeled to an unusually high specific activity. However, ligand binding studies have been reported for synaptosome preparations from brain. Early studies provided data that were difficult to accept, owing to the questionable purity of the ligand and to the relatively high concentrations added to membrane preparations, but later work has overcome these difficulties. The most recent studies indicate that the binding of botulinum neurotoxin to brain synaptosomes involves two classes of receptors. A high affinity site has an apparent K_d of 1 to 6 × 10^{-10} M, and a low affinity site has an apparent K_d of 5 × 10^{-8} M (31, 32).

There is evidence to suggest that the heavy chain of the neurotoxin molecule is responsible for binding. When added to neuromuscular preparations, the heavy chain does not paralyze transmission but it does protect tissues from the neuromuscular blocking actions of the intact molecule (L. L. Simpson and B. R. DasGupta, unpublished data). The proposed explanation for this finding is that the isolated heavy chain binds to and occludes receptors, thus preventing the intact molecule from binding. Evidence obtained from histological studies on the neuromuscular junction confirms that the heavy chain mediates binding (29, 30). Experiments on synaptosomes (28, 31–36) have shown that intact toxin binds to plasma membranes; the heavy chain competes for binding sites with the intact toxin; and monoclonal antibody directed against epitopes in the heavy chain prevents binding of the intact molecule. To date, no one has reported use of the labeled heavy chain as a ligand to characterize binding sites.

The receptor for botulinum neurotoxin has not been identified. Simpson & Rapport have shown that botulinum neurotoxin interacts with gangliosides, and this remains the only demonstration of a meaningful interactions between the toxin and a naturally occurring constituent of nerve tissue (37). The work has been reproduced by Kitamura et al, who reported that ganglioside G_{T1b} is most effective at inactivating the toxin (38). The ability of this species of ganglioside to produce inactivation is not equivalent for all serotypes. Of the six that have been tested, types A, B, E, and F were markedly inactivated, but types C and D were only mildly inactivated (39).

Various interpretations can be assigned to the finding that botulinum neurotoxin interacts with gangliosides; they include the following: (a) Gangliosides are merely acceptors and have no real role in the neuroparalytic process; (b) gangliosides are true receptors that mediate the first step in the neuroparalytic process; (c) a sialic acid-containing molecule other than ganglioside, such as a sialoglycoprotein, is the true receptor, and gangliosides partially mimic the behavior of the true receptor; or (d) gangliosides or sialoglycoproteins are involved in something other than the binding step, such as clustering and/or internalization.

Relatively little work is being done to further characterize the interaction between botulinum neurotoxin and gangliosides. Indeed, there is no research program that is entirely devoted to isolating and identifying the toxin receptor. In part, this absence of effort is related to the proposed mechanism of toxin action. It is widely acknowledged that poisoning is due to an intracellular action rather than to membrane binding; therefore, research interest has shifted to the cell interior. However, this shift in focus does not detract from the data that show that binding is the first step in the overall paralytic process, that binding does not have observable effects on cell function, and that binding is mediated by the heavy chain of the toxin molecule.

The literature on the binding of tetanus toxin has evolved quite differently from that on botulinum neurotoxin. Because the former substance is known for its effects on the central nervous system, it has received comparatively little attention as a neuromuscular blocking agent. There are no histological studies that demonstrate binding of tetanus toxin to nerve terminals of motor fibers, and there are few studies that characterize the pharmacological aspects of this binding. Schmitt et al have shown that tetanus toxin binds essentially irreversibly to nerve terminals before there is onset of neuromuscular blockade (14). Simpson has shown that the 50,000 dalton carboxyterminus of the heavy chain appears to mediate binding (40). This fragment will bind to and occlude receptors, thus affording protection against the neuroparalytic effects of the parent molecule.

The literature dealing with the binding of tetanus toxin to brain tissue is more extensive, and most of the reports predate those on neuromuscular transmission. The entire field of study began with the work of Wassermann & Takaki, who provided evidence that brain tissue has receptors for the toxin (41). They found that the residual toxicity in supernatants of solutions incubated with homogenates of brain was diminished, apparently because the toxin was absorbed by the brain. In the intervening years investigators have done radioligand studies to characterize the toxin receptor in brain synaptosomes. They have fractionated the toxin molecule to identify the binding component and have made a number of attempts to clarify the nature of the receptor.

Two different groups have reported that there is a high affinity tetanus toxin receptor in rat and bovine brain membranes. The reported dissociation constants were in reasonably good agreement and both were in the nanomolar range (17, 42). The binding of radiolabeled toxin to brain membranes was antagonized by unlabeled toxin, and radioligand that was already bound could be displaced by unlabeled material. A fragment representing the 50,000 dalton carboxyterminus of the heavy chain antagonized the binding of free toxin and displaced the binding of pre-bound toxin (16, 17).

The pharmacological studies on the neuromuscular junction (see above) and the ligand binding studies on brain membranes gave qualitatively similar results, but the quantitative aspects differed significantly. The apparent dissociation constant for tetanus toxin binding to the phrenic nerve-hemidiaphragm was about 100-fold higher than that reported for brain. This may be a reflection of the fact that a viable neuromuscular junction, unlike brain membranes, has permeability barriers and may also have mechanisms for sequestering toxin. It should be noted that there is a similar quantitative disparity between affinity constants for botulinum neurotoxin binding to brain membranes and neuromuscular junctions, and the underlying problems may be the same. The data suggest that the affinity constants obtained with brain membranes are authentic, but those obtained with functioning neuromuscular junctions are complicated by factors inherent in using a viable tissue. It is hoped that a paradigm will ultimately be developed that gives equivalent findings on inert membranes and on functioning tissues.

The receptor for tetanus toxin has not been unequivocally identified, but van Heyningen deserves credit for having isolated a component from nerve tissue that has receptor-like qualities. Using the original Wassermann-Takaki observations as the basis for his studies, van Heyningen proceeded to isolate the material(s) from brain responsible for adsorbing toxin. A series of reports (43–46) culminated in the discovery that certain classes of gangliosides could bind to and inactivate tetanus toxin. Later work has in some respects tended to support the idea that gangliosides could be tetanus toxin receptors (e.g. 47–51). For example, the 50,000 dalton carboxyterminus of the molecule, which is thought to mediate binding, has a high affinity for gangliosides, and gangliosides compete with brain membranes for binding of toxin (16, 17). Proteolytic agents such as trypsin and chymotrypsin and protein modifying agents such as iodoacetamide, ethoxyformic anhydride, N-ethylmaleimide, and N-bromosuccinimide do not abolish toxin binding sites, and these data support the belief that the toxin receptor is a lipid or complex lipid (i.e. ganglioside) as opposed to a protein (42). Finally, gangliosides can be inserted into non-neural membranes such as those of human erythrocytes, and the modified membranes bind tetanus toxin in a way that mimics nerve membranes (52, 53).

In spite of this suggestive evidence, compelling data that prove gangliosides are receptors have not been published. The various interpretations that were given to the interaction between botulinum neurotoxin and gangliosides are equally valid when discussing tetanus toxin and gangliosides. For both toxins there is evidence for an initial, nontoxic binding step, and there is evidence that the 50,000 dalton carboxyterminus of the heavy chain governs binding. Additional work is needed to isolate and definitively characterize the receptor.

Internalization Step

Expansion of the two-step model for botulinum neurotoxin action (e.g. binding step, poisoning step) to a three-step model (e.g. binding step, translocation step, poisoning step) was based on a specific observation. When phrenic nerve hemidiaphragms were incubated with toxin at 4° C and binding was allowed to go to completion, the membrane-bound toxin remained accessible to neutralizing antibody. However, when tissues were warmed and there was a short period of nerve stimulation, the toxin rapidly disappeared from accessibility to neutralizing antibody. This occurred long before onset of paralysis. These findings prompted the author to propose that a membrane translocation step was interposed between binding and poisoning (1, 2).

There are a variety of substances that cross membranes by the process of receptor-mediated endocytosis, and the process itself has been relatively well characterized (54–57). Those studies dealing with endocytosis of Semliki Forest virus and with diphtheria toxin may be most instructive in terms of providing an analogy. For both the virus and the toxin, there is an initial binding step at the plasma membrane. The receptor-bound material is internalized by structures variously referred to as endocytic vesicles or receptosomes. In most cases, these vesicles migrate toward lysosomes. A proton pump progressively lowers the vesicular pH to a value of 4.0 or lower. This fall in pH triggers a conformational change in the virus/toxin, the result of which is injection of material through the membrane and into the cytoplasm.

Three pieces of evidence support the idea that a pH-dependent step underlies the penetration of endosome membranes (58–62). First, drugs that raise the pH of endosomes and lysosomes (e.g. lysosomotropic agents, such as chloroquine) greatly diminish the activity of Semliki Forest virus and diphtheria toxin. Second, a pH gradient that is artificially created across the plasma membrane can cause direct injection of virus/toxin through the plasma membrane. As expected, lysosomotropic agents do not antagonize virus/toxin that penetrates directly into the cytoplasm and bypasses the endosome-lysosome pathway. Third, and of particularly relevance to diphtheria toxin, experiments on lipid bilayers show that a pH gradient causes the toxin to insert into the artificial membrane and form large channels (19, 63–66). Interestingly, these channels may be large enough to accommodate the passage of the distended form of a polypeptide.

The findings on Semliki Forest virus and on diphtheria toxin have been used to construct a hypothetical sequence that could account for internalization of botulinum neurotoxin and tetanus toxin (Figure 2). A number of recent discoveries encourage a belief that the model is correct. Pharmacological experiments on the mouse phrenic nerve-hemidiaphragm preparation have shown that drugs known to inhibit the actions of internalized substances (e.g. ammonium chloride and methylamine hydrochloride) also inhibit the neuromuscular blocking actions of clostridial toxins (67). In addition, at least one lysosomotropic agent has been shown to antagonize botulinum neurotoxin (e.g. chloroquine), although it did not antagonize tetanus toxin (68). The reason for this discrepancy is not clear.

Studies on lipid vesicles and on lipid bilayers have shown that the heavy chains of botulinum neurotoxin and tetanus toxin form pH-dependent channels (18, 19). More precisely, it is the 50,000 dalton aminoterminus of the heavy chains that is responsible for channel formation. This is a particularly interesting finding, because the aminoterminus of the tetanus toxin molecule has a hydrophobic domain, which could play a role in toxin insertion into membranes, and this hydrophobic domain is not exposed except at low pH (69).

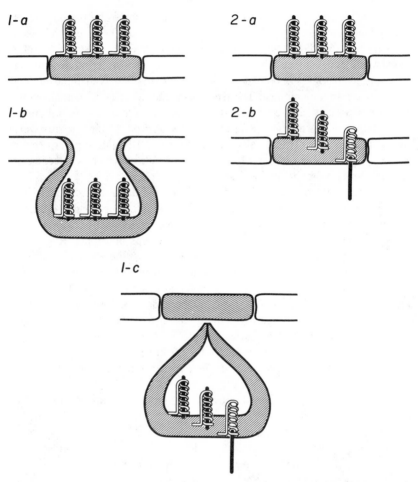

Figure 2   A mechanism for clostridial neurotoxin entry into cells can be built by analogy with other substances, such as Semliki Forest virus and diphtheria toxin. The proposed mechanism for translocation of neurotoxin involves two sequential events. The toxin binds to a specific class of receptors on the plasma membrane of cholinergic nerves (*1-a*). Either at that site or at some other specialized site (viz., caping), the toxin is internalized by the process of receptor mediated endocytosis (*1-b*). This represents the first half of the entry mechanism. The endocytic vesicle becomes progressively more acidic as it approaches the lysosome, and the fall in pH triggers a conformational change in the toxin molecule. A portion of the molecule, probably the aminoterminus, partitions into the membrane and forms channels. The passage of the light chain through the pH-induced channels may represent the second half of the entry mechanism (*1-c*).

By continuing the analogy with Semliki Forest virus and diphtheria toxin, one can propose an experimentally induced mechanism for clostridial neurotoxin entry into cells. This alternate mechanism begins with toxin binding to the plasma membrane (*2-a*). When the tissue is exposed to a medium with low pH, this triggers pH-dependent channel formation. The light chain can then be injected through the plasma membrane and directly into the cytoplasm (*2-b*).

The first study describing the channel forming properties of botulinum neurotoxin provided some comparisons between clostridial toxins and diphtheria toxin (19). Planar lipid bilayers were used to separate two compartments in which pH could be varied independently. In the presence of a symmetric pH of 7.0 or a symmetric pH of 4.0, botulinum neurotoxin, tetanus toxin, and diphtheria toxin fragments possessing the aminoterminus of the heavy chain had only modest channel forming activity. When a pH gradient was created that was equivalent to that across a prelysosomal membrane (i.e. 4.5 to 7.0), the toxin fragments were dramatically more active in forming channels. This result was obtained only when the toxin fragment was on the side of the membrane having a low pH; reversing the pH gradient effectively blocked channel formation.

Perhaps the most intriguing aspect of these channels is that sizing experiments suggest they are large enough to accommodate the passage of a polypeptide across a membrane. This could mean that the aminoterminus of the heavy chain acts like a tunnel protein through which the light chain might pass to reach the cytoplasm. But it is also possible that the channels are epiphenomena that are secondary to some other mechanism for toxin passage through the membrane.

The pharmacological and biophysical experiments pertaining to endocytosis and later penetration of an endosome membrane have been nicely complemented by the histological studies of Dolly and associates (29, 30). Using electron microscopic autoradiography of iodine-labeled toxin, they have shown that a substantial fraction of the material initially bound to cholinergic nerve endings is internalized. The internalization process is energy dependent and is inhibited by low temperature and by agents such as sodium azide and dinitrophenol. Ammonium chloride and methylamine hydrochloride antagonized the internalization process, and chloroquine appeared to trap the toxin inside vesicles. When taken in conjunction with the neuropharmacological studies, these histological data provide convincing evidence that botulinum neurotoxin must be internalized to produce its effects on neuromuscular transmission.

Comparable types of studies to show the internalization of tetanus toxin at the neuromuscular junction have not been published. However, work has been reported on other tissues, and the data are supportive of the concept of endocytosis (70).

The current state of the literature can be summarized in two statements reflecting the belief that internalization involves at least two events. There is widespread acceptance of the idea that clostridial neurotoxins must cross the plasma membrane, and receptor-mediated endocytosis is the most plausible mechanism to account for this. It is also thought that toxin molecules must reach the cytoplasm to exert their poisoning effect, but there is uncertainty about the underlying process. One possibility is that pH-induced channels act like tunnel proteins that permit the passage of active material into the cytoplasm, but other possibilities deserve to be considered.

Intracellular Poisoning Step

Botulinum neurotoxin and tetanus toxin block acetylcholine release from the neuromuscular junction (7, 71). Early studies on botulinum neurotoxin suggested a relatively simple outcome, in which the toxin blocked all transmitter release. Subsequent studies have provided a more complex picture.

Botulinum neurotoxin blocks nerve stimulus-induced release of transmitter, and the effect is virtually complete (26, 72). The toxin also blocks spontaneous quantal release, but the effect is not complete (73, 74). Even in severely poisoned tissues there is a residual population of spontaneous miniature endplate potentials (mepp's). These residual mepp's have a mean amplitude that is less than that seen at normal junctions. The effect of the toxin on spontaneous non-quantal release of acetylcholine is not clear. Two groups have reported that the toxin blocks non-quantal release (75, 76), while one group has reported no effect (77).

The action of the toxin on nerve stimulus-induced and on spontaneous quantal release of acetylcholine, and the putative action of the toxin on spontaneous non-quantal release, are all acute phenomena. Experiments on tissues that are chronically poisoned reveal an additional effect (78, 79). Several days after onset of toxin-induced blockade, there occurs with increasing frequency a spontaneous class of mepp's that are large in amplitude. The origin and mechanism of release of these unusually large mepp's is not known.

The effects of tetanus toxin at the mammalian neuromuscular junction are similar to those of botulinum neurotoxin (13–15, 80). Tetanus toxin blocks nerve stimulus-evoked release of acetylcholine, and it greatly diminishes the frequency of spontaneous mepp's. The effects of the toxin on spontaneous non-quantal release have not been reported. There are also no reports that describe the effects of chronic poisoning on a population of large amplitude mepps.

Some attention has been drawn to the fact that there are subtle differences between the effects of botulinum neurotoxin and tetanus toxin on transmitter release at the neuromuscular junction (e.g. 15, 80). These differences have been interpreted to mean that the two toxins have separate and distinct mechanisms for poisoning transmitter release. For example, Dreyer et al have proposed that tetanus toxin acts to influence the movement of synaptic vesicles toward the active zones, whereas botulinum neurotoxin acts at or within the active zones (80). This is an interesting idea that may ultimately prove to be true, but for the moment one should be cautious. In truth, the proposal that there are different mechanisms of action stems entirely from a comparison of botulinum neurotoxin type A and tetanus toxin. Comparisons with the six other botulinum neurotoxins have not been undertaken. This may be a critical issue, because data now show differences among the various botulinum neurotoxins (81, 82). It may be wise not to draw conclusions until all seven botulinum neurotoxins and tetanus toxin have been examined by the same experimental techniques. Such work may reveal that the seven botulinum neurotoxins are distinctly different from tetanus toxin, or it may reveal that all eight substances are merely variations on a common molecular theme.

No well-defined mechanism to account for the ability of clostridial toxins to block transmitter release has been advanced. A recent study hypothesizes that botulinum neurotoxin stimulates the intracellular metabolic systems that normally remove calcium from the vicinity of the active zones (83). One group has reported that tetanus toxin blocks calcium channels in nerve membranes (84); other groups have reported that neither botulinum neurotoxin nor tetanus toxin acts on calcium channels (85, 86).

The author has proposed that botulinum neurotoxin is an enzyme (2). This proposal was based on several clues, including the remarkable potency and long duration of action of the toxin, which are difficult to explain by a nonenzymatic mechanism. It was also based on a systematic comparison of botulinum neurotoxin with other toxins. The purpose of this comparison was to identify substances, sufficiently similar in structure and/or biological activity to botulinum neurotoxin, to serve as models. The outcome of this search was that no well-known neurotoxin could be found that was fundamentally similar in its structure-function relationships to botulinum neurotoxin. However, diphtheria toxin, a substance not ordinarily associated with the nervous system, appeared to share many features with botulinum neurotoxin. And it can now be added, there are many similarities between diptheria toxin and tetanus toxin as well.

As summarized in Table 1, the clostridial neurotoxins and diphtheria toxin (for reviews, see 87–89) are microbial in origin. The genetic material for each is thought to be in a virus particle or something derived from a virus, such as a plasmid. In the immediate post-translational stage, they are all single chain polypeptides that possess little toxicity (and see Figure 1). These inactive precursors are nicked by proteolytic cleavage to yield dichain molecules, with one heavy chain and one light chain. The tissue targeting domain is known to be in the carboxyterminus of the heavy chain, and the channel forming domain is in the aminoterminus of that chain. For diphtheria toxin, the light chain is an enzyme that has ADP-ribosylating activity.

The similarities between clostridial neurotoxins and diphtheria toxin are too numerous to overlook. It is noteworthy that all proceed through the same sequence of three steps in producing their poisoning effects. Each has a binding domain in one portion of the heavy chain and a channel forming domain in the other portion. It is difficult to avoid speculation that the clostridial neurotoxins, like diphtheria toxin, have an enzymatic domain in the light chain. This

Table 1 A Comparison of diphtheria toxin and clostridial neurotoxins

Characteristic	Diphtheria toxin	Botulinum neurotoxin	Tetanus toxin
Origin	Microbial *(Coryne-bacterium diph-theriae)*	Microbial *(Clostridi-um botulinum)*	Microbial *(Clostridi-um tetani)*
Source of genetic material	Virus	C&D: virus A,B,E,F&G: un-known	Plasmid
Post-translational structure	Single chain polypeptide	Single chain polypeptide	Single chain polypeptide
Active structure	Dichain polypeptide	Dichain polypeptide	Dichain polypeptide
Molecular weights of chains	Light $\sim$ 20,000 Heavy $\sim$ 40,000 (1:2 ratio)	Light $\sim$ 50,000 Heavy $\sim$ 100,000 (1:2 ratio)	Light $\sim$ 50,000 Heavy $\sim$ 100,000 (1:2 ratio)
Location of binding domain	Carboxyterminus of heavy chain	Carboxyterminus of heavy chain	Carboxyterminus of heavy chain
Location of channel forming domain	Aminoterminus of heavy chain	Aminoterminus of heavy chain	Aminoterminus of heavy chain
Location of enzyme domain	Light chain	?	?

speculation is especially hard to avoid when viewed in the context of recently published studies on the botulinum binary toxin.

The Mechanism Of Action Of The Binary Toxin

Efforts to isolate and characterize the eight botulinum toxins led to the discovery that one of them is unique. The serotype designated C_2 was found to be composed of two independent polypeptide chains (20, 21). There is a heavy chain and a light chain, but they are not linked by any covalent bonds. Neither of the chains possesses substantial toxicity, but the combination is very toxic (21, 22, 90, 91). In deference to the structural and toxicological data, the two chains can be regarded as a true binary toxin (22).

The botulinum binary toxin differs in the spectrum of its pharmacological actions from the botulinum neurotoxins (22, 90–92). The latter act rather exclusively on nerve endings to block release of transmitter. The binary toxin acts on a host of tissues, including brain, liver, lung, intestine, and vasculature.

When administered in vivo, the binary toxin and the neurotoxins produce respiratory failure, but the underlying mechanism is not the same. The neurotoxins block transmission between motoneurons and the muscles of respiration. The binary toxin evokes an array of cardiopulmonary effects, including increased vascular permeability, effusive secretions into the airway, pulmonary edema and bleeding, collection of fluids in the thoracic cavity, and extreme hypotension. Most of these effects appear to be related to the movement of fluids across membranes.

Although the manifestations of binary toxin and neurotoxin poisoning appear unrelated, the structure-activity relationships are quite similar. Studies involving chain-specific antibodies suggested that the heavy chain mediated binding and the light chain mediated poisoning (22). This proposed scheme has been verified by experimental evidence. Ohishi has published pharmacological experiments that implicate the heavy chain in binding (90, 91), and more recently he has complemented the work with histological experiments (23). Using fluorescent-labeled derivatives, he has convincingly shown that the heavy chain binds to the plasma membrane of vulnerable cells, and in the absence of this binding the light chain does not become associated with cells.

The light chain has been tested for a variety of enzymatic actions, and the result of this work has been a determination of the molecular basis for the action of the binary toxin. Two groups have shown that the light chain is an enzyme with ADP-ribosylating activity. Leppla (personal communication) has discovered that the chain ADP-ribosylates a protein found in Chinese hamster ovarian cells. The author has reported that the chain has ADP-ribosylating activity in two systems (24). In a model system, the toxin ADP-ribosylates homo-poly-L-arginine. In a system involving endogenous substrates, the toxin ADP-ribosylates a protein found in numerous eucaryotic cells.

The binary toxin is the first of the botulinum toxins for which a mechanism of action has been determined. Even so, there is a considerable amount of work remaining to be done. The substrate has yet to be isolated and characterized, and the role of the substrate in cell function is still unknown. These matters need to be resolved before a link can be made between the molecular action of the toxin and the cellular and systemic actions of the toxin.

The data on the binary toxin naturally raise the question whether botulinum neurotoxin or tetanus toxin have ADP-ribosylating activity. The author is aware of at least six laboratories that have tested this idea; although most of the results have not been published (but see 93), everyone is in agreement that the neurotoxins do not possess such activity, or if the neurotoxins do possess such activity it must be very difficult to demonstrate. The data on diphtheria toxin and on the binary toxin provide clues that the neurotoxins are enzymes, but the precise nature of that enzyme activity remains to be determined.

THE RIDDLE OF ORIGINS

There is one aspect of the study of botulinum toxin and tetanus toxin that has been extremely difficult to resolve. No one has been able to provide an explanation for the origin or the function of these molecules. Indeed, the question of origin and function has proved so baffling that no major article addressing the issue has been written during this century.

It may be helpful to clarify why these matters have been viewed as a riddle. Most neurotoxins of biological origin can be envisioned as serving one of two purposes: they are used by predators to immobilize prey (e.g. alpha-bungarotoxin), or they are used by potential prey to ward off predators (e.g. tetrodotoxin). In some cases it is possible to deduce the origin of a toxin used for these purposes. For example, certain components of snake venoms are enzymes (e.g. phospholipase A2 neurotoxins), and these neurotoxic enzymes may have evolved from digestive enzymes.

One can easily see why the clostridial neurotoxins are viewed as puzzling. To begin with, they do not serve any obvious function, either to advance predation or to ward off predation. And furthermore, there are no obvious predecessors from which they might have evolved. To make matters even more disconcerting, it must now be pointed out that this is only half the riddle.

Although clostridial toxins are named in accordance with the microorganisms that produce them, this practice results in what might be called misnomers. At least two of the botulinum neurotoxins (C and D) are encoded by genetic material that is not native to the host bacteria. The genetic material is found in a virus particle that enters the bacteria (94–96). Clostridia that are infected by the bacteriophage are capable of producing toxin, but when cured of the bacteriophage they lose the ability to make toxin.

The prevailing belief is that the genetic material responsible for synthesis of botulinum neurotoxin (94–96) and tetanus toxin (97) is found either in virus particles or in extrachromosomal elements that may have come from virus particles (e.g. plasmids). Aside from the fact that this raises questions about names like botulinum toxin and tetanus toxin, this information seems to make more obscure the reason for the existence of the molecules. On the one hand, the genetic information for the toxins is found in virus particles that infect procaryotes. But on the other hand, the toxins themselves affect eucaryotes, and in particular those highly developed eucaryotes that have a peripheral nervous system. By any standard of reasonableness, this is a puzzling state of affairs.

One advantage of the proposed model for clostridial neurotoxin action is that it has helped to explain the nature of the interaction between two remarkably potent toxins and the nervous system. It has served as a stimulus to move research from a phenomenological level, which describes toxin action in terms of outcome, to a mechanistic level, which describes toxin action in terms of cellular, subcellular, and even molecular events. Another advantage of the model, though perhaps less obvious at first, is that it provides tentative clues about the origin of clostridial neurotoxins. By combining certain elements of the molecular pharmacology of the toxins with certain principles of molecular biology, one can construct a hypothetical scheme to account for the origin of these substances.

THE CONCEPT OF SUPERFUNCTION

It must be stressed that the model discussed above is not unique to the clostridial toxins. As implied by the discussion and the data in Table 1, it is equally applicable to diphtheria toxin. In fact, the model is to varying degrees true for a host of bacterial toxins (e.g. *Pseudomonas aeruginosa* exotoxin, cholera toxin, *E. coli* enterotoxin, pertussis toxin) and for a number of plant lectins (e.g. abrin and ricin). In fairness to the accomplishments of others, one should note that many aspects of the model were developed before more recent work indicated that it could encompass the clostridial toxins (25).

An important implication arises from the finding that many protein toxins behave in accordance with the three-step model. The implication is that investigators should be seeking a general theory to account for the origin and function of a dozen or more protein toxins rather than a narrow explanation that pertains only to clostridial toxins. To be more precise, investigators should try to deduce the origin of a class of molecules that has two major properties: (*a*) The molecules are synthesized in one type of cell but act on another and remote type of cell, and (*b*) the molecules possess a receptor binding domain, a translocation domain, and an enzyme domain.

Pharmacologists will be quick to note that these two major properties are largely shared by another class of molecules that are ubiquitous among eucaryotes. Much of the terminology used to describe the protein toxins needs to be modified only slightly to become acceptable terminology for describing messenger systems. The most well understood messenger systems are those that have three components. (*a*) A first messenger or signal component (e.g. neurotransmitter, hormone) is synthesized in one cell type but is secreted to act on a remote cell type. (*b*) A transduction component is interposed between the extracellular first messenger and an intracellular second messenger. Typically, transduction can be attributed to the opening of ion channels and/or to the induction of an enzyme. (*c*) The intracellular enzyme (e.g. adenylate cyclase) or its product (e.g. cyclic-AMP) is a third component that initiates a cascade of events culminating in an organotypic response.

The similarities between toxins and messenger systems may be much more than merely semantic. To substantiate this claim, the author will introduce a novel term that may help to explain the relationships between protein toxins, messenger systems, and other complex molecular systems. The term is a corrollary of one that has been used to describe the immunoglobulin family; the term is superfunction.

Investigators studying the origin and genetic correlates of immunoglobulin proteins have coined the term supergene (98). Stated simply, a supergene is a set of individual genes or gene families that have sequence homology but that do not necessarily encode proteins with the same function. By contrast, one can envision superfunction as a set of individual functions or families of functions that are similar in terms of expressed activity but that do not necessarily stem from the same genes. Thus, there are messenger systems that involve a variety of transmitters and hormones as signals, a variety of ion channels or allosteric proteins as transducers, and a variety of enzymes and products as intracellular mediators; these messenger systems compose one functional family. The dozen or so protein toxins with binding, translocation, and enzyme domains compose another. These two families as well as others (see below) can be grouped together under the concept of superfunction.

The relatedness between toxins and messenger systems is far more extensive than can be considered here. However, three specific illustrations may help to make the point. There are examples of toxins whose tissue binding domain recognizes the same cell surface receptor as the signal component of messenger systems (99, 100). Another similarity is that toxins and messenger systems have been highly conservative with their intracellularly acting components. The former makes considerable use of ADP-ribosylating enzymes, and the latter makes considerable use of adenylate cyclase. Perhaps most provocatively, the two have numerous points of convergence. Cholera toxin ADP-ribosylates a regulatory protein that stimulates adenylate cyclase, and pertussis toxin ADP-ribosylates a regulatory protein that inhibits adenylate cyclase (101). Certainly the most striking example of convergence is anthrax toxin. The enzyme component of this toxin does not merely alter adenylate cyclase; the enzyme component of this toxin is adenylate cyclase (102).

Returning to the concept of superfunction, there is one last family that must be considered here. To do so begins to make clear the possible origin of botulinum and tetanus toxins. Many virus particles have components or can encode components that are essential to infection and that resemble the models discussed above. Of necessity, these particles must have a binding domain that can attach to receptors on the cell surface. They also have domains that mediate translocation. As discussed above, the mechanism of membrane translocation used by Semliki Forest virus has served to guide research on diphtheria toxin and clostridial toxins. And finally, virus particles encode the information for numerous enzymes that profoundly alter the behavior of infected cells.

Again, there are many examples that can be cited to show the relatedness between virus function and toxin function, but one is particularly illustrative in the present context. The multiple domain structure of viruses and toxins implies that all the domains must be present to obtain full expression of activity. In the absence of any particular domain, the virus or toxin loses its ability to exert its effects. Uchida et al have reported an interesting experiment in which an incomplete virus was mixed with an incomplete toxin to create a novel and completely functional unit (103). First, virus ghosts were produced by emptying Sendai virus particles of their normal contents. Next, a mutant of diphtheria toxin that possessed enzyme activity but lacked cell binding activity was isolated. The incomplete toxin was then loaded into the virus ghost. The newly constituted unit affected only those cells that had receptors for the virus, and it acted intracellularly only on those molecules susceptible to the ADP-ribosylating effects of diphtheria toxin.

This experiment sets the stage for putting forward two possible ideas to account for the origin of clostridial toxins. The first of these is rather straightforward and easy to grasp. Clostridial toxins may not have arisen *de novo* as unusual molecules synthesized in one cell and acting on another. Instead, the toxins may be variants on the proteins that viruses ordinarily synthesize. Virus particles are evolutionarily ancient, and therefore they could have served as the precursor for the functional property of originating in one place but acting remotely in another place. In addition, virus particles have or encode for binding domains, translocation domains, and enzyme domains. This means they could have been precursors for molecules such as toxins that possess similar domains. The clostridial toxins may be proteins encoded by nucleic acid that at one time served as a template for virus domains, but which through mutations and other modifications now serve as a template for toxin domains.

The second proposal is a variant on the first, and it attempts to address the fact that substrates for many of the potent protein toxins are found mainly or exclusively in eucaryotic cells. The essence of the proposal, which is illustrated in Figure 3, is as follows. Eucaryotic cells carry the genetic information for the binding, transduction, and enzyme-messenger functions, and virus particles carry the information for binding, translocation, and enzyme functions. It is conceivable that a recombinant event could have allowed a virus to capture a eucaryotic gene segment encoding an enzyme that participated in a messenger system. Or to make the proposal broader, the recombinant event could have resulted in capture of almost any eucaryotic enzyme. The product would be a gene segment of non-eucaryotic origin that encodes binding and translocation domains linked to a gene segment of eucaryotic origin that encodes an enzyme domain.

These two proposals certainly should not be viewed as rigid. To the contrary, they are conceptual models that are representative of the two most logical sources of the toxins, i.e. a modified viral origin, or a modified viral and

EUCARYOTIC DNA

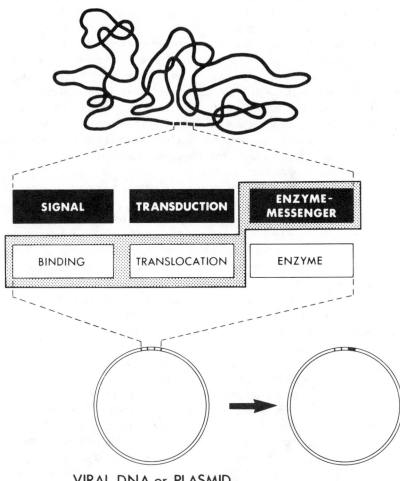

VIRAL DNA or PLASMID

Figure 3   One possible explanation for the origin of clostridial toxins involves the mechanism of recombination. Eucaryotic genes carry the information for signal, transduction, and enzyme components of messenger systems. Viral or other extrachromosomal elements carry the information for binding, translocation, and enzyme components associated with infectivity. Through a recombinant event, viral gene segments for binding and translocation may have become linked to a eucaryotic gene segment for enzyme activity. This newly constituted element could encode a multiple domain molecule similar to a protein toxin that acts on substrates in eucaryotic cells.

eucaryotic origin. Either of these origins, when viewed in the context of superfunction, could explain the two major properties of protein toxins (e.g. different sites for synthesis and activity; multiple domains).

For reasons that are clear, it is difficult to test the idea that a gene encoding the structural proteins of a virus evolved into a gene encoding a protein toxin. There is however a method for deducing whether the enzyme component of a protein toxin is the same as or similar to an enzyme normally occurring in eucaryotic cells. Investigators can search eucaryotic cells to determine whether there are enzymes that are indistinguishable from those in toxins. Only a limited amount of work has been done, but it is interesting to report that eucaryotic sources of cholera toxin-like (104, 105) and diphtheria toxin-like (106) enzymes have been reported. The workers who have made these exciting discoveries are continuing their efforts to compare enzymes in toxins and in nucleated cells.

Much more work must be done before one can say with certainty whether the two proposals just described can explain the origin of clostridial toxins. An important ingredient will be continued effort to determine the function of the light chains of botulinum neurotoxin and tetanus toxin. In the meantime, work is already in progress to locate a eucaryotic source of the enzyme found in the light chain of the botulinum binary toxin.

MERGING MOLECULAR PHARMACOLOGY AND MOLECULAR BIOLOGY: UTILIZING THE CONCEPT OF SUPERFUNCTION

The concept of superfunction implies that when a functional domain from one complex molecule is substituted for the equivalent domain in another molecule, the newly created structure may be biologically active. It would be desirable to obtain evidence to support this idea from naturally occurring events, but the chances of detecting a spontaneous recombination are rare. There is one exception to this rule. Botulinum neurotoxin occurs in at least seven serotypes. Individual types are usually synthesized by individual strains of bacteria, but there are strains that produce more than one type. A single strain that produces more than one botulinum neurotoxin greatly increases the possibility of detecting recombination.

In a series of interesting papers, a Japanese group has provided data that are indicative of a recombinant event (107–109). They have isolated a botulinum neurotoxin that behaves much like a hybrid, with a heavy chain apparently derived from one serotype and a light chain derived from another. Neurotoxin molecules with hybrid qualities possessed the same potency as non-hybrid molecules. The group that did the work has itself speculated that the hybrid toxin could be the result of recombination (107).

An alternate method to genetic recombination can be used to show that functional domains may be exchangeable between molecules that belong to the same family. Posttranslational products can be dissociated into their respective components, and then these components can be reassociated into a novel hybrid. There are examples of this that are especially relevant to the clostridial toxins. Botulinum neurotoxin (BNT) and tetanus toxin (TT) are composed of heavy (H) and light (L) chains linked by a disulfide bond (S–S). Thus, botulinum neurotoxin type A could be written as $BNT_A(H)$–S–S–$BNT_A(L)$, and tetanus toxin would be written as TT(H)–S–S–TT(L). The concept of superfunction implies that hybrid molecules such as $BNT_A(H)$–S–S–$BNT_B(L)$ or $BNT_F(H)$–S–S–$BNT_G(L)$ should produce neuromuscular blockade. Even more provocatively, the concept implies that BNT(H)–S–S–TT(L) and TT(H)–S–S–BNT(L) should also be biologically active. The proposed model for clostridial toxin action suggests that low doses of the former should be tissue targeted to cholinergic nerve endings, where it will produce flaccid paralysis, and the latter should enter the central nervous system, where it will produce spastic paralysis. Three laboratories are working collaboratively to make these posttranslational hybrids and to use them to test current thinking about clostridial toxin action (J. R. Robinson, Vanderbilt University; B. R. DasGupta, University of Wisconsin; and the author).

This is but a narrow application of an idea that many investigators have already grasped. Hybrid toxins are immensely valuable for studying toxin action, but they may also be useful as therapeutic agents and as pharmacological tools. Readers who are not familiar with the field of hybrid toxin research may wish to consult the reviews by Olsnes & Pihl (110), Vitetta et al (111), and Thorpe & Ross (112).

The clostridial toxins are among those multiple domain molecules whose constituent parts could be used to form hybrids that would be therapeutic agents or pharmacological research tools. A hybrid molecule that retained the heavy chain of botulinum neurotoxin but that replaced the light chain with an anti-light chain antibody might well be a clinically useful drug for entering nerve endings and arresting the effect of internalized toxin. Conversely, hybrid molecules that retained the light chains but replaced the heavy chains with drugs that are tissue targeted for specific types of nerve endings (e.g. dopaminergic, serotonergic, enkephalinergic) might well be a family of substances for blocking mediator release from all chemically transmitting nerves. In these and other settings, hybrid clostridial toxins could become valuable drugs in the disciplines of experimental and clinical pharmacology.

Literature Cited

1. Simpson, L. L. 1980. Kinetic studies on the interaction between botulinum toxin type A and the cholinergic neuromuscular junction. *J. Pharmacol. Exp. Ther.* 212:16–21
2. Simpson, L. L. 1981. The origin, structure and pharmacological activity of botulinum toxin. *Pharmacol. Rev.* 33: 155–88
3. Smith, L. DS. 1977. *Botulism: The Organism, Its Toxins, The Disease.* Springfield, Ill.: Thomas. 236 pp.
4. DasGupta, B. R., Sugiyama, H. 1972. A common subunit structure in *Clostridium botulinum* type A, B and E toxins. *Biochem. Biophys. Res. Commun.* 48: 108–12
5. Bizzini, B. 1979. Tetanus toxin. *Microbiol. Rev.* 43:224–40
6. van Heyningen, S. 1981. Tetanus toxin. *Pharmacol. Ther.* 11:141–57
7. Wellhöner, H.-H. 1982. Tetanus neurotoxin. *Rev. Physiol. Biochem. Pharmacol.* 93:1–68
8. Robinson, J. P., Hash, J. H. 1982. A review of the molecular structure of tetanus toxin. *Mol. Cell. Biochem.* 48:33–44
9. Kaeser, H. E., Saner, A. 1970. The effect of tetanus toxin on neuromuscular transmission. *Eur. Neurol.* 3:193–205
10. Diamond, J., Mellanby, J. 1971. The effect of tetanus toxin in the goldfish. *J. Physiol.* 215:727–41
11. Duchen, L. W., Tonge, D. A. 1973. The effects of tetanus toxin on neuromuscular transmission and on the morphology of motor end-plates in slow and fast skeletal muscle of the mouse. *J. Physiol.* 228: 157–72
12. Bevan, S., Wendon, L. M. B. 1984. A study of the action of tetanus toxin at rat soleus neuromuscular junctions. *J. Physiol.* 348:1–17
13. Habermann, E., Dreyer, F., Bigalke, H. 1980. Tetanus toxin blocks the neuromuscular transmission in vitro like botulinum A toxin. *Naunyn-Schmiedeberg's Arch. Pharmacol.* 311:33–40
14. Schmitt, A., Dreyer, F., John, C. 1981. At least three sequential steps are involved in the tetanus toxin-induced block of neuromuscular transmission. *Naunyn-Schmiedeberg's Arch. Pharmacol.* 317: 326–30
15. Dreyer, F., Schmitt, A. 1983. Transmitter release in tetanus and botulinum A toxin-poisoned mammalian motor end-plates and its dependence on nerve stimulation and temperature. *Pflügers Arch.* 399:228–34
16. Morris, N. P., Consiglio, E., Kohn, L. D., Habig, W. H., Hardegree, M. C., Helting, T. B. 1980. Interaction of fragments B and C of tetanus toxin with neural and thyroid membranes and with gangliosides. *J. Biol. Chem.* 255:6071–76
17. Goldberg, R. L., Costa, T., Habig, W. H., Kohn, L. D., Hardegree, M. C. 1981. Characterization of fragment C and tetanus toxin binding to rat brain membranes. *Mol. Pharmacol.* 20:565–70
18. Boquet, P., Duflot, E. 1982. Tetanus toxin fragment forms channels in lipid vesicles at low pH. *Proc. Natl. Acad. Sci. USA* 79:7614–18
19. Hoch, D. H., Romero-Mira, M., Ehrlich, B. E., Finkelstein, A., DasGupta, B. R., Simpson, L. L. 1985. Channels formed by botulinum, tetanus and diphtheria toxins in planar lipid bilayers: Relevance to translocation of proteins across membranes. *Proc. Natl. Acad. Sci. USA* 82:1692–96
20. Iwasaki, M., Ohishi, I., Sakaguchi, G. 1980. Evidence that botulinum C_2 toxin has two dissimilar components. *Infect. Immun.* 29:390–94
21. Ohishi, I., Iwasaki, M., Sakaguchi, G. 1980. Purification and characterization of two components of botulinum C_2 toxin. *Infect. Immun.* 30:668–73
22. Simpson, L. L. 1982. A comparison of the pharmacological properties of *Clostridium botulinum* type C_1 and type C_2 toxins. *J. Pharmacol. Exp. Ther.* 223: 695–701
23. Ohishi, I., Miyake, M. 1985. Binding of the two components of C_2 toxin to epithelial cells and brush borders of mouse intestine. *Infect. Immun.* 48:769–75
24. Simpson, L. L. 1984. Molecular basis for the pharmacological actions of *Clostridium botulinum* type C_2 toxin. *J. Pharmacol. Exp. Ther.* 230:665–69
25. Gill, D. M. 1978. Seven toxic peptides that cross cell membranes. In *Bacterial Toxins and Cell Membranes*, ed. J. Jeljaszewica, T. Wadstrom, pp. 291–332. London: Academic
26. Burgen, A. S. V., Dickens, F., Zatman, L. J. 1949. The action of botulinum toxin on the neuromuscular junction. *J. Physiol.* 109:10–24
27. Hirokawa, N., Kitamura, M. 1975. Localization of radioactive ^{125}I-labelled

botulinus toxin at the neuromuscular junction of mouse diaphragm. *Naunyn-Schmiedeberg's Arch. Pharmacol.* 287:107–10

28. Dolly, J. O., Williams, R. S., Black, J. D., Tse, C. K., Hambleton, P., Melling, J. 1982. Localization of sites for ^{125}I-labelled botulinum neurotoxin at murine neuromuscular junction and its binding to rat brain synaptosomes. *Toxicon* 20:141–48

29. Dolly, J. O., Black, J., Williams, R. S., Melling, J. 1984. Acceptors for botulinum neurotoxin reside on motor nerve terminals and mediate its internalization. *Nature* 307:457–60

30. Dolly, J. O., Halliwell, J. V., Black, J. D., Williams, R. S., Pelchen-Matthews, A., et al. 1984. Botulinum neurotoxin and dendrotoxin as probes for studies on transmitter release. *J. Physiol.* 79:280–303

31. Agui, T., Syuto, B., Oguma, K., Iida, H., Kubo, S. 1983. Binding of *Clostridium botulinum* type C neurotoxin to rat brain synaptosomes. *J. Biochem.* 94:521–27

32. Williams, R. S., Tse, C.-K., Dolly, J. O., Hambleton, P., Melling, J. 1983. Radioiodination of botulinum neurotoxin type A with retention of biological activity and its binding to brain synaptosomes. *Eur. J. Biochem.* 131:437–45

33. Kitamura, M. 1976. Binding of botulinum neurotoxin to the synaptosome fraction of rat brain. *Naunyn-Schmiedeberg's Arch. Pharmacol.* 295:171–75

34. Kozaki, S. 1979. Interaction of botulinum type A, B and E derivative toxins with synaptosomes of rat brain. *Naunyn-Schmiedeberg's Arch. Pharmacol.* 308:67–70

35. Hirokawa, N., Kitamura, M. 1979. Binding of *Clostridium botulinum* neurotoxin to the presynaptic membrane in the central nervous system. *J. Cell Biol.* 81:43–49

36. Kozaki, S., Sakaguchi, G. 1982. Binding to mouse brain synaptosomes of *Clostridium botulinum* type E derivative toxin before and after tryptic activation. *Toxicon* 20:841–46

37. Simpson, L. L., Rapport, M. M. 1971. The binding of botulinum toxin to membrane lipids: Sphingolipids, steroids and fatty acids. *J. Neurochem.* 18:1751–59

38. Kitamura, M., Iwamori, M., Nagai, Y. 1980. Interaction between *Clostridium botulinum* neurotoxin and gangliosides. *Biochim. Biophys. Acta* 628:328–35

39. Kozaki, S., Sakaguchi, G., Nishimura, M., Iwamori, M., Nagai, Y. 1984. In-

hibitory effect of ganglioside G_{T1B} on the activities of *Clostridium botulinum* toxins. *FEMS Microbiol. Lett.* 21:219–23

40. Simpson, L. L. 1984. Fragment C of tetanus toxin antagonizes the neuromuscular blocking properties of native tetanus toxin. *J. Pharmacol. Exp. Ther.* 228:600–4

41. Wassermann, A., Takaki, T. 1898. Über tetanus antitoxishe Eigenschaften des normalen Zentralnerven systems. *Berl. Klin. Wochenschr.* 35:5–6

42. Rogers, T. B., Snyder, S. H. 1981. High affinity binding of tetanus toxin to mammalian brain membranes. *J. Biol. Chem.* 256:2402–7

43. van Heyningen, W. E. 1959. The fixation of tetanus toxin by nervous tissue. *J. Gen. Microbiol.* 20:291–300

44. van Heyningen, W. E. 1959. Tentative identification of the tetanus toxin receptor in nervous tissue. *J. Gen. Microbiol.* 20:310–20

45. van Heyningen, W. E., Miller, P. A. 1961. The fixation of tetanus toxin by ganglioside. *J. Gen. Microbiol.* 24:107–19

46. van Heyningen, W. E. 1963. The fixation of tetanus toxin, strychnine, serotonin and other substances by ganglioside. *J. Gen. Microbiol.* 31:375–87

47. Clowes, A. W., Cherry, R. J., Chapman, D. 1972. Physical effects of tetanus toxin on model membranes containing gangliosides. *J. Mol. Biol.* 67:49–57

48. Dimpfel, W., Huang, R. T. C., Haberman, E. 1977. Gangliosides in nervous tissue cultures and binding of ^{125}I-labelled tetanus toxin, a neuronal marker. *J. Neurochem.* 29:329–34

49. Yavin, E., Yavin, Z., Kohn, L. D. 1983. Temperature-mediated interaction of tetanus toxin with cerebral neuron cultures: Characterization of a neuraminidase-insensitive toxin-receptor complex. *J. Neurochem.* 40:1212–19

50. Yavin, E. 1984. Gangliosides mediate association of tetanus toxin with neural cells in culture. *Arch. Biochem. Biophys.* 230:129–37

51. Yavin, E., Habig, W. H. 1984. Binding of tetanus toxin to somatic neural hybrid cells with varying ganglioside composition. *J. Neurochem.* 42:1313–20

52. Lazarovici, P., Yavin, E. 1985. Tetanus toxin interaction with human erythrocytes. 1. Properties of polysialoganglioside association with the cell surface. *Biochim. Biophys. Acta* 812:523–31

53. Lazarovici, P., Yavin, E. 1985. Tetanus toxin interaction with human erythro-

cytes. 2. Kinetic properties of toxin association and evidence for a ganglioside-toxin macromolecular complex formation. *Biochim. Biophys. Acta* 812: 532–42

54. Neville, D. M. Jr., Chang, T. 1978. Receptor-mediated protein transport into cells. Entry mechanisms for toxins, hormones, antibodies, viruses, lysosomal hydrolases, asialoglycoproteins, and carrier proteins. *Curr. Top. Membr. Transp.* 10:65–150

55. Goldstein, J. L., Anderson, R. G. W., Brown, M. S. 1979. Coated pits, coated vesicles, and receptor-mediated endocytosis. *Nature* 279:679–85

56. Pastan, I. H., Willingham, M. C. 1981. Receptor-mediated endocytosis of hormones in cultured cells. *Ann. Rev. Physiol.* 43:239–50

57. Anderson, R. G. W., Kaplan, J. 1983. Receptor-mediated endocytosis. *Modern Cell Biol.* 1:1–52

58. Helenius, A., Kartenbeck, J., Simons, K., Fries, E. 1980. On the entry of Semliki Forest virus into BHK-21 cells. *J. Cell Biol.* 84:404–20

59. White, J., Kartenbeck, J., Helenius, A. 1980. Fusion of Semliki Forest virus with the plasma membrane can be induced by low pH. *J. Cell Biol.* 87:264–72

60. Leppla, S. H., Dorland, R. B., Middlebrook, J. L. 1980. Inhibition of diphtheria toxin degradation and cytotoxic action by chloroquine. *J. Biol. Chem.* 255:2247–50

61. Sandvig, K., Olsnes, S. 1980. Diphtheria toxin entry into cells is facilitated by low pH. *J. Cell Biol.* 87:828–32

62. Draper, R. K., Simon, M. I. 1980. The entry of diphtheria toxin into the mammalian cell cytoplasm: Evidence for lysosomal involvement. *J. Cell Biol.* 87:849–54

63. Donovan, J. J., Simon, M. I., Draper, R. K., Montal, M. 1981. Diphtheria toxin forms transmembrane channels in planar lipid bilayers. *Proc. Natl. Acad. Sci. USA* 78:172–76

64. Kagan, B. L., Finkelstein, A., Colombini, M. 1981. Diphtheria toxin fragment forms large pores in phospholipid bilayer membranes. *Proc. Natl. Acad. Sci. USA* 78:4950–54

65. Misler, S. 1983. Gating of ion channels made by a diphtheria toxin fragment in phospholipid bilayer membranes. *Proc. Natl. Acad. Sci. USA* 80:4320–24

66. Zalman, L. S., Wisnieski, B. J. 1984. Mechanism of insertion of diphtheria toxin: Peptide entry and pore size determinations. *Proc. Natl. Acad. Sci. USA* 81:3341–45

67. Simpson, L. L. 1983. Ammonium chloride and methylamine hydrochloride antagonize clostridial neurotoxins. *J. Pharmacol. Exp. Ther.* 225:546–52

68. Simpson, L. L. 1982. The interaction between aminoquinolines and presynaptically acting neurotoxins. *J. Pharmacol. Exp. Ther.* 222:43–48

69. Boquet, P., Duflot, E., Hauttecoeur, B. 1984. Low pH induces a hydrophobic domain in the tetanus toxin molecule. *Eur. J. Biochem.* 144:339–44

70. Montesano, R., Roth, J., Robert, A., Orci, L. 1982. Non-coated membrane invaginations are involved in binding and internalization of cholera and tetanus toxin. *Nature* 296:651–53

71. Gundersen, C. B. 1980. The effects of botulinum toxin on the synthesis, storage and release of acetylcholine. *Prog. Neurobiol.* 14:99–119

72. Brooks, V. B. 1956. An intracellular study of the action of repetitive nerve volleys and of botulinum toxin on miniature end-plate potentials. *J. Physiol.* 134:264–77

73. Harris, A. J., Miledi, R. 1971. The effect of type D botulinum toxin on frog neuromuscular junctions. *J. Physiol.* 217:497–515

74. Spitzer, N. 1972. Miniature end-plate potentials at mammalian neuromuscular junctions poisoned by botulinum toxin. *Nature* 237:26–27

75. Dolezal, V., Vyskocil, F., Tucek, S. 1983. Decrease of the spontaneous nonquantal release of acetyl-choline from the phrenic nerve in botulinum-poisoned rat diaphragm. *Pflügers Arch.* 397:319–22

76. Gundersen, C. B., Jenden, D. J. 1983. Spontaneous output of acetylcholine from rat diaphragm preparations declines after treatment with botulinum toxin. *J. Pharmacol. Exp. Ther.* 224:265–68

77. Stanley, E. F., Drachman, D. B. 1983. Botulinum toxin blocks quantal but not non-quantal release of ACh at the neuromuscular junction. *Brain Res.* 261:172–75

78. Kim, Y. I., Lomo, T., Lupa, M. T., Thesleff, S. 1984. Miniature end-plate potentials in rat skeletal muscle poisoned with botulinum toxin. *J. Physiol.* 356:587–99

79. Thesleff, S. 1984. Transmitter release in botulinum-poisoned muscles. *J. Physiol.* 79:192–95

80. Dreyer, F., Becker, C., Bigalke, H., Funk, J., Penner, R., et al. 1984. Action of botulinum A toxin and tetanus toxin on

synaptic transmission. *J. Physiol.* 79: 252–58

81. Sellin, L. C., Thesleff, S., DasGupta, B. R. 1983. Different effects of types A and B botulinum toxin on transmitter release at the rat neuromuscular junction. *Acta Physiol. Scand.* 119:127–33

82. Sellin, L. C., Kauffman, J. A., DasGupta, B. R. 1983. Comparison of the effects of botulinum neurotoxin types A and E at the rat neuromuscular junction. *Med. Biol.* 61:120–25

83. Molgo, J., Thesleff, S. 1984. Studies on the mode of action of botulinum toxin type A at the frog neuromuscular junction. *Brain Res.* 297:309–16

84. Higashida, J., Sugimoto, N., Ozutsumi, K., Miki, N., Matsuda, M. 1983. A rapid and selective blockade of the calcium, but not sodium, component of action potentials in cultured neuroblastoma N1E-115 cells. *Brain Res.* 279:363–68

85. Gundersen, C. B., Katz, B., Miledi, R. 1982. The antagonism between botulinum toxin and calcium in motor nerve terminals. *Proc. R. Soc. London Ser. B* 216:369–76

86. Dreyer, F., Mallart, A., Brigant, J. L. 1983. Botulinum A toxin and tetanus toxin do not affect presynaptic membrane currents in mammalian motor nerve endings. *Brain Res.* 270:373–75

87. Collier, R. J. 1977. Inhibition of protein synthesis by exotoxins from *Corynebacterium diphtheriae* and *Pseudomonas aeruginosa.* In *The Specificity and Action of Animal, Bacterial and Plant Toxins,* ed. P. Cuatrecasas, pp. 67–98. London: Chapman & Hall

88. Pappenheimer, A. M. Jr. 1977. Diphtheria toxin. *Ann. Rev. Biochem.* 46:69–94

89. Uchida, T. 1983. Diphtheria toxin. *Pharmacol. Ther.* 19:107–22

90. Ohishi, I. 1983. Lethal and vascular permeability activities of botulinum C_2 toxin induced by separate injections of the two toxin components. *Infect. Immun.* 40:336–39

91. Ohishi, I. 1983. Response of mouse intestinal loop to botulinum C_2 toxin: Enterotoxic activity induced by cooperation of nonlinked protein components. *Infect. Immun.* 40:691–95

92. Jensen, W. I., Duncan, R. M. 1980. The susceptibility of the mallard duck *(Anas platyrhynchos)* to *Clostridium botulinum* C_2 toxin. *Jpn. J. Med. Sci. Biol.* 33:81–86

93. Wendon, L. M. B., Gill, D. M. 1982. Tetanus toxin action on cultured nerve

cells: Does it modify a neuronal protein? *Brain Res.* 238:292–97

94. Inoue, K., Iida, H. 1970. Conversion of toxigenicity in *Clostridium botulinum* type C. *Jpn. J. Microbiol.* 14:87–89

95. Inoue, K., Iida, H. 1971. Phage-conversion toxigenicity in *Clostridium botulinum* types C and D. *Jpn. J. Med. Sci. Biol.* 24:53–56

96. Eklund, M. W., Poysky, F. T., Reed, S. M. 1972. Bacteriophage and the toxigenicity on *Clostridium botulinum* type D. *Nature* 235:16–17

97. Finn, C. W. Jr., Silver, R. P., Habig, W. H., Hardegree, M. C., Zon, G., Garon, C. F. 1984. The structural gene for tetanus neurotoxin is on a plasmid. *Science* 224:881–84

98. Hood, L., Kronenberg, M., Hunkapiller, T. 1985. T cell antigen receptors and the immunoglobulin supergene family. *Cell* 40:225–29

99. Ledley, F. D., Lee, G., Kohn, L. D., Habig, W. H., Hardegree, M. C. 1977. Tetanus toxin interactions with thyroid plasma membranes. *J. Biol. Chem.* 252:4049–55

100. Habig, W. H., Grollman, E. F., Ledley, F. D., Meldolesi, M. F., Aloj, S. M., et al. 1978. Tetanus toxin interactions with the thyroid: Decreased toxin binding to membranes from a thyroid tumor with a thyrotropin receptor defect and in vivo stimulation of thyroid function. *Endocrinology* 102:844–51

101. Hayaishi, O., Ueda, K. 1982. *ADP-Ribosylation Reactions.* New York: Academic. 698 pp.

102. Leppla, S. H. 1982. Anthrax toxin edema factor: A bacterial adenylate cyclase that increases cyclic AMP concentrations in eukaryotic cells. *Proc. Natl. Acad. Sci. USA* 79:3162–66

103. Uchida, T., Yamaizumi, M., Okada, Y. 1977. Reassembled HVJ (Sendai virus) envelopes containing non-toxic mutant proteins of diphtheria toxin show toxicity to mouse L cell. *Nature* 266:839–40

104. Moss, J., Vaughan, M. 1978. Isolation of an avian erythrocyte protein possessing ADP-ribosylatransferase activity and capable of activating adenylate cyclase. *Proc. Natl. Acad. Sci. USA* 75:3621–24

105. Moss, J., Stanley, S. J., Watkins, P. A. 1980. Isolation and properties of an NAD- and guanidine-dependent ADP-ribosyltransferase from turkey erythrocytes. *J. Biol. Chem.* 255:5838–40

106. Lee, H., Iglewski, W. J. 1984. Cellular ADP-ribosyltransferase with the same mechanism of action as diphtheria toxin

and Pseudomonas toxin A. *Proc. Natl. Acad. Sci. USA* 81:2703–7

107. Ochanda, H. O., Syuto, B., Oguma, K., Iida, H., Kubo, S. 1984. Comparison of antigenicity of toxins produced by *Clostridium botulinum* type C and D strains. *Appl. Environ. Microbiol.* 47:1319–22

108. Oguma, K., Murayama, S., Syuto, B., Iida, H., Kubo, S. 1984. Analysis of antigenicity of *Clostridium botulinum* type C_1 and D toxins by polyclonal and monoclonal antibodies. *Infect. Immun.* 43:584–88

109. Terajima, J., Syuto, B., Ochanda, J. O., Kubo, S. 1985. Purification and characterization of neurotoxin produced by *Clostridium botulinum* type C 6813. *Infect. Immun.* 48:312–17

110. Olsnes, S., Pihl, A. 1982. Chimeric toxins. *Pharmacol. Ther.* 15:355–81

111. Vitetta, E. S., Krolick, K. A., Miyama-Inaba, M., Cushley, W., Uhr, J. W. 1983. Immunotoxins: A new approach to cancer therapy. *Science* 219:644–50

112. Thorpe, P. E., Ross, W. 1982. The preparation and cytotoxic properties of antibody-toxin conjugates. *Immunol. Rev.* 62:119–58

Ann. Rev. Pharmacol. Toxicol. 1986 26:455–515

THE PHARMACOLOGY AND TOXICOLOGY OF THE INTERFERONS: An Overview[1]

Gilbert J. Mannering and Laurel B. Deloria

Department of Pharmacology, University of Minnesota School of Medicine, Minneapolis, Minnesota 55455

INTRODUCTION[2]

Early virologists observed that a patient or an experimental animal, once recovered from a virus infection usually resisted reinfection from the same or similar virus. Vaccination was one of the early applications of this phenomenon, which was termed *viral interference.* As immunology evolved, investigators recognized that the infected body produces specific antiviral antibodies which appear in the circulation and on mucous surfaces attacked by viruses (humoral immunity), or that sensitized cells (principally lymphocytes) appear which can attack both virus particles and cells infected by viruses (cell-mediated immunity). The requirement of specific antibodies for specific viruses limited the general clinical usefulness of humoral and cell-mediated immunity.

As experience with cell cultures evolved, it became apparent with several experimental models that infection of cells with one virus protected against reinfection with an antigenically unrelated virus. The groundwork for the discovery of interferon was laid by Henle & Henle (6) in 1943 when they demonstrated interference between inactive and active influenza viruses in the developing chick embryo, but the mechanism of this type of interference was not understood until Isaacs & Lindenmann (7) performed an unconventional experiment. They incubated small pieces of chicken chorioallantoic membrane

---

[1]The vast literature that has accumulated during the past decade has made it necessary in many cases to cite reviews here rather than individual publications, particularly in the tables.

[2]For reviews see 1–5.

0362-1642/86/0415-0455$02.00

with heat-inactivated influenza virus, recovered the cell- and virus-free medium, and incubated it with fresh membranes inoculated with live virus. The live virus did not grow. Interference had been transferred to the fresh membrane by something that had been produced in the first membrane in response to the heat-killed virus. A virus-inhibiting substance was also reported in 1958 by Nagano & Kojima (8).

Isaacs & Lindenmann called their substance *interferon*. The name was "coined as a convenient laboratory shorthand and not as a result of a deliberate taxonomic exercise" (4). Interferon research has persisted for three decades only because of the stubborn efforts of a small cadre of "interferonologists" who continued to believe in the reality and importance of interferon while enduring widespread skepticism and occasional ridicule. Only recently has the question evolved from "Interferon, does it exist?" to "Interferons, how many?"

Isaacs & Lindenmann (9) went on to demonstrate that interferon is a protein, stable within pH extremes of 2 and 10, stable when heated at 60°C for 1 hr, and not affected by incubation with antiserum prepared against the virus that induced its production. Their observation that incubation of a virus with interferon had no effect on viral infection led them to assert the novel concept that interferon exerted its interference by rendering cells incapable of supporting viral replication rather than by interacting directly with a virus particle. The concept of species specificity was introduced shortly thereafter when Tyrrell (10) showed that interferon prepared in chickens had no activity in calf cells. Interferon has been induced in cultured cells from a large variety of mammals and other animals, including fish, amphibia, reptiles and birds. Interferon-like factors have also been reported in plants (11).

Interferon is not the only inhibitor of virus. According to Lockhart (12) and Stewart (5), the following criteria must be met before a viral inhibitor can be accepted as an interferon: (*a*) It must be a protein. (*b*) Its antiviral effect must not result from a nonspecific toxic effect on cells. (*c*) It must be active against a wide range of unrelated viruses. (*d*) It must inhibit virus replication through an intracellular effect which must involve synthesis of both RNA and protein by the cells. (*e*) It must exhibit activity on a defined host range of cells. (*f*) It must induce the following non-antiviral alterations in cells: priming, blocking, enhancement of double-stranded RNA toxicity, and inhibition of cell-multiplication, always in constant ratios.

Had interferon not been discovered by virologists, it certainly would have been revealed through one or more of its other effects and named accordingly. In fact, γ-interferon is classified as a lymphokine as well as an interferon. Before the recent purification of natural interferon and the production of recombinant interferons, crude preparations for laboratory and clinical studies were employed that were little more than protein mixtures contaminated with small amounts of interferon. It is remarkable that so much was learned about interferon before its purification. However, the many non-antiviral effects produced in a variety of biological models by these crude preparations were ignored or discounted largely because virologists, obsessed with the conviction that antiviral activity was the single *raison d'être* for interferon, assumed that the other effects must be due to impurities. Recent studies with pure interferons, however, show that crude preparations produce their multiple effects by virtue of their interferon content. Interferon can no longer be defined simply as a cellular protein that confers antiviral activity to cells. In fact, certain of the non-antiviral effects of interferons may prove to be of equal or greater importance than the antiviral activity.

CLASSIFICATION OF INTERFERONS[3]

Two of the three major classes of interferons were recognized quite early as originating in leukocytes or fibroblasts (Table 1). The discovery of γ-interferon was delayed considerably by a definition that required interferons to be stable at pH 2, relatively heat stable, and inducible by virus or double-stranded RNA. None of these criteria apply to γ-interferon. An international committee of scientists decided recently that differences in antigenicity could form a basis for classification of leukocyte, fibroblast, and immune interferons with respective designations of IFN-α, IFN-β, and IFN-γ. This classification is not addressed to molecular, or even biological, characteristics of interferons; but it has been generally accepted for its convenience. Such a scheme may be the best that can be expected at this time because the amino acid sequencing of at least 15 human interferons has not revealed homologous sequences or secondary or tertiary structures that allow chemical classification. There is a fair amount of homology of amino acid sequences of human α- and β-interferons, but almost none between γ-interferon and α/β-interferons.

Until recently, glycosylation was considered to be a feature of all interferons. Many believed it determined species and receptor specificities. However, pure natural and recombinant human IFN-αs are not glycosylated, yet they exhibit both species specificity and individual patterns of biological activity.

The rapid progress made in the isolation and characterization of a host of subspecies of IFN-αs has given rise to impromptu classification of subspecies of IFN-αs. Some publications designate human interferon with an Hu (IFN-α becomes HuIFN-α). Subtypes of IFN-α have been designated a_1, a_2, etc. Pestka & Baron (13) propose that recombinant interferon be differentiated from natural interferon by use of a lower case "r" (HuIFNr-α or HuIFLr-α).

The creation of recombinant hybrid interferons will undoubtedly generate still other subclassifications. Several recombinant hybrid interferons have

[3]For reviews see 13–17.

Table 1 Classification and properties of human interferons[a]

Type	Other designations	Source	Induced by	Specific activity (U/mg)	Number of subspecies	Molecular weight	Functional unit	Chromosome location	pH stability	Glycosylation[b]
α (IFN-α)	leukocyte IF type I, IFNα, IFL, LeIF, LIF, ifnLe	β and null lymphocytes and macrophages; recombinant	virus; double-stranded RNA	$2-4 \times 10^8$	$\geqslant 15$	16,500–25,000	monomer	(a, . . . a >18) chr 9	+	−
β (IFN-β)	fibroblast IF, type I, FIF, INF, ifnF	Fibroblasts, lymphoblasts; epithelial cells; recombinant	virus; double-stranded RNA	$2-4 \times 10^8$	1	20,000	dimer	2,5,9	+	+
γ (IFN-γ)	immune, type II, IFI, ImIF	T lymphocytes; recombinant	foreign antigens; mitogens	$>10^8$	1–2	17,000	trimer	12	−	+

[a]Assembled from publications by Pestka & Baron (13), Sikora (14), Pestka (15), and Knight (16).
[b]Refers to natural interferon; recombinant interferons are not glycoslated.

already been constructed and others will certainly be engineered with additions, deletions, substitutions, and overlaps. Species specificity and function of individual interferons can be altered by hybridization; for example, HuIFNr-A and HuIFNr-D produce an antiviral state in human but not in murine cell lines. However, HuIFNr-AD, one of four hybrids formed from these two recombinant interferons, is antiviral in murine cells (18, 19). Hybridization offers the hope that interferons can be tailored to elicit desired cellular activities without producing many of the undesired effects.

CELLULAR SOURCES OF INTERFERON[4]

Although interferon appears in the lungs, liver, brains, and other tissues of animals treated with appropriate inducing agents, the major production of the three main types of interferon occurs in a few cell types: IFN-α in B and null lymphocytes and macrophages, IFN-β in epithelial and fibroblast cells, and IFN-γ in T lymphocytes with the support of macrophages. There are exceptions to this generalization; for example, IFN-γ can be induced in bone marrow T cells with T-cell mitogens, and some IFN-β can be induced in macrophages. With the appropriate inducer, large granular lymphocytes may produce all three major types of interferon. Relatively large amounts of crude IFN-α have been produced for clinical trials by the Finnish Red Cross from interferon-primed, Sendai virus–induced human leukocytes obtained from the buffy coat of donor transfusion blood (23). Clinical trials have been conducted with IFN-α and IFN-β isolated from Sendai virus–induced Namalwa cells (24) and polyriboinosinic acid·polyribocytidylic acid (poly IC)-induced human foreskin fibroblasts (25), respectively.

INDUCTION OF α/β INTERFERONS[5]

Three milestones mark the development of the induction of α/β-interferons. The first was the previously cited observation of Isaacs & Lindenmann (7) that led to the discovery of interferon. The second was the realization that interferon can be induced by substances other than viruses. The third was the discovery that microgram quantities of the synthetic double-stranded polyribonucleotide, polyriboinosinic·polyribocytidylic acid (poly IC), induce large amounts of interferon in rabbits and rabbit kidney cells (30).

Interferon inducers can be classified according to source, potency, molecular size, chemical structure, mechanism of induction, types of interferon induced, and the cells and animal species they induce. Baron et al (17) categorize

[4]For reviews see 17, 20–22.
[5]For reviews see 17, 23, 26–29.

interferon inducers into two major classes: α/β inducers and γ inducers. Class A α/β inducers are relatively potent; they include the RNA viruses of animal, plant, insect, fungal, or bacterial origin, DNA viruses, and synthetic double-stranded RNA polymers. Most, but not all, Class B α/β inducers are relatively weak; they include microbes, microbial products, and synthetic chemicals (nonRNA polymers and low-molecular-weight compounds). Inducers of IFN-γ (in immunocompetent cells) are comprised of antigens (in sensitized immunocytes), antibody to OKT3 antigen on mature T lymphocytes, and a variety of mitogens.

Five types of interferon inducers are considered in this section: viruses, microbes and microbial products, synthetic RNA polymers, synthetic nonRNA high-molecular-weight polymers, and synthetic low-molecular-weight chemicals.

Induction by Viruses

Perhaps the most general characteristic of viruses is that with few exceptions they induce interferon in vertebrates and cultures of vertebrate cells. Ho (29) lists 87 viruses representing 15 families and 5 unclassified viruses that have been shown to induce interferon in animals (mammals, birds, reptiles, or fish), cultured cells, or both. The amount of interferon detected depends on (a) the virus inoculum (species, type and strain of virus, the particle composition and concentration, and the presence of contaminating substances), (b) conditions for production in animal hosts (species, strain, age, sex, route of inoculation, time after inoculation, tissue sampled for assay, temperature of housing, and previous exposure to virus or other inducing agent), and (c) conditions for production in cell cultures (species, type of tissues, passage level, "ageing," and contamination by mycoplasma and other agents, whether the cell population is pure or mixed). Descriptions of viruses as "good" or "poor" inducers are not always applicable; manipulation of conditions may convert a "poor" inducer to a "good" inducer or vice versa. Nevertheless, double-stranded RNA viruses are considered to be the best viral inducers. The best single-stranded RNA virus inducers of interferon are the paramyxoviruses, especially Newcastle disease virus or Sendai virus.

A virus need not be infective or (in many cases) even viable to be a good inducer of interferon. Blue-tongue virus, an orbivirus, is pathogenic for sheep but not for man. Both active and heat-killed blue-tongue virus produce high titers of interferon in a large number of cell and animal systems, and therapeutic uses of the virus have been proposed.

A large number of viruses from fungi, bacteria, and plants induce interferon in animals. Many of these nonanimal viruses have double-stranded RNA as their genome. Some are potent inducers.

Induction by Microbes and Microbial Products

A great variety of bacteria, chlamydia, rickettsia, mycoplasma, and protozoa are interferon inducers. Unicellular inducers are commonly intracellular parasites. Their mechanisms of induction are not clear. In the case of gram-negative bacteria, released endotoxin is believed to play a role. Double-stranded RNA can also be a microbial product responsible for interferon induction; for example, the antiviral properties of extracts of *Penicillium funiculosum* were shown to be due to double-stranded RNA found in the fungus. Mannan, a polysaccharide from *Candida albicans,* induces circulating interferon (probably IFN-γ) in mice. Other microbial interferon inducers include a capsular polysaccharide from *K. pneumoniae,* a B-cell mitogen from *Nocardia,* glycoprotein from Sendai virus, and the cell wall and ribosomal fractions of mycobacterium tuberculosis strain BCG.

Induction by Synthetic RNA Polymers

The synthetic RNA polymers rival the viruses as potent inducers of interferon. Although many of these polymers have been synthesized and tested, the molecular requirements for activity have not been completely defined (31–33). A double helix of high molecular weight (10^5daltons) is important. Sequences of the primary bases may be critical, but the 2'OH position on the ribose is crucial. Substitution at the purine N-7 and the pyrimidine C-5 positions diminishes activity. A high melting point is also important. Poly IC is an excellent inducer of interferon in laboratory rodents but a poor inducer in monkeys, chimpanzees, and humans because they possess high levels of serum ribonuclease. High titers of interferon are induced with poly ICLC, a hydrophilic complex of poly IC with poly-L-lysine and carboxymethylcellulose, because it resists hydrolysis by ribonuclease (34, 35).

The toxicity and refractiveness of the double-stranded RNA polymers have restricted their clinical application. Many of the toxic manifestations (leukopenia, fever, headache, nausea, lethargy, insomnia, and changes in hematopoietic and liver functions) are those that occur after administration of interferon (36, 37). However, Ts'o and colleagues (38, 39) have synthesized "mismatched" analogs of poly IC that induce high interferon titers with relatively low toxicity. They found that uracil or guanine interspersed into the poly (C) strand retained the ability to induce interferon if the frequency of random insertions did not exceed 1 residue in 12, a condition that preserves the 0.5–1 helical structure required for the triggering of interferon synthesis. Poly (I)-poly ($C_{12}U$) is undergoing clinical trials (39).

Induction by nonRNA Polymers[6]

Polycarboxylic polymers (pyran, polyacrylic acid, polymethacrylic acid), polysulfates (polyvinyl sulfate), and polyphosphates (polyphosphorylated polysaccharides) induce interferon in mice. The most studied of these polymers is pyran, a polymer of maleic anhydride and divinyl ether with a molecular weight of about 17,000. Its antiviral activity is much greater than can be explained by the small amount of interferon it induces. It is not degraded or excreted and it is prohibitively toxic. The diverse effects of these polymers, including the induction of interferon and its disproportionate antiviral activity relative to interferon induction, may result from the activation of macrophages.

Induction by Low-Molecular-Weight Chemicals[7]

Low-molecular-weight interferon inducers are an odd assortment of chemically diverse agents. Except for the antimetabolites (cycloheximide, streptovitacin A, streptimidone, and tenauzonic acid), little is known about their mode of action. Cyclohexane and other compounds that inhibit RNA synthesis are believed to induce interferon by reducing the critical concentration of a repressor that normally prevents the expression of an interferon gene. Many of the structurally unrelated chemical inducers are active in cell cultures, usually of macrophages or lymphocytes.

Tilorone is the best known of 800 bis-basic low-molecular-weight compounds synthesized in an unsuccessful attempt to create a clinically useful interferon inducer (43). High serum interferon titers were observed after the oral administration of tilorone to mice; a lesser inductive effect was seen in rats, and very little effect was seen in rabbits, hamsters, ferrets, cats, dogs, and unfortunately, humans. It is highly reactive in immunoregulation, but toxic. Tilorone intercalcates into DNA (44), an observation that could lead to an understanding of its mechanism of action. Tilorone is not effective intravenously. Other tricyclic compounds that have received considerable attention as interferon inducers are quinoline derivatives [e.g. BL-20803, 1,3-dimethyl-4-(3-dimethylaminopropylamino)-1H-pyrazolo-(3,4-b)-quinoline], anthraquinone derivatives e.g. 1-5-bis[(2-(diethylamino)ethyl)amino]-anthraquinone, and cationic dyes (e.g. toluidine blue, methylene blue, trypaflavine, and acridine orange). 10-Carboxymethyl-9-acridanone is a potent inducer of interferon that can be administered parenterally or orally.

Of substituted pyrimidines tested, 7 proved to be relatively good inducers of interferon in mice when given either parenterally or orally. Of these, 2-amino-5-bromo-6-methyl-4-pyrimidine (U-25;166) offered some promise as a therapeutic agent.

[6]See reviews in 17, 40–42.
[7]See reviews in 17, 26, 27, 29, 43.

Nasal applications of the propanediamine CP-20,961 and the xylenediamine CP-28,888 were effective in humans challenged with rhinovirus; interferon was detected in their nasal secretions.

Several radioprotective thiols induce interferon, the most active of which are 5,2-aminoethylisothiouronium (AET) and 3-aminopropylisothiourea.

INDUCTION OF γ-INTERFERON[8]

The target cells for induction, chromosomal affiliation, and the structural and physical nature of IFN-γ differ markedly from those of IFN-α and IFN-β. It is therefore not unexpected that the inducers of IFN-γ should also differ markedly. Far fewer substances are known to induce IFN-γ; they include mitogens, bacterial and viral antigens, allogeneic cells, and antisera directed against surface components.

Early work showed that exposure of animals or lymphocytes from animals that had been sensitized to specific antigens resulted in the production of IFN-γ. Later work showed that the target cells are specific subsets of T cells—e.g. specific cytotoxic T cells. These cells produce IFN-γ in culture when they are derived from animals previously sensitized to a viral or nonviral antigen (e.g. tetanus toxoid, diphtheria toxoid, tubercular PPD). Cell membrane–active substances that induce IFN-γ include phytohemagglutinin, concanavalin A, pokeweed antigen, streptolysin O, bacterial lipopolysaccharides, anti-lymphocyte serum, monoclones against OKT-3, staphylococcal enterotoxin, staphylococcal protein A, phorbol esters, calcium ionophore, and galactase.

"SPONTANEOUS" INDUCTION OF INTERFERON

Interferon has slowly become recognized as a hormone-like messenger that induces metabolic changes in distant cells (46–48). Since the production of interferon involves the switching on of transcription of interferon genes that otherwise remain dormant, the "hormonal" function of interferon must implicate a true induction process.

The lungs and intestines present vast "external" surfaces that come in contact with exogenous interferon inducers such as heterologous proteins, bacteria, viruses, toxins, allergens, and chemicals (49). Although these substances do not generally elicit detectable levels of serum interferon, interferon produced in this way may be taken up by circulating leukocytes and transported to other sites. Low levels of endogenous interferon are not readily detectable in blood; Bocci and associates (50) found antiviral activity in the abdominal and thoracic lymph of untreated rabbits but not in the plasma or lymph collected from the

[8]For reviews see 17, 20, 45.

hind leg. Evidence for the maintenance of low levels of both endogenously and exogenously induced interferon has been published recently by Galabru and associates (51), who measured serum, spleen, and lung interferon levels in untreated conventional and germ-free mice. They also measured normal and interferon-induced levels of spleen (2'5')oligo(A) synthetase (2-5A synthetase) and lung protein kinase. As will be discussed later, 2-5A synthetase and protein kinase are antiviral proteins induced by interferon and activated by double-stranded RNA. The assays of 2-5A synthetase and protein kinase, which have much longer lives than interferon, are convenient indirect ways of assessing interferon production. Serum interferon levels were not measurable in the great majority of either conventional or germ-free mice, but about 10% showed low levels of IFN-α and IFN-β; these mice also possessed the higher tissue levels of 2-5A synthetase and protein kinase. Relatively high levels of the two enzymes were present in the spleens and lungs of conventional mice; they were about doubled after interferon administration. On the other hand, levels of spleen 2-5A synthetase and lung protein kinase in the tissues of germ-free mice were only about 10 and 7%, respectively, of those seen in conventional mice. Moreover, administered interferon raised the levels of 2-5A synthetase and protein kinase activities in germ-free mice to only 15 and 40%, respectively, of those seen in untreated conventional mice. Thus it would appear that low tissue levels of interferon are induced continuously by both internal and external agents. Perhaps more importantly, these studies suggest that external agents may be required for full inductive responses of 2-5A synthetase and protein kinase to interferon.

Low levels of IFN-α have been detected consistently in human amniotic fluid in the absence of viral or other infections (52–54). Lebon and associates (53) reported the presence of interferon in the amniotic fluid of 60 women during their 16th to 38th week of pregnancy. The absence of detectable levels of interferon in the sera of mothers not only tends to exclude a maternal contribution of interferon to amniotic fluid but suggests that amniotic interferon is not transported into the mother's blood.

Relatively high levels of interferon have been detected in the uterus, placenta, and fetus of healthy, pregnant mice (52). Levels of placental interferon increase throughout gestation; the level in the uterus peaks at 13 days and disappears by parturition. Interferon was not detectable in the fetus except at 10 days of gestation when contamination from extra-embryonic tissues is difficult to avoid.

The suggestion has been made that amniotic interferon is more involved in the regulation of fetal development and the immunoregulation of fetal acceptance than as an antiviral agent. The presence of interferons in the placenta and amniotic fluid supports the view that the most important role for some species of interferon could be the regulation of normal (or even abnormal) cellular processes (55).

Circulating interferon has been detected in acquired immune deficiency syndrome (AIDS), systemic lupus erythematosus, rheumatoid arthritis, and multiple sclerosis in cases where virus does not appear to be the inducer (56). Levels of interferon of 90–159 units/ml of plasma have been found in apparently normal, healthy humans (57).

PRODUCTION OF INTERFERON BY TUMOR CELLS

Tumor cells, like normal cells, produce interferon when exposed to viruses and other interferon inducers (58–60). In fact, lymphoblastoid cells induced with Sendai virus are used commercially for the large-scale production of interferon (61). Of 19 lymphoblastoid cell lines tested, 11 were found to produce interferon spontaneously; of the remaining 8, 4 did not produce interferon in response to Sendai virus (62). The spontaneously produced interferons were shown to differ from virus-induced interferons in molecular weight and antigenicity. β-Lymphoblasts and other leukocyte cell lines also generate interferon spontaneously. While the mechanism of spontaneous induction of interferon in tumor cells is not known, one might postulate that many of the genes that remain dormant in normal cells, including interferon genes, are derepressed in the poorly differentiated tumor cell. Alternatively, tumor cells may produce interferon inducers. That this may be the case is suggested by the observation of Trinchieri and associates (63) that peripheral blood lymphocytes produce interferon when cultured with tumor cells. Although several investigators have suggested that natural killer (NK) cells are responsible for tumor-induced interferon, Weigent et al (64) showed that enriched human B-cells, cultured with xenogeneic or allogeneic tumor cells, produced 1,000–10,000 units of interferon per milliliter. Lackovic and co-workers (64a) identified IFN-α in the peritoneal cavities of mice inoculated with allogeneic Ehrlich ascites cells. They suggested that the interferon was produced by macrophages. Djeu and associates (65) showed that conventional or nude mice inoculated with syngeneic or allogeneic tumor cells rapidly develop serum interferon levels that peak within 24 hr. Timonen and associates (66) conclude that NK cells are responsible for the interferon induced in human lymphocytes by tumor cell contact.

Relatively high levels of interferon in the plasma of malignancy patients have been reported recently (57).

MECHANISM OF INDUCTION OF IFN-α AND IFN-β BY VIRUSES AND POLYRIBONUCLEOTIDES[9]

Isaacs (72) postulated in 1963 that a "foreign nucleic acid" was responsible for interferon induction. Four years later, Field et al (73) discovered that synthetic

[9]For reviews see 67–71.

polyribonucleotides were comparable to viruses in their ability to induce interferon. It is now generally accepted that viruses and polyribonucleotides induce interferon by the same mechanism. While there are still many unanswered questions regarding the mechanism, it is firmly established that interferon synthesis results from the switching on of transcription that occurs when dormant interferon genes are derepressed.

Space restrictions do not allow a discussion of the several hypothetical models that have been proposed through the years for the induction of interferon. The recent working model (Figure 1) of Marcus (71) was selected for this overview because it accommodates many of the contradictions that have pervaded earlier hypotheses and because it is likely to stimulate research that will challenge its many speculative features. The major divergence of this model from its predecessors is the assignment of a role of inducer-receptor to (2'5')oligo(A) synthetase (2-5A synthetase) and protein kinase, the two enzymes directly involved in the impairment of viral replication.

Credibility of the working model depends on several observations and speculations:

1. Induction requires new cellular RNA and protein synthesis.

2. Double-stranded RNA of viral or synthetic origin introduced to or formed in the cell, is the proximal inducer.

3. A single molecule of double-stranded RNA provides the threshold for the induction of a quantum (finite) yield of interferon. This important observation was made by Marcus and associates in carefully conducted and interpreted dose (virus)-response (interferon production) studies. These dose-response curves showed that the simultaneous introduction of a second virus particle suppressed the interferon-inducing activity of the first virus particle. This would explain why cells become refractive to interferon induction by viruses and other inducers, why a large amount of exogenous interferon can prevent induction, and why some double-stranded viruses do not induce measurable amounts of interferon (they induce too much interferon too rapidly).

4. An interferon inducer-receptor is formed when double-stranded RNA interacts reversibly with 2-5A synthetase or protein kinase. The interferon inducer-receptors are the actual inducers; they derepress interferon genes. The synthetase and kinase interferon receptors may function specifically for IFN-α and IFN-β gene banks, respectively.

5. The cell must harbor basal levels of 2-5A synthetase and protein kinase. Helical regions of heterologous nuclear (hn) RNA may induce low levels of "endogenous" interferon, thereby maintaining basal levels of the two receptor enzymes. Low basal levels of 2-5A synthetase and 2-5A per se have been observed in normal and regenerating livers of non-induced rats. A radioimmune assay has been used to show the presence of 2-5A in the liver, kidney, and spleen of untreated and germ-free mice (51). Basal levels of interferon inducer-

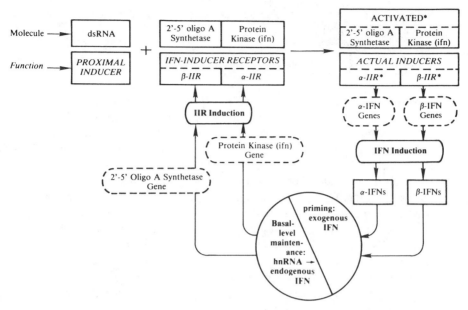

Figure 1   A schematic representation of the working model proposed for the mechanism of interferon induction by viruses (double-stranded RNA). The various elements of the model and their postulated functions are described in the text. Reprinted with permission from (71).

receptors and turnover rates must be high enough that induction occurs even in the presence of only one molecule of double-stranded RNA per cell.

When cells are treated with small amounts of interferon prior to exposure to viruses, induction occurs earlier and much larger amounts of interferon are produced. The procedure, known as "priming," has been used to increase the amounts of interferon produced by human leukocytes for use in clinical trials. Priming is attributed to a shortened induction phase because transcription of mRNA occurs earlier than in control cells. The concentrations of both 2-5A and protein kinase are increased in cells primed with interferon. In accordance with the model (Figure 1), the consequences of this would be an accelerated production of activated 2-5A synthetase and protein kinase and therefore a shortened lag phase for interferon induction.

MECHANISM OF INDUCTION OF γ-INTERFERON[10]

The mechanism of induction of IFN-γ is not known. Perhaps the molecules that induce IFN-γ (mitogens, antigens, etc) substitute for double-stranded RNA as

[10]For review see 45.

the proximate inducers in systems similar to those involved in the induction of IFN-α and IFN-β.

INTERFERON RECEPTORS[11]

When molecules of interferon leave a cell they attach to receptors in the adjacent cells or they enter the circulation and combine with receptors of distant cells. Receptors are localized randomly on the cell surface (75) or on coated pits (76). Estimates of the number of receptors range from 650 to 20,000 per cell (77). There is conflicting evidence about whether interferon must be internalized to act, but the consensus is that even if this does occur it is not a requirement. Interferon may bind directly or produce aggregates of receptors. Mouse IFN-α and IFN-β share and compete for the same receptors, but IFN-γ occupies different receptors. Nevertheless, genes for the receptors for all three major types of human interferon are located on the distal segment of the long arm of chromosome 21 (45, 77). The degree of sensitivity to interferon relates to the number of duplications of chromosome 21; thus children with Down's syndrome (trisomy 21) have an exaggerated sensitivity to the effects of interferon (77).

The role of gangliosides in interferon binding is not established but is suggested by the observations that Sepharose-bound interferon loses its antiviral properties when preincubated with gangliosides and that the addition of gangliosides to ganglioside-deficient mouse cells prior to treatment with interferon increases antiviral response (78). Inhibition of the antiviral properties of Sepharose-bound interferon is reversed by sialyl lactose, which indicates that interferon does not bind to the ceramide portion of gangliosides but to the polysaccharide end residues containing sialic acid and lactose. Gangliosides may function as low-affinity discriminators that may be involved in some interferon functions and not in others.

Interferon increases the concentration of cAMP in cells, but not in every cell type in which interferon is induced (79, 80). This suggests that the elevation of cAMP content is a consequence rather than a component of induction.

MECHANISMS OF ANTIVIRAL ACTIVITY OF INTERFERON[12]

Almost everything known about the biochemical mechanisms of the antiviral action of interferons has been derived from experiments with cell extracts. One

[11]For reviews see 17, 55, 74.
[12]For reviews see 68, 70, 81–84.

of the most provocative of these studies was made by Friedman and associates (85, 86), who suggested that interferon may create a latent antiviral state in cells that can be triggered by virus infection. These studies were relevant to the earlier observation by Kerr et al (87) that cell-free extracts from interferon-treated cells were extremely sensitive to inhibition of protein synthesis by double-stranded RNA. Since double-stranded RNA circumvented the need of viral infection for an interferon-induced translational blockade, it raised speculation that it might signal the antiviral state. Roberts et al (88) reported that a low-molecular-weight inhibitor of protein synthesis was generated when extracts of interferon-treated mouse L cells were incubated with ATP and double-stranded RNA. Kerr & Brown (89) determined the low-molecular-weight inhibitor to be 2-5A, a member of a new class of 2'5' isoadenylates that have novel 2'5' phosphodiester linkages between the riboses of the adenylic acid rather than the usual 3'5' linkages. This class of oligonucleotides promises to have regulatory functions that extend far beyond its involvement in antiviral activity. The 2-5A-dependent endonucleases also appear to be a ubiquitous component of mammalian cells, whether cultured or obtained directly from the animal. A variety of chemicals and glucocorticoids that do not induce interferon increase levels of 2-5A synthetase (e.g. butyrate, DMSO, phenobarbital, hydrocortisone, dexamethasone, and cortisol).

2-5A-Dependent antiviral activity involves at least three enzymes: 2-5A synthetase, 2' phosphodiesterase and endonuclease (Figure 2). Two activation steps occur; double-stranded RNA-activation of 2-5A synthetase and activation of inactive endonuclease by the 2-5A released by the activated synthetase. Two synthetases have been identified, one in the cytoplasm, the other in the nucleus; conceivably, they may regulate different events, depending on whether the activating double-stranded RNA is nuclear or cytoplasmic. Phosphodiesterase is present in nonlimiting concentrations relative to 2-5A but it is also induced by interferon in some systems.

One of the first questions raised by the discovery of the 2-5A system was whether it degrades viral RNA specifically. Some reports support one side, some the other, and still others support both sides of this question. However, while the question is not resolved, the preponderance of available evidence suggests that the 2-5A-dependent endonuclease cleaves both host and viral RNAs. If interferon can affect both nucleic acid and protein synthesis, why does it not kill cells as well as prevent virus multiplication? Burke (90) offers three explanations that do not require a specific biochemical action of the 2-5A system: (a) Virus replication is an exponential process; therefore a small effect on an early event can have a magnified effect on subsequent stages; (b) Interferon is induced in large amounts only in cells that are infected with virus; these cells may in fact die because the synthesis of host proteins is impaired, but most cells are not infected with virus and will not die. Interferon-inflicted cell

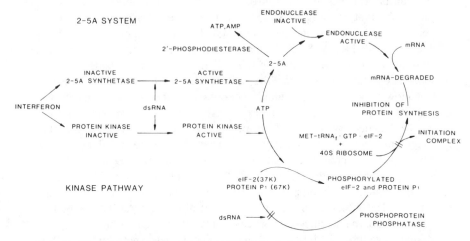

Figure 2   The role of induced enzymes in the inhibition of translation caused by double-stranded RNA. Reprinted with permission from (84).

death may in fact be a first line of defense against the spread of a virus infection; (*c*) Viral mRNAs may have a higher affinity than cellular RNAs for components of the protein-synthesis machinery of the cell and may therefore be more strongly affected by interferon treatment. To this may be added the comment that the RNAs involved in an exponentially expanding process are turning over more rapidly than those involved in processes that have achieved a steady-state status (normal cellular processes) and therefore might be expected to be more involved in the antiviral process than cellular macromolecules. This could also explain putative differential effects of interferon on exponentially replicating tumor and fetal cells in vivo.

Discovery of a second double-stranded mediated inhibitor of protein synthesis occurred about the same time as that of the 2-5A system (69, 81, 84). Lysates from control or interferon-treated rabbit reticulocytes were incubated with or without double-stranded RNA and ATP. Enhanced phosphorylation of two proteins was seen only in lysates that had been exposed to both interferon and double-stranded RNA. The smaller (37K) of the two was identified in several laboratories as the smallest subunit (α) of initiation factor eIF2. The larger (67K) proved to be a cAMP-independent protein kinase. As shown in Figure 2, initiation factor eIF2 is phosphorylated when protein kinase is activated by double-stranded RNA. This impairs the participation of eIF2 in the formation of the 40S initiation complex, and protein initiation synthesis is inhibited.

All three major classes of interferon induce the kinase. Kinase activity is enhanced in the liver, spleen, and plasma of mice injected with Newcastle disease virus, EMC virus, poly IC or polyriboadenylic acid·polyribouridylic acid (poly AU). The enhancement of kinase activity by poly AU is of interest because this polyribonucleotide does not induce interferon (91, 92).

Enzymes other than 2-5A and protein kinase may be involved in antiviral and other effects of interferon. One- and two-dimensional gel electrophoreses have revealed a number of unidentified polypeptides in cells that appear simultaneously with the antiviral state (84).

An antagonist of 2-5A such as p5'A2'p5'a2'p5'A might be useful in the treatment of what have been termed "interferon-induced diseases" if it were able to penetrate the eukaryotic cell and not be rapidly degraded by the 2'5' diesterase. If antagonists of this type can be chemically modified to overcome these problems, they must also be able to bind to the endonuclease.

PHARMACOKINETICS[13]

The fate of endogenous or exogenous interferons is determined largely by the type of interferon, the site of its induction or administration, and the amount. The very small amounts of interferon produced more or less continuously in organs such as the lung probably do not enter the circulation unless perhaps, they are transported by leukocytes. Interferon is probably diffused through extracellular fluid (paracrine excretion) to neighboring cells and catabolized. Some of this interferon appears to enter the lymph system. Viral infections induce large amounts of interferon which flood most of the body fluid pools. This interferon has a short half-life in the circulation owing to its binding to cellular receptors throughout the body and its catabolism by the kidney and liver. The immediate delivery of interferon to target cells must be paracrine in nature.

Intravenously administered IFN-α disappears rapidly from the plasma, with less than 0.1% of large doses remaining in the circulation after 24 hr. The relatively small size of the interferon molecule allows it to be filtered by the renal glomerulus; it is reabsorbed almost quantitatively by the tubules, where it is destroyed by proteolysis (97). Bocci (96) estimates that the kidneys eliminate at least 2% of the plasma IFN-α/min, thus clearing the plasma pool in less than an hour. Megadoses of interferon can overcome this rapid loss, but high plasma levels produce severe central nervous system toxicity. Moreover, high interferon levels suppress the immune system, which in some cases may compromise therapy. Intramuscular administration has therefore been the preferred route for IFN-α in clinical trials. Because intramuscular IFN-α enters the

---

[13]For reviews see 49, 93–96.

circulation primarily through capillaries, plasma levels are less transient and catabolism is less rapid than with intravenous interferon. Peak plasma levels occur in 1–6 hr, remain fairly stable for 6–12 hr and slowly disappear between 18 and 36 hr (96).

The pharmacokinetics of IFN-β and IFN-γ differ markedly from that of IFN-α. IFN-β and IFN-γ do not appear in significant concentrations in the plasma after intramuscular injection, and they are catabolized mainly by the liver rather than by the kidney (98–104). These interferons appear to reach target organs despite their apparent lack of transport by the circulatory system. Thus natural killer (NK) cells are activated as readily by intramuscular IFN-β and IFN-γ as by intramuscular IFN-α (105). This could mean that these interferons are removed slowly from the injection site by the lymphoid system or that circulating NK cells are activated while passing through the injection site. Antiviral activities measured in spleen and lung are similar after the intramuscular injection of IFN-α and IFN-β, despite a 10- to 30-fold difference in their serum levels (98).

The pharmacokinetics of IFN-β and IFN-γ were once believed to differ from that of IFN-α because IFN-β and IFN-γ are glycosylated and therefore attracted to tissues whereas IFN-α is not glycosylated and is therefore more capable of moving into the plasma pool (104). However, it has been shown in rats that the pharmacokinetics of recombinant HuIFNr-β and HuIFNr-γ, which are not glycosylated, do not differ from that of their natural glycosylated counterparts (106). However, in very thorough studies with the rabbit, Satoh and collaborators (103) observed differences in the pharmacokinetic parameters of recombinant and fibroblast-derived human IFN-β which they attributed to glycosylation. Differences in the pharmacokinetics of interferons are probably related to their hydrophobicity (106). All three IFN types of interferon are secretory proteins and have a hydrophobic signal peptide 20–23 amino acids long (107–109), but IFN-α is less hydrophobic than either IFN-β or IFN-γ.

Bocci (96) favors a strategy of delivering interferons via the lymph pool. This would minimize direct transfer of interferon into the blood and thereby maintain more constant tissue levels. The result would approximate that seen with continuous infusion. An estimated half of subcutaneously injected, and even more of intraperitoneally administered interferon would enter the lymph pool.

Only traces of serum interferon reach the central nervous system. Human IFN-β injected intrathecally in monkeys diffused throughout the cerebrospinal canal and reached the serum compartment (98). Some interferon was recovered from the pia mater surrounding the brain hemispheres, but none was found in the deeper layers of the brain. IFN-β injected into patients intrathecally or intraventricularly did not evoke central nervous system toxicity (110–111).

Intraperitoneal injection of partially purified mouse IFN-α + IFN-β produced concentrations in the spleen, liver, and lungs of mice that were about

100-fold greater than could be expected from the amount of serum in these organs (112). The recent availability of large amounts of human interferons has allowed the determination of conventional pharmacokinetic parameters of a variety of interferons administered intravenously to laboratory animals (108, 113). Results are compatible with earlier observations showing that interferon leaves the circulation rapidly, is cleared rapidly by the kidney, and is readily taken up by tissues.

One third of a dose of human recombinant IFN-α (HuIFNr-αA) labeled with ^{125}I was found in the kidney of mice 5 min after its intravenous administration; liver and stomach contained 5.5% and 1.4% of the dose, respectively (114). Sixty minutes after the injection, the kidney had lost three fourths and the liver about half of its interferon. The distribution of ^{125}I-labeled HuIFNr-A/D, a recombinant intramolecular hybrid of HuIFNr-αA and HuIFNr-αD was quite different from that of HuIFNr-αA; e.g., the amount in the liver (24%) was greater than in the kidney (15%). Moreover, not only was the initial concentration of HuIFNrα-A/D in the stomach several fold higher than that of HuIFNr-αA, but unlike that of HuIFNr-αA, it increased with time. This study raises hopes that it may be possible to tailor recombinant interferons to seek out target organs with some selectivity.

The therapeutic usefulness of interferon would be improved considerably if its clearance from the serum could be delayed. This has been accomplished recently by Rosenblum and associates (115) through the use of a murine interferon-specific monoclonal antibody that binds to HuIFNr-αA without altering its in vitro antiproliferative or antiviral properties. The interferon-antibody complex disappeared from the plasma of the intact rat three times more slowly than the free interferon.

NON-ANTIVIRAL EFFECTS[14]

Interferons modify a multitude of seemingly unrelated biological functions both in cultured cells and *in vivo* (Table 2). Some of these effects may be mediated through indiscriminating actions of the antiviral enzymes, 2-5A synthetase and protein kinase, whereas other functions may be elicited by still unidentified mechanisms, possibly triggered by binding to receptors not associated with antiviral activity. These functions may be enhanced or depressed by interferon depending on the biological model, temporal factors, or the concentration of interferon. Enhanced activity need not exclude the participation of the antiviral enzymes. Steady-state levels of enzymes are determined by the net activities of synthetic and degradative enzymes; an apparent increase in synthesis could be due to an interferon-induced depression of degradative processes.

[14]For reviews see 17, 20, 116–127.

Consideration of all, or even many, of the pleiotropic effects of interferon listed in Table 2 is not possible in this overview. The effects of interferon on cell proliferation, cell differentiation, activation of certain leukocytes, and drug metabolism are selected for brief discussion because of their relevance to prevalent therapeutic uses of interferon.

Cell Proliferation[15]

Six years after the discovery of interferon, Paucker and associates (231) described the first non-antiviral effect of interferon when they showed that the growth of mouse fibroblasts was inhibited by crude preparations of mouse interferon. Their observation was greeted with some skepticism because impurities in the crude preparation could have produced the effect. However, when highly purified interferon became available, it was demonstrated in several laboratories that interferon molecules inhibit the proliferation of a wide variety of cell types. Gresser & Tovey (232) were the first to demonstrate that chemically induced, transplantable, and spontaneous tumors of nonviral etiology were inhibited by interferon.

Cell lines have been used for most of the studies of the antiproliferative effects of interferon. Since they are derived from different sources and many have undergone changes during their continuous culture, it is not unexpected that they should exhibit widely different sensitivities to interferon. The concentrations of interferon required to inhibit their proliferation ranges between 0.2 and 10,000 units/ml (roughly 0.002 and 50 ng/ml) (117).

Few controlled studies have been made of the comparative antiproliferative effectiveness of the three major types of interferon. Based on units derived from their antiviral activity, IFN-γ has a greater antiproliferative effect than IFN-β, but this comparison can only be meaningful if IFN-β and IFN-γ have the same antiviral activity in the cells in which they were tested (117). The observation that IFN-γ synergizes the antitumor activity of IFN-α and IFN-β may have clinical significance (233). Several cloned human IFN-α subtypes differ in both their antiproliferative and antiviral activities (15). Interferon has an antiproliferative effect on normal human diploid fibroblasts, human mammary epithelium, and hematopoietic cells of laboratory animals; however, comparisons have not been made of the selective sensitivities of these cells to interferon with those of tumor cells taken from the same human or animal (117).

Most of the studies using asynchronously growing mouse or human tumor cell lines show that interferon lengthens all phases of the cell cycle, with G1 and G2 usually extended more than S. Quiescent cells stimulated to grow by serum or mitogenic factors show extended G1 and G2 or a slowing of entry into S from G1 (117).

---

[15]For reviews see 116, 117, 127.

Interferon inhibits the synthesis of enzymes and other proteins (Table 2). Induced systems may be particularly affected; for example, steroid- or DMSO-induced hemoglobin synthesis and steroid-induced enzyme synthesis in Friend cells. The inhibition by interferon of ornithine decarboxylase, an enzyme induced by mitogens, growth factors, and tumor promoters, may suggest that interferons can depress the growth and proliferation of cells and modify some of the more complex functions listed in Table 2 by inhibiting the synthesis of proteins and enzymes induced by growth factors (155). This could also contribute to interferon-induced modification of cell differentiation.

Gresser and associates (234) showed that the proliferation of interferon-resistant L1210 cells (later shown to lack IFN-α and IFN-β receptors) was inhibited by interferon in vivo but not in vitro. This was an important observation not only because it revealed that factors other than a direct action of interferon can be involved in the in vivo depression of cell proliferation but also because it led to the demonstration that interferon markedly potentiates natural and immunization-dependent lymphocyte cytotoxicity (128, 235, 236). This experiment and a similar study that used another interferon-resistant cell line (118) suggested that the antiproliferative effect of interferon in vivo was primarily, if not entirely, host-mediated. However, support for a direct action of interferon on cell proliferation came from the observation that interferon affects human tumors transplanted in athymic nude mice, which lack the immunoresponsive cells involved in the antiproliferative process. This experiment does not exclude the possibility that interferon may act primarily by some yet unidentified mechanism (118).

Since a major contribution of the antiproliferative effect of interferon in vivo is host-mediated, the in vitro testing of the antiproliferative effect of interferon on human tumor cells may not contribute much to therapeutic predictability.

Although the antiviral enzymes 2-5A synthetase and protein kinase may depress replication of viruses and cellular proteins indiscriminately, the destruction of viruses may be favored simply because they are replicating more rapidly than macromolecules of nonreplicating or slowly replicating cells. By analogy, tumor cells, which grow and proliferate more rapidly than most normal cells in vivo, would be affected preferentially by interferon. Although interferon has been shown to have an antiproliferative effect on normal cells in vitro, its depression of proliferation in vivo when administered to adult animals for relatively short periods has not been demonstrated. However, newborn mice injected for 6 days with large doses of interferon died of diffuse liver cell necrosis (217, 218). Liver damage did not occur if interferon injections were begun when the mice were 8 days old. The liver of the newborn mouse is comprised largely of hematopoietic cells, which are replaced by rapidly proliferating hepatocytes during the first week after parturition. The inhibition of liver regeneration in partially hepatectomized adult rats is another example of a preferential effect of interferon on rapidly dividing cells (132).

Table 2   Effects of interferon and interferon inducers[a]

Effect upon:	Change in vivo	Change in vitro	References
A. Cell Physiology			
Cell growth		↓	127–29
Induction of cell differentiation		↑↓	125, 127
Bone marrow cell proliferation		↓	130
Hematopoietic colony formation	↓	↓	131
Mitotic response to partial hepatectomy	↓		132
Expression of malignant phenotype		↓	133
Expression of carcinoembryonic antigen		↑	134
Cell locomotion		↓	135, 136
Pinocytosis		↓	136
Negative electrophoretic mobility		↑	137
Beat frequency of myocardial cells		↑↓	138, 139
Excitability of cultured neurones		↑	140
Thymidine uptake		↓	141
Iodine uptake in thyroid cells		↑	142
Saturation of 18-carbon fatty acids		↑	143, 144
Cholesterol and phosphatidylcholine synthesis		↑	145
Lipid synthesis		↓	146
Phospholipid synthesis	↓		147
Prostaglandin synthesis		↑	148, 149
HLA synthesis in melanoma cells		↑	150
Melanogenesis in melanoma cells		↓	151
Priming for interferon synthesis		↑	129, 152
Synthesis of new proteins		↑	153
"Overall" protein synthesis		↓	153
DNA synthesis		↓	154, 155
Globin mRNA		↑	156
Degradation of mRNA		↑	89
Degradation of c-MYC mRNA		↑	157
Release of plasminogen activator		↓	158
Induction of autoimmune disease	↑		159
Radioprotective activity (X or gamma rays)	↑		160, 161
Cytotoxicity of dsRNA	↑	↑	129
B. Enzyme Systems			
Xanthine oxidase	↑		162–164
Aldehyde oxidase	↓		165
2'5' Oligoadenylate synthetase		↑	89
Poly(ADP-ribose) polymerase		↓	166
Creatine kinase	↑		167
Thymidine kinase	↓		141
Glycerol-3-phosphate dehydrogenase	↓		168
Δ^4_3 Ketosteroid synthesis		↑	80
tRNA methylase	↑		169
Prostaglandin E synthetase		↑	170, 171

	Change		
Effect upon:	in vivo	in vitro	References
Steroid-inducible tyrosine amino transferase	↑ ↓		172, 173
Glutamine synthetase		↓	174
Ornithine decarboxylase		↓	155
Guanylate cyclase	↑	↑	175, 176
Adenylate cyclase activity		↑ ↓	79, 177
Indoleamine 2,3,dioxygenase	↑		178, 179
Tryptophan dioxygenase	↑		180
Cytochrome P-450 (uninduced, phenobarbital-induced, 3-methylcholanthrene-induced)		↓	181–183
Cytochrome b_5		↓	180, 181
NADPH cytochrome P-450 reductase		↓	184
Aryl hydrocarbon hydroxylase	↓	↓ ↑	185–187
Aminopyrine N-demethylase	↓	↓ ↑	183, 186, 188
Ethylmorphine N-demethylase	↓		181, 184, 188
Aniline hydroxylase	↓		181, 184, 188
p-Nitrophenetole deethylase	↓		183
Heme oxygenase	↑		180
ALA synthetase	↑		180
Catalase	↓		180

C. Cell Membrane

Density of plasma membrane		↓	189
Microfilament network in submembrane		↑	135
Rigidity of membrane		↑	135
Association of actin in membrane		↑	136
Number of intermembrane particles		↑	189
Movement of membrane receptors		↓	135
Expression of surface antigens		↑	190, 191
Proportion of saturated acyl side chains in membrane phospholipid		↑	143
Cholera toxin and TSH binding		↓	192
Lectin binding		↑	193
Transport of small ions and molecules		↑	194
Transport of thymidine and uridine across membranes		↓	195, 196
Net negative charge		↑	137

D. Immune Systems

Fc receptor expression		↑	197, 198
Natural killer cell activity	↑	↑	129, 199, 200
H-2 antigen expression	↑	↑	201
HLA + β_2 antigen expression		↑	202, 203
I-region antigen		↑	204
Antibody formation	↓	↓	129, 201, 205
Delayed-type hyperactivity	↓		206

Table 2 *(continued)*

Effect upon:	Change		References
	in vivo	in vitro	
Experimental allergic encephalomyelitis		↓	207
Fc receptor–mediated macrophage phagocytosis	↑	↑	208
Cytotoxicity of sensitized T cells		↑	209
Cytotoxicity of monocytes		↑	210, 211
Cytotoxicity of M. L. R.		↑	212
Graft vs host reaction	↑ ↓		206, 213
Generation of allospecific suppressor T lymphocytes		↓	214
E. Whole Animal			
Embryo toxicity	↑		187, 215, 216
Neonatal mortality	↑		216, 217
Liver glycogen	↓		172
Progressive glomerulonephritis	↑		218, 219
Abnormal tubular profiles in hepatic endoplasmic reticulum	↑		220
Neonatal liver necrosis	↑		216
Mitotic activity of hepatectomized livers	↓		132
Regeneration of hepatectomized liver	↓		221
Steroid dependence	↑		222
Survival time of lethally X- and γ-irradiated mice	↑		160, 161
Hexobarbital sleeping time	↑		184, 223, 224
Globules in kidney tubule	↑		49, 95, 219
Autoimmune disease	↑		159
Ascorbate synthesis	↓		182
Chemical carcinogenesis	↓		225
EMC virus–induced diabetes	↓		226, 227
Morphine addiction	↓		228
Analgesia + catalepsy	↑		229
Amplitude of EEG waves	↑		230

[a]For reviews see 116–27.

Cell Differentiation[16]

The earliest demonstration of the effect of interferon on cell differentiation was made by Chany & Vignal in 1968 (133) when they observed that a mouse cell line transformed by a Maloney strain of Sarcoma virus (MSV) reverted to its normal phenotype after prolonged culture with a crude interferon preparation. These reverted cells no longer form colonies in agarose nor do they induce tumors in mice.

[16]For reviews see 123–127.

Depending on the experimental model, interferon can inhibit or enhance spontaneous or induced differentiation of normal cells or tumor cells (Table 2). In some cases this can be accomplished with very low concentrations of interferon; for example, morphological differentiation of insulin-induced murine 3T3 cells can be inhibited with a concentration of interferon as low as 1 unit/ml (123). Differentiation requires a programmed change in gene expression that produces specific proteins associated with particular, terminally differentiated cell types. An example of this was seen during the conversion of mouse fibroblast 3T3-L1 cells to adipocyte cells (123). Levels of 10 proteins were increased and 2 were decreased; interferon prevented these changes. Total protein synthesis was not affected by interferon. Thus interferon appears to arrest the pattern of increases and decreases in synthesis of specific proteins without affecting total protein synthesis. The effects of certain enzymes and other proteins that are known to increase or decrease during spontaneous or induced differentiation of normal and tumor cells have been reviewed recently by Grossberg & Taylor (123) and Sreevalsan (122).

The detection of interferon in the amniotic fluid, uterus, and placenta of normal individuals raises the suspicion that interferon may play a role in the differentiation of developing fetal cells (53, 54).

Immunoresponsive Cells[17]

Interferon modifies the functions of NK cells, T cells, B cells, and monocytes. Interferon and interferon inducers such as poly IC, bacteria, and alloantigens enhance NK activity by a protein synthesis–dependent mechanism that increases the ability of NK cells to bind to and lyse virus-infected and tumor targets (241). Interferon increases NK activity by recruiting NK precursors and by increasing the lytic rate and recycling capacity of target-binding cells (197–198). This increased human NK cell activity is enhanced by interferon both in vivo and in vitro (199).

Interferon enhances target-specific T-cell cytotoxicity (209) and the cytotoxic phase of the mixed leukocyte reaction (212, 242); the proliferative phase of the reaction is inhibited. Similar antiproliferative but cytotoxicity-enhancing effects of interferon occur in mitogen-stimulated cell cultures (147, 243). Interferon inhibits the generation of T suppressor cells from mixed leukocyte cultures (214) but activates those that act on concanavalin A–stimulated cell cultures, immunoglobulin (Ig) production, and mixed leukocyte cultures (244).

Low doses enhance and high doses suppress Ig synthesis during activation of polyclonal B cells by pokeweed mitogen (245–246). Pretreatment of the lymphocytes with interferon enhances Ig production, but treatment after exposure to the mitogen has the opposite effect (247–249).

Cytotoxic (209, 210, 250) and phagocytic functions (208) of monocytes are

[17]For reviews see 17, 237–240.

enhanced by interferon in normal cells; as with T cells, suppressor function is depressed. Suppression of NK activity by monocytes is highly sensitive to interferon (211). The net effect of in vivo enhancement and suppression of T cells and monocytes remains to be delineated; the outcome may depend on the time and dose of interferon.

The nature and variety of the immunostimulatory and immunoresponsive effects of interferon (Table 2) justify the inclusion of all three major types of interferon as bona fide components of the immune system. In fact, immunomodulation of immunoreceptive cells may be the principal function of IFN-γ, which by definition qualifies both as a lymphokine and an interferon. IFN-γ may in fact be required for the maintenance of the physiological level of NK cell activity (238).

Drug Metabolism[18]

The biotransformation of drugs and other xenobiotics occurs primarily in the liver through oxidation, reduction, hydrolysis and conjugation. The oxidations are mediated principally by the cytochrome P-450 (P-450, monooxygenase; mixed function oxidase; MFO) system, which is comprised of NADPH P-450 reductase, NADH-cytochrome b_5 reductase, cytochrome b_5 and several P-450 isozymes of low substrate selectivity (254). The products formed by P-450-linked oxidations are usually more polar, water soluble, and excretable by the kidney than their antecedents. They are therefore less therapeutically effective or toxic, although in a few cases they may be more active (e.g. increased carcinogenicity of certain polycyclic hydrocarbons). The duration and intensity of action of individual drugs are determined largely by the activity of the P-450 system. A large number of xenobiotics induce their own oxidative biotransformation and that of other xenobiotics. A few others depress the P-450 system via suicidal reactions, through the formation of reactive intermediate metabolites that bind strongly to P-450, by acting as substrate inhibitors, or more relevantly to this overview by responding to immunomodulatory agents. Induction and depression of the P-450 system can alter the therapeutic effectiveness or toxicity of drugs markedly.

The concept of a special mechanism for the detoxification of foreign chemicals developed about the turn of this century at a time when there was a great deal of excitement over the new disciplines of microbiology and immunology. The concept, termed the "chemical defense hypothesis" (255), envisioned a general protective mechanism that dealt with toxic chemicals in a manner comparable to those involved in natural resistance to invading microorganisms and viruses. The hypothesis was challenged when it was found that certain xenobiotics became more toxic through biotransformation. (In this context,

[18]For reviews see 251–253.

note that allergies and autoimmune diseases are adverse immune responses.) Not only does the P-450 system qualify as a "chemical defense" mechanism of sorts, it also responds to a variety of modulators of the immune system (Table 3). In addition to inducing interferon, the immunomodulators listed in Table 3 exhibit a broad spectrum of biological activities, many of which are related to host immunity: (*a*) alteration of reticuloendothelial activity; (*b*) antiviral, antifungal, antibacterial, and antineoplastic activity; (*c*) sensitization of bacterial endotoxin; and (*d*) inhibition of adjuvant-induced arthritis (42). Although all of these agents are interferon inducers, it would seem unlikely that all would depress the P-450 system by the same mechanism. However, it would be a mistake to dismiss interferon as the cause of the depression of drug biotransformation simply on the basis that a given agent is a poor inducer of serum interferon; serum interferon levels are not necessarily reliable indicators of the interferon content of the liver and other organs (256, 301). All of these agents alter drug metabolism when administered in vivo but have no effect when added to microsomal preparations that biotransform drugs.

The first example of the impairment of the elimination of a drug by a host-defense mechanism was provided by Samaras & Deitz (302) in 1953 before P-450 was discovered. They observed that trypan blue, a depressant of the reticuloendothelial system, greatly prolonged the hypnotic effect of pentobarbital. Almost two decades later Munson and associates (223, 224, 280) reported that poly IC, pyran, and zymosan depressed in vivo and in vitro P-450-dependent drug biotransformation. Pyran induced little or no serum interferon and poly IC induced large titers of serum interferon, yet both agents depressed drug biotransformation about equally. This was interpreted to mean that modification of the reticuloendothelial system was indirectly involved in the depression of hepatic drug metabolism rather than a more direct action of interferon. Renton & Mannering (184) and Leeson & associates (303), showed that tilorone, a potent interferon inducer, markedly depressed the P-450 system when administered to rats. The question of whether the depression was due to some unknown property of tilorone or to the ability of tilorone to induce interferon was approached indirectly by studying the effects of a variety of known interferon inducers of widely different structures and molecular weights. All of these agents depressed the hepatic P-450 system (181). The authors suggested that the depression of the P-450 system is a general property of interferon inducers. Immunomodulators that have been shown to affect P-450 systems are listed in Table 3.

Other indirect evidence supports the view that interferon per se is involved in the depression of drug biotransformation. Peak serum levels of interferon appear about 2 hr, 12 hr, and 7 days after the administration of poly IC (304), tilorone (305), and *C. parvum* (306), respectively. The time required for the first indications of depression of drug biotransformation by each of these agents

Table 3 Depression of hepatic cytochrome P-450 systems by immunomodulators

Immunomodulator	Cytochrome or drug biotransformed[a]	Species	Reference
Poly IC	Ethylmorphine, benzo[a]pyrene, aniline, p-nitrophenetole, aminopyrine, hexobarbital S. T., P-450	rat or mouse	180, 181, 183, 187, 188, 223, 224, 251
Poly I and Poly C	ethylmorphine, P-450	mouse	256
Tilorone	ethylmorphine, aniline, aminopyrine, hexobarbital S. T. benzo[a]pyrene, P-450	rat	180, 181, 184, 187, 188
Quinacrine	ethoxyresorufin, ethylmorphine, aniline, P-450	rat	181, 257
Statolon	ethylmorphine, aniline, P-450	rat	181
Endotoxin	ethylmorphine, aniline, benzo[a]pyrene, nitroreductase, aminopyrine, azoreductase, biphenyl, ethoxyresorufin, benzyloxyphenoxazone, hexobarbital S. T., zoxazolamine P. T.	rat or mouse	181, 258, 260–262
CP 20,961	ethylmorphine, aniline, P-450	rat	181
CMA	ethylmorphine, P-450	mouse	unpublished
Maleic anhydride Divinyl ether copolymer (PYRAN)	aminopyrine, aniline, hexobarbital S. T., P-450	mouse	42, 223, 263
Freunds adjuvant (*mycobacterium butyricum*)	benzo[a]pyrene, pentobarbital S. T., ketamine, aminopyrine, paracetamol, P-450	rat, mouse	259, 264–267
Corynebacterium Parvum	p-nitroanisole, hexobarbital, aminopyrine, aniline, antipyrine, benzo[a]pyrene, P-450	mouse or rat	268, 269
Bacillus Calmette-Guerin (BCG)	aminopyrine, aniline, DICD, ethoxycoumarin, benzo[a]pyrene, P-450	rat, mouse	270–272
Bordetella pertussis	ethylmorphine, aniline, aminopyrine, phenytoin, P-450	mouse, rat	181, 273, 274
OK-432	aniline, aminopyrine, pentobarbital S. T., P-450	mouse	275
Lipid A	aminopyrine, aniline	mouse	276
Nocardia cell wall skeleton	aminopyrine, aniline, P-450	rat	277
N-acetylmuramyl-l-analyl-D-isoglutamine (MDP)	aniline, ethoxycoumarin, ethylmorphine, P-450	rat or mouse	278
Peptidoglycan monomer (PGM)	P-450, ethoxycoumarin	mouse	279

Methyl palmitate	hexobarbital S. T.	mouse	280
Zymosan	pentobarbital S. T., hexobarbital S. T.	mouse	280
Dextran sulfate	benzo[a]pyrene, aminopyrine, P-450	mouse	281
Latex	P-450	mouse	252
Colloidal carbon	ethylmorphine, carbon tetrachloride, P-450	rat	282, 283
Schistosoma mansoni	aminopyrine, aniline, benzo[a]pyrene, hexobarbital S. T., zoxazolamine P. T., P-450	mouse	284, 285
Trypanosoma brucei	aniline, p-nitroanisole, anthracene, P-450	mouse	286
Plasmodium berghei	hexobarbital S. T., aniline, p-nitroanisole, P-450	rat	287
Fasciola hepatica	hexobarbital S. T., zoxazolamine P. T., aniline, aminopyrine, P-450	rat	288
Viruses			
Mouse hepatitis virus	aniline, hexobarbital, strychnine, P-450	mouse	289, 290
Mengo virus	ethylmorphine, aniline, P-450	rat	181
Encephalomyocarditis virus (EMC)	aminopyrine, P-450	mouse	291
Newcastle Disease virus (NDV)	aminopyrine, ethylmorphine P-450	mouse	165, 292
Duck hepatitis virus	ethylmorphine	duck	293
Influenza vaccine	benzo[a]pyrene	human, mouse	294
Sindbis virus	tryptophane	mouse	295
Interferons			
Crude mouse Gamma (2000 × 3)	P-450 aminopyrine, diphenylhydantoin	mouse	271, 296
HuIFLr-αA,D or -αAD (50,000)	aminopyrine, P-450	mouse	297, 298
HuIFLr-αA,D or -AD (0.06–48 μg)	zoxazolamine P. T., hexobarbital S. T., ethoxycoumarin, benzphetamine, benzo[a]pyrene	mouse	19
IFN-α crude mouse (50,000)	aminopyrine, benzo[a]pyrene, P-450	mouse	297
IFN-β Calbiochem mouse (50,000)	aminopyrine, benzo[a]pyrene, P-450	mouse	297
IFN-α/β mouse (10,000 × 5 weeks)	ethoxyresorufin, ethoxycoumarin	mouse	299
rIFN-γ mouse (50,000 × 3 days)	p-nitroanisole, P-450	mouse	300
rIFN-γ mouse (5,000 × 3)	ethylmorphine, aminopyrine, P-450	mouse	162

[a]All immunomodulators were administered to animals, and preparations of their livers were assayed for cytochrome P-450 content or drug biotransformation activities, except when indicated by S. T. or P. T., in which cases animals were injected with the immunomodulator and their sleeping time after pentobarbital or hexobarbital, or the paralysis time after zoxazolamine was measured.

corresponds well with the appearance of these peak serum interferon levels (180, 184, 268). A temporal coincidence of interferon production and depressed drug biotransformation was also observed after mice were infected with encephalomyocarditis virus (291). Neither polyriboinosinic acid (poly I) nor polyribocytidylic acid (poly C) induces appreciable amounts of interferon nor do they depress P-450 systems (181). However, when an injection of poly I was followed an hour later with an injection of poly C, as much serum interferon was induced as by poly IC and drug biotransformation was depressed (256, 307). When the order of injection of poly I and poly C was reversed, neither interferon induction nor depression of the P-450 system occurred. Poly IC induces about equal serum interferon titers in C57B1/6J and C3H/HeJ mice, but Newcastle disease virus (NDV) induces only about one tenth as much serum interferon in C3H/HeJ mice as in C57B1/6J mice (308). As anticipated, NDV depressed the P-450 system in C57B1/6J mice but not in C3H/HeJ mice (165, 292).

Proof of the involvement of interferon in the depression of hepatic P-450 awaited the availability of a pure interferon that is active in a laboratory animal. This came in the form of HuIFNr-AD, a recombinant hybrid of HuIFNr-A and HuIFNr-D, which possesses antiviral activity in the mouse (18). HuIFNr-AD depressed the P-450 system in the mouse; HuIFNr-A and HuIFNr-D, which do not induce antiviral activity in the mouse, had little or no effect (19, 297). Pure recombinant mouse IFN-γ also depresses the P-450 systems (162, 300), possibly by a mechanism different from that initiated by IFN-α and IFN-β. When IFN-γ was used, three intraperitoneal injections spaced 3 hr apart were required (162).

The mechanism for the depression of the P-450 system by interferon remains unknown. The involvement of 2-5A synthetase or protein kinase would seem likely. This would require at least a small amount of endogenous double-stranded RNA (Figure 1); but, as discussed earlier, that is not an improbability. P-450 is only one of many examples in a growing list of enzymes and other proteins that are depressed by interferon (Table 2). It is conceivable that the same mechanism may be involved in the depression of most if not all of these proteins. Patterns of biotransformation of substrates and SDS-polyacrylamide gel electrophoresis of apoP-450 show that not all P-450 isozymes are depressed equally by interferon (309) or interferon inducers (310). The turnover rate of P-450 heme was used as an index of the turnover of P-450 to show that poly IC and tilorone depress only the more rapidly turning-over forms of P-450 (311).

Ghezzi and associates have recently proposed a novel mechanism for the depression of the P-450 system by interferon and interferon-inducing agents (163, 164). They observed that these agents increase xanthine oxidase activity in the liver and other tissues several fold. Because xanthine oxidase generates free oxygen radicals and oxygen radicals destroy P-450 (312), they proposed that interferon depresses the P-450 system because it induces xanthine oxidase activity. Allopurinol, an in vivo inhibitor of xanthine oxidase, partially protected mice against P-450 depression. However, in a more recent study from our laboratory (G. J. Mannering, L. B. Deloria, V. S. Abbott & N. J. Gooderman, unpublished data) the P-450 systems of untreated mice and mice whose hepatic xanthine oxidase activity had been lowered to less than 10% of normal by tungstate treatment responded equally to poly IC.

Studies of the mechanism of depression of the P-450 system are hampered by the lack of an experimental cell model. P-450 is not found in significant concentrations in replicating cells. Moreover, the P-450 present in these cells does not biotransform the xenobiotics of usual interest. This leaves nonreplicating primary hepatocytes as the only practical cell model. Only recently has it been possible to culture hepatocytes for 24 hr or more without great loss of P-450. In an early study, Renton et al (186) reported that a crude interferon preparation induced P-450 in cultured hepatocytes that had lost about 80% of their P-450. In a recent study (S. K. Kuwahara & G. J. Mannering, unpublished data), we showed that poly IC, a partially purified α/β mouse interferon, and recombinant HuIFNrAD did not affect the P-450 system of cultured mouse hepatocytes that had been cultured for 24 hr without appreciable loss of P-450. On the other hand, P-450 (P_1-450) that had been induced by 3-methylcholanthrene while the hepatocytes were being cultured was depressed by mouse interferon and poly IC. The failure of interferon to depress uninduced P-450 in cultured hepatocytes might be explained in two ways.

First, humoral factors not present in hepatocytes but supplied by other cells may be required. Kupffer cells may supply the humoral factor. Dextran sulfate, like pyran and several other insoluble polymers, depresses drug biotransformation (252). The effect is believed to be initiated as a consequence of phagocytosis by macrophages. Peterson & Renton (281) showed that levels of P-450 and aryl hydrocarbon hydroxylase (AHH) activity are not affected when freshly isolated hepatocytes are incubated for 30 min with dextran sulfate. However, when isolated Kupffer cells (sequestered macrophages) were added to the incubation mixture, the P-450 content and AHH activity of the hepatocytes were depressed markedly. The same effect was produced by the supernatant fraction from Kupffer cells that had been incubated with dextran sulfate. The low molecular weight of the humoral factor (less than 12,000 daltons) excluded interferon as the active component of the supernatant fraction. It was not determined whether interferon would have produced the same results in hepatocytes incubated for 30 min (a time increment too short to have had any appreciable effect on the enzymes regulating the steady-state of P-450 in hepatocytes) or whether the humoral factor from macrophages induced interferon in these hepatocytes.

Second, the maintenance of near normal levels of P-450 in hepatocytes may result from stabilization of the enzyme rather than an enzymically controlled steady state. In this case, the P-450 would not be turning over and its synthesis could not be affected by interferon-induced 2-5A synthetase or protein kinase. The observation that P_1-450 induced by 3-methylcholanthrene during culture was depressed by interferon whereas preexisting P-450 was not (S. K. Kuwahara & G. J. Mannering, unpublished data) supports the suggestion that endogenous P-450 in cultured hepatocytes is not turning over fast enough to be affected by interferon-induced mechanisms that depress protein synthesis.

Evaluation of the effects of interferon and other immunomodulators on drug biotransformation in humans has not received much attention. Interferon has been used clinically for the most part on advanced cancer patients. Under the circumstance, the inclusion of a drug metabolism study during treatment of these patients might seem frivolous. Moreover, the disease itself could complicate interpretation of the results; for example, tumors release "toxohormone" that greatly depresses P-450-dependent drug biotransformation (313–316). However, it is inevitable that chemical antitumor agents will be used in combination with interferon with increasing frequency. These drugs have such notoriously unfavorable therapeutic indexes that even a small depression of their biotransformation could produce toxicity with dire consequences.

Mouse interferon stimulated benzanthracene-induced aryl hydrocarbon hydrolyase activity in fetal mouse secondary cell cultures (185).

Viral and bacterial infections that produce immunomodulatory agents (e.g. endotoxins) are known to depress drug biotransformation (Table 3). It was originally assumed that hepatitis virus depressed P-450 (289, 290) because of associated morphological and biochemical changes in the liver. While this may be the case during advanced stages of the disease, the effect on drug biotransformation seen during early infection is likely due to the interferon induced by the virus. Viruses that do not inflict primary pathological effects also depress drug metabolism (165, 192). There is strong suspicion that much of the considerable day-by-day variation in levels of the P-450 systems seen in laboratory animals may be due to viruses that produce none of the usual overt signs of viral infections. This becomes particularly apparent when unusually low values are not further depressed by poly IC or other immunomodulators.

P-450-dependent benzo[a]pyrene hydroxylase activity in the lungs of mice infected with mouse-adapted influenza virus was only 10% of that of uninfected control mice, whereas no change was seen in the activity of this enzyme in the livers of the infected animals (294). This is of interest not only because it demonstrates that drug metabolism can be affected by an immunomodulator in an organ other than the liver but also because it shows that the effect can be localized.

Viral infections often occur in subjects who are receiving medication for reasons unrelated to the infection or to ameliorate the unpleasant effects of the infection. Several cases are now on record where virus infection has enhanced drug toxicity. The infecting agents have not always been identified, but the decreased ability to eliminate theophylline appears to be a common occurrence among patients suffering from upper respiratory infections (317). During an epidemic of influenza B infection in Seattle in 1980, theophylline toxicity was observed in 11 children; 6 of these patients had been maintained on the same dose of theophylline prior to the infection without exhibiting theophylline toxicity (318). The half-life of theophylline was increased in 4 young patients suffering from acute upper respiratory influenza A viral illness. Acute theophylline toxicity was observed in one of these patients (319). The half-life of theophylline was more than doubled 24 hr after the vaccination of 4 healthy volunteers with trivalent influenza vaccine (320). The vaccine also impaired the clearance of aminopyrine in healthy human subjects (321). The vaccine had no significant effect on biotransformation of theophylline and warfarin by elderly residents of rest homes (322). Activity of the immune system declines with age. Does this mean that the depressant effect of the vaccine on drug metabolism is inversely related to the activity of the immune system? Is it only a coincidence that activities of the immune system and the P-450 system decline with age (323–325)?

Depression of the P-450 system by interferon may influence chemical carcinogenesis. Many procarcinogenic polycyclic hydrocarbons are converted by the P-450 system to reactive metabolites that initiate carcinogenesis after they bind covalently to cellular macromolecules (326). Kishida et al (327) observed a delay in the development of carcinogenesis in 3-methyl cholanthrene (3-MC)-treated mice. Salerno et al (225) observed that none of the 3-MC-treated mice that received both 3-MC and interferon developed tumors whereas tumors developed in all of the animals that received 3-MC only. How much of the protective effect was due to inhibition of biotransformation of 3-MC and how much was due to an antiproliferative effect of interferon on the early formation of aberrant cells has not been determined.

CLINICAL APPLICATIONS[19]

The promise of a "magic bullet" that would eliminate viral diseases began with the discovery of interferon in 1957. Here was a natural therapeutic agent that would destroy almost all viruses as effectively as penicillin had killed bacteria. Best of all, it would do so without producing undesirable side effects. Enthusiasm, as unrealistic as it was unbounded, was heightened with the discovery that interferon worked against cancer in experimental animals. Now all that was needed was enough human interferon for clinical trials. This opportunity arrived when Cantell (23) produced large (for those days) amounts of crude

[19]For reviews see 328–335.

Table 4   Antiviral activity of exogenous interferon in humans

Disease	Interferon Type	Dose ($\times 10^6$)[a]	Response	Reference
Acute fulminant hepatitis	IFN-α	3 qd	3/6	337
Fulminant hepatitis B	IFN-β	3–6 qd	2/4	338, 339
Hepatitis B	IFN-β	10 qd × 19	2/2	340
	IFN-α	900	4/16	341
Herpes simplex	IFN-α	3 qd	4/4	337
	IFN-α	0.07/kg/5d	14/19	342
Herpes zoster	IFN-α	0.25/kg/4×	1/17	343
	IFN-α	0.5 kg/14×	5/5	344
Ocular dendritic keratitis	IFN-α	0.6 + trifluorothymidine	?/54	345 346
Human warts	IFN-α	1.2	2/2	347
	IFN-β	2.7 qd	0/1	348
Encephalitis	IFN-α	3 qd	2/3	337
Postmeasles dermatitis	IFN-α	3 qd	1/1	337
Cytomegalovirus (renal transplant patients)	IFN-α	3 qd × 15	0/41	349 350
Viral infections (renal transplant patients)	IFN-β	3/2 × 10/90d	0/16	351
Varicella in cancer patients	IFN-α	0.35/6×	13/21	352

[a] Units of interferon; qd = daily; d = number of days; × = number of times.

interferon from induced human leukocytes. Early trials with this material, both as an antiviral agent and as an antitumor agent, were encouraging (336). Genetic engineering, fostered by commercial enterprise, produced several molecular species of human recombinant IFN-α in the abundant quantities required for clinical testing. The results of these clinical trials, summarized in Tables 4 and 5, have had a sobering effect on those who had expected miracles. On the other hand, they have not discouraged those whose expectations had been tempered by their knowledge of interferon experiments with mice and by their experience with chemical antitumor and antiviral agents in general. The results of these initial trials should not be minimized even though they may not fulfill the expectations of the press, the lay public, and some clinicians.

IFN-α was effective in the treatment of several virus pathologies (Table 4), including chronic active hepatitis resulting from hepatitis B virus; life-threatening, virus-induced juvenile laryngeal papillomatosis; herpes zoster and simplex infections; acute epidemic keratoconjuntivitis; and warts. Twelve of 15 patients suffering from life-threatening viral illness (acute fulminant hepatitis, spreading herpes simplex in immunosuppressed patients, encephalitis, juvenile laryngeal papillomatosis, postmeasles dermatitis) recovered after being treated with IFN-α. All of these patients were critically ill, and many were near death

Table 5 Antitumor activity of exogenous interferon in humans

Tumor	Type	Dose[a]	Route of administration	Response	Reference
Brain	β human	3 qd	i.v., i.c.	2/4	353
	β human	3 qd		4/6	333
Breast	αA Recombinant	50/m², tiw × 28d		0/17	354
	α Cantell	3 qd × 28d		5/23	355
	α Cantell	3–9 qd × 28d		8/17	356
	α Lymphoblastoid	2 or 5–18/m² qd × 10d		1/27	357
	β Roswell Park	1 qd 34d	i.m., i.v.	1/6	358
	αA Recombinant	200–600/total		0/3	359
	αA Leuk(crude)	1 prior to surgery	i.t.	3/4	360
	rIFN-α2	10 + doxorubicin	i.m. + i.v.	2/2	334
Cervical	HuLeuk (crude)	2 qd in pressary prior to surgery		12/15	361
	rIFN-α2	2/2 × w	topical gel	5/7	362
	rIFN-α2	10 + doxorubicin	i.v. + i.m.	13/13	334
Colon	α Cantell	3 qd × 5		0/19	363
	αA Recombinant	50/m² tiw		1/18	364
	α Lymphoblastoid	3/m² tiw		0/19	365
	rIFN-α2	3–100 qd	i.m.	0/4	366
	α Cantell	?		2/32	367
	β Roswell Park	1/40 ×		0	358
	β Bioferon	?		0	368
	rIFN-α2	10 + doxorubicin	i.m. + i.v.	1/4	334
Chronic myelogenous leukemia	α Cantell	9–15 qd		22/25	369

(continued)

Table 5 (continued)

Tumor	Interferon Type	Dose[a]	Route of administration	Response	Reference
Hairy cell leukemia	α Cantell	3	i.m.	19/20	370
	rIFN-α2	10/3 × w		7/8	334
	rIFN-α2	2/m² tiw	s.c.	13/13	371
Kaposi's sarcoma	αA Recombinant	36–54 qd × 28		14/34	372
	rIFN-α2	50/5d		8/20	373
	rIFN-α2	1–50/m²		10/11 early stage	334
				12/29 late stage	334
Liver	α Cantell	3 qd × 60d		0/5	374
	IFLr-A	12–850/m²/tiw		0/16	375
Lung (nonsmall cell)	α Cantell	3 qd × 30 d	i.m. + i.v.	1/37	376
	rIFL-α2	10 + doxorubicin		3/3	334
Lymphoma	α Cantell	3–9 qd		6/11	356
	αA Recombinant	50 m² tiw		17/46	377
	α	?		35/51	378
	β Bioferon	4–6/qd		1/7	378
	α Cantell	1 qd/30d	i.m.	6/18	379
Melanoma	α Lymphoblastoid	2.5/m² qd		1/17	380
	αA Recombinant	50/m² tiw		7/31	381
	α Cantell	1,3,9 qd/42d		1/45	382
	α2 Recombinant	10–100 qd × 20		2/16	383
	HuLeuk (crude)	2	i.t.	1/2	360
	α Lymphoblastoid	15/m² every other day		3/33	384
	β Bioferon	?		1/2	368
	α	4–12 + cimentidine	i.m. or i.t.	3/6	385

Cancer	Interferon	Dose	Route	Response	Ref.
Myeloma	α Cantell	3–9 qd		6/10	356
	α Cantell	3–6 qd × 6 mo		3/11	386
	rIFN-α2	2–100	i.v., s.c.	20/38	334
	β Bioferon	3–10/29d		0/3	387
	rIFN-α2	3–100/qd	i.m./i.v.	5/16	366
	IFN-α2 (high-grade lymphoma)	50/m²/5d		4/27	334
Non-Hodgkin's lymphoma	IFN-α2 (low-grade lymphoma)	10/m²/tiw	s.c.	3/12	334
	IFL-rA	3–118		8/11	24
	β	4.5–9 qd/6 weeks		2/8	368
	α	2.5–5 qd/30	i.m.	4/6	388
Osteogenic sarcoma	α Cantell	3/tiw		16/30	389
Ovary	α Cantell	1–6 qd		1/15	390
	α Lymphoblastoid	2 or 5–18/m² qd × 10		1/13	391
	β	3/2 × w		0/8	392
	rIFN-α2	5–50/qd × 16	i.p.	7/11	393
	α lymphoblastoid	5/5d × 6	i.p.	19/28	394
Renal	α Cantell	3 qd		5/19	395
	αA Recombinant	50/m²qd		2/19	382
	αA Recombinant	2/m² qd		0/8	396
	αA Recombinant	20/m²qd		2/8	397
	α Cantell	1 qd		0/14	398
	α Cantell	10 qd		3/16	398
	α Lymphoblastoid	3/m²/tiw		2/21	399

ªDose, 10^6 units of interferon; qd = daily; tiw = three times a week; number = injections; response: stable, partial, or complete remission; i.t. = intratumor, i.c. = intracranial.

when interferon therapy was begun (337). Interferon has good potential for the treatment of other viral infections, including rabies (400–402).

The first and longest ongoing trial of interferon as an antitumor agent is that by Strander (389, 403), who has used crude human leukocyte interferon to treat postsurgical osteogenic sarcoma patients. Some of these patients have been followed for more than a decade. Fifty percent of those who received interferon have survived for 5 years as opposed to 25% in the control group. Results of more recent clinical trials, which usually employed huge doses of recombinant interferon, have reached the current literature. As can be seen in Table 5, these results do not encourage unbridled optimism that interferon will prove to be the ultimate antitumor agent. Nevertheless, various degrees of tumor regression have been observed in breast carcinoma, malignant lymphoma, multiple myeloma, acute leukemia, malignant melanoma, Kaposi's sarcoma, chronic leukemias, bladder carcinoma, malignant gliomas, and nasopharyngeal carcinoma. Responses have been recorded as tumor shrinkage, stabilization of tumor size, remissions, survival time, and other measures of antitumor activity but rarely as a "cure". Of 38 patients with breast cancer, multiple myeloma, and lymphoma treated with 3–9 × 10^6 units of IFN-α daily, 50% had some kind of favorable response, 34% experienced complete or partial remission, and 16% showed limited responses (355, 356). The effect of interferon on hairy cell leukemia is the most dramatic recorded to date; complete remissions were observed in 19 of the 20 patients treated with IFN-α (334, 370, 371).

Ikic and associates (360) have used crude IFN-α as an adjunct to surgical removal of tumors. Eight patients with bladder cancer, four with breast cancer, and two with malignant melanoma, all with poor prognoses, were treated with crude IFN-α injected either into the tumor, into its adjacent tissue, or in some cases, intramuscularly. All tumors showed complete or partial regression for up to 6 months. Two patients with bladder papillomatosis, who were unsuited for conventional therapeutic procedures, were treated with transurethral and intramuscular interferon. The reduction of tumor mass that resulted permitted resection, and complete regression was achieved. Topical application of interferon to tumors in two breast cancer patients led to more than 50% regression of the tumors, which were then removed by surgery. In another study, crude IFN-α produced substantial or total remissions in patients with cancers of the head and neck; 10 of 30 patients were considered completely cured (404). Similar encouraging results were obtained with presurgical injection of crude IFN-α in cervical cancer (361). IFN-α (1 × 10^6 units) applied in a gel with a vaginal applicator to areas of cervical intraepithelial neoplasm in 7 patients produced complete response in 2 patients and partial responses in 3 others (334).

In retrospect, mouse studies have largely predicted what has been found clinically. Gresser (405) has summarized the mouse studies as follows: (a)

Interferon is most effective when injected repeatedly and during the period of tumor growth; (b) efficacy is inversely related to the tumor load; (c) efficacy is roughly proportional to the dose; (d) antitumor effects are maximal when the direct contact between tumor cells and interferon is maximal; and (e) in most systems, interferon inhibits tumor growth, but regression of established tumors has not been reported. Although these studies were conducted in highly artificial systems, a great deal that can be used in the treatment of patients can be learned from mice. This is particularly true of pharmacokinetics, which does not differ among animal species as much as most of the other factors that influence treatment. Clearly there is need for recombinant mouse interferons, not only for pharmacokinetic studies but also for studies of the mechanisms of antiproliferative and other pleiotropic actions of interferon, most of which are not understood.

Combinations of interferon with known antitumor agents or modulators of the immune system have not been undertaken in earnest largely because of the need for preliminary evaluation of the effectiveness of interferon in the absence of agents that would complicate interpretation of results. Combination of the antiviral agent adenine arabinoside (Ara A) with interferon was more effective in the treatment of chronic hepatitis B virus infection than with either agent alone (328, 406, 407). This strategy had to be discontinued because the patients developed acute Ara A neurotoxicity. Attempts to treat dendritic keratitis with IFN-α were disappointing. However, results were excellent when interferon was combined with the antiviral agent trifluorothymidine (345, 346).

Cimetidine, a histamine$_2$ antagonist used in the treatment of gastric ulcers, was administered with IFN-α to 6 patients with metastatic melanoma on the basis that it would inhibit suppressor T cells, which bear histamine receptors (385). Since suppressor cells suppress helper T cells, and helper T cells promote the activities of macrophages and NK cells, which are believed to be involved in the antiproliferative effect of interferon, cimetidine should in theory enhance the antiproliferative action of interferon. No tumor regression was observed in these patients during the 3–8 weeks they received interferon alone. In contrast, coadministration of interferon and cimetidine was associated with complete remissions in two patients, partial remission in a third, and stationary disease status in a fourth. In a more recent report, complete regression was seen in an additional 5 of 8 patients (408). Complete remission was achieved in a patient with acute myelogenous leukemia treated with 4×10^6 units of intramuscular IFN-α and 1 g of oral cimetidine daily for 6 weeks (409).

In vitro studies that showed synergistic cytotoxic effects of recombinant IFN-α when used with 8 standard chemotherapeutic agents led to the selection of doxorubicin for Phase I clinical trials (234, 410). Partial responses were seen with several tumor types; complete responses were obtained in 3 cases of ovarian cancer (334).

Transformed cells are less sensitive to interferon than normal cells in vitro

(411–412). Any agent that makes tumor cells as responsive to interferon as normal cells are would be expected to enhance the antitumor activity of interferon. Butyrate is such a substance (413). Arginine butyrate coadministered with IFN-α reduced tumor incidence in mice inoculated with 180 TG Crocker tumor cells. When *C. parvum* was administered with either interferon or arginine butyrate alone, significant protection of the animals was achieved. However, optimal results were obtained when a single injection of *C. parvum* was followed by nine daily alternating injections of arginine butyrate and interferon. This combination of agents has not yet been tested clinically.

The story of the clinical use of the interferons has just begun. Few of the numerous recombinant IFN-αs have been tested; there have been few trials with IFN-β, probably because early results have been less encouraging than those obtained with IFN-α; the testing of IFN-γ has only reached the Phase I level (414). The concept of using recombinant hybrid interferons or interferons with altered amino acid sequences is still on the drawing board. The dose, frequency, and route of administration of interferon have been derived empirically. Serum levels of interferon have proven of little predictive value, particularly when the interferon has been injected intramuscularly. The intraperitoneal route, which Bocci (96) believes may be the preferred mode of administration, has received only preliminary evaluation (360, 385). Few trials have been made with direct injection of interferon into solid tumors. There is still no information on how much of the interferon reaches the tumors.

These early clinical trials predict that the future of interferon as an antineoplastic agent will depend largely on multiple factors: the kind of tumor (whether it is growing or quiescent, its size and age, its access to interferon), the patient (many have been in a profound state of immunodepression as a result of their malignancy or previous chemotherapy), and the kind, amount, frequency, and mode of administration of interferon. The bullet may acquire some magic status when it is the proper type and caliber and is aimed in the right direction at the right target at the right time.

TOXICOLOGY[20]

The early belief that interferon would not elicit untoward side effects was based largely on the philosophy that interferon existed only in response to, and to protect against, viral infections. Accordingly, the pleiotropic effects observed were attributed to impurities in the crude interferon preparations used at that time. When pure interferon was made available, it became apparent that most if not all of the multiple effects observed with the crude preparations were due to their interferon content (129). Moreover, when large amounts of recombinant

[20]For reviews see 94, 415–420.

interferon came into use, some new and more severe toxic manifestations surfaced.

The recording of side effects by clinicians has been remarkably consistent. Similar toxic effects have been reported for all three major types of interferon, although not always to the same extent. Since individual subspecies of IFN-α have different spectra of activities (18), it can be predicted that they will also exhibit different spectra of toxicities. Some of the toxic symptoms are dose related, some are not; tachyphylaxis develops in some patients, but not in others. All of the toxic signs and symptoms disappear when interferon treatment is discontinued or doses are reduced. It is now recognized that the unpleasant flu symptoms experienced with viral diseases are in fact due to the interferon induced by the virus.

Pyrexia, the earliest sign of toxicity observed with commonly used doses of interferon, appears in all patients within 3 hr after injection. Temperatures return to normal spontaneously within 12–24 hr after a single dose of interferon, and tachyphylaxis usually develops after about two weeks of therapy. The effect is not dose related. Headache and myalgia occur in most patients between 8 and 12 hr after injection. These symptoms are largely not dose dependent, and tachyphylaxis is commonly observed.

Reported cardiovascular effects include hypotension, cardiac dysrhythmia, tachycardia, and premature ventricular extrasystole.

Leukopenia has been observed in most patients 24 hr after the initiation of interferon therapy; it is transient and rarely causes the white count to fall below 2000 cells/ml of blood. The degree of leukopenia seems to relate to the degree of therapeutic effectiveness of interferon. Transient declines in platelet counts may accompany leukopenia. Hemoglobin levels are not usually affected, although mild anemia has been reported. Bone marrow depression, reminiscent of that seen with chemical neoplastic agents, has been observed after prolonged treatment. The hair loss seen after extensive interferon therapy is also remindful of that seen with chemical antineoplastic agents. The loss of hair is not uniform; in fact, eyelash growth is increased—in one case, to 6.5 cm (421)!

Although frank liver pathology has not been reported, interferon-induced elevation of serum transaminase levels indicates some hepatic dysfunction.

The effects of interferon on the central nervous system are the most problematical and can be dose limiting. Many patients receiving large doses of interferon complain of fatigue after 4–7 days of treatment. They become extremely lethargic and anorexic and in danger of further complicating a catabolic state that may in many cases already exist. Fatigue, often associated with nausea, can be a dose-limiting toxicity. An impressive number of CNS side effects have been reported: coma, confusion, conceptual disorganization, increased EEC wave activity, malaise, paresthesia, psychomotor slowing, speech stoppage, thought blocking, and visuospatial disorientation (422–24).

Recent evidence for the function of IFN-α as a regulatory polypeptide in both neuroendocrine and immune systems suggests a modus operandi for the neurotoxicity of interferon (228–230, 425–430). Human leukocyte interferon possesses immunological and biological endorphin- and ACTH-like activities (425). The antiviral activity of human IFN-α is neutralized by anti-ACTH, anti-IFN-α, and anti-γ-endorphin antisera; anti-IFN-α serum neutralizes ACTH activity. Neutralization of IFN-α activity by anti-ACTH and anti-γ-endorphin is prevented with ACTH and γ-endorphin, respectively. IFN-β and IFN-γ do not share these antigenic properties with IFN-α. Pro-opiomelanocortin is a polyprotein that generates several hormones, including ACTH and endorphin (431). Structural commonalities suggested by the immunological cross-reactivities between ACTH endorphin and interferon were verified by the revelation that 6 amino acid sequences are common to both pro-opiomelanocortin and IFN-α (432).

The intracerebral injection of HuIFNr-α, γ-endorphin, or morphine produce analgesia, catalepsy, and immobilization in mice (229); naloxone, a morphine antagonist, reverses these effects. Interferon mitigates opiate addiction liability and eliminates the withdrawal phenomenon initiated by naloxone in morphinized rats (228).

Whatever the relationship may be between the neurotoxicity and the opiate-like activities of interferon, at least one inconsistency requires explanation. The antigenic associations and some of the functional similarities that have been made between the interferon and the opiates in mice apply only to IFN-α, not IFN-β or IFN-γ, yet neurotoxicity is produced in humans by all three interferons (102, 358, 422–24).

As described earlier, Gresser and associates (216–220) produced severe liver necrosis in suckling mice when they injected them with large doses of interferon throughout the first 6 days postpartum. When smaller doses were given during the same early neonatal period, livers were damaged but in time they recovered. However, all of these mice died several weeks later from glomerular nephritis. A very similar glomerulonephritis developed in mice that recovered from lymphocytic choriomeningitis (LCM) virus infection. Recognition of the similarity in the interferon- and LCM-induced kidney lesions led Gresser and associates to a classical experiment (417). Some of the mice that were injected with an increased amount of LCM virus were given potent sheep antimouse interferon globulin; other similarly infected mice received control immunoglobulin. All of the control mice showed extensive liver necrosis, but no liver pathology was seen in mice that received the interferon antibody. Antimouse interferon globulin reduced the incidence of mortality from 72% to 27% in one experiment and from 31% to 10% in a second experiment. Whereas all of the control mice rapidly developed severe glomerular lesions, a marked delay was observed in the development of these lesions in the mice that received the interferon antibody, and the lesions were less severe. The results clearly indicated that the endogenous interferon induced by LCM virus was largely responsible for inhibition of growth, liver cell necrosis, glomerular nephritis, and death.

This experiment suggests that some effects of viral infections in humans may appear long after the infection has subsided, that these effects may be due to the interferon induced by the virus, and that they may not be recognized as such. The question has been raised as to whether autoimmune diseases may have been triggered by interferon induced early in life by viral infections. Elevated titers of interferon have been found in the sera of patients with SLE, rheumatoid arthritis, scleroderma, and Sjögren's syndrome (56, 417). A good correlation was found between interferon titers and disease activity (433). In one report, "high therapeutic effectiveness" resulted from the injection of interferon antibody into patients with autoimmune or allergic diseases. Is the teratogenesis attributed to rubella due to the large amount of interferon known to be induced by this virus during early pregnancy?

Is the induction of interferon by virus in itself a pathological response? If one assumes that low levels of endogenous interferon are required for the regulation of a variety of vital cellular functions, and that this is controlled by delicately balanced levels of endogenous double-stranded RNA, any sudden large influx of double strandedness introduced by a viral infection would seem catastrophic. In short, do cells have a very low tolerance to double-stranded RNA?

SUMMARY

Interferon was discovered three decades ago. The next 20 or more years of research were directed largely toward an understanding of its antiviral activity. The persistent short supply of interferon hampered progress, and the impure preparations available throughout these years clouded interpretation of results. Many of the experiments and clinical studies that interferonologists had dreamed of for 20 or more years became realities when modern technology provided quantities of pure interferon that exceeded expectations. Studies with these pure recombinant interferons removed all doubts that the many pleiotropic effects that had been observed with impure interferon preparations were due to interferon and not to the impurities. The interferons are now acknowledged lymphokines that are involved in many cellular processes. In fact, the antiviral activity of interferon, which led to its discovery, may be an exaggerated adaptive utilization of an interferon-regulated function that plays a more general role in cellular physiology.

The ability to isolate, purify, and produce pure interferon has led to the discovery of multiple species of leukocyte interferon. These interferons display different patterns of activity when tested by a variety of systems. This suggests that specific leukocyte interferons may be involved in specific physiological functions.

Results of preliminary trials of the interferons as antiviral and antitumor agents have been encouraging and occasionally dramatic. The overall clinical picture is expected to improve when more is learned about the pharmacokinetics of the interferons and which of the interferons are best suited for the treatment of specific tumors and antiviral diseases. There are indications that coadministration of interferons with chemical antineoplastic and antiviral agents may increase the effectiveness of interferon in clinical situations. As might be expected of agents that influence a large number of physiological functions, interferons produce numerous toxic side effects, some of which resemble those inflicted by viral diseases. These side effects are reversible and not life threatening.

Literature Cited

1. Tyrrell, D. A. J. 1976. *Interferon and its Clinical Potential*, pp. 1–101. London: Heineman Med. Books.
2. Billiau, A. 1984. The main concepts and achievements in interferon research: a historical account. In *Interferon*, Vol. 1, *General and Applied Aspects*, ed. A. Billiau, pp. 23–58. Amsterdam: Elsevier
3. Henle, W., Henle, G., 1984. The road to interferon: interference by inactivated influenza virus. See Ref. 2, pp. 3–22
4. Lindenmann, J. 1982. From Interference to interferon: a brief historical introduction. *Philos. Trans. R. Soc. London, Ser. B* 299:3–6
5. Stewart, W. E. II. 1981. *The Interferon System*. New York: Springer-Verlag. 493 pp. 2nd ed.
6. Henle, W., Henle, G., 1943. Interference of inactive virus with the propagation of virus of influenza. *Science* 98:87–89
7. Isaacs, A., Lindenmann, J. 1957. Virus Interference. I. The interferon. *Proc. R. Soc. London, Ser. B* 147:258–67
8. Nagano, Y., Kojima, Y. 1958. Inhibition de l'infection vaccinale par le virus homologue. *C. R. Soc. Biol.* 152:1627–30
9. Isaacs, A., Lindenmann, J., Valentine, R. C. 1957. Virus Interference. II. Some properties of interferon. *Proc. R. Soc. London, Ser. B* 147:268–73
10. Tyrrell, D. A. J. 1959. Interferon produced by cultures of calf kidney cells. *Nature* 184:452–53
11. Sela, I. 1984. Interferon and interferon-like factors in plants. In *Antiviral Drugs*

and *Interferon: The Molecular Basis of their Activity*, ed. Y. Becker, pp. 336–56. Boston: Nijhoff
12. Lockhart, R. Z. 1973. Criteria for acceptance of a viral inhibitor as an interferon and a general description of the biological properties of known interferons. In *Interferons and Interferon Inducers*, ed. N. B. Finter, pp. 11–28. New York: Am. Elsevier. 2nd ed.
13. Pestka, S., Baron, S. 1981. Definition and classification of the interferons. In *Methods in Enzymology*, Vol. 78, ed. S. Pestka, pp. 3–14. New York: Academic
14. Sikora, K. 1983. Introduction. In *Interferon and Cancer*, ed. K. Sikora, pp. 1–9. New York: Plenum
15. Pestka, S. 1983. The human interferons—from protein purification and sequence to cloning and expression in bacteria: before, between and beyond. *Arch. Biochem. Biophys.* 221:1–37
16. Knight, E. Jr. 1984. The Molecular structure of interferons. See Ref. 2, pp. 61–78
17. Baron, S., Grossberg, S. E., Klimpel, G. R., Brunell, P. A. 1984. Immune and interferon systems. In *Antiviral Agents and Viral Diseases of Man*, ed. G. J. Galasso, T. C. Merigan, R. A. Buchanan, pp. 123–78. New York: Raven. 2nd ed.
18. Weck, P. K., Apperson, S., Stebbing, N., Gray, P. W., Leung, D., et al. 1981. Antiviral activities of hybrids of two major human leukocyte interferons. *Nucleic Acids Res.* 9:6153–66

19. Parkinson, A., Lasker, J., Kramer, M. J., Huang, M.-T., Thomas, P. E., et al. 1982. Effects of three recombinant human leukocyte interferons on drug metabolism in mice. *Drug Metab. Dispos.* 10:579–85

20. Epstein, L. 1979. The comparative biology of immune & classical interferons. In *Biology of the Lymphokines*, ed. S. Cohen, E. Pick, J. J. Oppenheim, pp. 443–514. New York: Academic

21. Kirchner, H., Marcucci, F. 1984. Interferon production by leukocytes. In *Interferon*, Vol. 2, *Interferons and the Immune System*, ed. J. Vilcek, E. De-Maeyer, pp. 7–34. Amsterdam: Elsevier

22. Gordon, J., Minks, M. A. 1981. The interferon renaissance: molecular aspects of induction and action. *Microbiol. Rev.* 45:244–66

23. Cantell, K. 1979. Why is interferon not in clinical use today? In *Interferon*, 1, ed I. Gresser, pp. 2–28. New York: Academic

24. Sherwin, S. A., Fein, S., Whisnant, J., Oldham, R. 1982. Phase 1 trials of recombinant and non-recombinant alpha interferons in cancer patients. In *Interferons*, ed. T. C. Merigan, R. M. Friedman, pp. 433–47. New York: Academic

25. Horoszewicz, J. S., Leong, S. S., Ito, M., Buffett, R. F., Karakousis, C., et al. 1978. Human fibroblast interferon in human neoplasia: clinical and laboratory study. *Cancer Treat. Rep.* 62:1899–1906

26. Torrence, P. F., DeClercq, E. 1977. Inducers and induction of interferon. *Pharmacol. Ther.* 2:1–88

27. Stringfellow, D. A., ed. 1980. *Interferon and Interferon Inducers: Clinical Application*. New York: Dekker. 329 pp.

28. Pollard, R. B. 1982. Interferon and interferon inducers: development of clinical usefulness and therapeutic promise. *Drugs* 23:37–55

29. Ho, M. 1984. Induction and inducers of interferon. See Ref. 2, pp. 79–124

30. Field, A. K., Lampson, G. P., Tytell, A. A., Nemes, M. M., Hilleman, M. R. 1967. Inducers of interferon and host resistance. IV. Double-stranded replicative RNA from *E. coli* MS2 coliphage. *Proc. Natl. Acad. Sci. USA* 58:2102–107

31. Bobst, A. M., Torrence, P. F., Kouidou, S., Witkop, B. 1976. Dependence of interferon induction on nucleic acid conformation. *Proc. Natl. Acad. Sci. USA* 73:3788–92

32. DeClercq, E., Torrence, P. F. 1982. Structure activity relationships for interferon induction and inhibition of pro-

tein synthesis by polynucleotides. *Tex. Rep. Biol. Med.* 41:76–83

33. Torrence, P. F., De Clercq, E. 1984. Interferon induction by nucleic acids: structure-activity relationships. In *Interferons and their Applications*, ed. P. E. Came, W. A. Carter, pp. 233–58. New York: Springer-Verlag

34. Levy, H. B., 1981. Induction of interferon in vivo and in vitro by polynucleotides and derivatives and preparation of derivatives. See Ref. 13, pp. 291–99

35. Levy, H. B., Levine, A. S. 1982. Antitumor effects of interferon and poly ICLC and their possible utility as antineoplastic agents in man. *Tex. Rep. Biol. Med.* 41:653–61

36. Stringfellow, D. A. 1980. Interferon Inducers: Theory and experimental application. See Ref. 27, pp. 145–65

37. Levy, H. B. 1980. Induction of interferon by polynucleotides. See Ref. 27, pp. 167–86

38. Ts'o, P. O. P., Alderfer, J. L., Levy, J., Marshall, L. W., O'Malley, J., et al. 1976. An integrated and comparative study of the antiviral effects and other biological properties of the polyinosinic acid-polycytidylic acid and its mismatched analogues. *Mol. Pharmacol.* 12:299–312

39. Greene, J. J., Ts'o, P. O. P., Strayer, D. R., Carter, W. A. 1984. Therapeutic applications of double-stranded RNAs. See Ref. 33, pp. 535–55

40. Breinig, M. C., Munson, A. E., Morahan, P. S. 1980. Antiviral activity of synthetic polyanions. In *Anionic Polymeric Drugs*, ed. L. G. Donoruma, R. M. Ottenbrite, D. Vogl, pp. 211–26. New York: Wiley

41. Ottenbrite, R. M., Butler, G. B. 1984. *Anticancer and Interferon Agents: Synthesis and Properties*, ed. R. M. Ottenbrite, G. B. Butler, pp. 248–86. New York: Dekker

42. Barnes, D. W. 1980. Effects of anionic polymeric drugs and other immunoactive agents on microsomal mixed function oxidases. See Ref. 40, pp. 255–75

43. Mayer, G. D., Krueger, R. F. 1980. Tilorone hydrochloride and related molecules. See Ref. 27, pp. 187–221

44. Chandra, P., Woltersdorf, M. 1976. Tilorone hydrochloride—a specific probe for A-T regions of duplex deoxyribonucleic acid. *Biochem. Pharmacol.* 25:877–80

45. Epstein, L. 1981. Interferon–Gamma: Is it really different from the other interferons? In *Interferon*, 3, ed. I. Gresser, pp. 13–44. New York: Academic.

46. Baron, S. 1966. The biological significance of the interferon system. In *Interferons*, ed. N. Finter, pp. 268–313. Amsterdam: North Holland

47. Chany, C. 1976. Membrane-bound interferon specific cell receptor system: role in the establishment and amplification of the antiviral state. *Biomedicine* 24:148–57

48. Inglot, A. D. 1983. The hormonal concept of interferon. Brief review. *Arch. Virol.* 76:1–13

49. Bocci, V. 1981. Production and role of interferon in physiological conditions. *Biol. Rev. Cambridge Philos. Soc.* 56: 49–85

50. Bocci, V., Muscettola, M., Paulesu, L., Grasso, G. 1984. The physiological interferon response. II. Interferon is present in lymph but not plasma of healthy rabbits. *J. Gen. Virol.* 65:101–8

51. Galabru, J., Robert, N., Buffet-Janvresse, C., Riviere, Y., Hovanessian, A. G. 1985. Continuous production of interferon in normal mice: Effect of anti-interferon globulin, sex, age, strain, and environment on the levels of 2-5A synthetase and p67K kinase. *J. Gen. Virol.* 66:711–18

52. Fowler, A. K., Reed, C. D., Giron, D. J. 1980. Identification of an interferon in murine placentas. *Nature* 286:266–67

53. Lebon, P., Girard, S., Thepot, F., Chany, C. 1982. The presence of α-interferon in human amniotic fluid. *J. Gen. Virol.* 59:393–96

54. Chany, C., Duc-Goiran, P., Robert-Galliot, B., Lebon, P. 1982. Study of human amniotic interferon. See Ref. 24, pp. 241–48

55. Chany, C. 1984. Interferon receptors and interferon binding. In *Interferon*, Vol. 3, *Mechanisms of Production and Action*, ed. R. M. Friedman, pp. 11–32. Amsterdam: Elsevier

56. Hooks, J. J., Detrick-Hooks, B. 1984. Interferon in autoimmune diseases and other immunoregulatory disorders. See Ref. 21, pp. 165–83

57. Forti, R. L., Moldovan, R. A., Mitchell, W. M., Callicoat, P., Schuttman, S. S., et al. 1985. Application of objective biological assay of human interferons to clinical specimens and a survey of a normal population. *J. Clin. Microbiol.* 21:689–93

58. Billiau, A., Edy, V. G., Heremans, H., VanDamme, J., Desmyter, J., et al. 1977. Human interferon: mass production in a newly established cell line, MG63. *Antimicrob. Agents Chemother.* 12:11–14

59. Kawakita, M., Cabrer, B., Taira, H., Rebello, M., Slattery, E., et al. 1978. Purification of interferon from mouse Ehrlich ascites tumor cells. *J. Biol. Chem.* 253:598–602

60. Jameson, P., Grossberg, S. E. 1979. Production of interferon by human tumor cell lines. *Arch. Virol.* 62:209–20

61. Finter, N. B., Fantes, K. H. 1980. The purity and safety of interferons prepared for clinical use: the case for lymphoblastoid interferon. *Interferon*, 2, ed. I. Gresser, pp. 65–80. New York: Academic

62. Pickering, L. A., Kronenberg, L. H., Stewart, W. E. II. 1980. Spontaneous production of human interferon. *Proc. Natl. Acad. Sci. USA.* 77:5938–42

63. Trinchieri, G., Santoli, D., Knowles, B. B. 1977. Tumor cell lines induce interferon in human lymphocytes. *Nature* 270:611–13

64. Weigent, D. A., Langford, M. P., Smith, E. M., Blalock, J. E., Stanton, G. J. 1981. Human B lymphocytes produce leukocyte interferon after interaction with foreign cells. *Infect. Immun.* 32: 508–12

64a. Lackovic, V., Borecky, L., Zschiesche, W., Fahlbusch, B., Schumann, I. 1980. Production of interferon and other lymphokines during murine tumor growth. II. Induction of an interferon by Ehrlich ascites cells in outbred mice. *Acta Virol.* 24:45–54

65. Djeu, J. Y., Huang, K. Y., Herberman, R. B. 1980. Augmentation of natural killer activity and induction of interferon by tumor cells in vivo. *J. Exp. Med.* 151:781–89

66. Timonen, T., Saksela, E., Virtanen, I., Cantell, K. 1980. Natural killer cells are responsible for the interferon production induced in human lymphocytes by tumor cell contact. *Eur. J. Immunol.* 10:422–27

67. Williams, B. R. G. 1983. Biochemical actions. See Ref. 14, pp. 33–52

68. Kerr, I. M., Rice, A., Roberts, W. K., Cayley, P. J., Reid, A., et al. 1984. The 2-5A and protein kinase systems in interferon-treated and control cells. In *Gene Expression*, ed. B. F. C. Clark, H. U. Petersen, pp. 487–99. Copenhagen: Munksgaard

69. Revel, M. 1984. The interferon system in man: Nature of the interferon molecules and mode of action. See Ref. 11, pp. 357–433

70. Shannon, W. M. 1984. Mechanisms of action and pharmacology: chemical agents. See Ref. 17, pp. 55–121

71. Marcus, P. I. 1984. Interferon Induction

by Viruses: Double stranded ribonucleic acid as the proximal inducer molecule. See Ref. 55, pp. 113–75

72. Isaacs, A., Cox, R. A., Rotem, Z. 1963. Foreign nucleic acids as the stimulants to make interferon. *Lancet* 2:113–16

73. Field, A. K., Tytell, A. A., Lampson, G. P., Hilleman, M. R. 1967. Inducers of interferon and host resistance. II. Multi-stranded synthetic polynucleotide complexes. *Proc. Natl. Acad. Sci. USA* 58:1004–9

74. Aguet, M., Mogensen, K. E., 1983. Interferon Receptors. In *Interferon*, 5, ed. I. Gresser, pp. 1–22. New York: Academic

75. Kushnaryov, V. M., Sedmak, J. J., Bendler, J. W. III, Grossberg, S. E. 1982. Ultrastructural localization of interferon receptors on the surfaces of cultured cells and erythrocytes. *Infect. Immun.* 36:811–21

76. Kushnaryov, V. M., MacDonald, H. S., Sedmak, J. J., Grossberg, S. E. 1983. Ultrastructural distribution of interferon receptor sites on mouse L fibroblasts grown in suspension. Ganglioside blockade of ligand binding. *Infect. Immun.* 40:320–29

77. Epstein, C. J., Epstein, L. B. 1982. Genetic control of the response to interferon. *Tex. Rep. Biol. Med.* 41:324–31

78. Besancon, F., Ankel, H., Basu, S. 1976. Specificity and reversibility of interferon ganglioside interaction. *Nature* 259:576–78

79. Friedman, R. M., Pastan, I. 1969. Interferon and cyclic 3'5' adenosine monophosphate: potentiation of antiviral activity. *Biochem. Biophys. Res. Commun.* 36:735–39

80. Chany, C., Mathieu, D., Gregoire, D. 1980. Induction of delta-4-3-keto steroid synthesis by interferon in mouse adrenal tumor cell cultures. *J. Gen. Virol.* 50:447–50

81. Lebleu, B., Content, J. 1982. Mechanisms of interferon action: Biochemical and genetic approaches. In *Interferon, 4*, ed. I. Gresser, pp. 48–94. New York: Academic

82. Marcus, P. I. 1983. Interferon induction by viruses: One molecule of dsRNA as the threshold for interferon induction. See Ref. 74, pp. 116–80

83. Content, J. 1984. The antiviral effect of interferon on cells. See Ref. 2, pp. 125–38

84. Johnston, M. L., Torrence, P. F. 1984. The role of interferon-induced proteins, double-stranded RNA and 2',5' oligo-denylate in the interferon mediated inhibition of viral translation. See Ref. 55, pp. 189–298

85. Friedman, R. M., Esteban, R. M., Metz, D. H., Tovell, D. R., Kerr, I. M. 1972. Translation of RNA by L cell extracts: effects of interferon. *FEBS Lett.* 24:273–77

86. Friedman, R. M., Metz, D. H., Esteban, R. M., Tovell, D. R., Ball, L. A., Kerr, I. M. 1972. Mechanisms of interferon action: inhibition of viral messenger ribonucleic acid translation in L-cell extracts. *J. Virol.* 10:1184–98

87. Kerr, I. M., Brown, R. E., Ball, L. A. 1974. Increased sensitivity of cell free protein synthesis to double-stranded RNA after interferon treatment. *Nature* 250:57–59

88. Roberts, W. K., Clemens, M. J., Kerr, I. M. 1976. Interferon-induced inhibition of protein synthesis in L-cell extracts: an ATP-dependent step on the activation of an inhibitor by double-stranded RNA. *Proc. Natl. Acad. Sci. USA* 73:3136–40

89. Kerr, I. M., Brown, R. E. 1978. pppA2'p5'A2'p5'A: an inhibitor of protein synthesis synthesized with an enzyme fraction from interferon treated cells. *Proc. Natl. Acad. Sci. USA* 75:256–60

90. Burke, D. C. 1970. The status of interferon. *Sci. Am.* 236:42–48

91. Hovanessian, A. R., Riviere, Y., Montagnier, L., Michelson, M., Lacour, J., Lacour, F. 1982. Enhancement of interferon-mediated protein kinase in mouse and human plasma in response to treatment with polyadencylic·polyuridylic acid. *J. Interferon Res.* 2:209–15

92. Johnson, A. G. 1979. Modulation of the immune system by synthetic polynucleotides. *Springer Semin. Immunopathol.* 2:149–168

93. Billiau, A. 1981. Interferon therapy: Pharmacokinetic and pharmacological aspects. *Arch. Virol.* 67:121–133

94. Scott, G. M. 1982. Interferon: pharmacokinetics and toxicity. *Philos. Trans. R. Soc. London Ser. B* 299:91–107

95. Bocci, V. 1981. Pharmacokinetic studies of interferon. *Pharmacol. Ther.* 13:421–40

96. Bocci, V. 1984. Evaluation of routes of administration of interferon in cancer: a review and a proposal. *Cancer Drug Delivery* 1:337–51

97. Bino, T., Edery, H., Gertler, A., Rosenberg, H. 1982. Involvement of the kidney in catabolism of human leukocyte interferon. *J. Gen. Virol.* 59:39–45

98. Billiau, A., Heremans, H., Ververken,

D., VanDamme, J., Carton, H., De-
Somer, P. 1981. Tissue distribution of
human interferons after exogenous administration in rabbits, monkeys, and
mice. *Arch. Virol.* 68:19–25

99. Bocci, V., Pacini, A., Bandinelli, L.,
Pessina, G. P., Muscettola, M., Paulesu,
L. 1982. The role of liver in the catabo-
lism of human α & β interferon. *J. Gen.
Virol.* 60:397–400

100. Abreu, S. L. 1983. Pharmacokinetics of
rat fibroblast interferon. *J. Pharmacol.
Exp. Ther.* 226:197–200

101. Cantell, K., Fiers, W., Hirvonen, S.,
Pyhala, L. 1984. Circulating interferon
in rabbits after simultaneous intramuscular administration of human alpha and
gamma interferons. *J. Interferon Res.*
4:291–93

102. Gutterman, J. U., Rosenblum, M. G.,
Rios, A., Fritsche, H. A., Quesada, J. R.
1984. Pharmacokinetic study of partially
pure γ-interferon in cancer patients. *Cancer Res.* 44:4164–71

103. Satoh, Y. L., Kasama, K., Kajita, A.,
Shimizu, H., Ida, M. 1984. Different
pharmacokinetics between natural and
recombinant human interferon beta in
rabbits. *J. Interferon Res.* 4:411–22

104. Bocci, V., Pacini, A., Pessina, G. P.,
Paulesu, L., Muscettola, M., Lunghetti,
G. 1985. Catabolic sites of human in-
terferon-γ. *J. Gen. Virol.* 66:887–91

105. Lucero, M. A., Magdelenat, H., Fridman, W. H., Pouillart, P., Billardon, C.,
et al. 1982. Comparison of effects of
leukocyte and fibroblast interferon on immunological parameters in cancer patients. *Eur. J. Cancer Clin. Oncol.*
18:243–51

106. Tokazewski-Chen, S. A., Marafino, B.
J. Jr, Stebbing, N. 1983. Effects of
nephrectomy on the pharmacokinetics of
various human interferons in the rat. *J.
Pharmacol. Exp. Therap.* 227:9–15

107. Derynck, R., Content, J., DeClercq, E.,
Volckaert, G., Tavernier, J., et al.
1980. Isolation and structure of a human
fibroblast interferon gene. *Nature* 285:
542–47

108. Taniguchi, T., Mantei, N., Schwarz-
stein, M., Nogata, S., Muramatsu, M.,
Weissmann, C. 1980. Human leukocyte
and fibroblast interferons are structurally
related. *Nature* 285:547–49

109. Simonsen, C. C., Shepard, H. M., Gray,
P. W., Leung, D. W., Pennica, D., et al.
1982. Plasmid directed synthesis of human immune interferon in *E. coli*
and monkey cells. See Ref. 24, pp. 1–
14

110. Nagai, H., Arai, T., Kohno, S., Kohase,
M. 1982. Interferon therapy for malignant brain tumors. In *The Clinical Potential of Interferons*, ed. R. Kono, J. Vilcek, pp. 257–73. Tokyo: Univ. Tokyo
Press

111. Ueda, S., Hirakawa, K., Nakagawa, Y.,
Suzuki, K., Kishida, T. 1982. Brain
tumors. See Ref. 14, pp. 129–39

112. Heremans, H., Billiau, A., DeSomer, P.
1980. Interferon in experimental viral infections in mice: tissue interferon levels
resulting from the virus infection and
from exogeneous interferon therapy. *Infect. Immun.* 30:513–22

113. Bocci, V., Pessina, G. P., Pacini, A.,
Paulesu, L., Muscettola, M., Naldini,
A., Lunghetti, G. 1985. Pharmacokinetics of human lymphoblastoid interferon
in rabbits. *Gen. Pharmacol.* 16:277–79

114. Palleroni, A. V., Bohoslawec, O. 1984.
Use of ^{125}I-interferons in pharmacokinetic and tissue distribution studies. *J. Interferon Res.* 4:493–98

115. Rosenblum, M. G., Unger, B. W.,
Gutterman, J. U., Hersh, E. M., David,
G. S., Frincke, J. M. 1985. Modification
of human leukocyte interferon pharmacology with a monoclonal antibody. *Cancer Res.* 45:2421–24

116. Stewart, W. E. II. 1979. Varied biologic
effects of interferon. See Ref. 23, pp.
29–51

117. Taylor-Papadimitriou, J. 1984. Effects
of interferons on cell growth and function. See Ref. 2, pp. 139–66

118. Gresser, I. 1984. The effect of interferon
on the expression of surface antigens. See
Ref. 21, pp. 113–32

119. Sonnenfeld, G. 1984. Effects of interferon on antibody formation. See Ref.
21, pp. 85–99

120. Herberman, R. B. 1984. Interferon and
cytotoxic effector cells. See Ref. 21, pp.
61–84

121. Vogel, S. N., Friedman, R. M. 1984.
Interferon and macrophages: activation
and cell surface changes. See Ref. 21,
pp. 35–59

122. Sreevalsan, T. 1984. Effects of interferons on cell physiology. See Ref. 55,
pp. 343–87

123. Grossberg, S. E., Taylor, J. L. 1984.
Interferon effects on cell differentiation.
See Ref. 55, pp. 299–317

124. Djeu, J. Y. 1984. Regulation of cell function by interferon. In *Interferon: Research, Clinical Application, and Regulatory Considerations*. ed. K. C. Zoon,
P. D. Noguchi, T.-L. Liu, pp. 125–31.
Amsterdam: Elsevier

125. Fisher, P. B., Grant, S. 1985. Effects of
interferon on differentiation of normal

and tumor cells. *Pharmacol. Ther.* 27: 143–166

126. Rossi, G. B. 1985. Interferons and cell differentiation. In *Interferon*, 6, ed. I. Gresser, pp. 31–68. New York: Academic

127. Clemens, M. J., McNurlan, M. A. 1985. Regulation of cell proliferation and differentiation by interferons. *Biochem. J.* 226:345–60

128. Gresser, I. 1977. On the varied biological effects of interferon. *Cell Immunol.* 34: 406–15

129. Gresser, I., DeMaeyer-Guignard, J., Tovey, M. G., DeMaeyer, E. 1979. Electrophoretically pure mouse interferon exerts multiple biological effects. *Proc. Natl. Acad. Sci. USA* 76:5308–12

130. van't Hull, E., Schellekens, H., Lowenberg, B., deVries, M. J. 1978. Influence of interferon preparations on the proliferative capacity of human and mouse bone marrow cells in vitro. *Cancer Res.* 38:911–14

131. Zoumbos, N. C., Gascon, P., Djeu, J. Y., Young, N. S. 1985. Interferon as a mediator of hematopoietic suppression in aplastic anemia in vitro and possibly in vivo. *Proc. Natl. Acad. Sci. USA* 82: 188–92

132. Jahiel, R. L., Taylor, D., Rainford, N., Herschberg, S. E., Kroman, R. 1971. Inducers of interferon inhibit the mitotic response of liver cells to partial hepatectomy. *Proc. Natl. Acad. Sci. USA* 68:740–42

133. Chany, C., Vignal, M. 1968. Etude du mecanisme de l'etat refractaire des cellules à la production d'interferon, après inductions répétées, *C. R. Acad. Sci.* 267:1798–1800

134. Attallah, A. M., Needy, C. F., Noguchi, P. D., Elisberg, B. L. 1979. Enhancement of carcinoembryonic antigen expression. *Int. J. Cancer* 24:49–52

135. Tamm, I., Pfeffer, L. M., Wang, E., Landsberger, F. R., Murphy, J. S. 1981. Inhibition of cell proliferation and locomotion by interferon: membrane and cytoskeletal changes in treated cells. In *Cellular Responses to Molecular Modulators*, ed. L. W. Moses, J. Schultz, W. A. Scott, R. Werner, pp. 417–42. New York: Academic

136. Tamm, I., Pfeffer, L. M., Wang, E., Murphy, J. S. 1984. Interferon-induced changes in cell motility and structure. *Lymphokines* 9:37–70

137. Knight, E. Jr., Korant, B. D. 1977. A cell surface alteration in mouse L cells induced by interferon. *Biochem. Biophys. Res. Commun.* 74:707–13

138. Lampidis, T. J., Brouty-Boyé, D. 1981. Interferon inhibits cardiac cell function in vitro. *Proc. Soc. Exp. Biol. Med.* 166: 181–85

139. Blalock, J. E., Stanton, J. D. 1980. Common pathways of interferon and hormonal action. *Nature* 283:406–8

140. Calvet, M. C., Gresser, I. 1979. Interferon enhances the excitability of cultured neurones. *Nature* 278:558–60

141. Gewert, D. R., Shah, S., Clements, M. J. 1981. Inhibition of cell division by interferons. Changes in the transport and intracellular metabolism of thymidine in human lymphoblastoid cells. *Eur. J. Biochem.* 116:487–92

142. Friedman, R. M., Lee, G., Shifrin, S., Ambesi-Impiombato, S., Epstein, D., et al. 1982. Interferon interactions with thyroid cells. *J. Interferon Res.* 2:387–400

143. Chandrabose, K., Cuatrecasas, P., Pottathil, R. 1981. Changes in fatty acyl chains of phospholipids induced by interferon in mouse sarcoma S-180 cells. *Biochem. Biophys. Res. Commun.* 98: 661–68

144. Apostolov, K., Barker, W. 1984. Cyclic effects of interferon and its antagonist on the saturation of 18-carbon fatty acids. *Ann. Virol.* 135E:245–56

145. Pfeffer, L. M., Kwok, B. C. P., Lansberger, F. R., Tamm, I. 1985. Interferon stimulates cholesterol and phosphatidylcholine synthesis but inhibits cholesterol ester synthesis in HeLa-S3 cells. *Proc. Natl. Acad. Sci. USA* 82:2417–21

146. Grossberg, S. E., Keay, S. 1980. The effects of interferon on 3T3-L1 cell differentiation. *Ann. N.Y. Acad. Sci.* 350:294–300

147. Zwingelstein, G., Meister, R., Malak, N. A., Maury, C., Gresser, I. 1985. Interferon alters the composition and metabolism of lipids in the liver of suckling mice. *J. Interferon Res.* 5:315–25

148. Schultz, R. 1980. E-type prostaglandins and interferons: Yin-Yang modulation of macrophage tumorcidal activity. *Medical Hypothesis* 6:831–43

149. Grimm, W., Seitz, M., Kirchner, H., Gemsa, D. 1978. Prostaglandin synthesis in spleen cell cultures of mice injected with Corynebacterium Parvum. *Cell. Immunol.* 40:419–26

150. Basham, T. Y., Bourgeade, M. F., Creasey, A. A., Merigan, T. C. 1982. Interferon increases HLA synthesis in melanoma cells: interferon resistant and sensitive cell lines. *Proc. Natl. Acad. Sci. USA* 79:3265–69

151. Fisher, P. B., Mufson, R. A., Weinstein,

I. B. 1981. Interferon inhibits melanogenesis in B-16 mouse melanoma cells. *Biochem. Biophys. Res. Commun.* 100:823–30

152. DeMaeyer-Guignard, J., Cachard, A., DeMaeyer, E. 1980. Electrophoretically pure mouse interferon has priming but no blocking activity in poly (I.C.) induced cells. *Virology* 102:222–25

153. Cooper, H. L., Fagnani, R., London, J., Trepel, J., Lester, E. P. 1982. Effects of interferons on protein synthesis in human lymphocytes: enhanced synthesis of eight specific peptides in T cells and activation dependent inhibition of overall protein synthesis. *J. Immunol.* 126:828–33

154. Miorner, H., Landstrom, E., Larner, E., Larsson, I., Lundgren, E. A., Strannegard, O. 1978. Regulation of mitogen-induced lymphocyte DNA synthesis by human interferon of different origins. *Cell Immunol.* 35:15–24

155. Sreevalsan, T., Rosengurt, E., Taylor-Papadimitriou, J., Burchell, J. 1980. Differential effect of interferon on DNA synthesis, 2-deoxyglucose uptake and ornithine decarboxylase activity in 3T3 cells stimulated by polypeptide growth factors and tumor promoters. *J. Cell Physiol.* 104:1–9

156. Luftig, R. B., Conscience, J.-F., Skoultchi, A., McMillan, P., Revel, M., Ruddle, F. H. 1977. Effect of interferon on dimethyl sulfoxide-stimulated friend erythroleukemic cells: ultrastructural and biochemical study. *J. Virol.* 23:799–810

157. Dani, Ch., Mechti, N., Piechaczyh, M., LeBleu, B., Jeanteur, Ph., Blanchard, J. M. 1985. Increased rate of degradation of c-Myc on RNA in interferon-treated Daudi cells. *Proc. Natl. Acad. Sci. USA* 82:4896–99

158. Schroeder, E. W., Chou, L. N., Jaken, S., Black, P. H. 1978. Interferon inhibits the release of plasminogen activator for SV3T3 cells. *Nature* 276:828–29

159. Heremans, H., Billiau, A., Colombatti, A., Hilgers, J., DeSomer, P. 1978. Interferon treatment of NZB mice: accelerated progression of autoimmune disease. *Infect. Immun.* 21:925–30

160. Talas, M., Szolgay, E. 1978. Radioprotective activity of interferon inducers. *Arch. Virol.* 56:309–15

161. Ortaldo, J. R., McCoy, J. L. 1980. Protective effects of interferon in mice previously exposed to lethal irradiation. *Radiat. Res.* 81:262–66

162. Mannering, G. J., Abbott, V. S., Deloria, L. B., Gooderham, N. J. 1985. Correlation of the effects of interferon inducers on the depression of hepatic

cytochrome P-450 systems and the induction of xanthine oxidase. *Pharmacologist* 27:114

163. Ghezzi, P., Branchi, M., Mantovani, A., Spreafico, F., Salmona, M. 1984. Enhanced xanthine oxidase activity in mice treated with interferon and interferon inducers. *Biochem. Biophys. Res. Commun.* 119:144–49

164. Ghezzi, P., Bianchi, M., Gianera, L., Landolfo, S., Salmona, M. 1985. Role of reactive oxygen intermediates in the interferon-mediated depression of hepatic drug metabolism and protective effect of N-acetylcysteine. *Cancer Res.* 45:3444–47

165. Deloria, L. B., Abbott, V., Gooderham, N., Mannering, G. J. 1985. Induction of xanthine oxidase and depression of cytochrome P-450 by interferon inducers: genetic difference in the responses of mice. *Biochem. Biophys. Res. Commun.* 131:109–14

166. Butt, T. A., Sreevalsan, T. 1983. Interferon and sodium butyrate inhibit the stimulation of poly (ADP-ribose) synthetase in mouse cells stimulated to divide. *Exp. Cell Res.* 148:449–59

167. Fisher, P. B., Miranda, A. F., Bobiss, L. E., Pestka, S., Weinstein, I. B. 1983. Opposing effects of interferon produced in bacteria and of tumor promoters on myogenesis in human myoblast cultures. *Proc. Natl. Acad. Sci. USA* 80:2961–65

168. Illinger, D., Coupin, G., Richards, M., Poindron, P. 1976. Rat interferon inhibits steroid-inducible glycerol-3-phosphate dehydrogenase synthesis in rat glial cell line. *FEBS Lett.* 64:391–95

169. Rozee, K. R., Katz, L. J., McFarlane, E. S. 1969. Interferon stimulation of methylase activity in L-cells. *Can. J. Microbiol.* 15:969–74

170. Yaron, M., Yaron, I., Gurari-Rotman, D., Revel, M., Lindner, H. R., Zor, U. 1977. Stimulation of prostaglandin E production in cultured human fibroblasts by poly (I)·poly (C) and human interferon. *Nature* 267:457–59

171. Fitzpatrick, F. A., Stringfellow, D. A. 1980. Virus and interferon effects on cellular prostaglandin biosynthesis. *J. Immunol.* 125:431–37

172. Berry, L. J., Smythe, D. S., Colwell, L. S., Schoengold, R. J., Actor, P. 1971. Comparison of the effects of a synthetic polyribonucleotide with the effects of endotoxin on selected host responses. *Infect. Immun.* 3:444–48

173. Beck, G., Poindron, P., Illinger, D., Beck, J.-P., Ebel, J.-P., Falcoff, R. 1974. Inhibition of steroid inducible tyro-

sine aminotransferase by mouse and rat interferon in hepatoma tissue culture cells. *FEBS Lett.* 48:297–300

174. Matsuno, T., Shirasawa, N., Kohno, S. 1976. Interferon suppresses glutamine synthetase induction in chick embryonic neural retina. *Biochem. Biophys. Res. Commun.* 70:310–14

175. Vesely, D. L., Cantell, K. 1980. Human interferon enhances guanylate cyclase activity. *Biochem. Biophys. Res. Commun.* 96:574–79

176. Rochette-Egly, C., Tovey, M. G. 1982. Interferon enhances guanylate cyclase activity in human lymphoma cells. *Biochem. Biophys. Res. Commun.* 107:150–56

177. Banerjee, D. K., Baksi, K., Friedman, R. M. 1982. Interferon mediated inhibition of adenylate cyclase in mouse cells. *J. Interferon Res.* 2:501–10

178. Yoshida, R., Hayaishi, O. 1978. Induction of pulmonary indoleamine 2,3, dioxygenase by intraperitoneal injection of bacterial lipopolysaccharide. *Proc. Natl. Acad. Sci. USA* 75:3998–4000

179. Yoshida, R., Imanishi, J., Oku, T., Kishida, T., Hayaishi, O. 1981. Induction of pulmonary indoleamine 2,3, dioxygenase by interferon. *Proc. Natl. Acad. Sci. USA* 78:129–32

180. el Azhary, R., Mannering, G. J. 1979. Effects of interferon inducing agents (polyriboinosinic · polyribocytidylic acid, tilorone) in hepatic hemoproteins (cytochrome P-450, catalase, tryptophan 2,3 dioxygenase, mitochondrial cytochromes), heme metabolism and cytochrome P-450 linked monooxygenase systems. *Mol. Pharmacol.* 15:698–707

181. Renton, K. W., Mannering, G. J. 1976. Depression of hepatic cytochrome P-450 dependent monooxygenase system with administered interferon inducing agents. *Biochem. Biophys. Res. Commun.* 73: 343–48

182. Renton, K. W., Keyler, D. E., Mannering, G. J. 1979. Suppression of the inductive effects of phenobarbital and 3-methylcholanthrene in ascorbic acid synthesis and hepatic cytochrome P-450 linked monooxygenase systems by the interferon inducers, poly rI·rC and tilorone. *Biochem. Biophys. Res. Commun.* 88:1017–23

183. Mannering, G. J., Deloria, L. B., Abbott, V. S. 1981. Evaluation of hepatic mixed function oxidase (MFO) systems after administration of allylisopropylacetamide, CC1₄, CS₂ or polyriboinosinic · polyribocytidylic acid to mice. In *Industrial and Environmental Xenobiotics,* ed. I. Gut, M. Cikrt, G. L. Plaa, pp. 133–146. Berlin: Springer-Verlag

184. Renton, K. W., Mannering, G. J. 1976. Depression of the hepatic cytochrome P-450 monooxygenase system by administered tilorone. *Drug Metab. Dispos.* 4:223–31

185. Nebert, D. W., Friedman, R. M., 1973. Stimulation of aryl hydrocarbon hydroxylase induction in cell cultures by interferon. *J. Virol.* 11:193–97

186. Renton, K. W., Deloria, L. B., Mannering, G. J. 1978. Effect of polyribinosinic acid·polyribocytidylic acid and a mouse interferon preparation in cytochrome P-450 dependent monooxygenase systems in cultures of primary mouse hepatocytes. *Mol. Pharmacol.* 14:672–81

187. Robbins, M. S., Mannering, G. J. 1984. Effects of the interferon inducing agents tilorone and polyriboinosinic acid·polyribocytidylic acid on the hepatic monooxygenase systems of pregnant and fetal rats. *Biochem. Pharmacol.* 33:1213–22

188. Robbins, M. S., Mannering, G. J. 1984. Effects of the interferon inducing agents tilorone and polyriboinosinic acid·polyribocytidylic acid on the hepatic monooxygenase systems of the developing neonatal rat. *Biochem. Pharmacol.* 33:1223–27

189. Chang, E. H., Jay, F. T., Friedman, R. M. 1978. Physical, morphological and biochemical alterations in the membrane of AKR mouse cells after interferon treatment. *Proc. Natl. Acad. Sci. USA* 75:1859–63

190. Lindahl, P., Leary, P., Gresser, I. 1973. Enhancement by interferon of the expression of surface antigen in murine leukemia L1210 cells. *Proc. Natl. Acad. Sci. USA* 70:2785–88

191. Lindahl, P., Gresser, I., Leary, P., Tovey, M. 1976. Enhanced expression of histocompatability antigens of lymphoid cells in mice treated with interferon. *J. Infect. Dis.* 133S:A66–68

192. Kohn, L. D., Friedman, R. M., Holmes, J. M., Lee, G. 1976. Use of thyrotropin and cholera toxin to probe the mechanism by which interferon initiates its antiviral activity. *Proc. Natl. Acad. Sci. USA* 73:3695–99

193. Huet, C., Gresser, I., Bandu, M. T., Lindahl, P. 1974. Increased binding of concanavalin A to interferon-treated murine leukemia L1210 cells. *Proc. Soc. Exp. Biol. Med.* 147:52–57

194. Grollman, E. F., Lee, G., Ramos, S., Lazo, P. S., Kuback, R., et al. 1978. Relationships of the structure and func-

tion of the interferon receptor to hormone receptors and establishment of the antiviral state. *Cancer Res.* 38:4172–85
195. Degre, M., Hovig, T. 1976. Functional and ultrastructural studies on the effects of human interferon in cell membranes of in vitro cultured cells. *Acta Pathol. Microbiol. Scand. Sect. B* 84:347–49
196. Brouty-Boyé, D., Tovey, M. G. 1978. Inhibition by interferon of thymidine uptake in chemostat cultures of L1210 cells. *Intervirology* 9:243–52
197. Fridman, W. H., Gresser, I., Bandu, M. T., Aguet, M., Neauport-Sautes, C. 1980. Interferon enhances the expression of Fc receptors. *J. Immunol.* 124:2436–41
198. Itoh, K., Inoue, M., Kataoka, S., Kumagai, K. 1980. Differential effect of interferon on expression of IgG and IgM Fc γ receptors on human lymphocyte. *J. Immunol.* 124:2589–95
199. Einhorn, S., Blomgren, H., Strander, H., Troye, M. 1981. Enhanced human NK cell activity following treatment with interferon in vitro and in vivo. In *Mediation of Cellular Immunity in Cancer by Immune Modifiers*, ed. M. A. Chirigos, pp. 193–204. New York: Raven
200. Weigent, D. A., Stanton, G. J., Johnson, H. M. 1983. Recombinant gamma interferon enhances natural killer cell activity similar to murine gamma interferon. *Biochem. Biophys. Res. Commun.* 111:525–29
201. Gisler, R. H., Lindahl, P., Gresser, I. 1974. Effects of interferon on antibody synthesis in vitro. *J. Immunol.* 113:438–44
202. Heron, I., Hokland, M., Berg, K. 1978. Enhanced expression of beta-2-microglobulin and HLA antigens on human lymphoid cells by interferon. *Proc. Natl. Acad. Sci. USA* 75:6215–19
203. Fellous, M., Kamoun, M., Gresser, I., Bono, R. 1979. Enhanced expression of HLA antigens and β2-microglobulin on interferon-treated human lymphoid cells. *Eur. J. Immunol.* 9:446–49
204. Nakamura, M., Manser, T., Pearson, G. D. N., Daley, M. J., Gefter, M. L. 1984. Effect of IFN-γ on the immune response in vivo and on gene expression in vitro. *Nature* 307:381–82
205. Vignaux, F., Gresser, I., Fridman, W. H. 1980. Effect of virus induced interferon on the antibody response of suckling and adult mice. *Eur. J. Immunol.* 10:767–72
206. DeMaeyer, E., DeMaeyer-Guignard, J. 1980. Effects of interferon on sensitization and expression of delayed hypersen-

sitivity in the mouse. In *Biochemical Characterization of the Lymphokine*, ed. A. de Weck, K. Kristensen, M. Landy, pp. 383–91. New York: Academic
207. Abreu, S. L. 1982. Suppression of experimental allergic encephalomyelites by interferon. *Immunol. Commun.* 11:1–7
208. Huang, K. Y., Donahue, R. M., Gordon, F. B., Dressler, H. R. 1971. Enhancement of phagocytosis by interferon containing preparations. *Infect. Immun.* 4:581–88
209. Zarling, J. M., Sosmon, J., Eskra, L., Borden, E., Horoszowicz, J. S., Carter, W. A. 1978. Enhancement of T cell cytotoxic responses by purified human fibroblast interferon. *J. Immunol.* 121:2002–4
210. Jett, J. R., Mantovani, A., Herberman, R. B. 1980. Augmentation of human monocyte-mediated cytolysis by interferon. *Cell Immunol.* 54:425–34
211. Koren, H. S., Anderson, S. J., Fischer, D. G., Copeland, C. S., Jensen, P. J. 1980. Regulation of human natural killing. I. The role of monocytes, interferon, and prostaglandins. *J. Immunol.* 127:2007–14
212. Heron, I., Berg, K. 1979. Human leukocyte interferon: analyses of effect on MLC and effector cell generation. *Scand. J. Immunol.* 9:517–26
213. Levy, H. B., Riley, F. L. 1983. A comparison of immune modulating effects of interferon and interferon-inducers. *Lymphokines* 8:303–22
214. Fradelizi, D., Gresser, I. 1982. Interferon inhibits the generation of allospecific suppressor lymphocytes. *J. Exp. Med.* 155:1610–22
215. Adamson, R. H., Fabro, S. 1969. Embryotoxic effect of poly I·poly C. *Nature* 223:718
216. Gresser, I., Aguet, M., Morel-Maroger, L., Woodrow, D., Puvion-Dutilleul, F., et al. 1981. Electrophoretically pure mouse interferon inhibits growth, induces liver and kidney lesions, and kills suckling mice. *Am. J. Pathol.* 102:396–402
217. Gresser, I., Tovey, M. G., Maury, C., Chouroulinkov, L. 1975. Lethality of interferon preparations for newborn mice. *Nature* 258:76–78
218. Gresser, I., Maury, C., Tovey, M., Morel-Maroger, L., Pontillon, F. 1976. Progressive glomerulonephritis in mice treated with interferon preparations at birth. *Nature* 263:420–22
219. Morel-Maroger, L. 1982. Glomerular le-

sions induced by interferon. *Transplant. Proc.* 14:499–505
220. Moss, J., Woodrow, D. F., Sloper, J. C., Riviere, Y., Guillon, J. C., Gresser, I. 1982. Interferon as a cause of endoplasmic reticulum abnormalities within hepatocytes in newborn mice. *Br. J. Exp. Pathol.* 63:43–49
221. Frayssinet, C., Gresser, I., Tovey, M., Lindahl, P. 1973. Inhibitory effect of potent interferon preparations on the regeneration of mouse liver after partial hepatectomy. *Nature* 245:146–47
222. Knost, J. A., Sherwin, S. A., Abraham, P., Oldham, R. 1981. Increased steroid dependence after recombinant leukocyte interferon therapy. *Lancet* 1287–88
223. Morahan, P. S., Regelson, W., Munson, A. E. 1972. Pyran and polynucleotides: differences in biological activities. *Antimicrob. Agents Chemother.* 2:16–22
224. Morahan, P. S., Munson, A. E., Regelson, W., Commerford, S. L., Hamilton, L. D. 1972. Antiviral activity and side effects of polyriboinosinic-cytidylic acid complexes as affected by molecular size. *Proc. Natl. Acad. Sci. USA* 69:482–86
225. Salerno, R. A., Whitmire, C. E., Garcia, I. M., Huebner, R. J. 1972. Chemical carcinogensis in mice inhibited by interferon. *Nature* 239:31–32
226. Yoon, J.-W., Cha, C.-Y., Jordan, G. W. 1983. The role of interferon in virus-induced diabetes. *J. Infect. Dis.* 147:155–59
227. Vialettes, B., Baume, D., Charpin, C., DeMaeyer-Guignard, J., Vague, Ph. 1983. Assessment of viral and immune factors in EMC virus-induced diabetes: effects of cyclosporin A and interferon. *J. Clin. Lab. Immunol.* 10:35–40
228. Dafny, N., Zielinksi, M., Reyes-Vazquez, C. 1983. Alteration of morphine withdrawal to naloxone by interferon. *Neuropeptides* 3:453–63
229. Blalock, J. E., Smith, E. M. 1981. Human leukocyte interferon (HuIFN-α): potent endorphin-like opioid activity. *Biochem. Biophys. Res. Commun.* 101:472–78
230. Dafny, N. 1983. Interferon modifies EEG and EEG-like activity recorded from sensory, motor and limbic system structures in freely behaving rats. *Neurotoxicol.* 4:235–40
231. Paucker, K., Cantell, K., Henle, W. 1962. Quantitative studies on viral interference in suspended L cells. III. Effect of interfering viruses and interferon on the growth rate of cells. *Virology* 17:324–334

232. Gresser, I., Tovey, M. G. 1978. Antitumor effects of interferon. *Biochim. Biophys. Acta* 516:231–47
233. Fleischman, W. R., Kleyn, K. M., Bron, S. 1980. Potentiation of antitumor effect of virus induced interferon by mouse immune interferon. *J. Natl. Cancer Inst.* 65:963–66
234. Gresser, I., Maury, C., Brouty-Boyé, D. 1972. Mechanism of antitumor effect of interferon in mice. *Nature* 239:167–68
235. Balkwill, F. R. 1979. Interferons as cell regulatory molecules. *Cancer Immunol. Immunother.* 7:7–14
236. Lindahl, P., Leary, P., Gresser, I. 1972. Enhancement by interferon of the specific cytotoxicity of sensitized lymphocytes. *Proc. Natl. Acad. Sci. USA* 69:721–25
237. Cohen, S., Bigazzi, P. E. 1980. Lymphokines, cytokines, and interferons. See Ref. 61, pp. 81–95
238. Saksela, E. 1981. Interferon and natural killer cells. See Ref. 45, pp. 45–63
239. DeMaeyer, E. 1984. Interferons and the Immune system. See Ref. 2, pp. 167–85
240. Vilcek, J., DeMaeyer, E., eds. 1984. See Ref. 21, 268 pp.
241. Timonen, T., Ortaldo, J. R., Herberman, R. B. 1982. Characteristics of human large granular lymphocytes and relationship to natural killer and K cells. *J. Exp. Med.* 153:569–82
242. Heron, I., Hokland, M., Berg, K. 1983. 13 native human interferon alpha species assessed for immunoregulatory properties. *J. Interferon Res.* 3:231–39
243. Blomgren, H., Strander, H., Cantell, K. 1974. Effect of human leukocyte interferon on the response of lymphocytes to mitogenic stimuli in vitro. *Scand. J. Immunol.* 3:697–705
244. Schnapper, H. W., Aune, T. M., Pierce, C. W. 1983. Suppressor T cell activation by human leukocyte interferon. *J. Immunol.* 131:2301–6
245. Choi, Y. S., Lim, K. H., Sanders, F. K. 1981. Effect of interferon alpha on pokeweed mitogen-induced differentiation of human peripheral blood B lymphocytes. *Cell Immunol.* 64:20–28
246. Fleischer, T. A., Attallah, A. M., Tosato, G., Blaese, R. M., Greene, W. C. 1982. Interferon-mediated inhibition of polyclonal immunoglobulin synthesis. *J. Immunol.* 129:1099–103
247. Harfast, B., Huddlestone, J. R., Casali, P., Merigan, T. C., Oldstone, M. B. 1981. Interferon acts directly on human B lymphocytes to modulate immuno-

globulin synthesis. *J. Immunol.* 127: 2146–50

248. Rodriguez, M. A., Prinz, W. A., Sibbett, W. L., Bankhurst, A. D., Williams, R. C. 1983. α Interferon increases immunoglobulin production in cultured human mononuclear leukocytes. *J. Immunol.* 130:1215–19

249. Nathan, C. F., Murray, H. W., Wieba, M. E., Rubin, B. Y. 1983. Identification of interferon γ as the lymphokine that activates human macrophage oxidative metabolism and antimicrobial activity. *J. Exp. Med.* 158:670–89

250. Fischer, D. G., Golightly, M. G., Koren, H. S. 1983. Potentiation of the cytolytic activity of peripheral blood monocytes by lymphokines and interferon. *J. Immunol.* 130:1220–25

251. Mannering, G. J., Renton, K. W., el Azhary, R., Deloria, L. B. 1980. Effects of interferon-inducing agents on hepatic cytochrome P-450 drug metabolizing systems. *Ann. N.Y. Acad. Sci.* 350:314–331

252. Renton, K. W. 1981. Effects of interferon inducers and viral infection on the metabolism of drugs. In *Advances in Immunopharmacology*, ed. J. Hadden, L. Chedid, P. Mullen, F. Spreafico, pp. 17–24. New York: Pergamon

253. Renton, K. W. 1983. Relationships between the enzymes of detoxication and host defense mechanisms. In *Biological Basis of Detoxication*, ed. J. Caldwell, W. B. Jacoby, pp. 307–24. New York: Academic

254. Mannering, G. J. 1981. Hepatic cytochrome P-450 linked drug-metabolising systems. In *Concepts in Drug Metabolism*, ed. P. Jenner, B. Testa, pp. 53–166. New York: Dekker

255. Williams, T. C. 1959. *Detoxication Mechanisms.* New York: Wiley. 796 pp. 2nd ed.

256. Deloria, L. B., Mannering, G. J. 1982. Sequential administrations of polyriboinosinic acid and polyribocytidylic acid induce interferon and depress the hepatic cytochrome P-450 dependent monooxygenase system. *Biochem. Biophys. Res. Commun.* 106:947–52

257. Thabrew, M. I., Ioannides, C. 1984. Inhibition of rat hepatic mixed function oxidases by antimalarial drugs: selectivity for cytochrome P-450 and P-448. *Chem. Biol. Interactions* 51:285–294

258. Gorodischer, K., Krasner, J., McDevitt, J. J., Nolan, J. P., Yaffe, S. J. 1976. Hepatic microsomal drug metabolism after administration of endotoxin to rats. *Biochem. Pharmacol.* 25:351–353

259. Barbieri, E. J., Ciaccio, E. L. 1979. Depression of drug metabolism in the mouse by a combination of mycobacterium and anesthetics. *Br. J. Pharmacol.* 65:111–15

260. Abernathy, C. O., Zimmerman, H. J., Utili, R. 1980. Effects of endotoxin-tolerance on in vivo drug metabolism in mice. *Res. Commun. Chem. Pathol. Pharmacol.* 29:193–96

261. Williams, J. F., Lowitt, S., Szentivanyi, A. 1980. Endotoxin depression of hepatic mixed function oxidase system in C3H/HeJ and C3H/HeN mice. *Immunopharmacol.* 2:285–91

262. Falzon, M., Milton, A. S., Burke, M. D. 1984. Are decreases in hepatic cytochrome P-450 and other drug-metabolising enzymes caused by indomethacin in vivo mediated by intestinal bacterial endotoxins? *Biochem. Pharmacol.* 33:1285–92

263. Barnes, D. W., Morahan, P. S., Loveless, S., Munson, A. E. 1979. The effects of maleic anhydride-divinyl ether (MVE) copolymers on hepatic microsomal mixed-function oxidases and other biological activities. *J. Pharmacol. Exp. Ther.* 208:392–98

264. Morton, D. M., Chatfield, D. H. 1970. The effect of adjuvant-induced arthritis on the liver metabolism of drugs in rats. *Biochem. Pharmacol.* 19:473–81

265. Dipasquale, G., Welaj, P., Rassaert, C. L. 1974. Prolonged pentobarbital sleeping time in adjuvant-induced polyarthritic rats. *Res. Commun. Chem. Pathol. Pharmacol.* 9:253–64

266. Carlson, R. P., Ciaccio, E. L. 1975. Effect of benzo(a)pyrene induction of liver and lung metabolism in adjuvant-diseased rats. *Biochem. Pharmacol.* 24:1893–95

267. Cawthorne, M. A., Palmer, E. D., Green, J. 1976. Adjuvant-induced arthritis and drug-metabolising enzymes. *Biochem. Pharmacol.* 25:2683–88

268. Soyka, L. F., Hunt, W. G., Knight, S. E., Foster, R. S. 1976. Decreased liver and lung drug-metabolising activity in mice treated with Corynebacterium Parvum. *Cancer Res.* 36:4425–28

269. Farquhar, D., Benvenuto, J. A., Kuttesch, N., Loo, T. L. 1983. Inhibition of hepatic drug metabolism in the rat after Corynebacterium Parvum treatment. *Biochem. Pharmacol.* 32:1275–80

270. Farquhar, D., Loo, T. L., Gutterman, J. U., Hersh, E. M., Luna, M. A. 1976. Inhibition of drug-metabolising enzymes in the rat after Bacillus Calmette-Guerin

treatment. *Biochem. Pharmacol.* 25: 1529–35

271. Sonnenfeld, G., Harned, C. L., Thaniyavarn, S., Huff, T., Mandel, A. D., Nerland, D. E. 1980. Type II Interferon induction and passive transfer depress the murine cytochrome P-450 drug metabolism system. *Antimicrob. Agents Chemother.* 17:969–72

272. Ruzicka, T., Goerz, G., Vizethum, W., Kratka, J. 1980. Effects of intravenous and intracutaneous Bacillus Calmette-Guerin application on the drug metabolising system of the liver. *Dermatol.* 160: 135–41

273. Williams, J. F., Szentivanyi, A. 1977. Depression of hepatic drug metabolising enzyme activity by B. Pertussis vaccination. *Eur. J. Pharmacol.* 43:281–84

274. Renton, K. W. 1979. The deleterious effect of Bordetella Pertussis vaccine and poly (rI·rC) on the metabolism and disposition of phenytoin. *J. Pharmacol. Exp. Ther.* 208:267–70

275. Hojo, H., Hashimoto, Y. 1977. Inhibition of drug-metabolising enzymes in the mouse after treatment with host-mediating anti-tumor drugs. *Toxicol. Lett.* 1:89–93

276. Egawa, K., Kasai, N. 1979. Endotoxic glycolipid as a potent depressor of the hepatic drug-metabolising enzyme system in mice. *Microbiol. Immunol.* 23: 87–94

277. Iwasaki, K., Noguchi, H. 1982. Effect of hepatic microsomal mixed function oxidase activities in rats pretreated with Nocardia rubra cell wall skeleton. *Res. Commun. Chem. Pathol. Pharmacol.* 37:267–277

278. Williams, J. F., Szentivanyi, A. 1983. Continued studies on the effect of interferon inducers in the hepatic microsomal mixed-function oxidase system of rats and mice. *J. Interferon Res.* 3:211–17

279. Trescec, A., Iskric, S., Hrsak, I., Tomasic, J. 1983. Effect of immunoadjuvant peptidoglycan monomer on liver cytochrome P-450. *Biochem. Pharmacol.* 32:2354–57

280. Wooles, W. R., Munson, A. E. 1971. The effect of stimulants and depressants of reticuloendothelial activity on drug metabolism. *J. Reticuloendothel. Soc.* 9:108–19

281. Peterson, T. C., Renton, K. W. 1984. Depression of cytochrome P-450 dependent drug biotransformation in hepatocytes after activation of the reticuloendothial system by dextran sulfate.

J. Pharmacol. Exp. Ther. 229:299–304

282. Stenger, R. J., Petrelli, M., Segel, A., Williamson, J. N., Johnson, E. A. 1969. Modification of carbon tetrachloride hepatotoxicity by prior loading of the reticulendothelial system with carbon particles. *Am. J. Pathol.* 57:689–706

283. Leterrier, F., Reynier, M., Mariaud, J.-F. 1973. Effect of intracellular accumulation of inert carbon particles on the cytochromes P-450 and b5 levels of rat liver microsomes. *Biochem. Pharmacol.* 22:2206–8

284. Cha, Y.-N., Edwards, R. 1976. Effect of Schistosoma Mansoni infection on the hepatic drug-metabolising capacity of mice. *J. Pharmacol. Exp. Therap.* 199: 432–40

285. Cha, Y.-N., Byram, J. E., Heine, H. S., Bueding, E. 1980. Effect of Schistosoma Mansoni infection on hepatic drug-metabolising capacity of athymic nude mice. *Am. J. Trop. Med. Hyg.* 29:234–38

286. Shertzer, H. G., Hall, J. E., Seed, J. R. 1981. Hepatic mixed-function oxidase activity in mice infected with Trypanosoma Brucei Gambiense or treated with trypanocides. *Mol. Biochem. Parasitol.* 3: 199–204

287. McCarthy, J. S., Furner, R. L., VanDyke, K., Stitzel, R. E. 1970. Effects of malarial infection on host microsomal drug-metabolizing enzymes. *Biochem. Pharmacol.* 19:1341–49

288. Facino, R. M., Carini, M., Bertulelli, R., Genchi, C., Malchiodi, A. 1981. Decrease of the in vitro drug metabolizing activity of the hepatic mixed function-oxidase systems in rats infected experimentally with Fasciola Hepatica. *Pharmacol. Res. Commun.* 13:731–42

289. Kato, R., Nakamura, Y., Chiesara, E. 1963. Enhanced phenobarbital induction of liver microsomal drug-metabolizing enzymes in mice infected with murine hepatitis virus. *Biochem. Pharmacol.* 12:365–70

290. Budillon, G., Carrella, M., Coltorti, M. 1972. Phenobarbital liver microsomal induction in MHV-3 viral hepatitis of the mouse. *Experientia* 28:1011–12

291. Renton, K. W. 1981. The depression of hepatic cytochrome P-450-dependent mixed function oxidase during infection with EMC virus. *Biochem. Pharmacol.* 16:2333–36

292. Singh, G., Renton, K. W. 1981. Interferon-mediated depression of cytochrome P-450-dependent drug biotrans-

formation. *Mol. Pharmacol.* 20:681–84
293. Ragland, W. L., Friend, M., Trainer, D. O., Sladek, N. E. 1971. Interaction between duck hepatitis viruses and DDT in ducks. *Res. Commun. Chem. Pathol. Pharmacol.* 2:236–44
294. Corbett, T. H., Nettesheim, P. 1973. Effect of PR-8 viral respiratory infection on benzo[a]pyrene hydroxylase activity in BALB/c mice. *J. Natl. Cancer Inst.* 50:779–82
295. Moore, R. N., Berry, L. J., Garry, R. F., Waite, M. R. F. 1978. Effect of Sindbis virus infection on hydrocortisone-induced hepatic enzymes in mice. *Proc. Soc. Exp. Biol. Med.* 157:125–28
296. Harned, C. L., Nerland, D. E., Sonnenfeld, G. 1982. Effects of passive transfer and induction of gamma (type II immune) interferon preparations in the metabolism of diphenylhydantoin by murine cytochrome P-450. *J. Interferon Res.* 2:5–10
297. Singh, G., Renton, K. W., Stebbing, N. 1982. Homogeneous interferon from *E. coli* depresses hepatic cytochrome P-450 and drug biotransformation. *Biochem. Biophys. Res. Commun.* 106:1256–61
298. Renton, K. W., Singh, K., Stebbing, N. 1984. Relationship between the antiviral effects of interferons and their abilities to depress cytochrome P-450. *Biochem. Pharmacol.* 33:3899–902
299. Balkwill, F. R., Mowshowitz, S., Seilman, S. S., Moodie, E. M., Griffin, D. B., et al. 1984. Positive interactions between interferon and chemotherapy due to direct tumor action rather than effects on host drug-metabolizing enzymes. *Cancer Res.* 44:5249–55
300. Franklin, M. R., Finkle, B. S. 1985. Effect of murine gamma-interferon on the mouse liver and its drug-metabolizing enzymes: Comparison with human hybrid alpha-interferon. *J. Interferon Res.* 5:265–72
301. Sharpe, T. J., Birch, P. J., Planterose, D. N. 1971. Resistance to virus infection during the hyporeactive state of interferon induction. *J. Gen. Virol.* 12:331–33
302. Samaras, S. C., Dietz, N. 1953. Physiopathology of detoxification of pentobarbital sodium. *Fed. Proc.* 12:122
303. Leeson, G. A., Biedenbach, S. A., Chan, K. Y., Gibson, J. P., Wright, G. J. 1976. Decrease in activity of the drug metabolizing enzymes of rat liver following the administration of tilorone HCl. *Drug Metab. Dispos.* 4:232–38
304. Campbell, J. B., White, S. L., 1976. A comparison of the prophylactic and

therapeutic effects of poly I·C and endotoxin in mice infected with Mengo virus. *Can. J. Microbiol.* 22:1595–1602
305. DeClercq, E., Merigan, T. C. 1971. Bis-DEAE-fluorenone: mechanism of antiviral protection and stimulation of interferon production in the mouse. *J. Infect. Dis.* 123:190–99
306. Kirchner, H., Scott, M. T., Hirt, H. M., Munk, K. 1978. Protection of mice against viral infection by Corynebacterium Parvum and Bordetella Pertussis. *J. Gen. Virol.* 41:97–104
307. DeClercq, E., DeSomer, P. 1971. Antiviral activity of polyribocytidylic acid in cells primed with polyriboinosinic acid. *Science* 173:260–62
308. DeMaeyer, E., DeMaeyer-Guignard, J. 1979. Considerations on mouse genes influencing interferon production and action. See Ref. 23, pp. 75–100
309. Mannering, G. J., Deloria, L. B., Kuwahara, S. K. 1983. Depression of allylisopropylacetamide induced hepatic ethylmorphine N-demethylase activity in mice by polyriboinosinic acid·polyribocytidylic acid and recombinant hydrid human leukocyte interferon. *Pharmacologist* 25:265
310. Barnes, D. W., Moy, L., Russ, R. 1985. Electrophoretic patterns of murine hepatic microsomal proteins after treatment with the immunomodulator MVE copolymer. *Pharmacologist* 27:201
311. el Azhary, R., Renton, K. W., Mannering, G. J. 1980. Effect of interferon inducing agents (polyriboinosinic acid·polyribocytidylic acid and tilorone) on the heme turnover of hepatic cytochrome P-450. *Mol. Pharmacol.* 17:395–99
312. Paine, A. J. 1978. Excited states of oxygen in biology: their possible involvement in cytochrome P-450 linked oxidation as well as in the induction of the P-450 by many diverse compounds. *Biochem. Pharmacol.* 27:1805–13
313. Schacter, B. A., Kurtz, P. 1982. Alterations in hepatic and splenic microsomal components, drug metabolism, heme-oxygenase activity, and cytochrome P-450 turnover in Murphy-Sturm Lymphosarcoma rats. *Cancer Res.* 42:3557–64
314. Nakahara, W. 1967. Toxohormone. In *Methods in Cancer Research*, Vol. II, ed. H. Busch, pp. 203–37. New York: Academic
315. Kato, R., Yamazoe, Y., Mita, S., Kamataki, T., Kubota, T., et al. 1982. Decrease in the activity of hepatic microsomal drug-metabolizing enzymes in

tumor-bearing nude mice. *Gann* 73:907–11

316. Sladek, N. E., Domeyer, B. E., Merriman, R. L., Brophy, G. T. 1978. Differential effects of Walker 256 carcinosarcoma cells growing subcutaneously, intramuscularly or intraperitoneally on hepatic microsomal mixed-function oxygenase activity. *Drug Metab. Dispos.* 6:412–17

317. Chang, K. C., Lauer, B. D., Bell, T. D., Chai, H. 1978. Altered theophylline pharmacokinetics during acute respiratory viral illness. *Lancet* 1132–33

318. Kraemer, M. J., Furukawa, C. T., Koup, J. R., Shapiro, G. G., Pierson, W. E., Fierman, C. W. 1982. Altered theophylline clearance during an influenza B outbreak. *Pediatrics* 69:476–80

319. Walker, S. B., Middelkamp, J. N. 1982. Theophylline toxicity and viral infections. *Pediatrics* 7:508–9

320. Renton, K. W., Gray, J. D., Hall, R. J. 1980. Decreased elimination of theophylline after influenza vaccination. *CMA Journal* 123:288–90

321. Kramer, P., McClain, C. J. 1981. Depression of aminopyrine metabolism by influenza vaccination. *N. Engl. J. Med.* 305:1262–64

322. Patriarca, P. A., Kendal, A. P., Stricof, R. L., Weber, J. A., Meissner, M. K., Dateno, B. 1983. Influenza vaccination and warfarin or theophylline toxicity in nursing-home residents. *N. Engl. J. Med.* 308:1601–2

323. Crooks, J., O'Malley, K., Stevenson, I. 1976. Pharmacokinetics in the elderly. *Clin. Pharmacokinet.* 1:280–96

324. Triggs, E. 1975. Pharmacokinetics in the aged: A review. *J. Pharmacokinet. Biopharm.* 3:387–418

325. Schmucker, D. 1979. Age-related changes in drug disposition. *Pharmacol. Rev.* 30:445–56

326. Miller, E. C., Miller, J. A. 1981. Mechanisms of chemical carcinogenesis. *Cancer* 47:1055–64

327. Kishida, T., Toda, S., Toida, A., Hattori, T. 1971. Effect de l'interferon sur le cellule maligne de la souris. *C. R. Soc. Biol.* 165:1489–92

328. Merigan, T. C. 1981. Chemotherapy for viral diseases. In *Perspectives in Virology* XI, ed. M. Pollard, pp. 249–66. New York: Alan Liss

329. Yabrov, A. A. 1982. Interferon: Anticancer agent having multifarious activity. In *Progress in Clinical Cancer*, Vol. 8, ed. I. M. Ariel, pp. 99–145. New York: Grune & Stratton

330. Borden, E. C. 1983. Interferons and cancer: How the promise is being kept. See Ref. 74, pp. 45–83

331. Strander, H. 1983. Interferons and disease: A survey. In *Interferons: from molecular biology to clinical application*, ed. D. C. Burke, A. G. Morris, pp. 7–33. London: Cambridge Univ. Press

332. Scott, G. M. 1983. The antiviral effects of interferon. See Ref. 331, pp. 277–311

333. Came, P. E., Carter, W. A. 1984. Interferon: Its application and future as an antineoplastic agent. See Ref. 41, pp. 301–19

334. Kisner, D. L., Smyth, J. F. 1984. *Interferon alpha-2: Pre-Clinical and Clinical Evaluation.* Boston: Nijhoff. 111 pp.

335. Oldham, R. K. 1985. Interferon: a model for future biologicals. In *Interferon*, 6, ed. I. Gresser, pp. 127–143. New York: Academic

336. Stewart, W. E. II, Lin, L. S. 1979. Antiviral activities of interferons. *Pharmacol. Ther.* 6:443–512

337. Levin, S., Hahn, T., Rosenberg, H., Bino, T. 1982. Treatment of life-threatening viral infections with interferon α: pharmacokinetic studies in a clinical trial. *Isr. J. Med. Sci.* 18:440–46

338. Billiau, A., Edy, V. G., DeSomer, P. 1979. The clinical use of fibroblast interferon. In *Antiviral Mechanisms in the Control of Neoplasia*, ed. P. Chandra, pp. 675–96. New York: Plenum

339. Billiau, A., DeSomer, P. 1980. Clinical use of interferons in viral infections. See Ref. 27, pp. 113–144

340. Kingham, J. G. C., Ganguly, N. K., Shaari, Z. D., Mendelson, R., McGuire, M. J., et al. 1978. Treatment of HBs Ag-positive chronic active hepatitis with human fibroblast interferon. *Gut* 19:91–94

341. Merigan, T. C., Robinson, W. S., Gregory, P. B. 1980. Interferon in chronic hepatitis B infection. *Lancet*, pp. 422–23

342. Pazin, G. J., Armstrong, J. A., Lam, M. T., Tarr, G. G., Jannetta, P. J., Ho, M. 1979. Prevention of reactivated herpes simplex infection by human leukocyte interferon. *N. Eng. J. Med.* 301:225–29

343. Merigan, T. C., Gallagher, J. G., Pollard, R. B., Arvin, A. M. 1981. Short-course human leukocyte interferon in treatment of herpes zoster in patients with cancer. *Antimicrob. Agents Chemother.* 19:193–95

344. Merigan, T. C., Rand, K. H., Pollard, R. B., Abdallah, P. S., Jordan, G. W., Fried, R. P. 1978. Human leukocyte interferon for the treatment of herpes zoster in patients with cancer. *N. Eng. J. Med.* 298:981–87

345. Sundmacher, R., Newmann-Haefelin, D., Cantell, K. 1981. The clinical value of interferon in ocular viral diseases. In *Interferon: Properties, Mode of Action, Production, Clinical Application,* ed. K. Munk, H. Kirchner, pp. 191–96, Basil: Karger

346. Sundmacher, R. 1982. Interferon in ocular viral diseases. See Ref. 81, pp. 177–200

347. Pazin, G. J., Ho, M., Haverkos, H. W., Armstrong, J. A., Breining, M. C., et al. 1982. Effect of interferon-alpha on human warts. *J. Interferon Res.* 2:235–43

348. Gobel, U., Arnold, W., Wahn, V., Treuner, J., Jurgens, H., Cantell, K. 1981. Comparison of human fibroblast and leukocyte interferon in the treatment of severe laryngeal papillomatoses in children. *Eur. J. Pediatr.* 137:175–76

349. Cheeseman, S. H., Rubin, R., Stewart, J. A., Talkoff-Rubin, N. E., Cosimi, A., et al. 1979. Controlled clinical trial of prophylactic human leukocyte interferon in renal transplantation. *N. Eng. J. Med.* 300:1345–49

350. Cheeseman, S. H., Henle, W., Rubin, R., Talkoff-Rubin, N. E., Cosimi, B., Cantell, K., et al. 1980. Epstein barr virus infection in renal transplant recipients. *Ann. Intern. Med.* 93:39–42

351. Weimar, W., Schellekens, H., Lameijer, L. D., Masurol, N., Edy, V. G. 1978. Double-blind study of interferon administration in renal transplant recipients. *Eur. J. Clin. Invest.* 8:255–58

352. Arvin, A. M., Martin, D. P., Gard, E., Merigan, T. C., Feldman, S., et al. 1982. Alpha-interferon in simian and human varicella. See Ref. 24, pp. 393–97

353. Nakamura, O., Takakura, K., Kobayaski, S. 1982. Effect of human interferon β in the treatment of malignant brain tumors. See Ref. 24, pp. 465–477

354. Sherwin, S. A., Knost, J. A., Fein, S., Abrams, P. G., Foon, K. A. et al. 1982. A multiple-dose phase I trial of recombinant leukocyte A interferon in cancer patients. *J. Am. Med. Assoc.* 248:2461–66

355. Borden, E. C., Holland, J. F., Dao, T. L., Gutterman, J. U., Weiner, L., et al. 1982. Leukocyte-derived interferon (alpha) in human breast carcinoma. *Ann. Intern. Med.* 97:1–6

356. Gutterman, J. U., Blumenschein, G. R., Alexanian, R., Yap, H. Y., Buzdar, A. U., et al. 1980. Leukocyte interferon-induced tumor regression in human metastatic breast cancer, multiple myeloma, and malignant lymphoma. *Ann. Intern. Med.* 93:399–406

357. Silver, H. K. B., Connors, S., Salinas, F., Spinelli, J. 1983. Treatment response in a prospectively randomized study of high vs low dose treatment with lymphoblastoid interferon. *Proc. Am. Soc. Clin. Oncol.* 2:51

358. Hawkins, M. J., Krown, S. E., Borden, E. C., Krim, M., Real, F. X., et al. 1984. American Cancer Society Phase 1 trial of naturally produced β-interferon. *Cancer Res.* 44:5934–38

359. Gutterman, J. U., Quesada, J. 1982. Clinical investigation of partially pure and recombinant DNA derived leukocyte interferon in human cancer. *Tex. Rep. Biol. Med.* 41:626–33

360. Ikic, D., Maricic, Z., Oresic, V., Rode, B., Nola, P., et al. 1981. Application of human leukocyte interferon in patients with urinary bladder papillomatosis, breast cancer and melanoma. *Lancet* 1022–1024

361. Ikic, D., Kirkmajer, V., Maricic, Z., Jusic, D., Krusic, J., et al. 1981. Application of human leukocyte interferon in patients with carcinoma of the uterine cervix. *Lancet,* pp. 1027–30

362. Choo, Y. C., Hsu, C., Seto, C., W. H., Miller, D. G., Merigan, T. C., Ng, M. H., Ma, H. F. 1985. Intravaginal application of leukocyte interferon gel in the treatment of cervical intraepithelial neoplasia. *Arch. Gynecol.* 237:51–54

363. Figlin, R. A., Callaghan, M., Sarna, G. 1983. Phase II trial of α (human leukocyte) interferon administered daily in adenocarcinoma of the colon/rectum. *Cancer Treat. Rep.* 67:493–94

364. Neefe, J., Smith, F., Fein, S., Ayoob, M., Schein, P. 1983. A phase II trial of genetically engineered clone A alpha interferon in previously untreated advanced colon cancer. *Proc. Am. Soc. Clin. Oncol.* 2:52

365. Chaplinsky, T., Laszlo, J., Moore, J., Schneider, W. 1983. Phase II trial of interferon in metastatic colon carcinoma. *Proc. Am. Soc. Clin. Oncol.* 2:130

366. Kirkwood, J. M., Ernstoff, M. S., Davis, C. A., Reiss, M., Ferraresi, R., Rudnick, S. A. 1985. Comparison of intramuscular and intravenous recombinant alpha-2 interferon in melanoma and other cancers. *Ann. Intern. Med.* 103:32–36

367. Gutterman, J. U., Fine, S., Quesada, J., Horning, S. J., Levine, J. F., et al. 1982. Recombinant leukocyte α interferon: pharmacokinetics, single-dose tolerance, and biologic effects in cancer patients. *Ann. Intern. Med.* 96:549–56

368. Obert, H.-J. 1982. Clinical trials and

pilot studies with beta-interferon in Germany. See Ref. 24, pp. 427–32

369. Talpaz, M., McCredie, K. B., Keating, M. J., Gutterman, J. U. 1983. Clinical investigations of leukocyte interferon (huIFN-α) in chronic myelogenous leukemia. *Blood* 62:209a

370. Quesada, J. R., Hersh, P. M., Gutterman, J. U. 1984. Treatment of hairy cell leukemia with alpha interferon. *Am. Soc. Clin. Oncol.* 3:207

371. Thompson, J. A., Brady, J., Kidd, P., Fefer, A. 1985. Recombinant alpha-2 interferon in the treatment of hairy cell leukemia. *Cancer Treat. Rep.* 69:791–93

372. Krown, S. E., Real, F. X., Cunningham-Rundles, S., Myskowski, P., Koziner, B. 1983. Preliminary observations on the effect of recombinant leukocyte A interferon in homosexual men with Kaposi's sarcoma. *N. Eng. J. Med.* 308:1071–76

373. Volberding, P., Moran, T., Abrams, D., Rothman, J., Valero, R. 1983. Recombinant alpha interferon therapy of Kaposi's sarcoma in acquired immunodeficiency syndrome. *Blood* 62:118a

374. Nair, P. V., Tong, M. J., Kempf, R., Co, R., Lee, S.-D., Venturi, C. L. 1985. Clinical, serologic and immunologic effects of human leukocyte interferon in HBsAg-positive primary hepatocellular carcinoma. *Cancer* 56:1018–22

375. Sachs, E., DiBisceglie, A. M., Dusheiko, G. M., Lyons, S. F., et al. 1985. Treatment of hepatocellular carcinoma with recombinant leukocyte interferons: A pilot study. *Br. J. Cancer* 52:105–9

376. Sarna, G., Figlin, R., Callaghan, M. 1983. α Human leukocyte interferon as treatment for non-small cell carcinoma of the lung: a phase II trial. *J. Biol. Resp. Modif.* 2:343–47

377. Foon, K. A., Sherwin, S. A., Abrams, P. G., Longo, D. L., Fer, M. F., et al. 1984. Treatment of advanced non-Hodgkin's lymphoma with recombinant leukocyte A interferon. *N. Eng. J. Med.* 311:1148–52

378. Huhn, D., Fink, U., Themi, H., Siegert, W., Reithmuller, G., Wilmanns, W. 1982. Interferon in non-Hodgkin's lymphoma of low malignancy. See Ref. 345, pp. 217–23

379. Horning, S. J., Merigan, T. C., Krown, S. E., Gutterman, J. U., Louie, A., Gallagher, J., et al. 1985. Human interferon alpha in malignant lymphoma and Hodgkin's disease. *Cancer* 56:1305–10

380. Retsas, S., Priestman, T. J., Newton, K. A., Westbury, G. 1983. Evaluation of human lymphoblastoid interferon in advanced malignant melanoma. *Cancer* 51:273–76

381. Cregan, E. T., Ahmann, D. L., Green, S. J., Schutt, A. J., Rubin, H. J., et al. 1983. Recombinant leukocyte A interferon in disseminated malignant melanoma (DMM). *Proc. Am. Soc. Clin. Oncol.* 2:58

382. Krown, S. E., Einzig, A. L., Abramson, J. D., Oettgen, H. F. 1983. Treatment of advanced renal cell cancer with recombinant leukocyte A interferon. *Proc. Am. Soc. Clin. Oncol.* 2:58

383. Ernstoff, M. S., Reiss, M., Davis, C. A., Rudneck, S. A., Kirkwood, J. M. 1983. Intravenous recombinant alpha-2 interferon in metastatic melanoma. *Proc. Am. Soc. Clin. Oncol.* 2:57

384. Goldberg, R. M., Ayoob, M., Silgals, R., Ahlgren, J. D., Neefe, J. R. 1985. Phase II trial of lymphoblastoid interferon in metastatic malignant melanoma. *Cancer Treat. Rep.* 69:813–16

385. Borgstrom, S., vonEyben, C. E., Flodgren, P., Axelson, B., Sjogren, H. O. 1982. Human leukocyte interferon and cimentidine for metastatic melanoma. *N. Eng. J. Med.* 307:1080–81

386. Osserman, E. T., Sherman, W. F., Alexanian, R., Gutterman, J. U., Humphrey, R. L. 1980. Preliminary results of the American Cancer Society sponsored trial of human leukocyte interferon in multiple melanoma. *Proc. Am. Assoc. Cancer Res.* 21:161

387. DeSomer, P. 1982. Perspectives for clinical use of fibroblast interferon. See Ref. 345, pp. 177–84

388. Merigan, T. C., Sikora, K., Breeden, J. H., Levy, R., Rosenberg, S. A. 1978. Preliminary observation on the effect of human leukocyte interferon as non-Hodgkin's lymphoma. *N. Eng. J. Med.* 299:1449–53

389. Strander, H. 1982. Antitumor effects of interferon and its possible use as an antineoplastic agent. *Tex. Rep. Biol. Med.* 41:621–24

390. Freedman, R. S., Gutterman, J. U., Wharton, J. T., Rutledge, F. N. 1983. Leukocyte interferon in patients with epithelial ovarian carcinoma. *J. Biol. Resp. Modif.* 2:133–38

391. Silver, H. K. B., Connors, J., Salinas, F., Spinelli, J. 1983. Treatment response in a prospectively randomized study of high vs. low dose treatment with lymphoblastoid interferon. *Proc. Am. Soc. Clin. Oncol.* 2:51

392. Rambaldi, A., Introna, M., Colotta, F., Landolfo, S., Colombo, N., Mangioni,

C., Mantovani, A. 1985. Intraperitoneal administration of interferon β in ovarian cancer patients. *Cancer* 56: 294–301

393. Berek, J. S., Hacker, N. F., Lichtenstein, A., Jung. T., Spina, C., et al. 1985. Intraperitoneal recombinant α interferon for salvage immunotherapy in stage III epithelal ovarian cancer: A gynecologic oncology group study. *Cancer Res.* 45:4447–53

394. Abdulhay, G., DiSaia, P. J., Blessing, J. A., Creasman, W. T. 1985. Human lymphoblastoid interferon in the treatment of advanced epithelial ovarian malignancies. A gynecologic oncology group study. *Am. J. Obstet. Gynecol.* 152:418–23

395. Quesada, J. R., Hersh, E. M., Gutterman, J. U. 1983. Hairy cell leukemia: induction of remission with alpha interferon. *Blood* 62:207a

396. Quesada, J. R., Gutterman, J. U., Rios, A. 1983. Investigational therapy of renal cell carcinoma with recombinant alpha interferon. *Proc. Am. Assoc. Cancer Res.* 24:195

397. Quesada, J. R., Swanson, D. A., Trendade, A., Gutterman, J. U. 1983. Renal cell carcinoma: Antitumor effects of leukocyte interferon. *Cancer Res.* 43: 940–47

398. Kirkwood, J. M., Ernstoff, M. S. 1984. Interferon in the treatment of cancer. *J. Clin. Oncol.* 2:336–52

399. Vugrin, D., Hood, L., Taylor, W., Laszlo, J. 1985. Phase II study of human lymphoblastoid interferon in patients with advanced renal carcinoma. *Cancer Treat. Rep.* 69:817–20

400. Hilfenhaus, J., Weinmann, E., Majer, M., Barth, R., Jaeger, O. 1977. Administration of human interferon to rabies virus-infected monkeys after exposure. *J. Infect. Dis.* 135:846–49

401. Weinmann, E., Mayer, M., Hilfenhaus, J. 1979. Intramuscular and/or intralumbar postexposure treatment of rabies virus-infected cynomologus monkeys with human interferon. *Infect. Immun.* 24:24–31

402. Moreno, J. A., Baughcum, S. D., Levy, H. B., Baer, G. M. 1979. Further studies on rabies post exposure prophylaxis in mice: a comparison of vaccine with interferon and vaccine. *J. Gen. Virol.* 42: 219–22

403. Strander, H. 1975. *Report of the international workshop in interferon in the treatment of cancer.* New York: Sloan-Kettering Institute for Cancer Research. 39 pp.

404. Ikic, D., Brodarec, L., Padovan, I.,

Knezevic, M., Soos, E. 1981. Application of human leukocyte interferon in patients with tumors of the head & neck. *Lancet* 1025–27

405. Gresser, I. 1983. The antitumor effects of interferon in mice. See Ref. 68, pp. 65–76

406. Scullard, G. H., Andres, L. L., Greenberg, H. B., Smith, J. S., Sawhney, V. K., et al. 1981. Antiviral treatment of chronic hepatitis B virus infection: improvement in liver disease with interferon and adenine arabinoside. *Hepatology* 1:228–32

407. Scullard, R. H., Pollard, R. B., Smith, J. L., Sacks, S. L., Gregory, P. B., et al. 1981. Antiviral treatment of chronic hepatitis B virus infection: 1. Changes in viral markers with interferon combined with adenine arabinoside. *J. Infect. Dis.* 143:772–83

408. Flodgren, P., Borgstrom, S., Jonsson, P. E., Lindstrom, C., Sjogren, H. O. 1983. Metastatic malignant melanoma: regression induced by combined treatment with interferon and cimetidine. *Int. J. Cancer* 32:657–65

409. Ankerst, J., Faldt, R., Nilsson, P. G., Flodgren, P., Sjogren, H. O. 1984. Complete remission in a patient with acute myelogenous leukemia treated with leukocyte α interferon and cimentidine. *Cancer Immunol. Immunother.* 17:69–71

410. Welander, C. E., Morgan, T. M., Homesley, H. D., Trotta, P. P., Spiegel, R. J. 1985. Combined recombinant human interferon alpha 2 and cytotoxic agents studied in a clonogenic assay. *Int. J. Cancer* 35:721–29

411. Chany, C. 1961. An interferon-like inhibitor of viral multiplication from malignant cells (the viral autoinhibition phenomenon). *Virology* 13:485–92

412. Chany, C., Robbe-Maredor, F. 1969. Enhancing effect of the murine sarcoma virus in the replication of the mouse hepatitis virus in vitro. *Proc. Soc. Exp. Biol. Med.* 131:30–35

413. Bourgeade, M. F., Cerutte, C., Chany, C. 1979. Enhancement of interferon antitumor action by sodium butyrate. *Cancer Res.* 39:4720–23

414. Sherwin, S. A., Foon, K. A., Abrams, P. G., Heyman, M., Ochs, J. J., et al. 1984. A preliminary phase I trial of partially purified interferon-gamma in patients with cancer. *J. Biol. Resp. Modif.* 3:599–607

415. Borecky, L., Lackovic, V., eds. 1984. *Physiology and Pathology of Interferon System.* Basel: Karger. 386 pp.

416. Scott, G. M., Secher, D. S., Flowers, D., Boti, J., Cantell, K., Tyrrell, D. A.

J. 1981. Toxicity of interferon. *Br. Med. J.* 282:1345–48

417. Gresser, I. 1982. Can interferon induce disease? See Ref. 346, pp. 95–127
418. Smedley, H. M., Wheeler, T. 1983. Toxicity of interferon. See Ref. 14, pp. 203–10
419. Gresser, I. 1983. Interferon-induced disease. In *The Biology of the Interferon System*, ed. E. DeMaeyer, H. Schellekens, pp. 363–68. New York: Elsevier
420. Vilcek, J. 1984. Adverse effects of interferon in virus infections, autoimmune disease, and acquired immune deficiency. *Prog. Med. Virol.* 30:62–77
421. Foon, K. A., Dougher, G. 1984. Increased growth of eyelashes in a patient given leukocyte A interferon. *N. Eng. J. Med.* 311:1259
422. Smedley, H., Katrah, M., Sikora, K., Wheeler, T. 1983. Neurological effects of recombinant human interferon. *Br. Med. J.* 286:262–64
423. Adams, F., Quesada, J. R., Gutterman, J. U. 1984. Neuropsychiatric manifestations of human leukocyte interferon therapy in patients with cancer. *J. Am. Med. Assoc.* 252:938–41
424. Rohatiner, A. Z. S., Prior, P. F., Burton, A. C., Smith, A. T., Balkwill, F. R., Lister, T. A. 1983. Central nervous system toxicity of interferon. *Br. J. Cancer* 47:419–22
425. Smith, E. M., Blalock, J. E. 1981. Human lymphocyte production of cortico-

tropin and endorphin-like substances: association with leukocyte interferon. *Proc. Natl. Acad. Sci.* 78:7530–34
426. Blalock, J. E., Smith, E. M. 1981. Structure and function relationship of interferon and neuroendocrine hormones. See Ref. 419, pp. 93–99
427. Blalock, J. E. 1984. Relationships between neuroendocrine hormones and lymphokines. *Lymphokines* 9:1–13
428. Chang, K.-W. 1984. Opioid peptides have actions on the immune system *Trend Neurosci.* 7:234–35
429. Blalock, J. E., Smith, E. M. 1985. A complete regulatory loop between the immune and neuroendocrine systems. *Fed. Proc.* 45:108–11
430. Wybran, J. 1985. Enkephalins and endorphins as modifiers of the immune system: present and future. *Fed. Proc.* 44:92–94
431. Nakanishi, S., Numa, S. 1982. Structural organization of the corticotropin-beta-lipotropin precursor gene. *Int. Symp. Princess Takamatsu Cancer Res. Fund* 12:23–29
432. Jornvall, H., Persson, M., Ekman, R. 1982. Structural comparisons of leukocyte interferon and pro-opiomelanocortin correlated with immunological similarities. *FEBS Lett.* 137:153–56
433. Skurkovich, S. V., Eremkina, E. I. 1975. The probable role of interferon in allergy. *Ann. Allergy* 35:356–60

Ann. Rev. Pharmacol. Toxicol. 1986. 26:517–45

ELECTROPHYSIOLOGICAL CORRELATES OF SENSORIMOTOR SYSTEM NEUROTOXICOLOGY

Thomas Baker

Department of Anesthesiology, St. Joseph's Medical Center, Paterson, New Jersey 07503

Herbert E. Lowndes

Department of Pharmacology and Toxicology, College of Pharmacy, Rutgers University, Piscataway, New Jersey 08854

INTRODUCTION

In this review we consider the electrophysiological consequences of neuropathological changes induced by toxic chemicals in sensorimotor systems. A large body of neurotoxicological data is not covered, including that derived from observations of the acute effects of toxic chemicals on neural systems. The toxicological and/or pharmacological effects of such chemical-neural interactions in many cases leave no residual pathology; such data are adequately reviewed elsewhere.

In most instances, too few studies using neurotoxic chemicals have been reported to permit structural-functional correlations. Hence, we have relied on analogous studies from other areas of neurological research, particularly axotomy, on the assumption that while the neuron may be injured in various ways, it can respond to diverse forms of injury in only a few stereotyped fashions.

Systemic exposure to toxic chemicals exposes all levels of the neuron: the perikaryon, the axon, the nerve endings, and the target organs. Possible multiple sites of chemical attack tend to confound cause-effect relationships in a system as dynamic as a neuron and its target(s) of innervation. Particular manifestations of neurotoxicity thus may depend on one or more of the follow-

517

0362-1642/86/0415-0517$02.00

ing: the extent of the neuron exposed (1), toxicokinetics of the compound (cf 2–4), duration and route of exposure (cf 5), and species or other variables.

There are instances in which electrophysiological alterations occur without corresponding neuropathological changes. This may reflect the inherent sensitivity of properly chosen electrophysiological techniques in detecting incipient neurotoxicity, or merely that the appropriate ultrastructural correlate has not been examined.

Here we focus on the electrophysiological-neuropathological correlates of neurotoxicology at the level of the neuron. Except for compounds of toxinological interest, we have placed no restrictions on the term "neurotoxic chemical." We have made no attempt to comprehensively review all neurotoxic chemicals; rather, we have selected examples principally on the basis that they have received the greatest research interest. Electrophysiological correlates at the level of neuronal systems can usually be inferred from an understanding of the neurotoxicology of their component parts; space does not permit such a review. Additional information on systems responses in neurotoxicology is available (6).

NEURONAL CELL BODIES IN NEUROTOXICOLOGY

Compared to peripheral axons, neuronal perikarya have received disproportionately little attention in neurotoxicology except from morphologists. This stems, in part, from the greater difficulties in recording from perikarya than from peripheral axons, coupled with a focus on the axonopathic aspects of neurotoxicology.

Exposure of a neuronal cell body, its axon, and its target of innervation to neuropathic agents precipitates a dynamic series of events which has been only partially unraveled. If, as occurs in many cases, the lesion occurs in the axon (or perhaps in the myelin or myelinating cells?), reactive changes are expected in the perikaryon as signals of a shift in metabolic priorities away from maintenance and toward repair mechanisms. The signal for reordering of priorities may be a change in trophic signals from the innervated target. Those reactive changes are presumably stereotypic responses of the cell body to injury, much like those after axotomy, with the specific manifestations a function of the nature and extent of the lesion. It is interesting to speculate that axonal changes might be secondary to or exacerbated by remodeling in the cell body (7).

In axotomy, the lesion is focal, but the situation is likely to be much more complicated when cell body and axon are exposed to toxic agents. A preexisting or coexisting biochemical lesion in the cell body, not detectable by microscopy, could be a triggering or catalytic event for functional or morphological alterations appearing elsewhere. With modifications, this is similar to the concept suggested by Cavanagh (8) some two decades ago.

Perikaryal Responses to Axotomy

HISTOLOGY   Injury of axons, or of any portion of the neuron, elicits perikaryal responses that are primarily regenerative (9). Postaxotomy changes, variously referred to as the axon or retrograde reaction, or chromatolysis (10–13), are triggered by an unknown signal from the injury site (14) that may be conveyed by retrograde transport (15, 16). Striking changes occur in DNA-dependent RNA synthesis, evidenced by alterations in RNA-carrying organelles (i.e. chromatolysis), which can be blocked by actinomycin (17). The cell body remodels, apparently shifting protein synthesis priorities away from functional materials (e.g. neurotransmitter-related enzymes) toward membrane and soluble matrix proteins (18–21). Altered demand for cytoskeletal proteins (e.g. neurofilaments) leads to a reduction in slow component a of axoplasm transport (20); this in turn causes proximal axonal atrophy (22–25) with correspondingly decreased neurofilament content (cf 26).

Morphologically, the basophilic Nissl substance [containing the ribonucleoprotein of the granular or rough endoplasmic reticulum (RER)] granulates and disperses into the cytoplasm while the cisternae of the RER vesiculate. Swelling is evident in mitochondria and perikarya. The nucleolus and the nucleus enlarge, followed by eccentricity of the nucleus. Lysosomes and Golgi complexes become more prominent (9, 27). Microglial and astrocytic processes cause synaptic reorganization of axosomatic synapses (28), resulting in disjunction of more proximal synapses (29, 30). Disjunction is reversed only if neuromuscular contact is reestablished (31, 32).

ELECTROPHYSIOLOGY   Pioneering electrophysiological studies of axotomy-induced changes in motoneurons by Eccles and co-workers (33) tended to emphasize membrane, particularly dendritic, excitability changes. Monosynaptically evoked excitatory postsynaptic potentials (EPSPs) in axotomized motoneurons have a lower peak amplitude and prolonged time to peak (33, 34); this alteration in synaptic efficacy may underlie the diminished monosynaptic reflex (MSR) responses following axotomy (33–35) reported earlier (36). Eccles et al (33) reported finding no change in resting membrane potentials (RMPs), input resistance, membrane capacitance, or afterhyperpolarization potentials (AHPs). In spite of diminished EPSP efficacy, motoneuron excitability, particularly in the dendrites, may be enhanced, evidenced by decreases in somal-dendritic threshold, initial-segment conduction time, greater velocity of action potential upstroke, and a larger than normal number of all-or-none responses in axotomized motoneurons (33). An altered dendritic excitability likely underlies the increased incidence of delayed depolarizations (37–39). Subsequent studies showed shallow initial-segment, somal-dendritic inflections (e.g. 39). Combined with a more rapid voltage upstroke, these lead to achievement of somal-dendritic threshold at a more negative voltage (40).

Findings in axotomized motoneurons were not always consistent. Unlike the finding by Eccles et al (33), later studies revealed the overshoot of action potentials to be increased (41, 42) and axonal conduction velocities decreased (41–43). Significantly, AHP amplitude, duration, and conductance were found to be decreased in soleus [slow; type S (see 44)] motoneurons but unaccompanied by change in RMP or input resistance (37, 39, 41). Conversely, fast motoneurons (i.e. type FF) show no change in AHP following axotomy (but see below) but exhibited decreased RMPs and larger input resistances. Taken in concert, these findings have led to the suggestion that axotomy causes electrophysiological differences between fast and slow motoneurons, particularly AHP and input resistances, to diminish (41, 45). In effect, axotomy causes a "dedifferentiation" of motoneuron electrical properties (42), presumably signaling a stereotyped perikaryal remodeling following axon injury.

Perikaryal Responses in Neurotoxicology

HISTOLOGY   The pathological features of neuronal cell bodies in a variety of toxic neuropathies, detailed elsewhere (46, 47), vary from none to complete cellular necrosis. At one extreme is the loss of dorsal root ganglion, but not anterior horn cells, in doxorubicin neuropathy (48). At the other, primary degenerative changes appear uncommon even in neuropathies characterized by widespread axonal involvement. For example, light-microscopic examination of cell bodies has revealed them to be essentially normal in intoxications by acrylamide (49), isoniazid (50), and β,β'-iminodipropionitrile (IDPN) (51, 52). Ultrastructural studies confirmed only mild involvement. Anterior horn and dorsal root ganglion cells showed only mild dispersion of granular endoplasmic reticulum with some dissociation of polyribosomes and single ribosomes in the case of acrylamide neuropathy. Fine structural changes in tri-o-cresyl phosphate intoxication are similarly only slightly more than would be expected from distal axon loss, making them difficult to classify as primary or reactive (cf 49).

Neurofilamentous accumulations in the neuronal cytoplasm, only modest in the above-mentioned neuropathies, are striking features of experimental poisoning with aluminum salts (53, 54). Shelanski & Wisniewski (55) noted the appearance of neurofibrillary tangles to be an early consequence of subarachnoid administration of vincristine. Accumulations of neurofilaments have been observed to engorge the initial segment, proximal dendrites, and cytoplasm of anterior horn cells in a case of fulminating IDPN neuropathy (56). The link between neurofilament derangements in neuronal perikarya and the ultimate expressions of neurotoxicity are unknown; they certainly signal that remodeling has taken place in the cell body.

The principal cell body changes noted in many toxic neuropathies are reactive, usually secondary to axonal degeneration. The reactive changes vary in intensity depending on severity and duration of intoxication, species, toxic agent, and the neuronal cell body examined. Similar variations in response are observed following surgical axotomy (11); hence the variety of responses in axonopathies is not surprising. Interestingly, axon swellings alone seem not to initiate reactive changes: perikarya remain unremarkable in spite of large axonal spheroids in IDPN neuropathy (51, 52).

Neither the presence of axon swellings nor degeneration may be required to initiate morphological alterations in cell bodies. Recent studies report extensive remodeling after only 6–8 days of intoxication with acrylamide (100–240 mg/kg total cumulative dose), at which time there is no evidence of axonal degeneration (57, 58). Examination of perikarya late in intoxications when axonal degeneration is present is of limited predictive value; initial neuronal alterations that may contribute to development of the neurotoxicity might well be obscured later.

ELECTROPHYSIOLOGY   There have been few electrophysiological studies of perikaryal function in neurotoxicity. Those that have been reported, or are in progress, have examined the action potential generating capacity of spinal ganglion cells or spinal motoneurons.

Somjen and co-workers (59) recorded intracellular action potentials from ganglion cells of rats with methyl mercury intoxication, the early manifestation of which is a peripheral sensory neuropathy (60). They reported a marked fragility of the ganglion cells in poisoned animals, leading to difficulty in obtaining successful intracellular impalements; similar difficulties have been experienced in motoneuron recordings from IDPN-intoxicated cats (H. E. Lowndes, D. A. Delio & M. G. Fiori, unpublished observations). Whether this fragility signals physical modifications in neural membranes is a matter of speculation.

Although the values of rheobase and input resistance in methyl mercury poisoned ganglion cells fell within the normal range, Somjen et al (59) noted a paucity of recordings with high rheobase and low input resistance. Based on geometric considerations of perikaryal size, these data suggest that the largest-diameter ganglion cells are the most severely affected. Direct correlation between ganglion cell size and physiological function has not been established. Intracellularly recorded action potentials tended to be markedly prolonged, with durations as great as 15 msec. The long potentials, often characterized by plateaus, appeared to result from delays during the repolarization phase. In addition, the ability of the ganglion cells to follow trains of repetitive stimuli was poor.

Several key features of methyl mercury neuropathy deserve comment. First, the electrophysiological recordings bear no similarity to those from motoneurons undergoing chromatolysis. This is corroborated by the lack of

Table 1 Changes in action potential parameters of motoneurons in IDPN neuropathy

Alteration	Reference
Prolonged latency to onset[a]	52, 63
Shallow initial segment–somal dendritic inflection	52,63
Decreased initial-segment conduction time	52, 63
Decreased somal-dendritic threshold	52,63
Increased overshoot	64
Prolonged M spike	64
Decreased AHP amplitude, duration, and conductance[b]	65
Increased incidence of delayed depolarizations and repetitive firing	63, 65
Increased input resistance[c]	64
Monotonic firing in the primary range	66

[a]Prolonged latencies may reflect the presence of proximal axon swellings that characterize this neuropathy.
[b]In type S motoneurons (see text).
[c]In all motoneuron types (see text).

morphological evidence of chromatolysis (61) and no findings of fiber loss in the neuropathy (60). Lack of early evidence of axon degeneration or chromatolysis, yet with significant alterations in perikaryal function, indicates a direct action of methyl mercury on ganglion cell bodies, the largest diameter cells being most susceptible.

There is similarly a striking lack of evidence of chromatolysis in lumbar motoneurons of rats (51) or cats (52) with IDPN neuropathy. Despite the lack of morphological evidence of chromatolysis, electrophysiological studies of the motoneurons point to numerous parallels in action potential features in axotomized motoneurons and those in IDPN neuropathy. Electrophysiological alterations in motoneurons of IDPN treated cats are summarized in Table 1 and elsewhere (62).

Preliminary studies were performed in motoneurons not identified as to physiological type. As in early axotomy studies, this tended to obscure differential responses of the motoneuron subtypes. Subsequent studies in type-identified motoneurons (S, FR, FI, FF) have, in general, supported the original supposition (63) that the electrophysiological changes in IDPN neuropathy are reminiscent of those in chromatolytic motoneurons.

Differences between slow and fast motoneurons (i.e. S vs FF) tend to become less apparent following interruption of the motor axon. Motoneurons to fast-twitch motor units have for example larger sizes, lower input resistances, and briefer AHPs (45). Axotomy results in a decrease in AHP duration in slow motoneurons and some increase in the normally briefer AHP responses in fast motoneurons (41, 45). Duration of AHP is reduced in types S and FR but unchanged in fast (FI and FF) motoneurons of cats with IDPN neuropathy (D. A. Delio, H. E. Lowndes, unpublished observations). It is noteworthy that AHP duration becomes significantly shorter in slow motoneurons as early as day 14 of the neuropathy.

A second feature showing convergence of electrophysiological characteristics in axotomized motoneurons is an increase in input resistance. Input resistance is significantly greater in all motoneuron types (except FI) by 35 days of IDPN neuropathy (D. A. Delio, H. E. Lowndes, unpublished observations). It has been argued that the change in this passive electrical property may reflect a postaxotomy reduction in perikaryal size and alterations in dendritic geometry as additional features of convergence of motoneuron characteristics (45). It is not profitable to speculate on the possibility of changes in passive motoneuron properties in IDPN neuropathy until further corroborative data (e.g. membrane time constants) are obtained. Further, the small changes in passive properties conferred by alterations in parikaryal size or dendritic geometry are almost certain to be obscured by the preponderant physical changes in the ventral horns resulting from the development of the massive axon swellings.

NEUROTOXICOLOGY AND THE AXON

Wallerian Degeneration

HISTOLOGY   Following separation from its parent axon, either by mechanical or chemical lesion, the axon undergoes a stereotypic response first described by Waller (67) and subsequently detailed by several authors (cf 68, 69). Although the following brief description is derived from transection studies in which the precise time and location of the lesion are known, there is no evidence to suggest that the sequence differs following a chemically induced lesion. Focal swelling, with fragmentation of endoplasmic reticulum and accumulation of mitochondria and other organelles, appears within 24 hr adjacent to the transection site (cf 70, 71). Shortly thereafter, neurotubules and neurofilaments lose their longitudinal orientation and fragment; mitochondria swell; and the axolemma becomes occasionally discontinuous. A beaded appearance, reflecting areas of axonal narrowing and swelling (varicosities), is evident by 3 days, followed by fragmentation, usually first observed between nodes of Ranvier. Axonal degeneration is independent of myelin changes, which follow those in the axon (see 72, 73).

Histological features of nerves just proximal to the injury site are similar to those distal to the lesion; their proximal extent is determined by the nature of the injury (69). It is interesting to note that acrylamide, which induces a "dying-back" neuropathy (8), causes histological changes to appear much more proximal to a nerve ligature than normally (74, 75), regardless of the proximal-distal location of the ligature (7). Isoniazid, 2,5-hexanedione and misonidazole, other neurotoxic agents that have similarly been described as causing a dying-back lesion, fail to augment lesions proximal to a ligature (74).

ELECTROPHYSIOLOGY   Cragg & Thomas (23) suggested that nerve fiber diameter may be reduced proximal to sites of axonal injury. This would be consistent with decreases in conduction velocities in this region (41, 76). Presumably, axonal atrophy reflects a diminished supply of cytoskeletal protein, the principal determinant of axonal caliber, following a reordering of protein synthesis priorities in the perikaryon. While atrophy and decreased conduction velocities proximal to a neurotoxic lesion have not been directly investigated, recent studies (5) reveal that exposure to acrylamide can lead to a region of decreased neurofilaments (and axon caliber) that passes centrifugally down the nerve with time.

In contrast to morphological changes which many investigators believe progress centrifugally, electrophysiological alterations appear to progress centripetally. Nerve terminal function, evidenced by loss of repetitive generating capacity (77) within 48 hr, followed by failure of neuromuscular transmission by 4–5 days, is the first compromised, followed by centripetally advancing conduction block (78). Lack of decline in conduction velocities prior to onset of conduction block suggests an all-or-none failure.

Demyelination

PRIMARY DEMYELINATION   Primary demyelination independent of axonal alterations or degeneration appears randomly in both proximal and distal portions of nerves, distinct from clusters of demyelinated segments on certain fibers. Primary myelotoxins have been divided into three groups (79):

1. Those that disrupt myelin prior to, or in the absence of changes in either the axons or myelinating cells. Examples include hexachlorophene, isoniazid, cyanate, acetylethyl tetramethyl tetralin, triethyltin, and the salicylanilides. Principal morphological features include edema and vacuolation of myelin.
2. Lysolecithin, which causes direct disruption of myelin without intramyelinic edema.
3. Chemicals that injure myelinating cells (Schwann cells or oligodendrocytes). Examples include pyrithiamine, biscyclohexanone oxalyldihydrazone (Cuprizone®) and chronic exposure to carbon monoxide and cyanide.

A subclass that affects both myelin and myelinating cells includes lead, tellurium, and the hypocholesteremic agents ethidium bromide and diphtheria toxin.

DEMYELINATION SECONDARY TO AXON LOSS   In toxic neuropathies in which the axon appears to be the primary target [axonopathies according to the nosology of Spencer & Schaumburg (80)], demyelination is thought to occur as a passive sequel to axonal degeneration.

Secondary demyelination presumably follows a pattern similar to that in Wallerian degeneration [cf (9) for a more detailed description]. The nodes of Ranvier widen and Schmidt-Lanterman incisures dilate distal to the lesion site, either simultaneously or centrifugally over the next 36 hr. Degenerating axon fragments are surrounded by myelin that is fragmented by closures at the incisures (73), forming rows of ellipsoids which subdivide into smaller spheroids. The debris is phagocytized by proliferating Schwann cells and macrophages.

More common in neurotoxic situations is partial demyelination, usually involving only a percentage of the fibers in an affected nerve trunk. This demyelination, which can vary from paranodal to segmental (often in the same nerve fiber and in the presence of ongoing remyelination), can be secondary to focal axon swellings (without degeneration of the parent axon) or a primary effect of myelotoxic chemicals.

Demyelination and Impulse Conduction

Assuming axonal patency, complete block of impulse conduction is an extreme consequence of demyelination, rarely encountered in neurotoxicology. Early work by Denny-Brown & Brenner (81) with compression-induced focal demyelination indicates that the axon remains electrically excitable distal to the site of the demyelinated lesion, in contrast to situations in which the axon is also involved (see 82). In less extreme cases, conduction is altered but preserved. Compound action potentials, reflecting the net electrical activity at the recording site, are reduced in amplitude, delayed, and temporally dispersed. This has been convincingly demonstrated in studies of experimental allergic neuritis (83) and diphtheric demyelination (84, 85).

Caution must be exercised in inferring nerve fiber susceptibility from compound action potential records unless the latter are supported by correlative morphological and, optimally, single-fiber studies. A net slowing of compound action potentials could result from selective involvement of the largest diameter (fastest conducting) axons due to their degeneration, a velocity decrement in all fibers without axonal loss, or a combination of the two. In experimental vincristine neuropathy in the cat, conduction velocity histograms of single soleus afferents retain a bimodal distribution but with lower average velocity

(75–85 m/sec) than normal (90–100 m/sec) in the fastest conducting fibers (86). Morphological studies (87) reveal a combination of proximal axonal swellings and demyelination, with some distal Wallerian degeneration, principally involving the largest diameter fibers. Hence a combination of factors contributed to the apparent conduction slowing in this study. This is frequently the case in neurotoxicology, especially when the animals are tested in advanced stages of the neuropathy. Additional details are available (88).

Conduction velocity slowing due to demyelination has been demonstrated for single fibers in both the peripheral (89, 90) and central nervous systems (91), where the results of demyelination are qualitatively similar.

It should be noted that studies of demyelination have usually focused on the segmental rather than paranodal variety. Even then, myelin alterations at successive internodes are variable (92), associated with variation in internodal conduction times (93). Paranodal demyelination is an early and frequent concomitant in numerous examples of neurotoxicology, particularly those involving axonal swelling (see below). The consequences of paranodal demyelination on conduction velocity are not known with certainty. Slight alterations in nodal morphology do not appear associated with significant changes in conduction velocity (94, 95). Further, conduction velocity returns to normal despite the persistence of myelin vacuolization in triethyltin neuropathy (96).

Numerous morphological alterations occur in cases of neurotoxicity. Not only are parameters of fiber geometrically distorted, but also the properties of excitable membranes, ion concentrations, capacitance and impedance of myelin, axolemma, and axoplasm, and resistance of extracellular pathways to current flow (97). The status of these other determinants of conduction velocities in toxic neuropathies is essentially unknown. Recent studies (98) suggest that retraction of myelin loops from the axolemma (paranodal demyelination), commonly seen in many examples of neurotoxicology, may provide a low-impedance shunt between intra- and extracellular spaces. This could theoretically make the impact of paranodal demyelination on conduction greater than previously suspected.

Computer simulations of impulse conduction in demyelinated axons (95, 99) reveal conduction block to occur only after loss of 97.3% of myelin from a single node or two successive nodes with myelin reduced to 4% of normal. These calculations are based on equivalent changes in cable properties distributed evenly over the length of internodes. Interestingly, the same simulations revealed paranodal demyelination to be more effective in slowing impulse conduction than equivalent changes resulting from myelin loss. Details are reviewed elsewhere (97, 100).

Conduction of impulses in demyelinated axons occurs via either saltatory conduction, albeit with increased delay between excitation of successive nodes, or continuous conduction in demyelinated internodes (93, 101). Bostock &

Sears (101) calculated the velocity of continuous conduction through demyelinated regions (about 0.5 mm) to be only 5% of normal.

The refractory period for impulse transmission, the minimal interval at which the second of two impulses can enter but not transverse a portion of a nerve fiber (91), is markedly prolonged in demyelinated axons (91, 93, 102, 103); the safety factor for transmission is thus reduced, leading to impaired fidelity of transmission of trains of impulses (91, 93, 104, 105). During repetitive transmission across affected internodes, internodal conduction times increase progressively, associated with a progressive decrease in current generation at the node proximal to the affected internode (93).

Axonal Swellings

A common pathological feature of many chemically induced neuropathies is the formation of axon swellings, resulting from abnormal accumulations of cytoskeletal proteins, particularly neurofilaments. These neurofilamentous axonopathies have been observed to result from a diverse group of chemicals (Table 2) and may represent a subset of stereotypic responses of the neuron to certain forms of chemical insult.

MORPHOLOGY OF AXONAL SWELLINGS   Although their spatio-temporal location varies with the particular neurotoxic chemical, axon swellings share several features. Their hallmark is an abnormal focal accumulation of 10-nm neurofilaments that first appear distally (acrylamide, hexacarbons, carbon disulfide), proximally (IDPN, vincristine), or occasionally both proximally and distally (IDPN). Aluminum, depending on route of administration, induces accumulations of neurofilaments in proximal axons (107) or in the perikaryon (53). In the neuropathy induced by 3,4-dimethyl,2,5-hexanedione, the locus of the axonal swellings is dose related (110, 111), with higher doses producing the most proximal swellings.

The swellings, containing maloriented skeins of neurofilaments and other organelles, distend progressively with the duration of the neuropathy, ultimately achieving diameters of 30–50 μm in hexacarbon intoxication. Swell-

Table 2   Chemicals causing neurofilamentous axonopathies

Chemical	Reference
Acrylamide	49, 106
Aluminum	53, 54, 107
Carbon disulfide	108, 109
Dimethylhexanedione	110, 111
Hexacarbons	112, 113
β,β'-iminodipropionitrile	51, 114, 115
Vinca alkaloids (vincristine)	87

ings with diameters of 100–150 μm have been observed in IDPN-treated cats (52). In hexacarbon neuropathy, swellings first develop on the proximal side of nodes of Ranvier (116).

As the axon swelling enlarges, myelin is altered at the involved node(s). Initially, terminal loops become detached from the axolemma (paranodal demyelination). Larger swellings and/or more severe intoxication result in slippage or remodeling of myelin, resulting in thin, patchy, or absent myelin (51, 117).

The axon distal to axonal swellings undergoes Wallerian-like degeneration in many, but not all, neurofilamentous axonopathies. Axon loss is a hallmark, at least in the advanced stages of intoxication with acrylamide (49, 106, 118), hexacarbons (47) and carbon disulfide (119), and dimethylhexanedione (110, 111). Apparently, the presence of axon swellings is a necessary but insufficient condition for axon degeneration. Fiber loss does not occur in rodents chronically exposed to IDPN, despite the presence of enormous proximal axonal enlargements (120, 121). On the other hand, IDPN intoxication of felines results in not only typical proximal swellings, but also occasional contemporaneous distal swellings; mild fiber loss appears to accompany coexisting proximal and distal swellings in this neuropathy (115).

ELECTROPHYSIOLOGICAL CONSEQUENCES OF AXONAL SWELLINGS

Conduction block   Block of impulse conduction could arise from one or more consequences of axonal swellings: (*a*) Wallerian degeneration distal to the swelling; (*b*) demyelination of several successive internodes; (*c*) compromise of axolemmal mechanisms supporting action potential generation and propagation; and (*d*) enlargement of the axoplasm to an extent inconsistent with impulse propagation.

When a neuropathy has progressed to the stage in which axons degenerate (i.e. Wallerian degeneration), profiles of compound action potentials reflect the influence of loss of subpopulations of susceptible fiber diameters (see above). In most toxic neuropathies, these tend to be the largest diameter fibers subserving proprioceptive and α-motor axon functions. The dying-back hypothesis (8) predicts that with continued intoxication, axon degeneration should progress centripetally; hence the profile of compound action potentials would reflect not only the duration of intoxication, but also the proximo-distal location of the recording. Sumner (82) has detailed an experimental procedure for evaluation of centripetally advancing Wallerian degeneration in peripheral nerves.

Wallerian degeneration associated with axon swellings induced with toxic chemicals is essentially similar to that following axotomy; the two differ only in the nature of the lesion. Similarly, demyelination at several successive internodes would be expected to have direct consequences analogous to those following demyelination with diphtheric toxin (reviewed in 97).

Axon swellings represent abrupt discontinuities in axonal caliber; their size could be principal determinants of their influence on impulse conduction. Small increases in axonal caliber, such as occur in the early stages of neurofilamentous axonopathies, might be predicted to slow impulse conduction (122; reviewed in 123). The net effect on conduction velocity is difficult to determine since paranodal or nodal demyelination often accompanies even small swellings, and the relative influences of small degrees of demyelination and axon swelling are unknown. For example, conduction latencies in single motor axons of cats with IDPN neuropathy are significantly prolonged as early as 7 days of intoxication, when the proximal axons are very mildly distended; however, internodal and paranodal myelin thickness appear modestly reduced (52), confounding interpretation of the influence of the axon swelling alone.

Very large swellings (e.g. greater than 60–70 μm) such as occur in IDPN intoxication (51, 52, 115) are predicted to block impulse conduction regardless of the influence of demyelination. Parnas et al (124) calculated that a 5 : 1 ratio between the diameters of the enlargement and normal adjacent axon would be the critical point at which longitudinal currents through the enlarged portion of the axon would become insufficient to support impulse propagation. At this point, the axon swelling would represent an impedance mismatch with the contiguous axon and impulse conduction would be blocked. Experimentally this has been tested by recording intracellularly from a spinal motoneuron of cat with IDPN neuropathy and attempting to evoke motoneuron action potentials via orthodromic, then antidromic stimulation. Orthodromic stimulation (via dorsal roots) was effective in eliciting a motoneuron action potential; but antidromic stimulation, with a presumed intervening axonal swelling, frequently was not (63). Since the incidence of such recordings increases with duration of intoxication, during which there is progressive enlargement of axon swellings, it is probable that impulse conduction is blocked in the largest swellings.

Later studies of single motor units confirmed that the incidence of impulse blockade increases with the duration of IDPN intoxication and that all motor unit types (FF, FR, S) are equally susceptible (D. A. Delio, H. E. Lowndes, unpublished observations).

Impulse reflection and repetitive discharge   At some critical size, an axon swelling retards impulse conduction sufficiently that the just depolarized (i.e. nonswollen) portion of the axon repolarizes while the impulse is still transversing the swelling. Under such conditions, action potentials can be initiated in both forward and reverse directions and, in effect, the impulse is reflected back to its origin (123). Impulse reflection has been demonstrated in a number of models and experimental situations (125–129). This has not been tested in neurotoxic states.

A possible sequel to the slowing of the impulse in an axonal swelling is repetitive activation of the adjacent, presumably normal, axon. Single stimulation of soleus or medial gastrocnemius afferents in cats with IDPN neuropathy gives rise, in certain instances, to multiple action potentials in the dorsal root input (130). Large axonal swellings occur in the stem processes of dorsal root ganglia in IDPN treated animals (51). The multiple dorsal root discharges may arise from repetitive activation of the afferent fiber in the region of these axon swellings. Repetitive activation, again perhaps reflecting the influence of proximal axon swellings in alpha-motor axons, are also observed in ventral root recordings even in the absence of multiple potentials in the dorsal root input (130).

While the repetitive discharges arising in the dorsal root ganglia are likely related to the axon swellings, it is less certain that swellings in motor axons are the sole contributors to repetitive action potential discharges recorded in motoneurons. A high incidence of delayed depolarizations is observed in motoneuron recordings (63, 65); their possible contribution to repetitive activation of the motoneuron cannot be overlooked.

Axonal/perikaryal crosstalk   Axon swellings, whether in nerve trunks or the spinal/CNS interparenchyma, are grossly distended structures which must compress and abut upon neighboring neuronal elements. Their physical size, coupled with concomitant demyelination that leaves them electrically "un-insulated," give rise to the possibility of abnormal electrical interactions. Granit and co-workers (131, 132) observed the formation of an "artificial synapse" at the site of acute cut or crush injury in cat sciatic nerve. Ephaptic transmission, or crosstalk, occurs between pairs of spontaneously active nerve fibers in dystrophic mice, in which the spinal root axons are devoid of myelin and closely opposed in midroot (133–136). Crosstalk has also been observed in experimental neuromas (137).

The only studies of crosstalk employing neurotoxic agents have involved tullidora (buckthorn) (138) and β,β'-iminodipropionitrile (52, 63).

The neuropathy caused by IDPN is characterized by large, demyelinated swellings which fill spinal ventral horns and abut on axons, motoneurons, and each other (52, 56, 115), giving rise to crosstalk between numerous neuronal elements. Preliminary estimates suggested that about 12% of motoneurons were capable of crosstalk at 5 weeks of the neuropathy (63). More detailed studies revealed that all motor unit types are approximately equally involved, the incidence of crosstalk increased with duration of the neuropathy (presumably reflecting ever-enlarging axon swellings), and crosstalk occurs between both cell bodies and axon swellings (139). In late (i.e. 70 days) stages of the neuropathy almost one half of neuronal elements tested exhibited crosstalk. True ephapse formation between neuronal elements does not occur in IDPN neuropathy (140), and the exact location where crosstalk is initiated (soma, dendrites, axon, axon swelling) has not been determined. It has been suggested that the axon–axon interactions in this neuropathy may be mediated by activity-driven accumulations of extracellular potassium (99, 138).

Axonal Atrophy

IDPN neuropathy presents a unique opportunity to examine the influence of true diminution of axon diameter on impulse conduction. Proximal giant axon swellings enlarge at the expense of cytoskeletal proteins destined for maintenance of axon caliber (141), leading to axonal atrophy (51). Maximum motor conduction velocities in rat sciatic nerve trunks are diminished in animals chronically administered IDPN, in direct correlation with the observation of a reduction in the number of large axons and an increase in small-diameter fibers (i.e. axonal atrophy) (142). Studies of conduction velocities in single soleus and gastrocnemius motor axons (B. G. Gold, H. E. Lowndes, unpublished; 62) at 50 and 100 days of the neuropathy reveal a progressive decline until at 100 days average conduction velocities are reduced to nearly one half normal. At early stages of the neuropathy (7–35 days) a progressive decline in single fiber conduction velocities is also observed in all types of motor axons (S, FR, FF), but the fastest conducting axons (innervating type FF motor units) tend to exhibit the earliest and most severe reduction in velocities (64). It is interesting that the extent of axon swelling in IDPN neuropathy covaries with axon caliber (143), perhaps related to the greater neurofilament density in larger-diameter axons.

Recent studies reveal that the caliber of proximal axons is reduced during chronic administration of acrylamide (5). These authors suggest that the diminished delivery of neurofilaments underlying the atrophy may reflect a reordering of slow axoplasmic transport as a neuronal response to toxin-induced axonal injury. The electrophysiological correlates of acrylamide-induced axonal atrophy have not been reported.

NERVE TERMINAL FUNCTION IN NEUROTOXICOLOGY

In almost all examples of neurotoxicity investigated, nerve terminal function appears somehow compromised, regardless of whether the primary lesion occurs in the soma, axon, or myelin. In the case of axonopathies, many of which are distal, impaired terminal function as an early manifestation of neurotoxicity is consonant with the dying-back hypothesis (8). While terminal dysfunction is an obvious sequel to axon degeneration, it is less clear why deficits in terminal function occur prior to the appearance of neuropathology, whether a causal relationship exists between the two, whether they share a common initiating event [e.g. impaired axoplasmic transport (144)], or whether one or both are consequences of interrupted bidirectional trophic maintenance between the nerve cell body and its target of innervation. These are some of the major unanswered questions in neurotoxicology.

Sensory Terminals

Subjective sensory impairment is often the earliest symptom of incipient neurotoxicity in man. This is exemplified by clinical reports of acrylamide intoxication (118) and is borne out by experimental studies which confirm that sensory impairment precedes motor involvement (145, 146). In some instances, sensory neuropathy is the first manifest but is inevitably followed by motor involvement with progression of the neuropathy. In other cases, profound sensory involvement occurs without an apparent motor counterpart, as in the cases of doxorubicin (147; see however 148) and cisplatin (149) neurotoxicity.

The apparently greater susceptibility of peripheral sensory structures to the neurotoxic effects of certain chemicals may reflect toxicokinetic influences. Jacobs (3, 4) described finestrae in the "blood-nerve barrier" surrounding the dorsal root ganglia. Such finestrae would result in potentially greater exposure of these sensory perikarya to neurotoxicants than their motor counterparts, which enjoy relatively greater protection behind the "blood-brain barrier" of the CNS. While this is an intuitively appealing argument, it fails to take into account chemicals that cause a predominantly motor neuropathy or the simultaneous appearance of sensory and motor impairments with still other toxic chemicals (150, 151).

Also unexplained are the electrophysiological consequences at higher integrating centers (i.e. the cerebellum and cerebrum) of impaired sensory terminal function. Clinically, the consequences appear as anesthesias, parethesias, and symptoms suggestive of deficits in proprioception typified by ataxia and areflexia. While the consequences of altered proprioceptive inputs on spinal reflexes have been examined in the experimental neuropathies induced by acrylamide (152, 153), vincristine (86), and IDPN (63, 130), their supraspinal influences remain unexplored.

Muscle Spindles

HISTOLOGY   The neuropathologic features of muscle spindles and Pacinian corpuscles in various neurotoxicities have been described in detail (106, 113, 154).

ELECTROPHYSIOLOGY   Muscle spindles provide two types of proprioceptive information concerning a muscle: the rate and amount of its extension. The rate of lengthening is signaled by a dynamic discharge frequency proportional to the velocity of extension (the velocity or dynamic component of spindle discharge) while the length per se is signaled by a more constant discharge rate reflecting muscle length (the length or static component). Information concerning both the static and dynamic state of the muscle are critical to proprioception.

Sumner & Asbury (155) first demonstrated spindle defects in acrylamide intoxication. Subsequent detailed studies revealed the static and dynamic sensitivities of muscle spindles to be reduced in striking correlation with the appearance of clinical signs of the intoxication, especially ataxia (145). Loss of static responsiveness, particularly in secondary endings, coincided with the appearance of neurological deficits after 7 days administration of 15 mg/kg/day acrylamide to cats; doubling the dose to 30 mg/kg/day halved the time to onset of equivalent neurological impairment. The amount of muscle extension necessary to elicit a given discharge from a spindle was greater at this time, indicating an elevation in threshold, along with the loss in fidelity of static sensitivity. While there are contemporaneous lesions in the cerebellum even at these early stages of the neuropathy (156), the temporal link between muscle spindle dysfunction and neurological impairment is apparent.

The tendon reflex (knee jerk) is initiated by the dynamic discharge from primary muscle spindle endings activating homonymous motoneurons via spinal monosynaptic reflexes. The attentuation of dynamic sensitivities of the spindle endings early in acrylamide neuropathy provides a rational explanation for the areflexia that accompanies this neurotoxicity (157).

In contrast to acrylamide neuropathy, the dynamic but not the static sensitivity of muscle spindles is attenuated in vincristine neuropathy (86). Static responsiveness is retained only by those endings capable of any discharge; as many as 80% of presumed spindle endings become totally afunctional during the course of vincristine intoxication.

Position sensitivity of spindle endings is also impaired in diisopropylfluorophosphate (DFP) neuropathy (151). As in the case of acrylamide poisoning, secondary endings appear more susceptible to the neuropathic effects of DFP than their primary counterparts. Dynamic sensitivities are not attenuated in cats chronically intoxicated with DFP (151) or subacutely poisoned with soman (158).

The mechanism underlying muscle spindle dysfunction in the toxic neuropathies is unknown. Among other possibilities are: early degenerative events in the nerve membrane subserving mechanical transduction (i.e. the generator potential); impaired impulse conduction in the preterminal, intramuscular branches of the sensory nerve ending; and pathological alterations in capsular tissue surrounding the spindle endings. The latter would result in incorrect or incomplete transmission of physical forces from the muscle to the spindle ending. Additional details are given elsewhere (159).

Pacinian Corpuscles and Other Peripheral Cutaneous Receptors

ELECTROPHYSIOLOGY   Pacinian corpuscles from cat mesentery lose the ability to initiate generator potentials in proportion to the severity of acrylamide poisoning (160). Total doses in excess of 60 mg/kg result in corpuscles unresponsive to mechanical stimuli. Analogous studies of cutaneous mechanoreceptors (field, rapidly adapting, and slowly adapting types 1 and 2) similarly show a greater incidence of failure during acrylamide intoxication (161). An apparent shift in the distribution of relative numbers of these receptors, with an increase in rapidly adapting but a decrease in slowly adapting types, likely results from loss of position sensitivity (static responsiveness) in slowly adapting receptors, making them appear functionally to be rapidly adapting [i.e. retaining a pseudodynamic response (159)].

Frequency-response relationships of mechanoreceptors are unaltered following subacute soman administration, but the total number capable of responding is reduced by one third (158). Slowly adapting type 1 receptors have elevated thresholds and more irregular firing patterns, following even a single dose of vincristine (162).

Central Projections of Sensory Receptors

HISTOLOGY   The central projections of peripheral sensory receptors, being distally located from their cell bodies, might be expected to be involved early in the course of neurotoxic events for the same reasons as their peripheral counterparts. For example, the projections of primary afferent fibers (i.e. from muscle spindles) projecting onto the cells of origin in the dorsal spinocerebellar tract (Clark's column) show changes early in the course of acrylamide neuropathy reminiscent of those in peripheral terminals. By 10 days of the intoxication, the synaptic boutons on cells in Clark's column contain modest accumulations of neurofilaments and a depleted number of synaptic vesicles (B. S. Jortner, H. E. Lowndes, unpublished observations). These consequences of this defect, coupled with the coexisting deficit in muscle spindle ending function, must further compromise transmission of proprioceptive information.

In a stereological examination of synaptic boutons on anterior horn cells (lumbar motoneurons) of rats intoxicated with 2,5-hexanedione, Sterman &

Sposito (163) noted morphological changes including partial and occasionally complete detachment of the boutons; some synaptic degeneration also occurred, with involvement of microglia and astrocytes. These boutons are the terminals of primary afferents subserving spinal monosynaptic reflexes. These findings could indicate a primary lesion in the sensory neuron or its terminals. Alternatively, they could result from a remodeling of the motoneuron itself following a neurotoxic lesion at some level of the motor axis. Synaptic disjunction of temporarily redundant synapses is known to occur following section of motor axons (28).

Clioquinol neuropathy has the remarkable neuropathological feature, at least in experimental animals, of principally involving the distal ends of centrally projecting sensory axons, with relative sparing of axons of the peripheral nervous system (164).

ELECTROPHYSIOLOGY   A number of electrophysiological studies of primary afferent terminal function in acrylamide intoxication reveal that these central projections to spinal reflexes are affected at doses that have no visible effect on peripheral terminal (muscle spindle ending) function. Greater sensitivity of central projections may reflect underlying differences in the neurochemical substrates supporting central and peripheral projections. Unconditioned but not conditioned (posttetanic) monosynaptic reflex responses are reduced in cats given acrylamide (152). This defect in the primary afferent terminals to spinal monosynaptic reflex pathway results partly from a diminution of transmitter turnover (153). A motoneuron (perikaryal) contribution to the decreased monosynaptic reflexes was ruled out by studies demonstrating motoneuron responses to quipazine to be unchanged in acrylamide-treated animals (165). Additional evidence for an afferent terminal deficit is that dorsal root potentials cannot be evoked even with very large stimuli (166).

Monosynaptic reflexes are also altered in IDPN neuropathy (130). While it is probable that a sensory defect occurs in this neuropathy, direct experimental proof is lacking. However, the motoneuron involvement in this neuropathy is so extensive as to confound interpretation of a possible primary afferent terminal contribution to overall dysfunction. Similarly, studies of the delayed neuropathy resulting from tri-ortho-cresyl phosphate revealed attenuation of monosynaptic reflex responses (167); determination of the status of terminal projections in this neuropathy awaits precise assessment of the motoneuron contribution. Additional details are given elsewhere (168).

Motor Nerve Endings

HISTOLOGY   Neurotoxic agents can cause morphological damage of nerve endings. Using a model in which a localized organophosphorus-induced neuropathy is produced in a hind limb of cats (150, 169), various investigators (170–173) found ultrastructural changes in motor nerve endings. In this context, motor nerve endings are the final portion of peripheral motor axons that extend from the distal or last node of Ranvier and include the unmyelinated terminals. Typical morphological alterations include the presence of extensive lamellar whorls in both the axons and intramuscular axons, the disruption and retraction of nerve terminals from the synaptic cleft, and a dispersion of the basal lamina.

ELECTROPHYSIOLOGY   The morphological damage occurs contemporaneously with the loss of electrophysiological responsiveness of the motor nerve endings: This is evidenced by the loss of the capacity of motor nerve endings to generate repetitive discharges after conditioning by high frequency stimulation or facilitatory drugs in DFP (150, 169), acrylamide (146), and IDPN (174) neuropathies.

The neurotoxic agent dithiobiuret also affects motor nerve terminal function: The quantal release of acetylcholine is depressed, as well as the minature end plate frequency (175). These prejunctional toxic effects adversely affect the posttetanic potentiation evoked by high frequency conditioning of motor nerves (176).

Lead presumably affects motor nerve ending function by competing with calcium for prejunctional sites. Calcium uptake into the nerve terminal is thereby blocked and transmitter release is interrupted (177–179).

Interestingly, in acute methyl mercury toxicity, an increase in the spontaneous release of transmitter first occurs followed by the cessation of all activity at the neuromuscular junction. This agent increases the probability of transmitter release while causing reduction in the quantal content and the immediately available store of transmitter (180). Miyamoto (181) has postulated that the mercury ion has a high affinity for intracellular sulfhydryl groups that are involved in transmitter releasing mechanisms. This bimodal type of activity of methyl mercury at the neuromuscular junction is similar to that caused by black widow spider venom (182). Morphological studies have shown that a disruption of the motor nerve terminal and an absence of synaptic vesicles within the nerve ending occur after black widow spider venom treatment while the postjunctional structures are unaffected. The effects of some other neurotoxic agents on neuromuscular function are listed in Table 3.

ACKNOWLEDGMENTS

The authors' work cited in this article has been supported by USPHS NIH grants NS-01447, NS-11948, NS-23325, and the Amyotrophic Lateral Sclerosis Society of America.

Table 3   Electrophysiologic effects of neurotoxic agents at the neuromuscular junction

Agent	Effect	Reference
Aliphatic alcohols	EPP amplitude ↑ and then ↓ → 0	199, 200
	quantal content (m) ↑	200
	immediately available store ↓	
	mepp amplitude ↑	
	EPP decay phase ↑	
	mepp decay phase ↑	
Dithiobiuret	EPP amplitude ↓	
	RMP no change	
	mepp frequency no change or ↓	175, 198
	quantal content (m) ↓	175
	mepp amplitude ↑	
2,5-Hexanedione	mepp frequency ↑ and then ↓	201
	mepp amplitude ↑	
	mean quantal content (m) ↓ or no change	
Lead	ACh output ↓	183
	mepp frequency ↑	178
	EPP amplitude ↓	177
	Ca uptake by nerve terminals ↓	184
	quantal content (m)	
	↓ immediate available stores	185
	mepp amplitude ↓	186
	RMP ↑	187
	slowing of recovery of RMP	
	↓ spontaneous spike activity	
	↓ input resistance	
Mercury	EPP amplitude, ↑ and then ↓ → 0	188
	mepp frequency ↑	181
	mepp frequency ↑ and then ↓ → 0	180
	mepp amplitude no change	
	RMP no change	
	quantal content (m) ↓	
	p (probability of release) ↑	
	immediately available store ↓	
Organophosphorus anti-cholinesterase agents	EPP decay phase ↑	192, 193
	EPC decay phase ↑	194, 195
	EPP amplitude ↑	196
	At high doses or long duration	195
	EPP and EPC ↓	197
	mepp frequency ↑	193

Table 3 *(continued)*

Agent	Effect	Reference
	mepp amplitude ↑	193
	quantal content (m) ↓	196
	mepp decay phase ↓	196
Organotin (triethyltin)	EPP ↓ amplitude	189
	mepp amplitude no change	
	mepp frequency no change	
	ACh release during tetany ↓	190
	RMP ↓	191

Abbreviations: ACh, acetylcholine; EPP, end plate potential; mepp, miniature end plate potential; RMP, resting membrane potential

Literature Cited

1. Lowndes, H. E., Baker, T. 1980. Toxic site of action in distal axonopathies. See Ref. 47, pp. 193–205
2. Jacobs, J. M. 1978. Vascular permeability and neurotoxicity. *Environ. Health Perspect.* 26:107–16
3. Jacobs, J. M. 1980. Vascular permeability and neural injury. See Ref. 47, pp. 102–17
4. Jacobs, J. M. 1982. Vascular permeability and neurotoxicity. In *Nervous System Toxicology*, ed. C. H. Mitchell, pp. 285–98. New York: Raven
5. Gold, B. G., Griffin, J. W., Price, D. L. 1985. Slow axonal transport in acrylamide neuropathy: different abnormalities produced by single-dose and continuous administration. *J. Neurosci.* 5:1755–68
6. Lowndes, H. E., ed. 1986. *Electrophysiology in Neurotoxicology*. Boca Raton: CRC. In press
7. Sharer, L. R., Lowndes, H. E. 1985. Acrylamide-induced ascending degeneration of ligated peripheral nerve: effect of ligature location. *Neuropathol. Appl. Neurobiol.* 11:191–200
8. Cavanagh, J. B. 1964. The significance of the "dying-back" process in experimental and human neurological disease. *Int. Rev. Exp. Pathol.* 3:219–64
9. Selzer, M. E. 1980. Regeneration of peripheral nerve. In *The Physiology of Peripheral Nerve Disease*, ed. A. J. Sumner, pp. 358–431. Philadelphia: Saunders
10. Lieberman, A. R. 1971. The axon reaction: A review of the principal features of perikaryal responses to axon injury. *Int. Rev. Neurobiol.* 14:49–124
11. Lieberman, A. R. 1974. Some factors affecting retrograde neuronal responses to axonal lesions. In *Essays on the Nervous System*, ed. R. Bellaus, E. G. Gray, pp. 71–105. Oxford: Clarendon
12. Grafstein, B., McQuarrie, E. I. 1978. Role of the nerve cell body in axonal regeneration. In *Neuronal Plasticity*, ed. C. W. Cotman, pp. 155–95. New York: Raven
13. Barron, K. D., Cheang, T. Y., Daniels, A. C., Doolon, P. F. 1971. Subcellular accompaniments of axon reaction in cervical motoneurons of the cat. In *Progress in Neuropathology*, Vol. 1, ed. H. M. Zimmerman, pp. 255–80. New York: Grune & Stratton
14. Cragg, B. G. 1970. What is the signal for chromatolysis? *Brain Res.* 23:1–21
15. Purves, D. 1976. Long-term regulation in the vertebrate peripheral nervous system. *Int. Rev. Physiol.* 10:125–78
16. Singer, P. A., Mehler, S., Fernandez, H. L. 1984. Blockade of retrograde axonal transport delays the onset of metabolic and morphologic changes induced by axotomy. *J. Neurosci.* 2:1299–1306
17. Torvik, A., Heding, A. 1969. Effect of actinomycin D on retrograde nerve cell reaction: further observations. *Acta Neuropathol.* 14:62–71
18. Watson, W. E. 1976. *Cell Biology of Brain*. London: Chapman & Hall
19. Ross, R. A., Joh, G. H., Reis, D. J. 1975. Reversible changes in the ac-

cumulation and activities of tyrosine hydroxylase and dopamine-α-hydroxylase in neurons of locus coeruleus during the retrograde reaction. *Brain Res.* 92:57–72

20. Hoffman, P. N., Lasek, R. J. 1980. Axonal transport of the cytoskeleton in regenerating motor neurons: constancy and change. *Brain Res.* 202:317–53

21. Hall, M. E., Wilson, D. L., Stone, G. C. 1978. Changes in synthesis of specific proteins following axotomy: detection with two-dimensional gel electrophoresis. *J. Neurobiol.* 9:353–66

22. Hoffman, P. N., Griffin, J. W., Price, D. L. 1984. Control of axonal caliber by neurofilament transport. *J. Cell Biol.* 99:705–14

23. Cragg, B. G., Thomas, P. K. 1961. Changes in conduction velocity and fiber size proximal to peripheral nerve lesions. *J. Physiol.* 157:315–27

24. Carlson, J., Lais, A. C., Dyck, P. J. 1979. Axonal atrophy from permanent peripheral axotomy in adult cat. *J. Neuropathol. Exp. Neurol.* 38:579–85

25. Aitkin, J. T., Thomas, P. K. 1962. Retrograde changes in fibre size following nerve section. *J. Anat.* 96:121–29

26. Berthold, C. H. 1978. Morphology of normal peripheral axons. In *Physiology and Pathobiology of Axons*, ed. S. G. Waxman, pp. 3–63. New York: Raven

27. Price, D. L., Porter, K. R. 1972. The response of ventral horn neurons to axonal transection. *J. Cell Biol.* 53:24–37

28. Blinzinger, K., Kreutzberg, G. W. 1968. Displacement of synaptic terminals from regenerating motoneurons by microglial cells. *Z. Zellforsch.* 85:145–57

29. Price, D. L., Griffin, J. W. 1980. Neurons and unsheathing cells as targets of disease processes. See Ref. 47, pp. 2–23

30. Price, D. L. 1972. The response of amphibian glial cells to axonal transection. *J. Neuropathol. Exp. Neurol.* 31: 267–77

31. Matthews, M. R., Nelson, V. H. 1975. Detachment of structurally intact nerve endings from chromatolytic neurons of rat superior cervical ganglion during depression of synaptic transmission induced by postganglionic axotomy. *J. Physiol.* 245:91–135

32. Purves, D. 1975. Functional and structural changes in mammalian sympathetic neurons following interruption of their axons. *J. Physiol.* 252:429–63

33. Eccles, J. C., Libet, B., Young, R. R. 1958. The behavior of chromatolysed

motoneurons studied by intracellular recording. *J. Physiol.* 143:11–40

34. Kuno, M., Llinas, R. 1970. Enhancement of synaptic transmission by dendritic potentials in chromatolysed motoneurons of the cat. *J. Physiol.* 211:807–21

35. Kuno, M., Llinas, R. 1970. Alterations in synaptic action in chromatolysed motoneurons of the cat. *J. Physiol.* 210:823–38

36. Downman, C. B. B., Eccles, J. C., McIntyre, A. K. 1953. Functional changes in chromatolysed motoneurons. *J. Comp. Neurol.* 98:9–36

37. Heyer, C. B., Llinas, R. 1977. Control of rhythmic firing in normal and axotomized cat spinal motoneurons. *J. Neurophysiol.* 40:480–88

38. Traub, R. D., Llinas, R. 1977. The spatial distribution of tonic conductances in normal and axotomized motoneurons. *Neuroscience* 2:829–49

39. Gustafsson, B. 1979. Changes in motoneurone electrical properties following axotomy. *J. Physiol.* 293:197–215

40. Takata, M., Shahara, E., Fujita, S. 1980. The excitability of hypoglossal motoneurons undergoing chromatolysis. *Neuroscience* 5:413–19

41. Kuno, M., Miyata, Y., Muñoz-Martinez, E. J. 1974. Differential reaction of fast and slow alpha motoneurons to axotomy. *J. Physiol.* 240:725–39

42. Huizar, P., Kuno, M., Kudo, N., Miyata, Y. 1977. Reaction of intact spinal motoneurons to partial denervation of the muscle. *J. Physiol.* 205:175–91

43. Cullheim, S., Risling, M., 1982. Observations on the morphology and axonal conduction velocity of axotomized and regenerating sciatic motoneurons in the kitten. *Exp. Brain Res.* 45:428–32

44. Burke, R. E. 1982. Motor units: anatomy, physiology and functional organization. In *Handbook of Physiology, Section 1: The Nervous System. II. Motor System*, ed. V. B. Brook, pp. 345–422. Bethesda, Md: Am. Physiol. Soc.

45. Gustafsson, B., Pinter, M. J. 1984. Effects of axotomy on the distribution of passive electrical properties of cat motoneurons. *J. Physiol.* 356:433–42

46. Prineas, J., Spencer, P. S. 1975. Pathology of the nerve cell body in disorders of the peripheral nervous system. In *Peripheral Neuropathy*, Vol. I, ed. P. J. Dyck, P. K. Thomas, E. H. Lambert, pp. 253–95. Philadelphia: W. B. Saunders

47. Spencer, P. S., Schaumburg, H. H.

1980. *Experimental and Clinical Neurotoxicology.* Baltimore: Williams & Wilkins

48. Cho, E.-S. 1977. Toxic effects of adriamycin on the ganglia of the peripheral nervous system: a neuropathological study. *J. Neuropathol. Exp. Neurol.* 36:907–15

49. Prineas, J. 1969. The pathogenesis of dying-back polyneuropathies. II. An ultrastructural study of experimental acrylamide intoxication in the cat. *J. Neuropathol. Exp. Neurol.* 28:598–621

50. Cavanagh, J. B. 1967. On the pattern of change in peripheral nerves produced by isoniazid intoxication in rats. *J. Neurol. Neurosurg. Psychiatry* 30:26–33

51. Clark, A. W., Griffin, J. W., Price, D. L. 1980. The axonal pathology in chronic IDPN intoxication. *J. Neuropathol. Exp. Neurol.* 39:42–55

52. Delio, D. A., Fiori, M. G., Sharer, L. R., Lowndes, H. E. 1985. Evolution of axonal swellings in cats intoxicated with β,β'-iminodipropionitrile (IDPN). An electrophysiological and morphological study. *Exp. Neurol.* 87:235–48

53. Wisniewski, H. M., Narkiewicz, O., Wisniewski, K. 1967. Topography and dynamics of neurofibrillar degeneration in aluminum encephalopathy. *Acta Neuropathol.* 9:127–33

54. Wisniewski, H. M., Sturman, J. A., Shek, J. W. 1980. Aluminum chloride induced neurofibrillary changes in the developing rabbit: a chronic animal model. *Ann. Neurol.* 8:479–90

55. Shelanski, M. L., Wisniewski, H. 1969. Neurofibrillary degeneration induced by vincristine therapy. *Arch. Neurol.* 20:194–206

56. Fiori, M. G., Lowndes, H. E. 1986. Unusual neurofibrillary accumulations induced by β,β'-iminodipropionitrile (IDPN). Submitted for publication

57. Cavanagh, J. B. 1982. The pathokinetics of acrylamide intoxication: a reassessment of the problem. *Neuropathol. Appl. Neurobiol.* 8:315–36

58. Sterman, A. B. 1982. Acrylamide induces early morphologic reorganization of the neuronal cell body. *Neurology* 32:1023–26

59. Somjen, G. G., Herman, S. P., Klein, R. 1973. Electrophysiology of methyl mercury poisoning. *J. Pharmacol. Exp. Ther.* 186:579–92

60. Cavanagh, J. B., Chen, F. C. K. 1971. The effects of methyl mercury dicyandiamide on the peripheral nerves and spinal cord of rats. *Acta Neuropathol.* 19:208–15

61. Herman, S. P., Klein, R., Talley, F. A., Krigman, M. R. 1973. An ultrastructural study of methyl mercury induced primary sensory neuropathy in the rat. *Lab. Invest.* 28:104–18

62. Lowndes, H. E., Delio, D. A., Gold, B. G. 1985. Electrophysiological investigation of IDPN neuropathy-initial studies. *Neurotoxicol.* 6:25–42

63. Gold, B. G., Lowndes, H. E. 1984. Electrophysiological investigation of β,β'-iminodipropionitrile neuropathy: intracellular recordings in spinal cord. *Brain Res.* 308:235–44

64. Delio, D. A., Lowndes, H. E. 1986. Changes in contractile properties of identified motor unit types during the evolution of axonal swellings in β,β'-iminodipropionitrile neuropathy. In preparation

65. Delio, D. A., Lowndes, H. E. 1986. Motoneuron afterhyperpolarization, delayed depolarization and repetitive firing during the evolution of β,β'-iminodipropionitrile neuropathy. Submitted for publication

66. Delio, D. A., Lowndes, H. E. 1986. Motoneuron frequency-current responses in IDPN neuropathy. Submitted for publication

67. Waller, A. V. 1850. Experiments on the section of the glossopharyngeal and hypoglossal nerves of the frog, and observation on the alterations produced thereby in the structure of their premature-fibers. *Philos. Trans. R. Soc. London, Ser B.* 140:423–29

68. Guth, L. 1956. Regeneration in the mammalian peripheral nervous system. *Physiol. Rev.* 36:441–78

69. Sunderland S. 1978. *Nerves and Nerve Injuries.* London: Chruchill Livingstone. 2nd ed.

70. Zelena, J., Lubinska, L., Gutmann, E. 1968. Accumulations of organelles at the ends of interrupted axons. *Z. Zellforsch. Microsk. Anat.* 91:200–19

71. Donat, J. R., Wisniewski, H. M. 1973. The spatio-temporal pattern of Wallerian degeneration in mammalian peripheral nerves. *Brain Res.* 53:41–53

72. Williams, P. L., Hall, S. M. 1971. Prolonged in vivo observations of normal peripheral nerve fibers and their acute reactions to crush and deliberate trauma. *J. Anat.* 108:397–408

73. William, P. L., Hall, S. M. 1971. Chronic Wallerian degeneration—an in vivo and ultrastructural study. *J. Anat.* 109:487–503

74. Cavanagh, J. B., Gysbers, M. F. 1980. "Dying-back" above a nerve ligature pro-

duced by acrylamide. *Acta Neuropathol.* 51:169–77

75. Cavanagh, J. B., Gysbers, M. F. 1981. Ultrastructural changes in axons caused by acrylamide above a nerve ligature. *Neuropathol. Appl. Neurobiol.* 7:315–26

76. Kiraly, J. K., Krnjevic, K. 1959. Some retrograde changes in function of nerves after peripheral section. *Q. J. Exp. Physiol.* 44:244–57

77. Riker, W. F., Jr., Okamoto, M., 1969. Pharmacology of motor nerve terminals. *Ann. Rev. Pharmacol.* 9:173–208

78. Gilliat R. N., Hjarth, R. J. 1972. Nerve conduction during Wallerian degeneration in the baboon. *J. Neurol. Neurosurg. Psychiatry* 35:335–41

79. Cammer, W. 1980. Toxic demyelination: biochemical studies and hypothetical mechanism. See Ref. 47, pp. 239–56

80. Spencer, P. S., Schaumburg, H. H. 1980. Classification of neurotoxic disease: a morphological approach. See Ref. 47, pp. 92–99

81. Denny-Brown, D., Brenner, C. 1944. Paralysis of nerve induced by direct pressure and tourniquet. *Arch. Neurol. Psychiatry* 51:1–26

82. Sumner, A. J. 1980. Axonal polyneuropathies. See Ref. 9, pp. 340–57

83. Cragg, B. G., Thomas, P. K. 1964. Changes in nerve conduction in experimental allergic neuritis. *J. Neurol. Neurosurg. Psychiatry* 27:106–15

84. Mayer, R. F., Denny-Brown, D. 1964. Conduction velocity in peripheral nerve during experimental demyelination in the cat. *Neurology* 14:714–26

85. McDonald, W. I. 1963. The effects of experimental demyelination on conduction in peripheral nerve: a histological and electrophysiological study. II. Electrophysiological observations. *Brain* 86:501–24

86. Goldstein, B. D., Lowndes, H. E., Cho, E. S. 1981. Neurotoxicology of vincristine in the cat. Electrophysiological studies. *Arch. Toxicol.* 48:253–64

87. Cho, E-S., Lowndes, H. E., Goldstein, B. D. 1983. Neurotoxicology of vincristine in the cat. Morphological study. *Arch. Toxicol.* 52:83–90

88. Anderson, R. J. 1986. Peripheral nerve conduction velocities and excitability. In *Electrophysiology in Neurotoxicology*. ed. H. E. Lowndes. Boca Raton: CRC. In press

89. Hall, J. I. 1967. Studies on demyelinated peripheral nerves in guinea pigs with experimental allergic neuritis, a histological and electrophysiological study. II.

Electrophysiological observations. *Brain* 90:313–32

90. McDonald, W. I., Gelman, S. 1968. Demyelination and muscle spindle function: Effect of diphtheritic polyneuritis on nerve conduction and muscle spindle function in the cat. *Arch. Neurol.* 18:508–19

91. McDonald, W. I., Sears, T. A. 1970. Effect of experimental demyelination on conduction in the central nervous system. *Brain* 93:583–98

92. Thomas, P. K., Lascelles, R. G. 1965. Schwann cell abnormalities in diabetic neuropathy. *Lancet* 1:1355–57

93. Rasminsky, M., Sears, T. 1972. Intranodal conduction in undissected demyelinated nerve fibres. *J. Physiol.* 277:323–50

94. Morgan-Hughes, J. A. 1968. Experimental diphtheritic neuropathy, a pathological and electrophysiological study. *J. Neurol. Sci.* 7:157–75

95. Koles, F. J., Rasminsky, M. 1972. A computer simulation of conduction on demyelinated nerve fibres. *J. Physiol.* 227:351–64

96. Graham, D. I., de Jesus, P. V., Pleasure, D. E., Gonatas, N. K. 1976. Triethyltin sulfate–induced neuropathy in rats: Electrophysiologic, morphologic and biochemical studies. *Arch. Neurol.* 33:40–48

97. Rasminsky, M. 1978. Physiology of conduction in demyelinated axons. See Ref. 26, pp. 361–76

98. Funch, P. G., Faber, D. S. 1984. Measurement of myelin sheath resistances: implications for axonal conduction and pathophysiology. *Science* 225:538–40

99. Smith, R. S., Koles, Z. J. 1970. Myelinated nerve fibers: computed effect of myelin thickness on conduction velocity. *Am. J. Physiol.* 219:1256–58

100. Bostock, H. 1984. Internodal conduction along undissected nerve fibers in experimental neuropathy. In *Peripheral Neuropathy*, Vol. 1, ed. P. J. Dyck, P. K. Thomas, E. H. Lambert, R. Bunge, pp. 900–910. Philadelphia: Saunders

101. Bostock, H., Sears, T. A. 1976. Continuous conduction in demyelinated mammalian nerve fibres. *Nature* 263:786–87

102. Lehmann, H. J. 1967. Zur Pathophysiologie der Retracturperiode peripherer Nerven. *Dtsch. Z. Nervenheilkd.* 192:185–92

103. Lehmann, H. J., Pretschner, D. P. 1966. Experimentelle Untersuchungen zum

Engpassyndrom peripherer Nerven. *Dtsch. Z. Nervenheilkd.* 188:308–30

104. Davis, F. A. 1972. Impairment of repetitive impulse conduction in experimentally demyelinated and pressure injured nerves. *J. Neurol. Neurosurg. Psychiatry* 35:537–44

105. Lehmann, H. J., Tackmann, W., Lehmann, G. 1971. Funktionsänderung markhältiger Nervenfasern in N-tibialis des Meerschweinchens bei post diphtherischer Polyneuritis. *Z. Neurol.* 199:86–104

106. Schaumburg, H. H., Wisniewski, H. M., Spencer, P. S. 1974. Ultrastructural studies of the dying-back process. I. Peripheral nerve terminal and axon degeneration in systemic acrylamide intoxication. *J. Neuropathol. Exp. Neurol.* 33:260–84

107. Troncoso, J. C., Price, D. L., Griffin, J. W., Pashach, I. M. 1982. Axonal pathology in aluminum intoxication. *Ann. Neurol.* 12:278–83

108. Linnoila, I., Haltia, M., Seppalainen, A. M., Polo, J. 1975. Experimental carbon disulphide poisoning: morphological and neurophysiological studies. In *Proceedings VIIth International Congress of Neuropathology, Budapest 1974*, Vol. II. ed. St. Kornyey, St. Tariska, G. Gasztanyi, 383A. Amsterdam: Exerpta Medica

109. Szendzikowski, S., Stetkiewicz, J., Wionska-Noter, T., Zdrajkowska, I. 1973. Structural aspects of experimental carbon disulfide neuropathy. I. Development of neurohistological changes in chronically intoxicated rats. *Int. Arch. Arbeitsmedizin* 31:135–49

110. Anthony, D. C., Bockleheide, K., Graham, D. G. 1983. The effect of 3,4-dimethyl substitution on the neurotoxicity of 2,5-hexanedione. I. Accelerated clinical neuropathy is accompanied by more proximal swellings. *Toxicol. Appl. Pharmacol.* 72:362–71

111. Anthony, D. C., Giangaspero, F., Graham, D. G. 1983. The spatiotemporal pattern of the axonopathy associated with the neurotoxicity of 3,4-dimethyl,2,5-hexanedione in the rat. *J. Neuropathol. Exp. Neurol.* 42:548–60

112. Spencer, P. S., Schaumburg, H. H. 1976. Feline nervous system response to chronic intoxication with commercial grades of methyl n-butyl ketone, methyl isobutyl ketone and methyl ethyl ketone. *Toxicol. Appl. Pharmacol.* 37:301–11

113. Spencer, P. S., Schaumburg, H. H. 1977. Ultrastructural studies of the dying-back process. IV. Differential vulnerability of PNS and CNS fibers in experimental centralperipheral distal axonopathies. *J. Neuropathol. Exp. Neurol.* 36:300–20

114. Chou, S. M., Hartmann, H. A. 1964. Axonal lesions and waltzing syndrome after IDPN administration in rats. With a concept—"Axostasis". *Acta Neuropathol.* 3:428–50

115. Griffin, J. W., Gold, B. G., Cork, L. C., Price, D. L., Lowndes, H. E. 1982. IDPN neuropathy in the cat: coexistence of proximal and distal axonal swellings. *Neuropathol. Appl. Neurobiol.* 8:351–64

116. Spencer, P. S., Couri, D., Schaumburg, H. H. 1980. n-Hexane and methyl n-butyl ketone. See Ref. 47, pp. 456–75

117. Griffin, J. W., Price, D. L. 1981. Demyelination in experimental IDPN and hexacarbon neuropathies: evidence for an axonal influence. *Lab. Invest.* 45:130–41

118. LeQuesne, P. M. 1980. Acrylamide. See Ref. 47, pp. 309–25

119. Seppalainen, A. M., Haltia, M. 1980. Carbon disulfide. See Ref. 47, pp. 356–73

120. Long, R. R., Griffin, J. W., Stanley, E. F., Price, D. L. 1980. Myelin sheath responses to alterations in axon caliber. *Neurology* 30:435A

121. Griffin, J. W., Cork, L. C., Hoffman, P. N., Price, D. L. 1984. Experimental models of motor neuron degeneration. See Ref. 100, pp. 621–35

122. Goldstein, S. S., Rall, W. 1974. Changes in action potential shape and velocity for changing core conduction geometry. *Biophys. J.* 14:731–57

123. Goldstein, S. S. 1978. Models of conduction in nonuniform axons. See Ref. 26, pp. 227–36

124. Parnas, I., Hochstein, S., Parnas, H. 1976. Theoretical analysis of parameters leading to frequency modulation along an inhomogeneous axon. *J. Neurophysiol.* 39:909–23

125. Ramon, F., Moore, J. W., Joyner, R. W., Westerfield, N. 1976. Squid giant axons: a model of the neuron soma? *Biophys. J.* 16:953–63

126. Grampp, W. 1966. Impulse activity in different parts of the slowly adapting stretch receptor of the lobster. *Acta Physiol. Scand.* 66: Suppl. 262:3–63

127. Calvin, W. H., Hartline, D. K. 1976. Retrograde invasion of lobster stretch receptor somata in control of firing rate and extraspike patterning. *J. Neurophysiol.* 39:106–18

128. Granit, R. 1972. *Mechanisms Regulating the Discharge of Motoneurons*, pp. 27–47. Springfield, Ill: C. C. Thomas

129. Nelson, P. G., Burke, R. E. 1967. Delayed depolarizations in cat motoneurons. *Exp. Neurol.* 17:16–26

130. Gold, B. G., Lowndes, H. E. 1984. Electrophysiological investigation of β, β'-iminodipropionitrile neurotoxicity: monosynaptic reflexes and recurrent inhibition. *Neurotoxicol.* 5:1–14

131. Granit, R., Leksell, L., Skogland, C. R. 1944. Fibre interaction in injured or compressed regions of nerve. *Brain* 67:125–40

132. Granit, R., Skogland, C. R. 1945. Facilitation, inhibition and depression at the artificial synapse formed by the cut end of a mammalian nerve. *J. Physiol.* 103:434–48

133. Huizar, P., Kuno, M., Miyoto, Y. 1975. Electrophysiological properties of spinal motoneurons of normal and dystrophic mice. *J. Physiol.* 248:231–46

134. Rasminsky, M. 1978. Ectopic generation of impulses and crosstalk in spinal nerve roots of "dystrophic" mice. *Ann. Neurol.* 3:351–57

135. Rasminsky, M. 1980. Ephaptic transmission between single nerve fibres in the spinal nerve roots of dystrophic mice. *J. Physiol.* 305:151–69

136. Rasminsky, M. 1982. Ectopic excitation, ephaptic excitation and auto-excitation in peripheral nerve fibers of mutant mice. In *Abnormal Nerves and Muscles as Impulse Generators*, ed. W. J. Culp, J. Ochoa, pp. 344–62. Oxford: Oxford Univ. Press

137. Devon, M., Bernstein, J. J. 1982. Abnormal impulse generation in neuromas: electrophysiology and ultrastructure. See Ref. 136, pp. 363–80

138. Hernandez-Cruz, A., Muñoz-Martinez, E. J. 1984. Axon-to-axon transmission in *Tullidora* (buckthorn) neuropathy. *Exp. Neurol.* 84:533–48

139. Delio, D. A., Lowndes, H. E. 1986. Electrical crosstalk between intraspinal elements during progression of IDPN neuropathy. *Exp. Neurol.* In press

140. Gold, B. G., Griffin, J. W., Price, D. L., Cork, L. C., Lowndes, H. E. 1985. Structural correlates of some physiological alterations in IDPN neuropathy. *Brain Res.* In press

141. Griffin, J. W., Cork, L. C., Troncoso, J. C., Price, D. L. 1982. Experimental neurotoxic disorders of motor neurons: neurofibrillary pathology. In *Advances in Neurology*, Vol. 36, *Human Motor Neuron Diseases*, ed. L. P. Rowland, pp. 419–431. New York: Raven

142. Hofinger, E., LeQuesne, P. M., Gajree, T. 1982. Conduction velocity in nerve fibres with axonal atrophy due to chronic β,β'-iminodipropionitrile (IDPN). *J. Neurol. Sci.* 53:159–67

143. Fahnestock, K., Griffin, J. W., Hoffman, P. N., Anthony, C. D., Graham, D. G. 1984. Caliber-dependent vulnerability in IDPN and DMHD neurotoxicity. *Neurotoxicology* 5:304–5

144. Brimijoin, S. 1984. The role of axonal transport in nerve disease. See Ref. 100, pp. 477–93

145. Lowndes, H. E., Baker, T., Cho, E. S., Jortner, B. S. 1978. Position sensitivity of de-efferented muscle spindles in experimental acrylamide neuropathy. *J. Pharmacol. Exp. Ther.* 205:40–48

146. Lowndes, H. E., Baker, T. 1976. Studies on drug-induced neuropathies. III. Motor nerve deficit in cats with acrylamide neuropathy. *Eur. J. Pharmacol.* 35:177–84

147. Cho, E-S., Spencer, P. S., Jortner, B. S. 1980. Doxorubicin. See Ref. 47, pp. 430–39

148. Yamamoto, T., Zwasaki, Y., Konno, H. 1984. Retrograde transport of adriamycin: an experimental form of motor neuron disease? *Neurology* 34:1299–1304

149. Thompson, S. W., Davis, L. E., Kornfeld, M., Hilgers, R. D., Standeter, J. C. 1984. Cisplatin neuropathy. Clinical, electrophysiologic, morphologic and toxicologic studies. *Cancer* 54:1269–75

150. Lowndes, H. E., Baker, T., Riker, W. F. Jr. 1974. Motor nerve dysfunction in delayed DFP neuropathy. *Eur. J. Pharmacol.* 29:66–73

151. Baker, T., Lowndes, H. E. 1980. Muscle spindle function in organophosphorus neuropathy. *Brain Res.* 185:77–84

152. Goldstein, B. D., Lowndes, H. E. 1979. Spinal cord defect in the peripheral neuropathy resulting from acrylamide. *Neurotoxicology* 1:75–87

153. Goldstein, B. D., Lowndes, H. E. 1981. Group Ia primary afferent terminal defect in cats with acrylamide neuropathy. *Neurotoxicol.* 2:297–312

154. Cavanagh, J. B. 1964. Peripheral nerve changes in ortho-cresyl phosphate poisoning in the cat. *J. Pathol. Bacteriol.* 87:365–82

155. Sumner, A. J., Asbury, A. K. 1975. Physiological studies of the dying-back phenomenon. Muscle stretch afferents in acrylamide neuropathy. *Brain* 98:91–100

156. Cavanagh, J. B., Nolan, C. C. 1982. Selective loss of Purkinje cells from the rat cerebellum caused by acrylamide and the responses of β-glucuronidase and β-

galactosidase. *Acta Neuropathol.* 58: 210–14

157. Lowndes, H. E., Baker, T., Michelson, L. P., Vincent-Ablazey, M. 1978. Attenuated dynamic responses of primary endings of muscle spindles: a basis for depressed tendon responses in acrylamide neuropathy. *Ann. Neurol.* 3:433–37

158. Goldstein, B. G. 1985. Electrophysiological changes in peripheral sensory receptors following sub-acute administration of soman. *Toxicologist* 5:85

159. Goldstein, B. G. 1986. Sensory nerve terminal function. In *Electrophysiology in Neurotoxicology*, ed. H. E. Lowndes. Boca Raton: CRC. In press

160. Spencer, P. S., Hanna, R., Sussman, M., Pappas, G. 1977. Inactivation of pacinian corpuscle mechano-sensitivity by acrylamide. *J. Gen. Physiol.* 70:17a

161. Goldstein, B. D. 1985. Cutaneous sensory receptors are reduced in number following acrylamide administration. *Toxicologist* 5:84

162. Leon, J., McComas, A. J. 1984. Effects of vincristine sulfate on touch dome function in the rat. *Exp. Neurol.* 84:283–91

163. Sterman, A. B., Sposito, N. 1984. Motoneuron axosomatic synapses are altered in axonopathy. *J. Neuropathol. Exp. Neurol.* 43:201–9

164. Schaumburg, H. H., Spencer, P. S. 1980. Clioquinol. See Ref. 47, pp. 395–406

165. Goldstein, B. D. 1985. Acrylamide neurotoxicity: altered spinal monosynaptic responses to quipazine, a serotonin agonist in cats. *Toxicol. Appl. Pharmacol.* 78:436–44

166. DeRojas, T., Goldstein, B. D. 1985. Acrylamide alters the function of the primary afferent terminal. *Soc. Neurosci. Abstr.* 11:995

167. Lapadula, D. M., Kinnes, C. G., Somjen, G. G., Abou-Donia, M. B. 1982. Monosynaptic reflex depression in cats with organophosphorous neuropathy: effects of tri-o-cresyl phosphate. *Neurotoxicology* 3:51–62

168. Goldstein, B. G. 1986. Spinal cord reflexes. In *Electrophysiology in Neurotoxicology*. ed. H. E. Lowndes, Boca Raton: CRC. In press

169. Lowndes, H. E., Baker, T., Riker, W. F. Jr. 1975. Motor nerve terminal responsiveness to edrophonium in delayed DFP neuropathy. *Eur. J. Pharmacol.* 30:66–72

170. Glazer, E., Baker, T., Riker, W. F. Jr. 1978. The neuropathology of DFP at cat soleus neuromuscular junction. *J. Neurocytol.* 7:741–58

171. Baker, T., Drakontides, A. B., Riker, W. F. Jr. 1982. Prevention of the organophosphorus neuropathy by glucocorticoids. *Exp. Neurol.* 78:397–408

172. Drakontides, A. B., Baker, T., Riker W. F. Jr. 1982. A morphological study of the effect of glucocorticoid treatment on delayed organophosphorus neuropathy. *Neurotoxicology* 3:167–78

173. Drakontides, A. B., Baker, T. 1983. An electrophysiologic and ultrastructural study of the phenylmethanesulfanyl fluoride protection against a delayed organophosphorous neuropathy. *Toxicol. Appl. Pharmacol.* 70:411–22

174. Baker, T., Lowndes, H. E. 1984. The effect of iminodipropionitrile on mammalian motor nerve endings. *Pharmacologist* 26:230 (Abstr.)

175. Weiler, M. H., Peterson, R. E. 1984. 2,4-Dithiobiuret depresses transmitter release at the rat neuromuscular junction. *Soc. Neurosci. Abstr.* 10:1197

176. Atchison, W. D., Lalley, P. M., Cassens, R. G., Peterson, R. 1981. Depression of neuromuscular function in the rat by chronic 2,4-dithiobiuret treatment. *Neurotoxicology* 2:(2)329–46

177. Manalis, R. S., Cooper, G. P. 1973. Presynaptic and postsynaptic effects of lead at the frog neuromuscular junction. *Nature* 243:354–56

178. Cooper, G. P., Manalis, R. S. 1984. Interactions of lead and cadmium on acetylcholine release at the frog neuromuscular junction. *Toxicol. Appl. Pharmacol.* 74: 411–16

179. Cooper, G. P., Manalis, R. S. 1984. Heavy metals: effects on synaptic transmission. *Neurotoxicology* 5:247–66

180. Atchison, W. D., Narahashi, T. 1982. Methyl mercury-induced depression of neuromuscular transmission in the rat. *Neurotoxicology* 3:(3)37–50

181. Miyamoto, M. D. 1983. Hg^{++} causes neurotoxicity at an intracellular site following entry through Na and Ca channels. *Brain Res.* 267:375–79

182. Okamoto, M., Longenecker, H. E., Riker, W. F., Long, S. K. 1971. Destruction of mammalian motor nerve terminals by black widow spider venom. *Science* 172:733–36

183. Kostial, K., Vouk, V. B. Lead ions and synaptic treatment in the superior cervical ganglion of the cat. *Br. J. Pharmacol.* 12:219–22

184. Kober, T. E., Cooper, G. P. 1976. Lead competitively inhibits calcium-dependent synaptic transmission in the bullfrog sympathetic ganglion. *Nature* 262:704–5

185. Atchison, W. D., Narahashi, T. 1984. Mechanism of action of lead on neuromuscular junctions. *Neurotoxicology* 5:(3)267–82

186. Manalis, R. S., Cooper, G. P., Pomeroy, S. E. 1984. Effect of lead on neuromuscular transmission in the frog. *Brain Res.* 294:95–109

187. Audesirk, G., Audesirk, T. 1983. Effects of chronic low level lead exposure on the physiology of individually identifiable neurons. *Neurotoxicology* 4(4):13–26

188. Manalis, R. S., Cooper, G. P. 1975. Evoked transmitter release increased by inorganic mercury at frog neuromuscular junction. *Nature* 257:690–91

189. Allen, J. E., Gage, P. W., Leaver, D. D., Leow, A. C. T. 1980. Triethyltin depresses evoked transmitter release at the mouse neuromuscular junction. *Chem. Biol. Interact.* 31:227–31

190. Bierkamper, G. G., Valdes, J. D. 1982. Triethyltin intoxication alters acetylcholine release from rat phrenic nerve-hemidiaphragm. *Neurobehav. Toxicol. Teratol.* 4:251–54

191. Millington, W. R., Bierkamper, G. G., 1982. Chronic triethyltin exposure reduces the resting membrane potential of rat soleus muscle. *Neurobehav. Toxicol. Teratol.* 4:255–57

192. Katz, B., Miledi, R. 1975. The nature of the prolonged endplate depolarization in anti-esterase treated muscle. *Proc. Roy. Soc. Lond. (B) J. Physiol.* 231:549–74

193. Bierkamper, G. G. 1981. Electrophysiological effects of diisopropylfluorophosphate on neuromuscular transmission. *Eur. J. Pharmacol.* 73:343–48

194. Kordas, M. 1977. On the role of junctional cholinesterase in determining the time course of end-plate current. *J. Physiol.* 270:133–50

195. Kuba, K., Albuquerque, E. X., Barnard, E. A. 1973. Diisopropylfluorophosphate: suppression of ionic conductance of the cholinergic receptor. *Science* 181: 853–56

196. Laskowski, M. B., Dethbarn, W-D. 1975. Presynaptic effects of neuromuscular cholinesterase inhibition. *J. Pharmacol. Exp. Ther.* 194:351–56

197. Fox, D. A., Lowndes, H. E., Bierkamper, G. G. 1982. Electrophysiological techniques in neurotoxicology. In *Nervous System Toxicology*, ed. C. L. Mitchell, pp. 299–335. New York: Raven

198. Atchison, W. D. 1984. Decreased quantal content associated with dithiobiuret-induced paralysis in the rat. *Soc. Neurosci. Abstr.* 10:201

199. Gage, P. W. 1965. The effect of methyl, ethyl and n-propyl-alcohol on neuromuscular transmission in the rat. *J. Pharmacol. Exp. Ther.* 150:236–43

200. Gage, P. W., McBurney, R. N., Schneider, G. T. 1975. Effects of some aliphatic alcohols on the conductance change caused by a quantum of acetylcholine at the toad end-plate. *J. Physiol.* 244:409–29

201. Cangiano, A., Lutzemberger, L., Rizzuto, N., Simonati, A., Rossi, A., Toschi, G. 1980. Neurotoxic effects of 2,5-hexanedione in rats: Early morphological and functional changes in nerve fibers and neuromuscular junctions. *Neurotoxicology* 2:25–32

Ann. Rev. Pharmacol. Toxicol. 1986. 26:547–65
Copyright © 1986 by Annual Reviews Inc. All rights reserved

TOXICOLOGICAL ASPECTS OF ALTERATIONS OF PULMONARY MACROPHAGE FUNCTION

Joseph D. Brain

Department of Environmental Science and Physiology, Harvard University School of Public Health, 665 Huntington Avenue, Boston, Massachusetts 02115

INTRODUCTION

Pulmonary macrophages are similar to mononuclear phagocytes throughout the body, such as those found in the peritoneal cavity or liver. Yet, pulmonary macrophages face unique challenges. Found on the inner surfaces of the respiratory tract, they come in direct contact with toxic particles and gases as well as pathogens contained in the inspired air. Their mobility, phagocytic capacity, and bactericidal properties are essential to the maintenance of clean and sterile alveoli.

Since these cells are accessible by bronchopulmonary lavage, they have been studied extensively in vitro. Our knowledge of the cell biology and toxicology of phagocytic cells has been extended by experiments with isolated pulmonary macrophages. These cells are of interest since their migratory patterns, phagocytic behavior, and secretory potential are pivotal events in the pathogenesis of pulmonary disease. Even though macrophages are an essential line of defense for airway and alveolar surfaces, they can also injure the host. For these reasons, the toxicology of pulmonary macrophages is an essential aspect of how toxic agents injure the lung (1).

Under certain conditions, macrophages are damaged as a consequence of particle ingestion, and the nature of that damage is relevant to pulmonary disease. In response to phagocytic stimuli, macrophages secrete lysosomal hydrolases, proteases, and antiproteases, chemotactic factors, interferon, and other mediators (2). Excessive or prolonged secretion, or secretion in an inappropriate site, can cause tissue damage. An imbalance between protease and antiprotease levels in the lungs can lead to emphysema [reviewed by P. J.

547

0362-1642/86/0415-0547$02.00

Stone (3)]. Macrophages may be involved in this process either by secretion of the neutral protease, elastase (4), or by binding and releasing the polymorphonuclear neutrophil elastase (5). In vitro studies show that macrophages, after stimulation with a variety of agents such as crystalline silica (6) or cold-insoluble globulin (7), produce factors that stimulate fibroblast proliferation and/or collagen production. The production of such factors in vivo are relevant to wound healing (8) and are important in fibrogenesis. Macrophages appear to be involved in the pathogenesis of atherosclerosis (9); they may also have a role in identifying and destroying neoplastic cells (10). Finally, pulmonary macrophages appear to present antigen in vivo to T cells and thereby trigger T cell–dependent immune responses (11). In turn, the phagocytic activity of macrophages may be modified by local antibody production (12).

In this review we describe the major classes of pulmonary macrophages and discuss their origin, function, and quantitation. After discussing how toxic particles and gases affect pulmonary macrophages, we summarize evidence that macrophages may contribute to the pathogenesis of pulmonary diseases.

CLASSES OF PULMONARY MACROPHAGES

Pulmonary macrophages encompass at least three types: the best known is the alveolar macrophage. Alveolar macrophages are large, mononuclear, phagocytic cells found on alveolar surfaces. They are not part of the continuous epithelial layer of Type 1 and Type 2 cells, rather, alveolar macrophages rest on this lining covered by surfactant. Figure 1 shows a hamster alveolar macrophage containing ingested iron oxide particles. Another kind of pulmonary macrophage is the airway macrophage (13). Airway macrophages can be found in the conducting airways, both large and small. They may be present as passengers on the mucus escalator, or they may be found beneath the mucus lining, adhering to the bronchial epithelium (14).

Interstitial macrophages comprise a third subdivision of pulmonary macrophages. They are found in the various connective tissue compartments of the lung, including alveolar walls, lymph nodes, and peribronchial and perivascular spaces. In addition to these three primary types, other minor macrophage compartments exist. For example, macrophages are found in the pleural space. In some species, there may also be intravascular macrophages similar to Kupffer cells in the hepatic sinusoids. In ruminants, these macrophages are very prominent (15).

Even macrophages from a single compartment need not be homogeneous. Both in structure and in function, heterogeneity is common. Many investigators have described considerable variability in macrophages recovered by bronchoalveolar lavage. For example, Godleski et al (16) have shown that hamster lung macrophages vary considerably in regard to the amount of antigen present

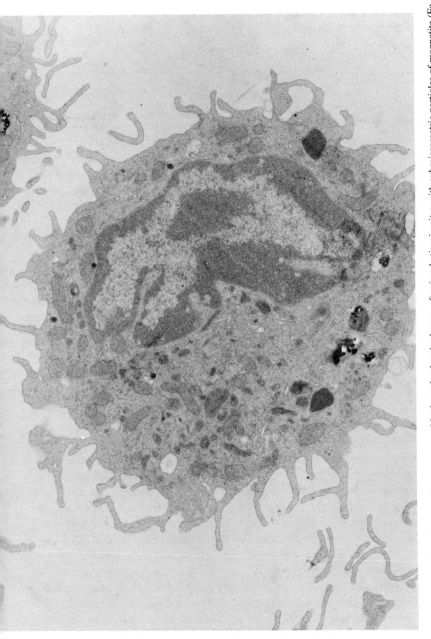

Figure 1 Hamster alveolar macrophages recovered by bronchoalveolar lavage after incubation in vitro with submicrometric particles of magnetite (Fe_3O_4). These electron-dense particles can be seen in the phagolysosomes on the lower left side of the nucleus and in the phagolysosome in part of another alveolar macrophage visible in the upper right corner. Many small pseudopods extend from the plasma membrane. 10,800 X. (Courtesy of Dr. Peter Valberg and Ms. Rebecca Stearns)

on their plasma membranes. This antigen is not present on macrophages in other organs, and increasing amounts of antigen on alveolar macrophages appear to correlate with the length of time that they have been resident in the alveolar space (17).

ORIGIN OF PULMONARY MACROPHAGES

The origin and kinetics of pulmonary macrophages have received extensive study (18, 19). The data demonstrate that multiple strategies for maintaining the macrophage population in the lungs exist. In normal unchallenged animals, the immediate precursors are supplied by a cell renewal system in the pulmonary interstitium. Division of existing alveolar macrophages may also contribute to the maintenance of a pool of free cells. Demand for more macrophages, as a result of infection or deposition of large numbers of inhaled particles, may be met by (a) increased multiplication of free macrophages, (b) release of preexisting cells from reservoirs within the lungs, (c) increased production from macrophage precursors in the lung interstitium, and (d) an increased flux of monocytes from the blood to the lung. Newborn animals have relatively few pulmonary macrophages; those present are immature. However, within a week or so normal numbers of fully activated macrophages develop in the lungs (20).

FUNCTION OF PULMONARY MACROPHAGES

Particle Clearance

Macrophages keep the surfaces of the lungs clean and sterile. They ingest inhaled pathogens and particles as well as endogenous effete cells and even "worn-out" surfactant (21). Several reviews of these functions are available (18, 19, 22–25).

Although large numbers of infectious particles are continuously deposited in the lungs, the alveolar surface is usually sterile. During acute infection or injury they are also supplemented by other leukocytes. Increased particles stimulate the recruitment of additional macrophages. Like other phagocytes, alveolar macrophages are rich in lysosomes, subcellular organelles 0.5 μm or less in diameter (see Figure 1). Among the enzymes known to be present in lysosomes are proteases (26), acid ribonuclease (26), β-glucuronidase (27), acid phosphatase (26, 27), lysozyme (28), β-galactosidase (29), and phospholipases (30). The lysosomes attach themselves to the phagosomal membrane surrounding the ingested pathogen. Then the lysosomal and phagosomal membranes become continuous, and the lytic enzymes kill and digest the bacteria. Macrophages also are responsible for the intracellular killing of parasites such as African trypanosomes and malarial parasites (31). Lung macrophages are also involved in the response to viral infections (32–34).

More important to the microbicidal activity of macrophages than lytic enzymes are the oxygen-dependent cytotoxic systems. Although best described in neutrophils (35, 36), these mechanisms are also present in pulmonary macrophages. Phagocytosis triggers increased oxygen consumption and the generation of oxygen radicals such as superoxide (O_2^-), hydroxyl radicals, singlet oxygen, and H_2O_2. These highly reactive oxygen derivatives modify macromolecules of pathogens. Lipids, proteins, and nucleic acids may be modified by (myelo)peroxidase and halide-mediated oxygen-dependent reactions (36). Damaging oxidizing agents can also include several halogen derivatives such as chlorine, chloridium ions, and hypochlorous acid. Macrophages also contain ingredients that can protect them against the damaging effects of these oxidizing agents. Protective substances include vitamin E, ascorbic acid, and the glutathione redox system as well as catalase and superoxide dismutase.

Not only do pulmonary macrophages ingest and kill pathogens but they also deal with nonliving, insoluble dust and debris. Figure 1 shows how iron oxide is taken up into membrane-bound vesicles in the macrophage cytoplasm. This function is essential, since rapid endocytosis of insoluble particles prevents particle penetration through alveolar epithelia and facilitates alveolar-bronchiolar transport (14).

Secretion and Regulation

Macrophages have many functions besides phagocytosis of particles and microbes. They secrete a variety of substances that interact with multi-enzyme cascades and with other cells such as lymphocytes, fibroblasts, neutrophils, and other macrophages. Thus, the macrophage both responds to and regulates its external environment. Werb (37) has recently reviewed materials secreted by macrophages. Interactions between alveolar macrophages and lymphocytes may be involved in the suppression or induction of immunologic pulmonary disease. Unanue (38) has reviewed other aspects of the immunoregulatory function of the macrophage and has described factors that regulate the expression of I-region-associated antigens (Ia) by macrophages. Macrophages are involved in the presentation of antigens and interact with the helper-inducer set of T lymphocytes. Finally, interactions between macrophages and lymphocytes are modified by exposure to inhaled particles such as tobacco smoke (39).

As we discuss below, some of these secretions are involved in connective tissue turnover, e.g. collagenase, elastase, and lysosomal enzymes; others affect lymphoid cells by helping to regulate mitogenesis and differentiation. Macrophages release additional products such as interferon, fibronectin, lysozyme, certain components of complement, and antiproteases. Other biologically active materials secreted by macrophages include an angiogenesis factor, plasminogen activator, prostaglandins, nucleosides, cyclic nucleotides, pyrogens, granulopoietins, and factors influencing fibroblast proliferation and tumor growth. Still other agents may interact with humoral enzyme systems such as the clotting, complement, fibrinolytic, and kinin-generating system. Macrophages are known to secrete plasminogen activator and a variety of arachidonic acid oxygenation products such as prostaglandins F_2 and E_2 and thromboxane B_2 (37). Finally, macrophages secrete interleukin-1 and a variety of mitogens for T and B cells.

MEASURING THE PHAGOCYTIC PROPERTIES OF PULMONARY MACROPHAGES IN SITU

The capacity of the lung to ingest and kill pathogens via its macrophages has been widely studied. After a bacterial aerosol exposure, the progress of intrapulmonary bacterial killing can be assayed by counting bacterial colony forming units (CFU) in pour plate cultures containing samples of lung homogenates from animals sacrificed at various times. The results are then compared to the number of CFU seen immediately after the bacterial challenge. This technique was first developed by Laurenzi, Berman, First & Kass (40) and has been used extensively to study the effects of toxic agents, clinical syndromes, and environmental factors on intrapulmonary killing. For example, Green & Kass (41) demonstrated the depressant effects of ethanol and hypoxia. Other depressants that have been studied include NO_2 (42) and cigarette smoke (43, 44). Goldstein et al (45) showed that the toxic effects of ozone on killing were more a consequence of defects in intracellular bactericidal activity than of impaired bacterial ingestion.

Brain & Corkery (46) have devised a technique for estimating the extent of in situ phagocytosis of radioactive particles administered to rodents by intratracheal (i.t.) instillation or by inhalation. Their approach is based on analysis of how particles and macrophages wash out of the lung during repeated lung lavage. They established that pulmonary lavage removes macrophages in a pattern distinctly different from that of free particles (those not associated with macrophages or fixed tissues).

Within hours after the i.t. instillation of an ^{198}Au colloid, Brain & Corkery (46) observed that the curve describing the washout of radioactivity began to lose the shape characteristic of free particles and started to mimic the washout of the macrophages; this suggests a transfer of particles from the free state to a cell-associated state. A mathematical curve fitting gave rise to an index, λ: the fraction of particles phagocytosed. In hamsters, λ is usually around 50–75% by 2 hr, more than 95% by 10 hr, and nearly 100% at 24 hr.

This assay has proven to be a useful way to examine the impact of particles on the function of pulmonary macrophages in vivo. Brain & Corkery (46) examined the effects of preexposure to iron oxide, colloidal carbon, and coal dust on the endocytosis of colloidal gold. For all three materials, endocytosis measured 2 hr postexposure was significantly depressed. However, when the hamsters were given the test gold particles 24 hr postexposure, only the coal dust group exhibited depressed endocytosis. Brain & Corkery concluded that all dusts can competitively inhibit endocytosis, but only some exhibit a sustained toxic effect on macrophage function. Beck et al (47) have incorporated the λ assay into a comprehensive in vivo hamster bioassay designed to assess the toxicity of particulates for the lungs. The λ assay discriminates between relatively nontoxic dusts like Fe_2O_3 and Al_2O_3 and the highly fibrogenic dust alpha quartz (silica). Its cytotoxicity for macrophages is reflected by the depression in λ. At the highest dose of alpha quartz studied, less than 30% of the gold was ingested in 90 min compared to more than 60% in the controls.

A novel approach to describing macrophage function in situ has recently been described. Brain et al (48) and Gehr et al (49) have described how both phagocytosis of iron oxide particles and macrophage motility can be monitored noninvasively with magnetometric methods. When magnetic forms of iron oxide are instilled or inhaled into the lungs, the retained particles can be used as an in vivo tracer for phagocytosis, cytoplasmic motility, and particle clearance [reviewed by Brain et al (50)]. These particles can be magnetized and aligned by an external magnetic field; the remanent magnetism coming from them can then be measured at the surface of a human's or animal's chest. Immediately following magnetization, the field from the lungs begins to decay (relaxation). Interestingly, the characteristics of this decay change with time after aerosol exposure. These time-dependent changes in relaxation are related to the progression of particle ingestion by macrophages in situ (48, 49).

Relaxation is caused by the random reorientation of particles away from their initially aligned state. Our in vivo experiments suggest that the rotational forces applied to the particles come largely from intracellular movements of phagosomes and lysosomes that contain the particles (48, 49). We believe that these movements arise from contractions of the cytoskeleton, which orchestrate cell motion required for functions such as phagocytosis, secretion, or ameboid movement. The hypothesis that organelle motion is a dominant mechanism for relaxation has now been confirmed in studies of hamster pulmonary macrophages observed in vitro (51, 52). Cultured macrophages that had previously ingested magnetic particles exhibited relaxation that was quantitatively similar to that seen in vivo, demonstrating that cardiac and respiratory movements are not essential for particle misalignment. Cytochalasin B (51) or D (52) slowed relaxation as did cold, formalin fixation, or nocodazole (52). Each of these interventions compromises the contractile capabilities of the cytoskeleton.

HARVESTING PULMONARY MACROPHAGES

Recovering macrophages from the lungs is important for two reasons: first, a change in macrophage number is one important index of response to inhaled particles and gases. Second, in vitro studies of pulmonary macrophages exposed to toxic agents require the isolation of pure populations of macrophages from the lungs of animals and humans, but success in isolating pulmonary macrophages depends on the particular subclass involved. Alveolar macrophages, for example, represent a relatively accessible cell population. Unfortunately, airway and connective tissue macrophages in the lungs cannot be recovered with the same ease and purity.

Alveolar macrophages are usually recovered by bronchoalveolar lavage. After filling all or part of the lungs with saline via the airways, one can withdraw the fluid. The recovered saline brings with it both cells and molecules that are contained in airway and alveolar lining fluid. Not all free cells recovered by lung lavage meet the definition of alveolar macrophages discussed earlier. Some Type 1 and Type 2 pneumonocytes, airway epithelial cells, and contaminating red and white blood cells may also be harvested. Airway macrophages are always present, being more prevalent in the initial washes, less so in the later washes.

Lung lavage to recover macrophages was first used by Gersing & Schumacher (53) and has been used extensively since (54–56). Brain & Frank (57) attempted to make the technique more sensitive and reproducible by utilizing multiple lung washings and by identifying and controlling the factors influencing macrophage yields.

Excised lungs, whole lungs in situ, or parts of lungs in situ can be lavaged. Usually, lungs of small animals are washed in situ since the possibility of causing leaks in the lungs is reduced. Following exsanguination, the neck is opened and the trachea cannulated. The chest wall or diaphragm should be opened to allow the lungs to empty themselves of as much air as possible. Washes are then carried out as just described. In most mammalian species, yields of 3–15 million cells/g lung are obtained when the lungs are washed 12 times (19).

Lungs of living animals, especially large ones such as calves and dogs, may also be lavaged. Instilled saline not recovered will be absorbed into the capillaries. Following topical anesthesia of the upper airways, a cuffed endotracheal tube is introduced through the larynx and placed in the left or right bronchus or even in smaller airways. The cuff is then inflated to create a tight seal. The intubated lung or lobe may then be lavaged while the remaining lung meets the ventilatory demands of the animal. Smaller subdivisions of the lung may be lavaged by using smaller-caliber endotracheal tubes; tubes without inflatable cuffs may be simply wedged in an appropriately sized airway. Since only a small percentage of the lungs is washed, the lavage of different lung segments can yield different results. This is more likely when injury or disease is nonuniformly distributed in the lungs. Recoveries of injected saline may be less in animals possessing considerable collateral ventilation (e.g. dog).

Similar procedures have been used to recover macrophages from human subjects. With the advent of flexible fiberoptic bronchoscopy, access to the lower respiratory tract has become relatively easy and nontraumatic. Segmental lobes can be lavaged to obtain evidence of particle exposure or to obtain human macrophages for in vitro study. Lung lavage in humans generally uses volumes ranging from 100 to 1000 ml (58, 59).

To obtain quantitatively consistent recoveries of macrophages it is necessary to control all aspects of the harvesting procedure. Gas-freeing the lungs, the length of the postmortem delay time, wash volume, leakage, pathological changes, and the number of washes all influence the results (19). So does age, sex, lung weight, and body weight (19). Additional observations (57) dealt with the effects of wash osmolarity and temperature, and duration of the washing cycle. Mechanical factors are also involved in the recovery of free cells from the alveolar surface and airways. Massage of the excised lungs or of the chest wall when the lungs are washed in situ increases macrophage recovery.

Lung lavage is often used to quantify changes in macrophage pool size following challenges with toxic materials, lung infection, or lung injury. Lung lavage is more reliable and sensitive with multiple washings. The mean cumulative yield increases at a faster rate than does the standard error (60). Even though individual washes vary, differences tend to cancel each other so that the cumulative total yield becomes less variable. Lungs should be washed at least six times to achieve maximum sensitivity.

It is not surprising that a cell system so intimately involved with inhaled materials responds to the quantity of particles presented to it. Brain exposed hamsters and rats (23, 60) to a wide variety of particulates, including carbon, coal dust, barium sulfate, triphenyl phosphate, chrysotile, iron oxide, and cigarette smoke, and observed increased macrophage numbers. Beck et al (47) have described changes in macrophage populations after exposing hamsters to iron oxide, aluminum oxide, volcanic ash, and silica. Macrophages in man also respond to chronic exposure to inhaled tobacco smoke (61). Brain (60) observed that smaller particles tend to be more effective stimuli than larger particles. The numbers of macrophages released may be related more to particle number or to particle surface area than to particle mass.

When interpreting changes in the numbers of macrophages present in the lungs, one must be aware of two assumptions. The ratio of the cells harvested to those actually present in situ is usually assumed to be the same in controls and in exposed groups, but the possibility exists that the treatment has influenced the efficiency of recovery. If toxic particles provoke an inflammatory response, bronchoconstriction, or atelectasis, altered cell harvest efficiency may occur.

One should also remember that the pool size of macrophages is dynamically determined. The equilibrium number of cells present at a point in time is a function of the input and output history of the pool. For example, if the pool size decreases, it may be due to decreased production or recruitment of free cells, or to accelerated clearance of macrophages in the lungs. If input and output of free cells both increase, the pool size can remain constant in spite of increased release of alveolar macrophages onto the lung surface. Accelerated or depressed lysis of macrophages also influences the equilibrium number of free cells.

MEASURING THE PHAGOCYTIC PROPERTIES OF PULMONARY MACROPHAGES IN VITRO

Many methods are available to assess in vitro endocytosis by macrophages. A review describing the merits and limitations of different approaches has been published by Kavet & Brain (62). Once harvested, phagocytic cells are usually studied as adherent monolayers or as cells in suspension. Certain principles apply to endocytic assays regardless of which type of culture system is employed. First, one should characterize the cell population introduced into the incubation medium. It is important to quantify (a) the number (or concentration) of cells present, (b) the percentage of each cell type present, and (c) the fraction of phagocytes that are viable. Particle uptake per cell (or per cell mass) will be improperly estimated if nonmacrophages or nonviable macrophages are included. The recovered cells should be purified or appropriate corrections should be made when the endocytic rates are calculated.

Second, in both suspension and monolayers, it is necessary to be able to (a) arrest phagocytosis and (b) separate the cells from unphagocytosed particles. With monolayers, these two aims are simultaneously achieved with a thorough rinse of the coverslip or culture dish. In a suspension system, arrest and separation usually require a two-step process. Phagocytic arrest can be accomplished by rapidly chilling the culture, by adding inhibitors such as iodoacetate, sodium fluoride, or N-ethylmaleimide, or by diluting suspensions to the point at which the probability of cell-particle contact approaches zero. When the cells and particles in suspension assays have different densities and/or sedimentation rates, separation of arrested cells from remaining free particles can be accomplished by centrifugation. Filtration can also be used to separate cells and free particles, provided that all cells are trapped by the filter and all free particles pass through.

A new assay for pulmonary macrophage endocytosis that uses flow cytometry was recently developed (63). Macrophages recovered by lung lavage are incubated with fluorescent latex particles. Then a cytofluorograph is used to characterize the uptake of particles by small samples of pulmonary macrophages. A linear relationship exists between the number of fluorescent particles associated with each cell and the intensity of fluorescent light emitted by each cell. Particle uptake is significantly inhibited by removing divalent cations with ethylenediaminetetraacetic acid and lowering the incubation temperature (64).

PATHOPHYSIOLOGY OF PULMONARY MACROPHAGES

In addition to protecting the host, macrophages also participate in the pathogenesis of lung disease. Because macrophages are actively phagocytic, inhaled toxic, radioactive, or carcinogenic particles become concentrated within pulmonary macrophages. What begins as a diffuse exposure becomes highly localized and nonuniform. "Hot spots" of high dosage are formed that may exceed the thresholds for certain effects and cause damage. Macrophages may also metabolize chemicals and change them to a more toxic form.

When macrophages adhere to the airway epithelium they may increase epithelial exposure to inhaled toxic materials. More importantly, this close association with the bronchial epithelium can lead to transbronchial transport of inhaled particles and subsequent reingestion by connective tissue macrophages (65). These cells, like their relatives in the alveolar and airway compartments, also segregate, retain, and perhaps metabolize carcinogenic and other toxic particles.

"Hot spots" may be associated with damage to the epithelial barriers and thus with enhanced epithelial transport. These, in turn, could lead to increased access of toxic particles to the connective tissue compartment. Epithelial defenses may also be breached at the alveolar level; because of lymphatic pathways, particles may arrive in similar sites. Particles gaining access to the lymphatics are cleared slowly, thus increasing their contribution to the pathogenesis of many lung diseases. Years after exposure to particles, these connective tissue burdens may constitute the major reservoir of retained particles. Connective tissue macrophages may contribute to progressive damage by concentrating and storing potent toxic particles for long periods.

Another way in which macrophages may be involved is through diminution or failure of their defensive role. A number of investigators, using both in vivo and in vitro bactericidal or phagocytic assays, have shown that macrophage function can be compromised by environmental insults and pathological changes. Such diverse agents as silica, immunosuppressives, ethanol intoxication, cigarette smoke, air pollution, and oxygen toxicity can depress the ability of pulmonary macrophages to protect their host. For example, diesel exhaust may depress the phagocytic activity of these cells (66). Sometimes the agent or factor acts directly on the macrophage, producing a damaged or even a dead cell. For example, the ingestion of lead oxide particles is followed by swelling of the mitochondria, nuclear membrane, and endoplasmic reticulum as well as the appearance of precipitation complexes within the nuclear chromatin and cytoplasm (67).

In other cases (e.g. high concentrations of inhaled particles) the mechanism can be competitive inhibition in which the phagocytic machinery becomes saturated even in the absence of cytotoxicity. Then again, particularly in those situations involving pulmonary edema or altered acid-base balance, the macrophages may be undamaged, but their activity may be depressed because of an indirect effect on their milieu, the airway, or alveolar microenvironment. However, macrophage failure or damage is not always a cause of the disease in question; sometimes changes in macrophages may simply reflect the onset and progression of the disease. For example, changes in macrophage activity during pulmonary edema associated with oxygen toxicity fall in this class. It is not the macrophage's failure to ingest particles or bacteria that causes the edema; rather, the presence of edema alters macrophage function.

There are situations in which pulmonary macrophages not only fail but contribute directly to the pathogenesis of pulmonary diseases. Two important examples involve pulmonary connective tissue (68, 69). Connective tissue proteins have an essential role in lung structure and function. Collagen and elastin help maintain alveolar, airway, and vascular stability, limit lung expansion, and contribute to lung recoil at all lung volumes. Two groups of lung disease are associated with aberrations of normal collagen and elastin balance: emphysematous and fibrotic disorders.

Emphysema

Studies of the pathogenesis of emphysema have focused attention on the balance between elastase and anti-elastase in the respiratory tract (70). Elastase is involved in wound healing and in the disposal of damaged cells and debris. Although these enzymes are useful, when chronically present their digestive capacity may damage pulmonary tissues. Release of lysosomal enzymes, particularly proteases, from activated macrophages and other leukocytes promotes the development of emphysema. Release occurs as a consequence of cell death, cell injury, exocytosis, or regurgitation while feeding. Increased deposition of particles acts to recruit additional macrophages; thus the effect may be reinforced. For example, Warheit et al (71) have recently demonstrated that inhaled chrysotile asbestos fibers that deposit at alveolar duct bifurcations activate complement. In turn, complement activation enhances the inflammatory response by attracting more macrophages into the region. Macrophages also secrete substances that are chemotaxic for neutrophils (72).

Interest in proteolytic injury was stimulated because of knowledge about pulmonary emphysema associated with inborn α_1-antitrypsin-inhibitor deficiency in humans (73). Imbalances between proteolytic activity and its inhibition have important implications as a general mechanism of lung injury. Macrophages secrete enzymes capable of connective tissue degradation. Both collagenase and elastase activity can be detected in fluids from macrophage cultures (74–77). The release of both enzymes is stimulated by cell activation and by phagocytosis. There is evidence that exposure to smoke causes increased synthesis and release of elastolytic enzymes from these cells (78–80). Importantly, culture media from alveolar macrophages of smokers contained greater elastase activity than media obtained from macrophages of nonsmokers. Smokers have higher levels of elastase activity in bronchoalveolar lavage fluid than do nonsmokers (81). These findings help confirm the suspected role of macrophages in the pathogenesis of pulmonary emphysema in smokers. Generally macrophages contribute less elastase to lavage fluid than do neutrophils. However, connective tissue macrophages that release elastase in direct contact with elastin may be very important.

Other pollutant particles characteristic of work and urban environments also act to recruit more cells, to activate them, and to release proteolytic enzymes. For all these situations, the extent of damage depends on the number of additional macrophages recruited, on the extent of their activation, and on the degree to which elastase and other toxic materials are secreted or released from macrophages. Pathogenesis of emphysema may also be facilitated by damage to epithelial barriers that provides greater access of alveolar elastase to elastin in the interstitium.

A number of animal models have been produced that support the proteolytic theory of emphysema. A lesion very similar to emphysema can be produced by intratracheal instillation or aerosolization of nonspecific proteolytic enzymes such as papain or by elastase (82–84). Homogenates of neutrophils or pulmonary macrophages have a similar effect (4, 85), as does elastase present in purulent sputum (86, 87). In all these models, the lesion is usually characterized by an initial phase of enzymatic degradation of elastin in the lungs, a subsequent resynthesis to control levels, and then a more gradual architectural derangement leading to expanded airspaces and/or destruction of alveoli.

The role of antiproteases should be noted. When porcine pancreatic elastase is instilled into hamsters with no serum or with serum from α_1-antitrypsin deficient people, the result is a lesion resembling emphysema. However, when identical amounts of pancreatic elastase are added with serum from normal individuals, no change occurs. Thus the maintenance of a normal balance between elastase and elastase inhibitors is critical. The body's defenses against excessive elastase levels include inhibitors present in alveolar and airway lining fluid and the ingestion and degradation of elastase by macrophages. Macrophages bind PMN elastase, although some of the enzyme may remain active.

We have previously described how reactive metabolites of oxygen such as superoxide anions, hydroxyl radicals, and hydrogen peroxide are used by macrophages and neutrophils to kill microorganisms. However, these agents may also cause damage. For example, they may damage cell membranes or essential metabolic enzymes. They may reduce the activity of endogenous protease inhibitors and thus allow the activity of extracellular proteases to go unchecked. Oxygen radicals may also have an indirect effect by damaging other phagocytic cells and causing additional release of toxic and proteolytic enzymes (88). Recently, Weitberg et al (89) have demonstrated that human phagocytes that produce oxygen radicals may also produce cytogenic damage in cultured mammalian cells. It is conceivable that chronic inflammatory states characterized by persistent increases in macrophages may contribute to cancer by this mechanism.

Fibrosis

Fibrogenesis also involves macrophage damage. Dead or dying macrophages may release substance(s) that can attract fibroblasts and elicit fibrogenic responses. Dust particles of appropriate size, shape, chemical composition, and durability may deposit on alveolar surfaces and stimulate production of excess collagen in the alveolar wall. In such fibrotic diseases as asbestosis and silicosis, progressive fibrogenesis may continue long after inhalation of dust particles has stopped. A continued influx of new macrophages is frequently a prominent feature of the fibrogenic process (90). Excessive collagen or alterations in types of collagen may make the lungs stiffer than normal, severely decreasing the vital capacity and increasing the muscular forces required for breathing.

Asbestos, glass, and other fibrous dusts have been shown to stimulate collagen synthesis (91, 92). Fibers over 5 μm in length are sometimes incompletely ingested by macrophages (93) and may lead to macrophage death or release of mediators. Growth of fibroblasts in vitro has been shown to require a solid supporting particle of critical minimum dimensions (94).

There is evidence that fibrogenesis involves macrophages and occurs as a two-step process (95, 96). Silica does not exert a direct stimulatory effect on fibroblasts (92). Rather, the interaction of a particle with a macrophage is thought to release factors that then stimulate local production of collagen by fibroblasts.

A number of investigators have produced evidence showing that macrophages can produce a factor or factors that, in turn, influence the proliferation (97) and biosynthetic activity (98) of fibroblasts. After adding silica particles to mouse macrophages, Heppleston & Styles (96) reported the presence of a factor that stimulated chick fibroblasts to produce collagen. Using rabbit pulmonary macrophages and WI-38 fibroblasts, Burrell & Anderson (99) showed the same response. Aalto & Kulonen (6) reported that macrophages damaged by quartz in vitro release factors that stimulate collagen synthesis by fibroblasts in culture. Using a diffusion chamber implanted into mouse peritoneal cavities, Bateman et al (100) observed that when mouse peritoneal macrophages were incubated with either chrysotile asbestos or silica, factors that diffused through a Nucleopore membrane produced fibrosis. It is possible that generation of similar fibrogenesis stimulating factors by quartz-damaged pulmonary macrophages in vivo may play a role in the development of fibrosis in the lungs, but such factors have not yet been isolated from the developing silicotic lung (101).

Emerging areas of research interest that may involve macrophages include the responses of the lung to inhaled antigens and allergens, and environmental allergic respiratory disease. Current evidence shows that inhaled organic chemicals, dusts, molds, and animal proteins can cause a variety of lung responses such as allergic asthma, extrinsic allergic alveolitis, immune complex disease, and other phenomena. Excellent discussions of these diseases are available (102); they suggest that macrophages may be involved.

CONCLUSION

Research in inhalation toxicology must not only delineate dose-response relationships, it must also elucidate mechanisms of lung injury. Pulmonary macrophages defend alveolar and airway surfaces, but they are also capable of injuring the host while exercising their defensive role. Further studies are needed of the ultrastructural and biochemical features of normal pulmonary macrophages as well as their alterations following exposure to physical, chemical, and infectious agents.

Literature Cited

1. Witschi H., Nettesheim, P., eds. 1982. *Mechanisms in Respiratory Toxicology*, Vol. II. Boca Raton, Fla: CRC
2. Hunninghake, G. W., Gadek, J. E., Szapiel, S. V., Strumpf, I. J., Kawanami, O., et al. 1980. The human alveolar macrophage. In *Methods in Cell Biology*, Vol. 21A, ed. C. C. Harris, B. F. Trump, G. D. Stoner, pp. 95–112. New York: Academic
3. Stone, P. J. 1983. The elastase-antielastase hypothesis of the pathogenesis of emphysema. See Ref. 70, pp. 405–12
4. Mass, B., Ikeda, I., Meranze, D. R., Weinbaum, G., Kimbel, P. 1972. Induction of experimental emphysema: cellular and species specificity. *Am. Rev. Respir. Dis.* 106:384–91
5. McGowan, S. E., Stone, P. J., Calore, J. D., Snider, G. L., Franzblau, C. 1983. The fate of neutrophil elastase incorporated by human alveolar macrophages. *Am. Rev. Respir. Dis.* 127:449–55
6. Aalto, M., Kulonen, E. 1979. Fractionation of connective-tissue-activating fac-

tors from the culture medium of silica-treated macrophages. *Acta Pathol. Microbiol. Scand. Sect. C.* 87:241–50
7. Martin, B. M., Gimbrone, M. A., Majeau, G. R., Unanue, E. R., Cotran, R. S. 1981. Monocyte/macrophage-derived growth factor production: modulation by cold insoluble globulin and extracellular matrix. *Arteriosclerosis* 1:361a
8. Diegelman, R. F., Cohen, I. K., Kaplan, A. M. 1981. The role of macrophages in wound repair: a review. *Plast. Reconstr. Surg.* 68:107–13
9. Watanabe, T., Hirata, M., Yoshikawa, Y., Nagafuchi, Y., Toyoshima, H., Watanabe, T. 1980. Role of macrophages in atherosclerosis: sequential observations of cholesterol-induced rabbit aortic lesion by the immunoperoxidase technique using monoclonal antimacrophage antibody. *Lab. Invest.* 53:80–90
10. Kan-Mitchell, J., Hengst, J. C. D., Kempf, R. A., Rothbart, R. K., Simons, S. M., et al. 1985. Cytotoxic activity of human pulmonary alveolar macrophages. *Cancer Res.* 45:453–58

11. Holt, P. G., Leivers, S. 1985. Alveolar macrophages: antigen presentation activity in vivo. *Aust. J. Exp. Biol. Med. Sci.* 63:33–39

12. Harmsen, A. G., Bice, D. E., Muggenburg, B. A. 1985. The effect of local antibody responses on in vivo and in vitro phagocytosis by pulmonary alveolar macrophages. *J. Leuk. Biol.* 37:483–92

13. Brain, J. D., Gehr, P., Kavet, R. I. 1984. Airway macrophages: The importance of the fixation method. *Am. Rev. Respir. Dis.* 129:823–26

14. Sorokin, S. P., Brain, J. D. 1975. Pathways of clearance in mouse lungs exposed to iron oxide aerosols. *Anat. Rec.* 181:581–626

15. Warner, A. P., Brain, J. D. 1984. Intravascular pulmonary macrophages: ruminants actively participate in reticuloendothelial clearance of particles. *Fed. Proc.* 43:1001 (Abstr.)

16. Godleski, J. J., Mortara, M., Joher, M. A., Kobzik, L., Brain, J. D. 1984. Monoclonal antibody to an alveolar macrophage surface antigen in hamsters. *Am. Rev. Respir. Dis.* 130:249–55

17. Harbison, M. L., Godleski, J. J., Mortara, M., Brain, J. D. 1984. Correlation of lung macrophage age and surface antigen in the hamster. *Lab. Invest.* 50:653–58

18. Brain, J. D. 1985. Macrophages in the respiratory tract. In *Handbook of Physiology—The Respiratory System I. Circulation and Nonrespiratory Functions,* ed. A. P. Fishman, A. B. Fisher, pp. 447–71. Bethesda, Md: American Physiological Society

19. Brain, J. D., Godleski, J. J., Sorokin, S. P. 1977. Structure, origin and fate of the macrophage, In *Respiratory Defense Mechanisms* (Lung Biology in Health and Disease, Monograph 5), ed. J. D. Brain, D. F. Proctor, L. Reid, pp. 849–52. New York: Marcel Dekker

20. Zeidler, R. B., Kim, H. D. 1985. Phagocytosis, chemiluminescence, and cell volume of alveolar macrophages from neonatal and adult pigs. *J. Leuk. Biol.* 37:29–43

21. Eckert, H., Lux, M., Lachmann, B. 1983. The role of alveolar macrophages in surfactant turnover. *Lung* 161:213–18

22. Bowden, D. H. 1973. The alveolar macrophage. *Curr. Top. Pathol.* 55:1–36

23. Brain, J. D. 1970. Free cells in the lungs: Some aspects of their role, quantitation, and regulation. *Arch. Intern. Med.* 126:447–87

24. Hocking, W. G., Golde, D. W. 1979. The pulmonary-alveolar macrophage. *N. Eng. J. Med.* 301:580–87

25. Hocking, W. G., Golde, D. W. 1979. The pulmonary-alveolar macrophage. *N. Eng. J. Med.* 301:639–45

26. Cohn, Z. A., Wiener, E. 1963. The particulate hydrolases of macrophages. I. Comparative enzymology, isolation, and properties. *J. Exp. Med.* 18:991–1008

27. Leake, E. S., Gonzalves-Ojeda, D., Myrvik, Q. N. 1964. Enzymatic difference between normal alveolar macrophages and oil-induced peritoneal macrophages obtained from rabbits. *Exp. Cell Res.* 33:553–61

28. Sorber, W. A., Leake, E. S., Myrvik, Q. N. 1974. Isolation and characterization of hydrolase-containing granules from rabbit lung macrophages. *J. Reticuloendothel. Soc.* 16:184–92

29. Yarborough, D. J., Meyer, O. T., Dannenberg, A. M. Jr., Pearson, B. 1967. Histochemistry of macrophage hydrolases. III. Studies of β-galactosidase, β-glucuronidase and aminopeptidase by inodolyl and naphthyl substrates. *J. Reticuloendothel. Soc.* 4:390–408

30. Franson, R. C., Waite, M. 1973. Lysosomal phospholipases A_1 and A_2 of normal and bacillus Calmette Guerin-induced alveolar macrophages. *J. Cell Biol.* 56:621–27

31. Sethi, K. K. 1982. Intracellular killing of parasites by macrophages. *Clin. Immunol. Allergy* 2:541–65

32. Rodgers, B. C., Mims, C. A. 1982. Role of macrophage activation and interferon in the resistance of alveolar macrophages from infected mice to influenza virus. *Infect. Immun.* 36:1154–59

33. Rose, R. M., Crumpacker, C., Waner, J. L., Brain, J. D. 1982. Murine cytomegalovirus pneumonia: Description of a model and investigation of pathogenesis. *Am. Rev. Respir. Dis.* 125:568–73

34. Rose, R. M., Crumpacker, C., Waner, J. L., Brain, J. D. 1983. Treatment of murine cytomegalovirus pneumonia with acyclovir and interferon. *Am. Rev. Respir. Dis.* 127:198–203

35. Babior, B. M. 1980. The role of oxygen radicals in microbial killing by phagocytes. In *The Reticuloendothelial System. A Comprehensive Treatise,* Vol. II, *Biochemistry and Metabolism,* ed. A. J. Sbarra, R. R. Strauss, pp. 339–54. New York: Plenum

36. Klebanoff, S. J. 1980. Myeloperoxidase-mediated cytotoxic systems. See Ref. 35, pp. 279–308

37. Werb, Z. 1983. How the macrophage

regulates its extracellular environment. *Am. J. Anat.* 166:237–56

38. Unanue, E. R. 1982. Symbiotic relationships between macrophages and lymphocytes. In *Macrophages and Natural Killer Cells*, ed. S. J. Normann, E. Sorkin, pp. 49–63. New York: Plenum

39. DeShazo, R. D., Banks, D. E., Diem, J. E., Nordberg, J. A., Baser, Y., et al. 1983. Bronchoalveolar lavage cell–lymphocyte interactions in normal nonsmokers and smokers. *Am. Rev. Respir. Dis.* 127:545–48

40. Laurenzi, G. A., Berman, L., First, M., Kass, E. H. 1964. A quantitative study of the deposition and clearance of bacteria in the murine lung. *J. Clin. Invest.* 43:759–68

41. Green, G. M., Kass, E. H. 1964. Factors influencing the clearance of bacteria by the lung. *J. Clin. Invest.* 43:769–76

42. Goldstein, E., Eagle, M. C., Hoeprich, P. D. 1973. Effect of nitrogen dioxide on pulmonary bacterial defense mechanisms. *Arch. Environ. Health.* 26:202–4

43. Laurenzi, G. A., Guarneri, J. J., Endriga, R. B., Carey, J. P. 1963. Clearance of bacteria by the lower respiratory tract. *Science* 142:1572–73

44. Spurgash, A., Ehrlich, R., Petzold, R. 1968. Effect of cigarette smoke on resistance to respiratory infection. *Arch. Environ. Health* 16:385–90

45. Goldstein, E., Lippert, W., Warshauer, D. 1974. Pulmonary alveolar macrophage. Defender against bacterial infection of the lung. *J. Clin. Invest.* 54:519–28

46. Brain, J. D., Corkery, G. C. 1977. The effect of increased particles on the endocytosis of radiocolloids by pulmonary macrophages *in vivo*: competitive and toxic effects. In *Inhaled Particles and Vapours*, IV, ed. W. H. Walton, pp. 551–64. London: Pergamon

47. Beck, B. D., Brain, J. D., Bohannon, D. 1982. An *in vivo* hamster bioassay to assess the toxicity of particulates for the lungs. *Toxicol. Appl. Pharmacol.* 66:9–29

48. Brain, J. D., Bloom, S. B., Valberg, P. A., Gehr, P. 1984. Behavior of magnetic dusts in the lungs of rabbits correlates with phagocytosis. *Exp. Lung Res.* 6:115–31

49. Gehr, P., Brain, J. D., Nemoto, I., Bloom, S. B. 1983. Behavior of magnetic particles in hamster lungs: estimates of clearance and cytoplasmic motility. *J. Appl. Physiol. Respir. Environ. Exercise Physiol.* 55:1196–202

50. Brain, J. D., Gehr, P., Valberg, P. A., Bloom, S. B., Nemoto, I. 1985. Biomagnetism in the study of lung function. In *Biomagnetism: Applications and Theory*, ed. H. Weinberg, G. Stroink, T. Kattila, pp. 378–87. New York: Pergamon

51. Gehr, P., Brain, J. D., Bloom, S. B. 1983. Magnetometry: a tool to study intracellular movement. *J. Cell Biol.* 97: 194a

52. Valberg, P. A. 1984. Magnetometry of ingested particles in pulmonary macrophages. *Science* 224:513–16

53. Gersing, R., Schumacher, H. 1955. Experimentelle Untersuchungen über die Staubphagozytose. *Beitr. Silikose-Forsch.* 25:31–34

54. LaBelle, C. W., Brieger, H. 1959. Synergistic effects on aerosols. II. Effects on rate of clearance from the lung. *Arch. Indust. Health* 20:100–5

55. LaBelle, C. W., Brieger, H. 1960. The fate of inhaled particles in the early postexposure period. 1:432–37

56. Myrvik, Q. N., Leake, E. S., Fariss, B. 1961. Studies on pulmonary alveolar macrophages from the normal rabbit: A technique to procure them in a high state of purity. *J. Immunol.* 86:128–32

57. Brain, J. D., Frank, R. 1973. Alveolar macrophage adhesion: wash electrolyte composition and free cell yield. *J. Appl. Physiol.* 34:75–80

58. Burns, D. M., Shure, D., Francoz, R., Kalafer, M., Harrel, J., et al. 1983. The physiologic consequences of saline lobar lavage in healthy human adults. *Am. Rev. Respir. Dis.* 127:695–701

59. Low, R. B., Davis, G. S., Giancola, M. S. 1978. Biochemical analyses of bronchoalveolar lavage fluids of normal healthy volunteers. *Am. Rev. Respir. Dis.* 118:863–76

60. Brain, J. D. 1971. The effects of increased particles on the number of alveolar macrophages. In *Inhaled Particles* III, ed. W. H. Walton, pp. 209–25. London: Unwin

61. Plowman, P. N. 1982. The pulmonary macrophage population of human smokers. *Ann. Occup. Hyg.* 25:393–405

62. Kavet, R. I., Brain, J. D. 1980. Methods to quantify endocytosis: a review. *J. Reticuloendothel. Soc.* 27:201–21

63. Parod, R. J., Brain, J. D. 1982. Uptake of latex particles by macrophages: characterization using flow cytometry. *Am. J. Physiol.* 245 *(Cell Physiol. 14)*: C220–26

64. Parod, R. J., Brain, J. D. 1983. Uptake of latex particles by pulmonary mac-

rophages: role of calcium. *Am. J. Physiol.* 245 *(Cell Physiol. 14):* C227–34

65. Watson, A. Y., Brain, J. D. 1979. Uptake of iron oxide aerosols by mouse airway epithelium. *Lab. Invest.* 40:450–59

66. Castranova, V., Bowman, L., Reasor, M. J., Lewis, T., Tucker, J., Miles, P. R. 1985. The response of rat alveolar macrophages to chronic inhalation of coal dust and/or diesel exhaust. *Environ. Res.* 36:405–19

67. DeVries, C. R., Ingram, P., Walker, S. R., Linton, R. W., Gutknecht, W. F., Shelburne, J. D. 1983. Acute toxicity of lead particulates on pulmonary alveolar macrophages. Ultrastructural and microanalytical studies. *Lab. Invest.* 48:35–44

68. Harington, J. S., Allison, A. C. 1977. Tissue and cellular reactions to particles, fibers, and aerosols retained after inhalation. In *Handbook of Physiology, Section 9, Reactions to Environmental Agents,* ed. H. L. Falk, S. D. Murphy, pp. 263–83. Bethesda, Md: Am. Physiol. Soc.

69. Turino, G. M., Rodriquez, J. R., Greenbaum, L. M., Mandl, I. 1974. Mechanisms of pulmonary injury. *Am. J. Med.* 57:493–505

70. Snider, G. L. 1983. *Emphysema.* In *Clinics in Chest Medicine,* Vol. 4. No. 3. Philadelphia: Saunders

71. Warheit, D. B., George, G., Hill, L. H., Snyderman, R., Brody, A. R. 1985. Inhaled asbestos activates a complement-dependent chemoattractant for macrophages. *Lab. Invest.* 52:505–14

72. Snella, M-C. 1985. Manganese dioxide induces alveolar macrophage chemotaxis for neutrophils in vitro. *Toxicology* 34:153–59

73. Laurell, C. B., Erikson, S. 1963. The electrophoretic α_1-globulin pattern of serum in α_1-antitrypsin deficiency. *Scand. J. Clin. Lab Invest.* 15:132–40

74. Wahl, L. M., Wahl, S. M., Mergenhagen, S. E., Martin, G. R. 1975. Collagenase production by lymphokine-activated macrophages. *Science* 187:261–63

75. Werb, Z., Gordon, S. 1975. Elastase secretion by stimulated macrophages. Characterization and regulation. *J. Exp. Med.* 142:361–77

76. Wharton, W. 1983. Human macrophage-like cell line U937-1 elaborates mitogenic activity for fibroblasts. *J. Reticuloendothel. Soc.* 33:151–56

77. White, R., Lin, H. S., Kuhn, C., III. 1977. Elastase secretion by peritoneal exudative and alveolar macrophages. *J. Exp. Med.* 146:802–8

78. Kuhn, C. III, Senior, R. M. 1978. The role of elastase in the development of emphysema. *Lung* 155:188–97

79. Kuhn, C. III, Senior, R. M., Pierce, J. A. 1982. The pathogenesis of emphysema. In *Mechanisms in Respiratory Toxicology,* Vol. 2, ed. H. Witschi, P. Nettesheim, pp. 155–211. Boca Raton, Fla: CRC

80. Rodriguez, F. J., White, R. R., Senior, R. M., Levine, E. A. 1977. Elastase release from human alveolar macrophages: comparison between smokers and nonsmokers. *Science* 198:313–14

81. Janoff, A., Raju, L., Dearing, R. 1983. Levels of elastase activity in bronchoalveolar lavage fluids of healthy smokers and nonsmokers. *Am. Rev. Respir. Dis.* 127:540–44

82. Johanson, W. G. Jr., Pierce, A. K. 1972. Effects of elastase, collagenase, and papain on structure and function of rat lungs in vitro. *J. Clin. Invest.* 51:288–93

83. Kaplan, P. D., Kuhn, C., Pierce, J. A. 1973. The induction of emphysema with elastase. I. The evolution of the lesion and the influence of serum. *J. Lab. Clin. Med.* 82:349–56

84. Snider, G. L., Hayes, J. A., Franzblau, C., Kagan, H. M., Stone, P. J., Korthy, A. K. 1974. Relationship between elastolytic activity and experimental emphysema-inducing properties of papain preparations. *Am. Rev. Respir. Dis.* 110:254–62

85. Weinbaum, G., Marco, V., Ikeda, T., Mass, B., Meranze, D. R., Kimbel, P. 1974. Enzymatic production of experimental emphysema in the dog: route of exposure. *Am. Rev. Respir. Dis.* 109: 351–57

86. Lieberman, J. 1973. Involvement of leukocytic proteases in emphysema and antitrypsin deficiency. *Arch. Environ. Health* 27:196–200

87. Lieberman, J., Gawad, M. A. 1971. Inhibitors and activators of leukocytic proteases in purulent sputum: digestion of human lung and inhibition by alpha$_1$-antitrypsin. *J. Lab. Clin. Med.* 77:713–27

88. Riley, D. J., Kerr, J. S. 1985. Oxidant injury of the extracellular matrix: potential role in the pathogenesis of pulmonary emphysema. *Lung* 163:1–13

89. Weitberg, A. B., Weitzman, S. A., Destrempes, M., Latt, S. A., Stossel, T. P. 1983. Stimulated human phagocytes produce cytogenetic changes in cultured mammalian cells. *N. Engl. J. Med.* 308:25–29

90. Tryka, A. F., Godleski, J. J., Brain, J.

D. 1984. Alterations in alveolar macrophages in hamsters developing pulmonary fibrosis. *Exp. Lung Res.* 7:41–52

91. Davis, J. K. G. 1973. Are ferruginous bodies an indication of atmospheric pollution by asbestos? In *Biological Effects of Asbestos*. ed. P. Bogovski, J. C. Gilson, V. Timbrell, J. C. Wagner, pp. 238–42. Lyons, France: IARC

92. Richards, R. J., Morris, T. G. 1973. Collagen and mucopolysaccharide production in growing lung fibroblasts exposed to chrysotile asbestos. *Life Sci.* 12:441–51

93. Allison, A. C. 1973. Effects of asbestos particles on macrophages, mesothelial cells and fibroblasts. See Ref. 91, pp. 89–93

94. Maroudas, N. G. 1973. Chemical and mechanical requirements for fibroblast adhesion. *Nature* 244:353–54

95. Allison, A. C., Harington, J. S., Birbeck, M. 1966. An examination of the cytotoxic effects of silica on macrophages. *J. Exp. Med.* 124:141–54

96. Heppleston, A. G., Styles, J. A. 1967. Activity of a macrophage factor in collagen formation by silica. *Nature* 214:521–24

97. Leibovich, S. J., Ross, R. 1976. A macrophage-dependent factor that stimulates the proliferation of fibroblasts *in vitro*. *Am. J. Pathol.* 84:501–4

98. Aho, S., Kulonen, E. 1977. Effect of silica-liberated macrophage factors on protein synthesis in cell-free systems. *Exp. Cell Res.* 104:31–38

99. Burrell, R., Anderson, M. 1973. The induction of fibrosis by silica-treated alveolar macrophages. *Environ. Res.* 6:389–94

100. Bateman, E. D., Emerson, R. J., Cole, P. J. 1982. A study of macrophage mediated initiation of fibrosis by asbestos and silica using a diffusion chamber technique. *Br. J. Exp. Pathol.* 63:414–25

101. Reiser, K. M., Last, J. A. 1979. Silicosis and fibrogenesis: Fact and artifact. *Toxicology* 13:51–72

102. Kirkpatrick, C. H., Reynolds, H. Y., eds. 1976. *Immunologic and Infectious Reactions in the Lung* (Lung Biology in Health and Disease, Monograph 1). New York: Dekker

Ann. Rev. Pharmacol. Toxicol. 1986. 26:567–76

REVIEW OF REVIEWS

E. Leong Way

Department of Pharmacology, University of California, San Francisco, California 94143

HERBAL MEDICINE

Within the past decade there has been a resurgence of interest in plant products with biologic activity. In large part, the stimulus has been provided by the People's Republic of China opening its doors. Successes there in preventive medicine, eradication of certain parasitic and venereal diseases, acupuncture, and burn therapy as well as extensive research projects in materia medica were a revelation to the West.

The massive program mentioned above was the consequence of political as well as practical considerations. During the early years after the Communist Party assumed control of China, there was dire need of physicians throughout the country, and particularly in rural areas. To Mao Zedong and the party planners the solution was simple: Mao deemed that "Chinese traditional medicine is a vast valuable national treasure which should be intensively exploited and improved." A ukase was issued, therefore, that Western-trained physicians and traditional Chinese practitioners should merge their knowledge and skills to serve the people. As a consequence, relative to other biologic sciences, pharmacology assumed an exalted position as an intensive program to justify established herbal remedies and to discover new ones was launched. Numerous projects were initiated at research institutes and universities throughout the country to isolate and identify active constituents of known herbal remedies and to screen other natural products for possible therapeutic application.

Concerted efforts were also made to provide a rational basis for Chinese traditional medicine. However, the basic conceptualizations of such a system cannot be buttressed or refuted by experimentation. Whatever the merits of these past theories, it is my personal view that these concepts have long outlived their usefulness. I am not alone in such views, but surprisingly few investigators have made such a flat assertion. Likely, most of the current in-

567

0362-1642/86/0415-0567$02.00

vestigators in this field do not believe it worth the bother to criticize openly the outmoded traditional theories. Perhaps many refrain either out of fear of offending or just fear. In any event, the scientifically trained pharmacologists in China obviously ignore the traditional theories by performing research on herbal remedies using the experimental approach. The new knowledge emanating from these projects has been truly impressive, and many reviews and monographs have dealt with these matters. Although the programs in more Westernized countries are not nearly so extensive, there is no state of dormancy as evidenced by several recent monographs describing ongoing research on plant products with biologic activity.

Balandrin et al provide a concise overview of extractable plant chemicals and their economic importance and cite some more recent examples of pesticides, alleochemicals, and potential medicinals (1). They point out, however, that most species of higher plants have never been described, much less surveyed, for chemical or biologically active constituents, and that new sources of commercially valuable materials remain to be discovered. Only about 5–15% of 250,000–750,000 species of higher plants have been surveyed for biologically active compounds. Balandrin et al anticipate that biologically active plant materials will play an increasingly significant role in the development of new products for regulating plant growth as well as for insect and weed control. Advances in the biotechnology of chromatographic and spectroscopic techniques as well as in methods of culturing plant cells and tissues should provide new means for the commercial processing of plants and the chemicals they produce. They gloom their predictions by warning that if the current trend of destruction of tropical forests continues at its present rate, plant scientists may have only a few decades remaining to investigate the plant kingdom for useful chemicals. On a more optimistic beat, I should point out that marine plants and animals, although by no means immune, are less likely to be affected by human machinations, and the surface has scarcely been scratched concerning the active constituents of these natural products.

Takemi and associates edit *Herbal Medicine: Kampo, Past and Present* (2). "Kampo" refers to Japanese herbal medicine in the Chinese tradition. This volume contains articles by invited speakers that were presented at a conference convened by the foremost commercial concern dealing with herbal remedies in Japan on the occasion of its ninetieth anniversary. The topics include a potpourri of history, philosophic concepts, political science, and pharmacology both basic and clinical. Of particular interest is the presentation by Hosoya on the pharmacology of Kampo prescriptions, in which he describes attempts to identify the optimal combination of the various ingredients that yields the desired pharmacologic activity. Qian traces traditional medicine in China from its early days to the current research programs to identify and isolate the active constituents in natural products. Nishioka's paper on the discovery of active components in rhubarb with novel biologic activities, and Shibata's on quality control of extract preparations are also worth reading.

Chang et al (3) have edited a volume containing the proceedings of an international symposium held recently in Hong Kong on Chinese medicinal products. In the symposium, there were 89 presentations with special emphasis given to 8 areas. Two of these were concerned with hepato-pharmacology and anticancer agents. Separate sessions were devoted to three drug topics, namely ginseng, gossypol, and abortifacient proteins. With respect to the latter agents, particularly impressive are the detailed studies by Pan and his associates establishing the chemistry and structure of trichosanthin. In the presentation of two general sessions, Hosoya reports studies on the construction of pre-scriptions in ancient Chinese medicine, Hsu on the processing of medicinal herbs, and Zimmerman on the possible mechanism of action of traditional oriental drugs for bronchitis. In a subject that is seldom discussed, Wang & Hu describe the toxicity and side effects of some Chinese medicinal herbs. With a more modern approach to systematizing the knowledge on Chinese medicines, Lee & Chang discuss the establishment of a computerized data base that provides on-line information with respect to botanical, chemical, pharmacolog-ical, and clinical reports on common Chinese medicinal materials.

Lien & Li describe Chinese plants with anticancer properties and provide an analysis of the structure-activity relationships of the active principles (4). In recent years over a thousand species of plants have been screened in China for either antitumor or cytotoxic activity, and many have been reported to be active experimentally. The authors list in their compilation 120 species of plants belonging to some 60 different families that have been shown to exhibit anticancer activity in established cell lines in vitro and animal models in vivo. Whenever available, clinical data are also included. Among the active chemical groups present in plants discussed are the sesquiterpenes, diterpenes, triterpenes, steroids, alkaloids, and others. This treatment of the subject in-cludes an examination of the structure of the active components and their possible mechanism of action.

DRUG DEPENDENCE

The Committee on Problems of Drug Dependence provides an updated au-thoritative monograph on the testing of drugs for physical dependence potential and abuse liability, terms that have been defined operationally for laboratory evaluation (5). Physical dependence refers to pharmacologic events that occur consequent to repeated drug administration, whereas abuse potential is used with reference to events that precede or accompany strong drug-seeking behavior. Even though both physical dependence and abuse potential frequently occur together, they are distinguishable and can be evaluated separately.

Some compounds can be observed to produce physical dependence (that is, withdrawal signs after repeated drug administration) and not be abused, while other agents can produce abuse with behavioral consequences at doses that do not necessarily produce tolerance and physical dependence (e.g. cocaine). Physical dependence potential of a substance can be quantified by measuring t'.e intensity of certain physiologic and biochemical events that appear upon immediate discontinuance of an agent following chronic administration. The abuse potential of a drug can be assessed by observing and analyzing the drug seeking, drug discrimination, and drug-taking behavior associated with self-administration of the pharmacologic agent.

The usefulness of the tests resides in their predictive value in human situations. Although the validity of animal testing procedures is subject to controversy, the debates do not negate the need for such methodology. There are instances in which drugs passing animal screens show abuse liability in humans, and street users have been able to discover abusable drugs or drug combinations that were never tested in animals or suspected of abuse liability even after extensive clinical use. Despite such deficiencies, laboratory procedures for assessment of liability potential are widely used in academic, governmental, and industrial research.

In general, the predictive value of testing procedures can be best demonstrated on drug classes that have a distinct pharmacologic profile and a long history of physical dependence and abuse liability. In such instances, an uncharacterized agent can be easily classified by comparison tests with prototypic drugs and further identified by substitution tests for cross-tolerance and cross-dependence. The best example of this is the opiate group, but even in this drug class problems surfaced when the mixed agonist-antagonists and partial agonists appeared on the scene. For rational explanations it then became necessary to utilize additional tests and to invoke the concept of multiple opioid receptors.

The battery of test procedures available now for identifying opioid drugs and quantifying their dependence liability is impressive. Such tests range from simple in vitro pharmacologic methods in excised organs, to chemical affinity binding measurements on homogenized tissues, to more complicated behavioral tests on intact animals and humans.

The ease of predicting physical dependence potential and abuse liability of other drug classes varies considerably. Tests for assessing general central nervous depressants are reasonably precise, especially when one considers the wide range of substances included in this category. Sleep induction, locomotor activity, electroencephalographic activity, and behavioral performance after acute drug administration are useful parameters for categorizing sedative/ hypnotics, anesthetics, anxiolytics, and antihistamines. These acute tests are greatly enhanced and complemented by tolerance, cross-tolerance, physical dependence, and cross-dependence data obtained after chronic administration that are coupled with drug self-administration tests.

Procedures for appraising stimulants also include behavioral self-administration tests after acute and chronic drug administration. Tolerance, but not physical dependence development, appears useful for characterizing this drug group. The self-administration tests, however, provide more precise information. Indeed, reinforcing efficacy analysis utilizing progressive ratio performance, rates of response, and discrete trial choice permits the detection of differences between CNS stimulants and reveals cocaine to be one of the most potent agents with respect to reinforcing efficacy.

The characterization of other types of agents for abuse liability is more difficult. Various reasons can be offered to excuse this deficiency. The newness and poor availability of compounds limit the amount of acquired information that can be retrieved. However, there may be even more complicating factors. For example, drugs of abuse that produce hallucinations can hardly be identified by this phenomenon in experimental animals. Rather, the investigator must rely on making behavioral profile comparisons of an unknown compound with a prototypic one; unfortunately there is relatively little information on such agents. Certainly, better test procedures are needed for assessing hallucinogens, anticholinergics, and dissociative anesthetics. This may not be wholly true for characterizing cannabinoid-like activity. With the isolation and identification of delta-9-tetrahydrocannabinol as the prime active principle in marihuana *(cannabis sativa)*, a standard for making comparisons became available, and since then considerable information has been amassed on its acute and chronic behavioral profile.

In the final analysis, abuse liability of chemical agents needs to be evaluated in humans. In general, the principles applied in animal methodology after acute and chronic drug administration can be extended to human situations. There are limitations imposed by pharmacologic, clinical, and ethical considerations, but these are offset in part by the information that can be furnished by the subject to the investigator in a well-designed experiment. Testing in humans is complicated by the fact that there is great interindividual variability in reactivity to and tolerance for various substances—the latter phenomenon can be drastically modified by prior drug experience. Simple random assignment to drug or control group is usually not sufficient to assure equivalent groups because most drug trials are based on small samples, and the attrition rate for the needed testing over an extended period is high. In addition to matching experimental and control groups, therefore, attention should be paid both to obtaining subjects who will represent the population likely to be administered the drug clinically and to finding methods for endpoint analysis to avoid loss of data for those who do not complete the test period.

GENERAL PHARMACOLOGY

The seventh edition of Goodman & Gilman's classic pharmacology textbook now appears with the names of four authors (6). The son of one of the original authors assumed the chief responsibility for editing the sixth edition although Goodman and Gilman remained as coauthors. With the death in 1984 of Alfred Gilman, who leaves behind the legacy of a great teacher and author, the succession of responsibility appears to be well planned.

The major revision of the text occurred in the sixth edition, in which new topics and different sequential presentations of the subject matter were made. The present revision retains this format, and the chapters in the main appear to be updated versions of the earlier presentation, even though some authors have been replaced.

The introductory material relevant to basic principles has been expanded and improved. Even though the intraspinal and intrathecal routes of drugs are discussed in the chapters on local anesthetics, these routes should also be mentioned in the general material. The discovery of opiate receptors in the spinal cord and the successful use of intrathecal or intraspinal morphine reinforces this notion.

A statement in Chapter 3, "Principles of Therapeutics," to which I take issue because it appears overly dogmatic is the assertion that "placebo is an indispensable element of the controlled clinical trial." The necessity for a placebo in clinical assessments of drug efficacy has become axiomatic, but I would argue on pharmacologic principles that its use is usually, if not always, unnecessary. If the dose-response relationship of the agent is evaluated double-blind, the low point of the dose-response curve would be in essence the placebo response. Not only is such an assessment scientifically sound but it is also justified ethically because the investigator needs to establish the safest effective dose of the agent tested, while not depriving the patient of needed medication. I would concede that in subjective evaluations, in which response sensitivity in subjects is low and the variation great, placebos may be necessary to establish drug efficacy; but in such instances the resulting data are usually not convincing.

In checking my previous review of the sixth edition (7), I note that one of my nitpickings had been dealt with. The term "tranquilizer" has now been dropped in the chapter on the history of the anesthetics. However, in the handling of the subject matter in this area I still note a lack of historical perspective. Although the discoveries of ether, nitrous oxide, and chloroform are discussed, the advancements made after World War II are ignored. I searched in vain for the names of the inventors of halothane, enflurane, and isoflurane, nor could I find information about when these gases were introduced or what concepts had led to their development.

In general, the section on the mechanism of action of the various drug classes appears to be informative, educational, and current. An exception is the chapter on the antipsychotic agents. There are many good basic data indicating that both the beneficial and undesirable effects of the agents used to treat schizophrenia can be attributed in large part to an antidopaminergic action. Even though dopamine may not have a causal relationship to the disease process, it appears to be involved in its manifestations. The rank order of binding affinities of the antischizophrenic compounds in the brain exhibits a surprisingly good correlation with the rank order therapeutic-efficacies and the production of extrapyramidal effects. The discussion on the mechanism of action of diazepam does not include references beyond 1982. Although the role of GABA is included, the recent exciting discovery of the receptor with distinct recognition sites for diazepam, GABA, and chloride is not cited. On the other hand, the chapter on opiates includes references as late as 1984, and the reader is clued to the most recent advancements made in identifying the precursor proteins of three opioid peptide families and the multiple opioid receptors.

However, the above noted shortcomings are not major. I accorded the sixth edition high praise, and this seventh one is an improvement.

OPIOPEPTINS

Undenfriend & Meienhofer's edited monograh brings us authoritative current information on the status of the opioid peptides (8). They were able to achieve their mission because they were highly successful in enticing leading busy contributors in the field to summarize and review their areas. Although the treatment of certain topics is not ideally balanced, the volume is well worth having. Particularly impressive is the opening chapter by Numa, who describes the Herculean efforts in his laboratory leading to the elucidation of two opiopeptin precursors, preproenkephalin A and preproenkephalin B. The structure of a third opiopeptin precursor, pro-opiomelanocortin, is discussed by Cibelli, Douglass & Herbert. Thus the application of recombinant DNA technology has enabled the elucidation of the primary structure of three opiopeptin precursors, and all endogenous opioid peptides identified to date are derived from these three precursors. The striking structural similarity of these three precursor proteins to their genes suggests their close evolutionary relationship. In other chapters, Undenfriend & Kilpatrick discuss the processing of proenkephalin B; Goldstein, the biology and chemistry of dynorphin; Paterson, Robson & Kosterlitz, the characterization of opioid receptors; Yamashiro & Li, the structure-activity relationships of β-endorphin including some native analogs with opioid antagonistic properties; Schiller, an extensive conformational analysis of enkephalins; and Hansen & Morgan, the structure-activity relationships of enkephalin peptides. The final chapter by Clement-Jones & Besser provides a fairly comprehensive review of the clinical pharmacology of the opiopeptins and covers investigations of their clinical application in pain, narcotic dependence, psychoses, and endocrine regulation. As yet, the clinical applications of the opiopeptins have been limited because their use is undoubtedly predicated upon a more thorough understanding of their physiologic roles. As one of the authors (S. Undenfriend) states:

> It is of interest that we know now far more about the chemistry and genetics of the enkephalin-containing peptides than we do about their physiological roles. It is likely that the same technologies will soon permit the full characterization of the various opiate receptors at the molecular level. At the moment, however, it appears that the application of good "old fashioned" physiology and pharmacology are still required to elucidate the role(s) of the opiate peptides in health and disease.

DOMESTICATION OF CHEMISTRY

In his review concerning the "domestication" of chemicals by design of safer substances for human use (9), Ariens coins some new terms that sometimes interfere with readability. Despite these linguistic forays, which are sometimes distracting and annoying, he has penned a thoughtful scholarly essay. "Domestication of chemistry" he defines as "the adoption of chemistry and chemical to intimate association with and to the advantage of man." Ariens points out that in today's chemistry-dependent society with more than 60,000 man-made chemicals and with about 1000 new products being introduced on the market annually, nobody can avoid exposure to chemicals at some level or escape the inherent health risks. To domesticate chemicals requires a good comprehension of the toxicodynamics and the toxicokinetics of compounds foreign to the body (xenobiotics). Risky leads can be minimized by recognizing unsafe types of chemical structure and by applying routine in vitro screening tests early. For example, mutagenic agents are likely to have carcinogenic potential, and the correlation between alkylating ability and mutagenicity of chemical agents is extremely high. Hence, the introduction of highly electrophilic or nucleophilic groups and unsaturated bonds should, if possible, be avoided in agents that are to be used commercially, especially those that might pollute the environment.

ANALGETICS

Kuhar & Pasternak have edited a monograph on analgetics with the object of integrating the latest concepts, methodology, and findings in the experimental laboratory and clinic for the development of new and better pain relievers (10). Apparently there were delays in getting the material to press, since the volume does not cover certain exciting developments that occurred before its publication in 1984.

Apart from a few 1981 and 1982 references, the citations in most chapters seldom extend beyond 1980, suggesting that the editors experienced trouble making some of the authors meet their deadlines. As a result, when the book was published, the journey on some of the pathways the authors suggested exploring had already been completed. None of the book's authors, including myself, mentions dynorphin, which was isolated and completely sequenced in 1981. Despite this criticism, the editors have provided a useful reference and abbreviated bible for workers in the field. Frederickson's coverage of the state of the endogenous opioids up to 1981 is informative and comprehensive. Goodman & Pasternak expose their expertise and their personal bias on the various opiate receptors. Basbaum discusses the anatomic aspects of pain related to drug action and makes a strong case for modulation of pain mechanisms by descending pathways from the periaqueductal gray and medulla, as well as for a spinal site. Michine covers structure-activity relationships of opiate agonists and antagonists. Brune & Lang provide some unfamiliar names and a textbook essay on nonopioid analgesics. Wood's listing of analgesic models in analgesic testing might have been flavored by a critique similar to that in Wallenstein's evaluation of analgesics in man. Haubrich and three others discuss nonendogenous opioid peptides in nociception with particular emphasis on substance P and neurotensin. The discussion of the management of pain with opiates (Inturrisi & Foley) is prefaced by a treatment of the pharmacologic basis for their application as were the nonsteroidal anti-inflammatory agents (Kantor). Finally, in projecting future vistas, I pontificate:

To remedy current deficiencies in the management of pain, proper communication is essential at all levels. This involves adequate orientation in the medical problems associated with pain in the curriculum for medical, dental, nursing, and pharmacy students and maintaining the education intensively for the practitioner on a continuing basis. In the treatment of the patient with severe pain, a holistic approach is, of course, essential but the advances from the experimental laboratory and the clinical must be appreciated. The major breakthroughs can only occur from the fundamental contribution emanating first from the experimental laboratory and this work can only flourish in an atmosphere that has economic, political, and philosophic support from an educated public at large.

Literature Cited

1. Balandrin, M. F., Klocke, J. A., Wurtele, E. S., Bollinger, W. H. 1985. Natural plant chemicals: Sources of industrial medicinal materials. *Science* 228:1154–60

2. Takemi, T., Hasegawa, M., Kumagai, A., Otsuka, Y., eds. 1985. *Herbal Medicine: Kampo, Past and Present.* Tokyo: Tsumura Jutendo. 148 pp.

3. Chang, H. M., Yeung, H. W., Tsu, W. W., Koo, A., eds. 1985. *Advances in Chinese Medicinal Materials Research.* Singapore/Philadelphia: World Scientific. 742 pp.

4. Lien, E. J., Li, W. Y. 1985. *Structure-Activity Relationship Analysis of Chinese Anticancer Drugs and Related Plants.* Long Beach, Calif. Oriental Healing Arts Institute.

5. The Committee on Problems of Drug Dependence, Inc. *Testing Drugs for Physical Dependence Potential and Abuse Liability,* ed. J. V. Brady, S. E. Lukas.

NIDA Res. Monogr. 52. Washington, DC: GPO. 153 pp.

6. Gilman, A. G., Goodman, L. S., Rall, T. W., Murad, F., eds. 1985. *The Pharmacological Basis of Therapeutics.* New York: MacMillan. 1839 pp. 7th ed.

7. Way, E. L. 1982. Review of reviews. *Ann. Rev. Pharmacol. Toxicol.* 21:605–13

8. Undenfriend, S., Meienhofer, J., eds. 1984. *The Peptides—Analysis, Synthesis, Biology,* Vol. 6. *Opioid Peptides, Biology, Chemistry and Genetics.* Orlando: Academic. 410 pp.

9. Ariens, E. J. 1984. Domestication of chemistry by design of safer chemicals: Structure-activity relationships. *Drug Metab. Rev.* 15(3):425–504

10. Kuhar, M. J., Pasternak, G. W., eds. 1984. *Analgesics: Neurochemical, Behavioral and Clinical Perspectives.* New York: Raven. 341 pp.

SUBJECT INDEX

A

Abortifacient proteins, 569
Abrin
  botulinum toxin and, 430
Acanthifolicin
  cytotoxicity of, 128-29
ACE
  See Angiotensin-converting
    enzyme
Acetaminophen
  nephrotoxicity of, 276-77
Acetazolamide
  potassium excretion and, 299
  urinary calcium excretion and,
    105-6
Acetylcholine, 2, 13-14, 40
  autonomium and, 124
  botulinum toxin and, 427, 438
  brevetoxin and, 131
  calcium channels and, 237-38,
    245-46
  dithiobiuret and, 536
  ethylcholine azaridinium ion
    and, 168-71
  intraocular pressure and, 403
  tetanus toxin and, 438
  thyrotropin-releasing hormone
    and, 315, 318
  vascular smooth muscle and,
    190
Acetylcholinesterase
  organophosphorus compounds
    and, 40, 42, 45
  salicylates and, 91
  soman toxicity and, 44
N-Acetylcysteine
  hexachloro-1,3-butadiene and,
    273
Acetylethylcholine azaridinium
    ion, 174
Acetylethyl tetramethyl tetralin
  demyelination and, 524
Acid-base balance
  pulmonary macrophages and,
    558
  urinary calcium excretion and,
    105
Acidosis
  potassium excretion and, 295
  urinary calcium excretion and,
    105
Acid phosphatase
  pulmonary macrophages and,
    550

Acid ribonuclease
  pulmonary macrophages and,
    550
Acquired immune deficiency
    syndrome
  interferon and, 465
Acrylamide
  areflexia and, 533
  axonal swellings and, 527-28
  monosynaptic reflex responses
    and, 535
  motor nerve endings and, 536
  neuronal cell bodies and, 520
  neuropathy and, 524
  Pacinian corpuscles and, 534
  peripheral neuropathy and, 49-
    50
  sensory impairment and, 532
ACTH
  See Corticotropin
Actinia equina
  biologically active peptides of,
    124
Actinomycin
  RNA synthesis and, 519
Active transport
  calcium
    acetazolamide and, 106
    mechanisms of, 102
Adenine arabinoside
  interferon and, 493
Adenine nucleotides
  lung removal of, 188-89
Adenosine
  cardiovascular effects of, 118
Adenosine kinase
  5'-deoxy-5-iodotubercidin
    and, 119
Adenylate cyclase
  calcitonin and, 104
  calcium channels and, 245
  cholera toxin and, 444
  cisplatin and, 92
  loop diuretics and, 89
  messenger systems and, 444
  parathyroid hormone and, 104
  pertussis toxin and, 444
  vanadate and, 417
ADH
  See Antidiuretic hormone
Adrenal medulla
  proenkephalin A and, 65-66
Adrenergic agents
  intraocular pressure and, 407-
    20

mechanism of action of, 408
α-Adrenergic agents
  intraocular pressure and, 410-
    12
ß-Adrenergic agents
  intraocular pressure and, 412-
    15
ß-Adrenergic blockers
  anthopleurins and, 122
Adrenergic receptors
  eye and, 407-8
ß-Adrenergic receptors
  buproprion and, 35
  calcium channels and, 244-45
  postsynaptic
    antidepressants and, 25
Aglycones, 120
Agonists
  hydrophobic loading and, 12
Agoraphobia
  alprazolam and, 35
AIDS
  See Acquired immune de-
    ficiency syndrome
Air pollution
  pulmonary macrophages and,
    557
Alcohol, 18
Aldehyde dehydrogenase
  cytochrome P-450 and, 338
Aldosterone
  potassium excretion and, 295,
    303-4
  spironolactone and, 300-1
  urinary calcium excretion and,
    111
Aliphatic alcohols
  neuromuscular junction and,
    537
Alkaloids, 569
  marine, 128
  pulmonary toxicity of, 268
  thyrotropin-releasing hormone
    and, 312
Alkalosis
  potassium excretion and, 295
  urinary calcium excretion and,
    105
Alkylammonium salts
  neuromuscular junction and,
    11
Allogeneic cells
  interferon and, 463
Allopurinol
  interferon and, 485

577

CUMULATIVE INDEXES

CONTRIBUTING AUTHORS, VOLUMES 22–26

CHAPTER TITLES, VOLUMES 22–26

Annual Reviews Inc. $\boxed{ORDER\ FORM}$
A NONPROFIT SCIENTIFIC PUBLISHER
4139 El Camino Way, Palo Alto, CA 94306-9981, USA • (415) 493-4400

Annual Reviews Inc. publications are available directly from our office by mail or telephone (paid by credit card or purchase order), through booksellers and subscription agents, worldwide, and through participating professional societies. Prices subject to change without notice.

- **Individuals:** Prepayment required on new accounts by check or money order (in U.S. dollars, check drawn on U.S. bank) or charge to credit card — American Express, VISA, MasterCard.
- **Institutional buyers:** Please include purchase order number.
- **Students:** $10.00 discount from retail price, per volume. Prepayment required. Proof of student status must be provided (photocopy of student I.D. or signature of department secretary is acceptable). Students must send orders direct to Annual Reviews. Orders received through bookstores and institutions requesting student rates will be returned.
- **Professional Society Members:** Members of professional societies that have a contractual arrangement with Annual Reviews may order books through their society at a reduced rate. Check with your society for information.

Regular orders: Please list the volumes you wish to order by volume number.
Standing orders: New volume in the series will be sent to you automatically each year upon publication. Cancellation may be made at any time. Please indicate volume number to begin standing order.
Prepublication orders: Volumes not yet published will be shipped in month and year indicated.
California orders: Add applicable sales tax.
Postage paid (4th class bookrate/surface mail) by **Annual Reviews Inc.** Airmail postage extra.

ANNUAL REVIEWS SERIES		Prices Postpaid per volume USA/elsewhere	Regular Order Please send:	Standing Order Begin with:
			Vol. number	Vol. number

Annual Review of **ANTHROPOLOGY** (Prices of Volumes in brackets effective until 12/31/85)

[Vols. 1-10	(1972-1981)	**$20.00/$21.00**]		
[Vol. 11	(1982)	**$22.00/$25.00**]		
[Vols. 12-14	(1983-1985)	**$27.00/$30.00**]		
Vols. 1-14	(1972-1985)	**$27.00/$30.00**		
Vol. 15	(avail. Oct. 1986)	**$31.00/$34.00**	Vol(s). _____	Vol. _____

Annual Review of **ASTRONOMY AND ASTROPHYSICS** (Prices of Volumes in brackets effective until 12/31/85)

[Vols. 1-2, 4-19	(1963-1964; 1966-1981)	**$20.00/$21.00**]		
[Vol. 20	(1982)	**$22.00/$25.00**]		
[Vols. 21-23	(1983-1985)	**$44.00/$47.00**]		
Vols. 1-2, 4-20	(1963-1964; 1966-1982)	**$27.00/$30.00**		
Vols. 21-23	(1983-1985)	**$44.00/$47.00**		
Vol. 24	(avail. Sept. 1986)	**$44.00/$47.00**	Vol(s). _____	Vol. _____

Annual Review of **BIOCHEMISTRY** (Prices of Volumes in brackets effective until 12/31/85)

[Vols. 30-34, 36-50	(1961-1965; 1967-1981)	**$21.00/$22.00**]		
[Vol. 51	(1982)	**$23.00/$26.00**]		
[Vols. 52-54	(1983-1985)	**$29.00/$32.00**]		
Vols. 30-34, 36-54	(1961-1965; 1967-1985)	**$29.00/$32.00**		
Vol. 55	(avail. July 1986)	**$33.00/$36.00**	Vol(s). _____	Vol. _____

Annual Review of **BIOPHYSICS AND BIOPHYSICAL CHEMISTRY** (Prices of Vols. in brackets effective until 12/31/85)
(Formerly Annual Review of Biophysics and Bioengineering)

[Vols. 1-10	(1972-1981)	**$20.00/$21.00**]		
[Vol. 11	(1982)	**$22.00/$25.00**]		
[Vols. 12-14	(1983-1985)	**$47.00/$50.00**]		
Vols. 1-11	(1972-1982)	**$27.00/$30.00**		
Vols. 12-14	(1983-1985)	**$47.00/$50.00**		
Vol. 15	(avail. June 1986)	**$47.00/$50.00**	Vol(s). _____	Vol. _____

Annual Review of **CELL BIOLOGY**

Vol. 1	(1985)	**$27.00/$30.00**		
Vol. 2	(avail. Nov. 1986)	**$31.00/$34.00**	Vol(s). _____	Vol. _____

Annual Review of **COMPUTER SCIENCE**

Vol. 1	(avail. late 1986)	**Price not yet established**	Vol. _____	Vol. _____

Annual Review of **EARTH AND PLANETARY SCIENCES** (Prices of Volumes in brackets effective until 12/31/85)

[Vols. 1-9	(1973-1981)	**$20.00/$21.00**]		
[Vol. 10	(1982)	**$22.00/$25.00**]		
[Vols. 11-13	(1983-1985)	**$44.00/$47.00**]		
Vols. 1-10	(1973-1982)	**$27.00/$30.00**		
Vols. 11-13	(1983-1985)	**$44.00/$47.00**		
Vol. 14	(avail. May 1986)	**$44.00/$47.00**	Vol(s). _____	Vol. _____

Annual Review of **ECOLOGY AND SYSTEMATICS** (Prices of Volumes in brackets effective until 12/31/85)

[Vols. 1-12	(1970-1981)................... $20.00/$21.00]		
[Vol. 13	(1982) .... $22.00/$25.00]		
[Vols. 14-16	(1983-1985)................... $27.00/$30.00]		
Vols. 1-16	(1970-1985)................... $27.00/$30.00		
Vol. 17	(avail. Nov. 1986)............. $31.00/$34.00	Vol(s). _____	Vol. _____

Annual Review of **ENERGY** (Prices of Volumes in brackets effective until 12/31/85)

[Vols. 1-6	(1976-1981)................... $20.00/$21.00]		
[Vol. 7	(1982)................... $22.00/$25.00]		
[Vols. 8-10	(1983-1985)................... $56.00/$59.00]		
Vols. 1-7	(1976-1982)................... $27.00/$30.00		
Vols. 8-10	(1983-1985)................... $56.00/$59.00		
Vol. 11	(avail. Oct. 1986)............. $56.00/$59.00	Vol(s). _____	Vol. _____

Annual Review of **ENTOMOLOGY** (Prices of Volumes in brackets effective until 12/31/85)

[Vols. 9-16, 18-26	(1964-1971; 1973-1981)........ $20.00/$21.00]		
[Vol. 27	(1982)................... $22.00/$25.00]		
[Vols. 28-30	(1983-1985)................... $27.00/$30.00]		
Vols. 9-16, 18-30	(1964-1971; 1973-1985)........ $27.00/$30.00		
Vol. 31	(avail. Jan. 1986)............. $31.00/$34.00	Vol(s). _____	Vol. _____

Annual Review of **FLUID MECHANICS** (Prices of Volumes in brackets effective until 12/31/85)

[Vols. 1-5, 7-13	(1969-1973; 1975-1981)........ $20.00/$21.00]		
[Vol. 14	(1982)................... $22.00/$25.00]		
[Vols. 15-17	(1983-1985)................... $28.00/$31.00]		
Vols. 1-5, 7-17	(1969-1973; 1975-1985)........ $28.00/$31.00		
Vol. 18	(avail. Jan. 1986)............. $32.00/$35.00	Vol(s). _____	Vol. _____

Annual Review of **GENETICS** (Prices of Volumes in brackets effective until 12/31/85)

[Vols. 1-15	(1967-1981)................... $20.00/$21.00]		
[Vol. 16	(1982)................... $22.00/$25.00]		
[Vols. 17-19	(1983-1985)................... $27.00/$30.00]		
Vols. 1-19	(1967-1985)................... $27.00/$30.00		
Vol. 20	(avail. Dec. 1986)............. $31.00/$34.00	Vol(s). _____	Vol. _____

Annual Review of **IMMUNOLOGY**

Vols. 1-3	(1983-1985)................... $27.00/$30.00		
Vol. 4	(avail. April 1986)............. $31.00/$34.00	Vol(s). _____	Vol. _____

Annual Review of **MATERIALS SCIENCE** (Prices of Volumes in brackets effective until 12/31/85)

[Vols. 1-11	(1971-1981)................... $20.00/$21.00]		
[Vol. 12	(1982)................... $22.00/$25.00]		
[Vols. 13-15	(1983-1985)................... $64.00/$67.00]		
Vols. 1-12	(1971-1982)................... $27.00/$30.00		
Vols. 13-15	(1983-1985)................... $64.00/$67.00		
Vol. 16	(avail. August 1986)............. $64.00/$67.00	Vol(s). _____	Vol. _____

Annual Review of **MEDICINE** (Prices of Volumes in brackets effective until 12/31/85)

[Vols. 1-3, 5-15, 17-32	(1950-52; 1954-64; 1966-81)...... $20.00/$21.00]		
[Vol. 33	(1982)................... $22.00/$25.00]		
[Vols. 34-36	(1983-1985)................... $27.00/$30.00]		
Vols. 1-3, 5-15, 17-36	(1950-52; 1954-64; 1966-85)..... $27.00/$30.00		
Vol. 37	(avail. April 1986)............. $31.00/$34.00	Vol(s). _____	Vol. _____

Annual Review of **MICROBIOLOGY** (Prices of Volumes in brackets effective until 12/31/85)

[Vols. 18-35	(1964-1981)................... $20.00/$21.00]		
[Vol. 36	(1982) .... $22.00/$25.00]		
[Vols. 37-39	(1983-1985)................... $27.00/$30.00]		
Vols. 18-39	(1964-1985)................... $27.00/$30.00		
Vol. 40	(avail. Oct. 1986)............. $31.00/$34.00	Vol(s). _____	Vol. _____

Annual Review of **NEUROSCIENCE** (Prices of Volumes in brackets effective until 12/31/85)

[Vols. 1-4	(1978-1981)................... $20.00/$21.00]		
[Vol. 5	(1982) .... $22.00/$25.00]		
[Vols. 6-8	(1983-1985)................... $27.00/$30.00]		
Vols. 1-8	(1978-1985)................... $27.00/$30.00		
Vol. 9	(avail. March 1986)............. $31.00/$34.00	Vol(s). _____	Vol. _____

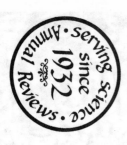